Electroencephalogram for Presurgical Epilepsy Evaluation

Electrical activity is foundation on which the brain network works. Abnormal activity occurs in patients with epilepsy. In 1912, a Russian scholar named Kaufmann first observed abnormal electrical activities in experimental epileptic seizures in an animal. The animal's cranium was opened and the examination findings revealed that the abnormal electrical activities were neither artifacts nor injury potentials. The abnormal activity originated from the cortex itself. Hans Berger, a German psychiatrist, made a great contribution to epileptology. In 1929, he reported the research results, and he was the first researcher who recorded spontaneous electrical activities from healthy human scalp and proved that such electrical activities would change during the interictal stage. In that year he also recorded spike and slow wave complex. In 1931, Jackson emphasized that the epileptic discharge was characterized by "a transient excessive discharge of highly unstable cells." Their findings laid an important foundation for epileptology. Clinically, the discharge phenomena in electroencephalography (EEG) are the only evidence for the diagnosis of epilepsy. Electroencephalography (EEG) has evolved from short-term 4-channel to 8-channel EEG, to multi-channel long-term EEG combined with video monitoring, and to subdural electrodes electroencephalography (SDEG), depth electronencephalography (DEEG), and stereoelectroencephalography (SEEG). All these new developments are of critical value to the diagnosis, follow-up, and preoperative localization. However, the design scheme of intracranial electrode is based on scalp EEG, clinical symptoms, neuroimaging, etc. Therefore, the importance of scalp EEG is self-evident. EEG may vary depending on specific seizure types. It is essential to have a detailed and in-depth understanding of scalp EEG to ensure accurate detection. One of the main intentions of this book is to vividly reveal the characteristics of electrical activity for each seizure type.

In the 1970s, ILAE classified epileptic seizures scientifically for the first time. The classification system has been revised several times after that and is still under continual discussion and revision. This demonstrates the complexity of epileptic symptoms and our incomplete understanding of the essence of the disease. Moreover, the descriptions and nomenclature of symptoms are also not unified. Almost every patient's seizure has its peculiar points different from other patients'. In other words, there are no two patients who have completely identical seizure types. For example, patients with tonic-clonic seizures have their own detailed posture characteristics, and patients with hypermotor seizures have different symptom sequences. We know nothing about what differences in anatomic foundation and the propagation of electrical activities contribute to these differences in details. We also cannot demonstrate what sites or how many neurons are involved. Therefore, documentation of the details and sequence of each patient's seizure is the basis for further investigations. In light of the changes in electroencephalograms at each stage and accumulation of experience, combining modern technology, the secrets in epilepsy may eventually be revealed.

This book is a fundamental book for further studies. The final results of any study that is based on incorrect original data can hardly be considered as convincing. So, the conclusion drawn from any genetic studies that are based on incorrect description of epileptic symptoms and/or misclassification of epilepsy is inevitably incorrect. In light of this, this book is more than a must-read for beginners. Clinically experienced physicians who want to further probe into epilepsy and researchers who are engaged in fundamental research of epilepsy may also benefit from reading it.

Here I'd like to share with you a quote from Henri Cartier-Bresson, the "father of modern photojournalism," who once said, "If your pictures aren't good enough, you aren't close enough."

Adviser, China Association Against Epilepsy

Beijing, China
September, 2021

Xun Wu

Introduction

Epilepsy is a common disease of the nervous system. In China, there are nearly ten million of epileptic patients, 30% of whom have drug-resistant epilepsy or refractory epilepsy, which means antiseizure medication cannot effectively control the seizures. Over the years, surgical operation has been an important approach to treat refractory epilepsy. The rapid development in the construction of epilepsy centers in China in recent years makes surgical treatment of epilepsy, which is centered on the resection of epileptogenic focus, more readily available for relieving the suffering of epileptic patients. Techniques for surgical treatment of epilepsy deserve further popularization and promotion. Standardized preoperative evaluation is a core component of epilepsy surgery. An important work in the evaluation is to identify the epileptogenic focus precisely. Electroencephalography is indispensable and irreplaceable for the localization of epileptogenic focus. It may be said that the important work in epilepsy centers is preoperative evaluation, and electroencephalography (EEG) is the soul of preoperative evaluation.

Scalp EEG plays an important role in the localization of epileptogenic focus. However, noninvasive technique is not adequate to identify the precise localization of the epileptogenic focus in about one-third of the patients. In such cases, it is necessary to implant intracranial electrodes to identify the epileptogenic focus. This is called intracranial EEG. Depending on the patient's specific situation, subdural electrodes may be embedded via cranial opening or drilling, and depth electrodes may be embedded using stereotactic technique. Intracranial EEG has been extensively applied in preoperative evaluation due to its clear signal and potential to effectively identify the epileptogenic focus.

However, epilepsy center staff may have mixed feelings for the application of intracranial EEG because of the complexity of the localization of epileptogenic focus. They are much interested in the dominance of the technique since it can clearly display the activity process accompanying the epileptic seizure but are at a loss when facing the uncertainty of the results from the technique. It takes a long training process to master the application of intracranial EEG. If there is a book on the skills and application knowledge of the localization of epileptogenic focus with intracranial EEG, it would undoubtedly benefit in their dealing with epilepsy quite a lot. In light of this, the idea of writing a book on EEG for preoperative evaluation emerged and I started to collect and sort out after multiple communication and consultation with my colleagues. The book gradually took shape after years of joint efforts with them. The representative cases of the book are meticulously selected. For each selected case, the patient's scalp EEG and intracranial EEG as well as detailed medical history, surgery protocol decision, and follow-up results are provided for reference. It is hoped that with this book readers will know how to design intracranial electrode implantation scheme in light of the patient's medical history, characteristics of seizure symptoms, scalp EEG, and seizure video. Furthermore, to facilitate understanding, a short comment and explanation about each case are provided to point out the generality and specificity of the case and experience from the success or failure for the reference of the readers. In order to help readers to better understand the characteristics of cases and EEG, we arranged and numbered several dozen of cases according to the anatomic site and provided corresponding introductions to the anatomy knowledge of the sites and the characteristics of the epileptic seizures.

With the transition of time and the continual progress of technology, the number of SEEG has been gradually increasing in recent years. However, more data need to be accumulated. This book only incorporates a few SEEG cases. But this does not impede the readers' understanding of the intracranial EEG.

The compilation of this book had been encouraged by professional colleagues. Professor Liu Xiaoyan at Peking University frequently asked for the compilation progress, and Professor Wu Xun and CAAE Honorary Chairman Li Shichao also paid much attention to this book. We want to express our thanks to them. Inspired by these experts, we sped up in the compilation of the book.

Many colleagues in Beijing Epilepsy Center took part in the compilation of this book. We are grateful to them for their dedication. The information accumulated in the preoperative evaluation of numerous cases in Beijing Epilepsy Center provides first-hand data for the compilation of this book, and the publication of the book is the best reward to the contribution made by our colleagues in the center.

Much of the content may not be fully included. There may be some defects or errors in the book. Thanks for your criticism. We hope that this book will promote the progress of preoperative evaluation.

Yuping Wang

Chief Neurologist, Department of Neurology
Xuanwu Hospital Capital Medical University
Director, Beijing Epilepsy Center
September 7, 2021

About the Editor

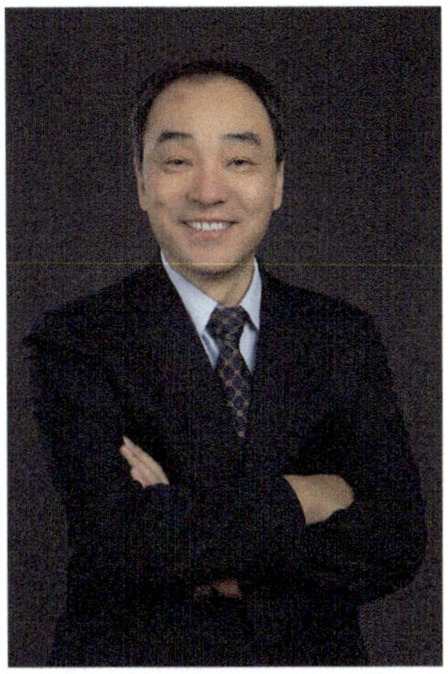

Yuping Wang MD, Chief Physician, Professor, Doctoral Supervisor, former Director of Department of Neurology, Xuanwu Hospital Capital Medical University, graduated from the Department of Medicine, Hebei Medical University. He received BMS in 1983 and MMSC in 1986, and graduated from Tottori University with a medical doctorate in 1996, and then completed his postdoctoral research at Chinese Academy of Medical Sciences and Peking Union Medical College Hospital (CAMS and PUMCH) in 1998. He worked in the Department of Neurology, Xuanwu Hospital Capital Medical University, and established specialized outpatient clinics including Involuntary Movement Clinic, Epilepsy Clinic, Center for Sleep Disorders. He established Beijing Comprehensive Epilepsy Center, Beijing Key Laboratory of Neuromodulation, Institute of Sleep and Consciousness Disorders, and Beijing Institute of Brain Disorders. He engaged in pathological and physiological studies of cerebrovascular diseases, epilepsy, sleep, cognitive, affective disorders, etc. He identified cognitive potential component N270, created a number of clinical diagnostics and treatment techniques, established standardized procedure for preoperative evaluation of epilepsy, formulated multiple neurostimulation treatment schemes for brain functional diseases, and developed multiple disease diagnostics and treatment devices. He completed a number of studies funded by National Natural Science Foundation of China (NSFC), the 863 Program, and/or other national special key study programs, was honored with Chinese Medical Science and Technology Award, Beijing Science and Technology Progress Award, Wu Jieping Medical Research Award, etc.

His incumbent academic positions include: Vice Chairman of China Association Against Epilepsy (CAAE); Chairman of CAAE Working Committee on Standardized Construction of Epilepsy Centers; Chairman-elect of Psychosomatic Medicine Branch of Chinese Medical Association (CMA); member of the standing committee of Neurology Branch of Chinese Medical Association (CMA);Leader of Sleep Disorder Expert Group; Chairman of Neurology Branch of China International Exchange and Promotive Association for Medical and Health Care (CPAM); Chairman of Neurology Professional Committee of Chinese Medical Education Association

(CMEA); Vice Chairman of Neurology Branch of Council, Chinese Medical Doctor Association (CMDA); member of the Steering Committee of International League Against Epilepsy (ILAE); member of the Steering Committee on Epileptic Seizure Autodetection Devices, International Federation of Clinical Neurophysiology (IFCN); associate editor of *Frontiers in Neurology* (epilepsy section); member of editorial board of *Sleep Medicine*, *Clinical Neurophysiology*, *Journal of Clinical Neurophysiology*, and *Chinese Journal of Neurology*.

Contents

1 Preoperative Epilepsy Surgery Evaluation

Lin Hua, Liankun Ren, and Yuping Wang

Epileptic Seizure and Its Classification

Epileptic seizures are transient brain disorders caused by abnormal discharge of cerebral neurons. Patients have varied clinical manifestations, including sensory, motor, conscious, mental, behavioral, and autonomic dysfunctions, or a combination of symptoms, depending on the specific location of abnormally discharging neurons and the brain network involved. A patient may have one or more epileptic seizure types.

Despite the variety and complexity of clinical manifestations, epileptic seizures are generally characterized by paroxysmal, transitory, recurrent, and stereotyped behaviors. A full understanding of the commonality of epileptic seizures and the clinical manifestations of various seizure types is of great significance for definite diagnosis of epileptic seizures. Definite diagnosis of epileptic seizures can be made on patient's seizure semiologies and epileptiform discharges.

The epileptic seizure classification, which is based on clinical symptoms and EEG findings, was first proposed by Gastaut in 1964, and has been recognized over time. The International League Against Epilepsy (ILAE) Commission on Classification and Terminology proposed an international epileptic seizures classification on the basis of this approach in 1981. The classification system is mainly based on the clinical manifestations and EEG features in line with the principle of dichotomy: An epileptic seizure is a partial seizure if the initial manifestations and EEG findings reveal it is originated from the abnormal local neurons discharge. If the initial manifestations and EEG findings reveal involvement of both hemispheres, the epileptic seizure is a generalized one. Furthermore, seizures that cannot be classified according to the current classification system due to insufficient or incomplete data are referred to as unclassified. ILAE 1981 Classification of the Epilepsies (Table 1.1) has been popularized and applied to date worldwide.

L. Hua · L. Ren · Y. Wang (✉)
Department of Neurology, Beijing, China
e-mail: linhua@ccmu.edu.cn

The understanding of epileptic seizures and epilepsy has been improved in recent years with the continual fundamental and clinical studies of epilepsy. Epileptologists gradually realized the ILAE 1981 Classification of the Epilepsies had some defects: ① The name "partial seizures" is ambiguous and might be taken for granted as the manifestation of seizures on a part of the body, making it hard for beginners to understand why a secondarily generalized tonic-clonic seizure is a partial seizure.

② Beginners might have difficulty in determining the presence/absence of disorders of consciousness (DOC) by the adjectives "simple" and "complex." ③ Due to the lack of complete symptomatologic information, sometimes it may be hard to classify a seizure according to the ILAE 1981 classification system. ④ Some new clinical seizure types (e.g., epileptic spasm and absence with eyelid myoclonus) are not included in the ILAE 1981 Classification of the Epilepsies. In light of these problems, ILAE proposed a new diagnostic scheme for seizures and epilepsy in 2001, which reclassified and supplemented seizures (Table 1.2).

In 2017, ILAE released a new epileptic seizure classification system which provides a reclassification of seizures by incorporating new developments and understandings in the field of epilepsy since 1981 and taking into account the opinions of experts and clinicians. The new classification system was still mainly based on clinical symptoms but partially taking into consideration EEG and/or other examinations. It was proposed in the ILAE 2017 Classification of Seizure Types (Table 1.3) that: some seizures, such as tonic seizure, clonic seizure, myoclonic seizure, atonic seizure, are either generalized seizures or focal seizures; therefore the above seizure types were added into the category of focal seizures. Epileptic spasm may be associated with focal pathological changes and may also display the characteristics of generalization in clinical manifestations or EEG. Therefore, an epileptic spasm, which may need further EEG and imaging data, may be categorized into focal seizure, or generalized seizure, or unknown seizure.

Y. Wang (ed.), *Electroencephalogram for Presurgical Epilepsy Evaluation*, https://doi.org/10.1007/978-981-95-8003-3_1

Table 1.1 ILAE 1981 classification of seizure types

Partial seizures			Generalized seizures	Unclassified seizures
Simple partial seizures	**Complex partial seizures**	**Partial seizures** **Secondarily generalized seizures**		
With motor signs Focal motor without march Focal motor with march (Jacksonian) Versive Postural Phonatory (vocalization or arrest of speech) With somatosensory or special-sensory symptoms Somatosensory Visual Auditory Olfactory Gustatory Vertiginous With autonomic symptoms or signs Epigastric sensation Pallor Sweating Flushing Piloerection Pupillary dilatation With psychic symptoms Dysphasic Dysmnesic (e.g., deja vu) Cognitive (e.g., dreamy states, distortions of time sense) Affective (fear, anger, etc.) Illusions (e.g., macropsia) Structured hallucinations (e.g., music, scenes)	Simple partial onset followed by impairment of consciousness With simple partial features followed by impaired consciousness With automatisms With impairment of consciousness at onset With impairment of consciousness only With automatisms	Simple partial seizures evolving to generalized seizures Complex partial seizures evolving to generalized seizures Simple partial seizures evolving to complex partial seizures evolving to generalized seizures	Absence seizures Atypical absence Myoclonic seizures Clonic seizure Tonic seizures Tonic-clonic seizure Atonic seizures	

Presently, ILAE Classification of the Epilepsies is the most extensively used for epileptic seizure classification. However, the classification system is dependent on more EEG and imaging results for definite classification of seizures. In case of the lack of the abovementioned examination results, it would be difficult to make this electro-clinical classification accurately or it is inconvenient to apply the classification in clinical process. H. Lüders in 1998 proposed a symptomatological classification system which is completely based on clinical symptoms for classification of epileptic seizures. Unlike ILAE Classification of the Epilepsies, this classification system is free of the dependence on EEG and clinical physicians can classify seizures in a "what you see is what you get" way. The symptomatological classification system of seizures has been used in Cleveland Clinic Epilepsy Center for more than 20 years for providing a easier-to-use way to understand the symptoms of epileptic seizures, especially focal epilepsies. The classification system is frequently used for preoperative evaluation nowadays.

The symptomatological classification system has been proposed step by step after the analysis of many video EEGs (VEEGs). It divides seizures into five major categories (Table 1.4) according to the most obvious symptoms and the four fields (sensory, autonomic, conscious, and behavioral) of epileptic seizures. Epileptic seizures seldom only involve a single field. Many epileptic seizures may present symptoms in all four fields. However, classification of seizures with the symptomatological classification system is based on the most obvious symptom. For example, if a seizure has loss of consciousness as its major symptom, it generally would be classified as a dialeptic seizure even though it is with concomitant autonomic symptoms such as salivation and palpitation, which are considered as subsidiary manifestations. A complete symptomatological classification consists of three parts, i.e., classification, symptomatology localization, and evolution of seizure.

Table 1.2 ILAE 2001 classification of epileptic seizure types (draft)

Generalized seizures	Focal seizures	Reflex seizures
Tonic-clonic seizure Clonic seizures Without tonic features With tonic features Typical absence seizure Atypical absence seizure Myoclonic absence seizure Tonic seizure Spasm Myoclonic seizure Eyelid myoclonus Without absences With absences Myoclonic atonic seizures Negative myoclonus Atonic seizures Reflex seizures in generalized epilepsy syndromes	Focal sensory seizures With elementary sensory symptoms (e.g., occipital lobe and parietal lobe seizures) With experiential sensory symptoms (e.g., temporoparietooccipital junction seizures) Focal motor seizures With elementary clonic motor symptoms With asymmetric tonic motor seizures (e.g., supplementary motor area seizures) With typical (temporal lobe) automatism (e.g., mesial temporal lobe seizures) With hyperkinetic automatisms With focal negative myoclonus With inhibitory motor seizures Gelastic seizures Hemiclonic seizures Secondarily generalized seizures Reflex seizures in focal epilepsy syndromes	Visual stimuli Flickering light: color and patterns should be specified whenever possible Other visual stimuli Thinking Music Eating Praxis Somatosensory Proprioceptive Reading Hot water Startle

Table 1.3 ILAE 2017 classification of seizure types

Focal onset		Generalized onset	Unknown onset
Aware	Impaired awareness	Motor Tonic-clonic Clonic Tonic Myoclonic Myoclonic-tonic-clonic Myoclonic-atonic Atonic Epileptic spasms Nonmotor (absence) Typical Atypical Myoclonic Eyelid myoclonia	Motor Tonic-clonic Epileptic spasms Nonmotor Behavior arrest
Motor onset			Unclassified
Automatism			
Atonic			
Clonic Epileptic spasms Hyperkinetic Myoclonic Tonic			
Nonmotor onset			
Autonomic			
Behavior arrest			
Cognitive Emotional Sensory			
Focal to bilateral tonic-clonic			

Table 1.4 Types of epileptic seizure

Seizure	Explanation
Aura	A subjective sensation, without any objective changes based on which autonomic seizures can be identified
Ictal symptomatology	Ictal symptomatology refers to objective autonomic functional changes, regardless of the subjective feeling of the individual patient himself/herself
Dialeptic seizures	Dialeptic seizures are mainly characterized by "alternation of consciousness," which can be described as "lapse of consciousness"
Motor seizures	The major manifestations of seizures are motor symptoms
Special seizures	Seizures do not fall in any of the above four classification fields. The majority of these seizures are mainly negative seizures in clinical

Table 1.5 Characterization classification of epileptic seizures

Seizure type		
Aura	Somatosensory	
	Visual	
	Auditory	
	Olfactory	
	Gustatory	
	Psychic	
	Abdominal	
	Autonomic nerve	
Autonomic seizure		
Dialeptic seizure		
Motor seizure	Simple motor seizure[a]	Myoclonic seizure
		Tonic seizure
		Epileptic spasm
		Clonic seizure
		Tonic-clonic seizure
		Versive seizure
	Complex motor seizure	Hypermotor seizure
		Automotor seizure
		Gelastic seizure
Special seizure	Atonic seizure	
	Hypomotor seizure	
	Kinetic seizure	
	Negative myoclonic seizure	
	Astatic seizure	
	Aphasic seizure	

Note: [a]If it is impossible to differentiate any simple motor seizures as clonic, tonic, or myoclonic seizures, then it is classified as "simple motor seizures." The classification of seizures should follow the most definite and most detailed procedures as far as possible. Unclassified seizures should not be classified reluctantly

Table 1.5 lists the overall architecture of the characterization and classification of seizure symptoms. ① Aura: It refers to epileptic seizures during which exclusively subjective symptoms occur in the patient. An aura seizure is identified only when the patient's EEG presents epileptiform discharges or the patient experiences subsequent motor seizure(s). ② Autonomic seizure: An autonomic seizure is demonstrated only with objective evidence showing that an epileptic seizure has given rise to autonomic symptoms (e.g., palpitation), and the patient's EEG has epileptiform discharges. Sometimes the patient who has an autonomic seizure does not necessarily have any subjective feelings. ③ Dialeptic seizure: Altered state of consciousness is the major manifestation of a dialeptic seizures. A patient experiencing dialeptic seizure shows almost no response or only limited response to external stimuli. He/she will totally have no memory of the seizure course afterward. In some cases, "automatism" that is hard to define may occur. Dialeptic seizures are exclusively based on clinically altered state of consciousness regardless of any abnormality in the patient's EEG. In ILAE Classification of the Seizure Types, "absence seizures" refers to seizures with EEG of 3Hz spike and slow complex waves. "Complex partial seizures" refers to seizures that show focal epileptiform discharge(s). Absence seizures and complex partial seizures consist of electro-clinical manifestations. ④ Motor seizures: Seizures characterized primarily by motor manifestations. Such seizures are subdivided into simple and complex motor seizures according to the morphological characteristics of the primary motor actions. Simple motor seizures are motor seizures characterized by some unnatural speed, sequence, or posture (e.g., convulsion). The motor actions in complex motor seizures are similar to normal physiological motor actions. However, the space-time of their occurrences is inappropriate. An example is the manifestations of automatism. The patient's state of consciousness is generally but not necessarily affected during the occurrence of a complex motor seizure. ⑤ Special seizures: Special seizures include atonic seizures, astatic seizures, hypomotor seizures, akinesia seizures, negative myoclonic seizures, and aphasic seizures. In clinical process, they are mostly negative seizures dominated by negative symptoms.

Table 1.6 Symptomatological lateralization of seizures

Lateralizing seizure phenomenon	Hemisphere
Head and eye deviation	Contralateral
Dystonic hand posturing	Contralateral
Figure-4 sign	Contralateral
Automatisms with preserved responsiveness	Non-dominant
Ictal speech	Non-dominant
Postictal aphasia	Dominant
Ictal vomiting	Non-dominant
Ictal spitting	Non-dominant
Peri-ictal urinary urge	Non-dominant
Postictal nose rubbing	Ipsilateral
Postictal coughing	Non-dominant
Unilateral clonic seizure	Contralateral
Unilateral tonic seizures	Contralateral
Unilateral eye blinking	Ipsilateral
Asymmetric ending	Ipsilateral

Characterization localization: Epileptic seizures have their distribution and involvement regions. It is essential to determine the lateralization and localization of epileptogenic focus. Generally, localization-related information (e.g., left face, right hand) should be recorded. Common recordings are as follows: left lateral (or right lateral), generalized, axial, and asymmetrical. For example, axial epileptic spasm seizures, bilateral asymmetrical tonic seizures. Some common symptomatological lateralization meanings are presented in Table 1.6.

Evolution of the seizures: many seizures may evolve from one type to other types. The evolution relation is indicated with the symbol →; for example, aura→ left hand clonic seizure→generalized tonic-clonic seizure. The onset symptoms are generally of great significance for localization and lateralization.

It is noteworthy that, any seizure symptoms that are narrated by patients or their relatives rather than videotaped or recorded with EEG can be indicated by the use of italic type or the attachment of quotation marks. By following this classification rule, most physicians and technicians will be able to describe a seizure in a "what you see is what you get" way.

Basic Methods for Epilepsy Preoperative Evaluation

Drug-resistant or refractory epilepsy refers to the condition that seizures cannot be effectively controlled with two standard antiseizure medication regimens. About 30% of epilepsy patients are drug-resistant. However, at least 50% of them can achieve complete seizure control through surgical procedures. Successful surgical treatment of refractory epilepsy requires a number of important considerations, including the following: ① Being familiar with the indications for surgery and selection of appropriate surgical procedures for the patient. ② Adequate preoperative evaluation, precise localization of epileptogenic focus, and preparation of a reasonable surgical protocol. ③ Careful implementation of surgical plan. ④ Rational adjustment of perioperative management and appropriate administration of postoperative antiseizure medication.

The preoperative evaluation of epilepsy is a complex procedure aimed at precisely locating the epileptogenic zone and functional area using integrated methods to achieve optimum response to surgical treatment and minimize functional impairment. The classic epileptogenic zone is defined as the minimum brain tissue to be resected to achieve seizure-free results of post-operation. In recent years, the network theory of epileptic seizure has garnered significant attention. According to the theory, a certain loop is involved in the origin and propagation of epileptic seizures. Electrophysiologically, SEEG suggests that the epileptogenic zone includes the origin zone and early fast propagation zone/primary early discharge tissue zone.

In current clinical practice, areas related to the epileptogenic zone are identified and eventually pinpointed for evaluation of the epilepsy network, since the epileptogenic zone is merely a theoretical concept. So far, there is no gold standard for the positioning of epileptogenic zone based on careful observation, analysis of seizure symptoms, evaluation by brain electromagnetic physiological, structural imaging and functional imaging from a variety of perspectives for a final comprehensive consideration.

In general, appropriate examination techniques should be selected for preoperative evaluations based on clinical, electrophysiological, anatomical, and functional characteristics. The basic methods currently available for preoperative evaluation include the following.

Basic Methods for Noninvasive Evaluation

Electroencephalography and *Magnetoencephalography*

1. *Video EEG (VEEG) monitoring* It involves an EEG device and a synchronous video device to monitor the behavioral and EEG manifestations of epileptic seizures. The objective of this technique is to identify more than three conventional seizures for facilitating the identification of the real-time relationship between epileptic seizure and EEG change and for lateralizing and positioning of epileptic seizures based on the site that displays epileptiform discharge in EEG.

   Electroencephalogram (EEG) is the foundation of preoperative evaluation and is used to locate the epileptogenic zone in epilepsy evaluation. The spatial distribution pattern of interictal abnormal discharges provides overall information on the normal and abnormal activities of the brain allowing for plotting the range of the irritation zone. The combination of the information on ictal electric discharges and the analysis of synchronously displayed seizure symptoms is used to identify the epileptogenic zone and propagation mode.
2. *Magnetoencephalography (MEG)* MEG is a noninvasive technique that reflects the electrical activity of the brain by detecting the magnetic field variations generated by the electric current of neuronal excitation. In particular, it can complement EEG by reflecting the activity of electric current on the brain surface. MEG has the merits of high sensitivity and spatial resolution for detecting abnormal electrical discharges. Unlike EEG, MEG signals are not distorted or attenuated when passing through tissue layers in the head. When combined with cerebral electric dipole positioning technique, MEG can provide three-dimensional visualization of signals collected from the brain surface, eliminating the volume conduction effect of electric current, which is helpful to determine the spatial position of interictal electric discharge over the cortex and the deep parts of the brain, providing more information on epileptic irritation zone in preoperative evaluation. Moreover, MEG can be used to locate speech cortex helping to reduce potential damage to the functional zone caused by surgical operations.

Structure Imaging

1. *Cranial CT* Although cranial CT has limitations in differentiating different brain tissues, it is still valuable in identifying certain intracranial pathological changes (e.g., intracranial hemorrhage, cerebral vascular malformation) and epileptogenic focus with calcification features (e.g., tuberous sclerosis, paraganglioma).

   Cranial CT also plays an auxiliary role in epilepsy evaluation and can accurately locate implanted intracranial electrodes, SEEG electrodes, and Deep Brain Stimulation (DBS) electrodes.

2. *Magnetic resonance imaging (MRI)* MRI scanning sequences, including T1WI, T2WI, and fluid attenuated inversion recovery (FLAIR), can yield high-resolution brain images that clearly display the anatomical structure of the brain and distinguish cerebral gray matter and white matter. It is capable of determining the anatomic position and range of a focus and the focus' relation to surrounding tissues. Its high resolution helps to identify minimal lesion(s) for providing a basis for further level diagnosis. MRI can accurately identify a variety of foci (e.g., hippocampal sclerosis, gray matter heterotopia, focal cortical dysplasia, and brain parenchymal damage). The scanning sequence for hippocampus MRI presents the long axis of hippocampus. The selection of short tau inversion recovery (STIR) sequence is helpful for better reflecting the internal structure of hippocampus and identifying minimal hippocampal lesions. High-resolution cranial MRI scans are recommended for all patients undergoing epilepsy evaluation.

   In epilepsy evaluation, MRI is used to identify epileptogenic lesion, and fast FLAIR sequence and diffusion-weighted imaging (DWI) help to further determine the focus. It is currently a challenge to locate the focus in patients who have negative examination results in conventional MRI examination. For them, image post-processing analysis is recommended, including the application of voxel-based morphometry (VBM) and quantitative measurement of cortical thickness will be beneficial to identify minimal structural lesion(s).

Functional Imaging

1. *Single photon emission computed tomography (SPECT)* SPECT is an imaging technique that reflects cerebral blood perfusion and brain functions. It is particularly useful in the evaluation of refractory epilepsy as the epileptogenic zone presents with interictal hypoperfusion and ictal hyperperfusion. Interictal and ictal SPECT provide valuable information in diagnosis of lateralization and determination of the range of the epileptogenic focus. While SPECT has lower detection sensitivity in interictal phase, it has high detection specificity in ictal phase for the detection of epileptogenic zone. Digital subtraction technique can help to reveal the change to hyperperfusion in epileptogenic zone during the ictal phase.

   Ictal SPECT examination, despite its operational difficulty, can be particularly helpful in identifying epileptogenic zone.

2. *Positron emission computed tomography (PET)* In clinical practice, metabolic imaging by 18F-fluorodeoxyglucose (18F-FDG) PET helps to find out the functional metabolism of nuclide tracer in different tissue sites. In the interictal phase, the activity of neuronal cells in epileptogenic focus decreases, resulting in decreased glucose metabolism and uptake of 18F-FDG, which is reflected as hypometabolism zone in PET images.

   During epilepsy evaluation, PET has higher sensitivity than SPECT in interictal phase, especially in patients with negative MRI and for the detection of focal cortical dysplasia. In light of this, PET is therefore crucial for locating epileptogenic zones. The integration of PET and MRI has further improved PET's ability to reveal spatial information. It is noteworthy that the hypometabolism zones in PET images may include epileptogenic foci, epileptogenic zones, and functional impairment zones, which must be carefully differentiated by various means.

Basic Methods for Invasive Evaluation

The second step of preoperative evaluation is invasive examination, which is required when the information obtained from noninvasive evaluations is inconsistent or when more precise positioning of the epileptogenic zone and functional zone is required. Invasive examinations mainly include surgical insertion of intracranial electrodes to record intracranial electrical signals. At present, clinical applications of electrodes include subdural electrodes and stereotactic electrodes, while epidural electrodes and oval foramen electrodes are less frequently used. Electrocorticograms (ECoG) and Stereoelectroencephalography (SEEG) in clinical applications directly record the field potential activity signals collected by subdural electrodes and stereotactic electrodes from brain tissues. Compared with scalp EEG, ECoG improved spatial and temporal resolution and provides clear evidence of early seizure.

It is noteworthy that intracranial electrodes are not primarily used for epileptic focus detection, but rather for verification. The implantation of intracranial electrodes, regardless of their types, should be based on definite theoretical hypothesis.

Interictal

Similar to scalp EEG, seizure discharges reveal an irritation zone but does not directly indicate the epileptogenic zone. However, intracranial EEG recordings directly capture the activity of the cerebral cortex. Localized phenomena of relative significance include the following.

1. Focal, rhythmic, or periodic discharge, periodic fast-rhythmic and localized delta brush pattern has high relevance to focal cortical dysplasia (FCD).
2. In recent years, interictal high-frequency oscillation observed through high-frequency sampling has high indicative significance of epileptogenic zone.

Ictal

During ictal recordings, intracranial EEG directly reflects the epileptic seizure.

1. *Typical paroxysmal discharge patterns are characterized by* ① Decreased focal voltage, with fast activities (beta-gamma), and dynamic evolution of frequency, voltage, and spatial distribution over time. ② Rare onset activities including other rhythms (δ, θ, α). ③ Wide-band sampling-based direct current shift (DC shift) that is helpful to the localization of the onset zone.
2. *Important notes* ① The onset of discharge in intracranial seizures must be earlier than the onset of clinical seizure. ② Even typical seizure pattern cannot eliminate the possibility that the electrodes fail to cover the true seizure onset zone and the collected cerebral electrical activities might spread to wider regions by conduction or activation. ③ Symptomatological-cerebral electrical-physiological-anatomic structural explanation of clinical seizure as a whole should be emphasized.

Brain Function Evaluation

Scales or Mental Task Tests

Scales or mental task tests are used to evaluate the cognitive and behavioral state of the patient comprehensively. The Wechsler Scales (WS) are commonly used for IQ testing, which can reflect the patient's intelligence level but cannot provide information for lateralizing and localizing epileptogenic focus. Cognitive task tests, including vocabulary-based verbal tests (e.g., naming test) and non-verbal tests, may be used for cognitive screening. Memory tests, including verbal and non-verbal learning match tests, are necessary. Executive function tests, which must include verbal and non-verbal fluency test and a problem-solving ability test, are also important. Psychomotor, sensory, visual perception, and speech ability tests can be selected as needed. Cognitive function evaluation is helpful for revealing the functional impairment zones.

Intracarotid Amobarbital Procedure (IAP)

In intracarotid amobarbital procedure (IAP), also known as Wada test, short-term anesthesia of the left/right cerebral hemisphere is induced through the injection of pentobarbital (amytal) into left/right internal carotid artery to evaluate the speech function and memory function of the non-anesthetized cerebral hemisphere. For lateralizing speech function, especially the separate evaluation of left and right hemispheres, the Wada test utilizes selective deactivation of cerebral hemisphere functions to simulate the surgical resection of a hemisphere optimally. In temporal lobe epilepsy (TLE), Wada test is helpful in assessing the risk of postoperative memory defect. Due to the global supply shortage of pentobarbital, propofol may be used as an alternative.

Evoked Potential

In consideration of the compensatory potential of the nervous system and the presence of functional compensation to a varying extent in some patients' cortex in the hemisphere opposite to their focal side, accurate evaluation of such compensation is essential to the prediction of the impact of the resection of focus on the limbs and speech functions of the patient. Motor evoked potential (MEP) is frequently used for evaluating the function of the focal cortex and the compensation by the opposite cortex. MEP records with the compound action potential of the corresponding muscles indicate the integrity of the motor conduction tract. MEP can be evoked by electrical or magnetic stimulation, with magnetic stimulation being economical, noninvasive, reproducible, and sensitive. Moreover, magnetic stimulation causes less pain than electric stimulation, making it very suitable for the evaluation of cortical function prior to hemispherectomy.

Functional Magnetic Resonance Imaging (fMRI)

Functional magnetic resonance imaging (fMRI) can display minute changes in MRI signals of different brain areas caused by changes in blood oxygen saturation of venous capillaries. After performing a task, fMRI can provide functional localization of motor cortex, sensory cortex, visual cortex, and speech cortex areas. A comparison of the functional evaluation results with the epileptogenic zone will be helpful to the preparation of surgical protocol and the protection of brain function.

Electric Stimulation of Cortex

After the implantation of intracranial electrodes, cortical mapping is carried out per routine. Cortical mapping is the gold standard for brain function localization. The following parameters and procedures are used for high-frequency stimulation with subdural electrodes.

1. *Stimulation parameters* The high-frequency stimulation parameters for subdural electrodes are as follows: 50 Hz, biphasic stimuli, wave width 0.2 ms, lasting 1–5 s (or shorter for localization of motor cortex, longer for testing speech and other cognitive tasks); intensity of stimuli: 1–15 mA; the intensity of electric current is gradually increased with a gradient of 1 mA. Since low current intensity in the application of SEEG can give rise to functional responses, the intensity of electric current stimuli could be increased gradually from 0.5 mA, with the step of 0.5 mA.
2. *Stimulation procedures* A distribution map of electrodes on cortex is plotted, with preliminary hypotheses on the responses that may be induced through a specific elec-

trode. The stimulation should be carried out when the patient is conscious and in good general state. The patient is placed at semi-reclined position or decubitus position and allowed to relax. The stimulation is videotaped for further analysis and a dedicated person records the responses to the stimuli. The stimuli are delivered by adjacent electrode pair, starting from the intensity of 1 mA/0.5 mA with gradual increase. The duration of a stimulation test should be limited to 1 hour as far as possible, and an interval of 24 h should be arranged before the next stimulation in order to prevent excessive stimulation.

Other Evaluation Methods

1. *Magnetic resonance spectroscopy (MRS)* Magnetic resonance spectrum (MRS) is the only noninvasive technique used to determine the chemical compound in a specific tissue area in a living body. It is used to identify pathological changes from the perspective of the metabolism in tissues and cells. The contents and ratios of N-acetyl aspartic acid (NAA), choline compound (Cho), and phosphocreatine creatinine (Cr) can help to localize the epileptogenic zone. MRS plays an important role in the diagnosis and evaluation of epilepsies, especially temporal lobe epilepsy (TLE).
2. *Cortico-cortical evoked potentials (CCEP)* Cortico-cortical evoked potentials (CCEP) through intracranial electrodes to stimulate localized areas of the brain, and responses in adjacent and/or distant sites to the potentials that have a time-locked relationship with the stimulus are recorded. Currently, classic stimulation parameters are as follows: 1 Hz, wave width 0.3 ms, stimulus intensity 4–8 mA; 50 biphasic repetitive stimuli are delivered by two adjacent electrodes (cathode and anode) in sequence, and response signal sampling rate is more than 2000 Hz. CCEP can provide information on the electrical conduction between brain areas, reflecting the connection between different brain areas. It is helpful in explaining epileptic seizure network and studying brain function.
3. *Multi-modality imaging technique* Multi-modality imaging integrates a variety of measuring modes of nervous activities to provide complementary imaging information by incorporating structural imaging and functional imaging techniques (MRI+PET, SISCOM), brain electromagnetic physiological and structural imaging techniques, and/or the incorporation of brain electromagnetic physiological and functional imaging techniques (EEG/fMRI).
4. *Intracranial event-related potentials (ERP) examination* The implantation of intracranial electrodes enables precise spatial and temporal resolution, making intracranial event-related potentials (ERP) test helpful for accurately localizing specific brain functions, such as visual/spatial perception, auditory cognition, speech function, memory function, and emotional cognitive function. It is also beneficial to understand the cognitive processing.
5. *Further analyses with digital signal processing techniques* The information gathered from electrophysiological records can be further analyzed by employing digital signal processing techniques and using software such as Matlab and Python, to investigate the electrophysiological patterns and underlying electrophysiological mechanisms of epileptic seizures.

Basic Principles and Strategies for Preoperative Evaluation of Epilepsy

Basic Principles for Preoperative Evaluation of Epilepsy

Concepts about epileptogenic focus and epilepsy network:

1. *Seizure zone* A zone which presents a series of clinical manifestations caused by neuron excessive synchronous discharge. A true epileptogenic focus should be an area where electric activity is abnormal that epileptic seizures may be triggered. Resection of this zone could eliminate epileptic seizures. Table 1.7 lists some basic concepts about epileptogenic focus. These zones are not equal to true epileptogenic foci. Therefore, all information regarding these should be collected prior to preoperative evaluation for determination of epileptogenic focus after multidisciplinary discussion and comprehensive analysis under the guidance of experts.

Table 1.7 Concepts and methods for localizing epileptogenic focus

Concept	Definition	Test method
Irritation zone	A zone where spikes or sharp waves occur in interictal phase	EEG, cortical electrode and depth electrode EEG, MEG, synchronous recording of EEG and functional MRI
Seizure onset zone	A zone which gives rise to epileptic seizures	EEG, cortical electrode and depth electrode EEG
Seizure symptomatic zone	A zone which gives rise to clinical seizure symptoms	Clinical observation, patient report, and electrophysiological examination
Functional deficit zone	Non-epileptic cerebral dysfunction zone	Physical examination of the nervous system, neuropsychological test, EEG, SPECT, PET
Lesion zone	Abnormal cerebral structure zone	Cerebral structure imaging (CT, MRI), histopathology

2. *Irritation zone* A zone where epileptiform discharges occur in interictal EEG/MEG. Continuous abnormal discharges and excessive synchronization can give rise to clinical seizure. Epileptiform discharge with spikes or sharp waves can be identified in EEG and MEG. Interictal spikes or sharp waves are not identical to epileptic seizures. Irritation zone is also not equal to epileptogenic focus, and not every patient's scalp EEG will display spikes or sharp waves.
3. *Seizure onset zone (SOZ)* The area where the first abnormal continuous discharge occurs and leads to subsequent clinical seizure. Throughout the entire process of epileptic seizure, EEG can record the gradual propagation of the typical abnormal discharge from the onset zone to other zones or the whole brain. The seizure onset zone could be determined by the ictal EEG, which is the best method to monitor abnormal discharge by video EEG or intracranial EEG. Scalp EEG is subject to the influence of the conduction medium and the artifacts of myoelectrical activity at the onset. Initial abnormal discharge site can be observed only in some patients. In other patients, the electrical activities recorded by scalp electrodes cannot be precisely localized. The cortical or depth electrodes (including stereoelectroencephalography) can display the temporal sequence of the abnormal discharges at different sites. This is the only method for precisely localizing the SOZ. The SOZ can be either localized or relatively extensive.
4. *Seizure symptomatic zone*

   When the abnormal discharges propagate to some specific functional brain regions, it could lead to clinical seizure symptoms. The zone that leads to the onset of clinical symptoms is referred to as the symptomatic zone. It is very important to localize the epileptogenic focus according to clinical symptoms. The localization of epileptogenic focus may have two results: one is that the symptomatic zone basically coincides with the epileptogenic focus, the other is that the symptomatic zone is not equal to the epileptogenic focus. However, the first symptom is of important reference significance for the localization of epileptogenic focus.
5. *Functional deficit zone* Functional brain imaging (PET, SPECT, fMRI) may reveal some areas with cerebral dysfunction. These abnormal areas may be functional brain regions involved by epileptic seizure in interictal phase and ictal phase. Patients in interictal phase generally present hypoperfusion or hypometabolism in focal cerebral zone; ictal SPECT may reveal hyperperfusion of focal cerebral zones. All abnormal functional areas identified by ictal and interictal SPECT-based SISCOM technique and coregistered PET and MRI technique are of suggestive significance for the localization of epileptogenic focus; these identified areas, together with the seizure symptoms and EEG, can help to localize the epileptogenic focus.
6. *Epileptogenic brain lesions* CT and MRI scans may find some structural lesions that are closely associated with epileptic seizures; however, this does not mean these lesions are necessarily the cause of epileptic seizures. When used to identify epileptogenic brain injury areas, MRI, especially high field intensity MRI, is superior to CT; the application of FLAIR imaging technique can identify many minimal pathological brain changes, such as hippocampal sclerosis and gray matter heterotopia. Voxel-based morphometry (VBM) may reveal minimal structural abnormality with very high sensitivity, and it is especially suitable for finding some focal cortical dysplasia that cannot be found by routine imaging techniques.

In conclusion, the localization of epileptogenic focus should be done in light of patient's specific conditions and with rationally selected examination methods. The precise location of epileptogenic focus can be identified only through proper and comprehensive analysis of all examination results. Generally speaking, the localization results are reliable when the structural imaging findings are in agreement with the clinical seizure symptoms and interictal and ictal scalp EEG findings. If these examinations yield inconsistent results, prolonged electroencephalography using intracranial electrodes might be needed to record the ictal intracranial EEG for the localization. About 1/3–1/2 of epileptic patients may need this technique for final and precise localization of the epileptogenic focus.

It is gradually recognized with the pathophysiological studies of epilepsy, especially in the extensive application process of SEEG, that the brain regions involved in an epileptic seizure are generally not limited to a specific area; rather, sometimes a number of widely separated brain regions may be involved and they affect, promote, alternatively activate each other, and these regions may have mutual causality. In most cases, it is impossible to identify which region is the true epileptogenic focus. In light of this, epilepsy network has been introduced to define the important epileptic cerebral zones. In practice, a comprehensive analysis on the basis of evidence from the abovementioned examinations is carried out to determine the closeness of the involvement of different brain regions in epileptic seizure, the activation sequence of these regions, and the epilepsy network, in order to guide the surgical resection of the epileptic zone.

The contribution of examination techniques to localization of epileptogenic focus varies (Table 1.8). Some techniques have higher localization reliability, others have higher localization sensitivity. Therefore, the relationship between the results from these techniques should be analyzed in an all-round way. When there is conflicting information during the localization process, two basic principles should be followed: first, examination results of higher reliability should take precedence over results of lower reliability; second, the principle of temporal sequence should be followed in the analysis of EEG and symptomatic information, i.e., the earlier the information, the more reliable site suggested by the information.

When it is impossible to get all reliable information, or when the contradiction between different important information makes it impossible to understand the process of the epileptic seizure, intracranial electrodes recording (including subdural electrode EEG and stereotactic EEG) should be considered (Table 1.9) to further localize the epileptogenic focus. The information available from intracranial EEG includes interictal spikes and sharp waves, interictal high-frequency oscillation, burst EEG, subclinical seizures and clinical seizures; for their localization significance, refer to Table 1.10.

A protocol should be prepared based on the semiologic features, the scalp EEG and the comprehensive analysis results of the MEG or PET to make the reasonable intracranial electrode implantation scheme. The information from intracranial EEG can be used to verify or reject the hypothesis on epileptic zones.

Table 1.8 Comparison of reliability and sensitivity among localization techniques

Technique	Reliability	Sensitivity
Symptomatology	+++	++
Scalp EEG/MEG (interictal)	++	+++
Scalp EEG (ictal)	+++	++
Intracranial EEG	++++	+++
MRI/CT	+++	+
Brain function imaging	+	++++

Note: ++++ highest priority; +++ high priority; ++ preferred priority; + ordinary priority

Table 1.10 Comparison of localization significance of the intracranial EEG

Intracranial EEG indicator	Characteristics	Application principles and precautions	Localization significance
Sharp waves	Protruded from the background, 70–200 ms	Collectible in a wide range which generally goes beyond the seizure onset zone	++
Spike waves	Protruded from the background, <70 ms	Collectible in a wide range which generally goes beyond the seizure onset zone	++
Gamma activity	30–80 Hz	First discharge channel is of high localization significance	+++
HFO-ripple	80–250 Hz oscillation	Pay more attention to the differentiation of physiological activities	+++
HFO-fast ripple	250–500 Hz oscillation	Pay more attention to the differentiation of physiological activities	+++
HFO burst/event DC shift	Temporary multi-channel burst activities Very slow monophasic or biphasic electrical activity	First discharge channel is of high localization significance First shift channel is of high localization significance	+++ +++
Subclinical seizures	Long-lasting, with ictal discharges but without clinical symptoms	Initial abnormal rhythmic activity is of importance	++++
Clinical seizure	Long-lasting, with ictal discharges and clinical symptoms	Initial abnormal rhythmic activity is of importance	++++

Table 1.9 Principles for phase II intracranial electrode implantation

Cranial MRI/CT	EEG/MEG	Symptomatology	Consistency of results	Evaluation conclusion
+	+	+	***	Phase I
+	+	–	**	Phase I
+	–	+	**	Phase I
–	+	+	**	Phase I
+	–	–	*	Phase II
–	+	–	*	Phase II
–	–	+	*	Phase II
			?	Phase II

Note: + information provided; – no information provided; ***in highly agreement, ** in agreement, * information inadequate, ? Contradictory information

Strategies for Preoperative Epilepsy Evaluation

The quality of preoperative evaluation decides the outcome of surgical treatment. More and more techniques for preoperative evaluation make the localization of epileptogenic focus precise. In spite of this, preoperative evaluation is still an extremely complicated systematic work at present; one has to determine the localization significance of multiple evaluation techniques, evaluate the sensitivity and reliability of the techniques, decide the application sequence of these evaluation techniques, in order to minimize the medical resources and workload needed for the evaluation. When there are contradictory examination results, one has to trade off the pros and cons of the techniques, identify their commonness, eliminate the false results, and retain the true results in order to localize the true epileptogenic focus. When one finds helpless and at a loss, you should break free from the fetters of preconceived conventional ideas, make use of invasive examination techniques, and find out the clues. The accumulation of experience is very critical. The following basic strategies are provided here for reference.

1. *Strategies for localization of hemispheric giant lesions* Imaging plays a crucial role in locating seizure focus. Results from structural imaging (mainly brain CT and MRI) are very intuitive and facilitate clinical understanding of seizure-related lesions. When any huge unilateral hemispherical focus is found in MRI or CT, consideration should be first given to the relationship between the focus and the seizure. The key point is to confirm that symptoms (including myoclonus, spasm, tonic, somatic sensory aura, visual aura) of epileptic seizure are in agreement with the lateralization of the lesion. If it is consistent, then the epileptogenic focus is localized to this side. Two noteworthy points: ① If interictal discharges and ictal abnormal rhythm are identified in scalp EEG, then the localization of the epileptogenic focus is further supported; however, even in cases where discharges occur in both sides or the bilateral rhythms are synchronous and basically symmetric, the possibility that the epileptogenic focus located on the lesion side cannot be rejected and this does not impede the resection or mutilation of the hemisphere. ② A rare scenario is that the epileptogenic zone localized to the side opposite to the lesion according to the symptoms of seizure. This seems to be incomprehensible; however, the possibility that the lesion hemisphere is the epileptogenic focus cannot be excluded and should be judged in light of other available information.
2. *Strategies for localization of solitary structural lesion* It has been found in imaging that solitary structural lesion is one of the most important and reliable information for localization. It is necessary to find any symptomatic clues and to demonstrate that lesions can explain the symptoms. If this is the case, the localization is generally reliable. In such cases, if the interictal and ictal EEG information is in agreement with the lesion, the reliability of the localization by imaging examination is further supported. Even if the interictal and ictal EEG information is not in agreement with the lesion, the localization value of the lesion cannot be denied. If the symptomatic information fails to show localization significance but the EEG is in agreement with the lesion, then the position of the lesion revealed by imaging examination is still very valuable. MEG has localization significance identical to that identified in interictal EEG, but the spatial positioning precision is higher. The voxel-based morphometry (VBM) technique has reliability in identifying minute structural changes and the application of the technique deserves promotion.
3. *Application strategy of EEG and MEG in patients with negative imaging* Highly synchronized abnormal discharges can be detected with EEG and MEG. The spatial sites suggested by the discharges are exceptionally excited, showing that these regions are generally in a highly active state and may give rise to persistent burst activity. Therefore, areas with abnormal discharges are of definite suggestive significance in the localization process. *Important notes* ① In case of multiple abnormal discharge zones being identified, the localization of epileptogenic focus should be based on the available ictal features and symptomatic information rather than merely based on the interictal discharges. ② The principle of temporal sequence should be followed during the analysis of ictal EEG. The earlier abnormal activities, the closer site to the epileptogenic focus; however, since the limitations of the EEG sampling, the network relationship between these spatial sites should be analyzed carefully in order to make clear the propagation route of epileptic activities. ③ Comparison of symptoms and EEG results is important, and video EEG should be read synchronously and carefully finding the occurrence sequence of multiple events. Cortical zones indicated by symptoms may overlap with those indicated by EEG characteristics. During the evaluation, full consideration should be given to the dynamic process of the propagation of epileptic activities and cortical dynamic propagation network map related to the seizure should be delineated.
4. *Strategies for reverse tracking of symptomatic clues in patients with negative imaging findings* It is very important to carry out in-depth semiology analysis in patients with negative imaging findings. Attention should be paid to the clues on two aspects: ① Repetitive communication with patients to get in-depth understanding of the auras. The auras could provide information of localization significance. For example, abnormal feelings in body parts

have the highest localization significance and may point to specific cortical regions: autonomic symptoms and emotional symptoms may suggest that the epileptogenic focus is located in limbic systems; cognitive symptoms suggest the epileptogenic focus is located in associative cortex. ② The initial motor symptoms should be analyzed carefully, and the epileptogenic focus might be indicated at corresponding cortex with motor symptoms. Furthermore, abnormal behavioral manifestations indicated that the epileptogenic focus is located in frontal-temporal lobe regions or insular lobe region. The principles for inverse look up should be followed during the semiology localization, that is to say, seizure motor action should be traced back to the earliest one. The earlier symptoms reveal the site of the epileptogenic focus. Symptomatology information plus functional brain imaging or MEG results could improve the reliability of localization.

5. *Strategies for functional brain imaging in patients with negative imaging findings* For patients with negative imaging findings, SISCOM results or PET hypometabolism are of important significance for localization. If the seizure symptoms indicate that a patient has temporal lobe epilepsy, and PET hypometabolism is in unilateral temporal lobe, then the PET lateralization is of important significance. The coregistered PET-MRI technique reveals cortical focal hypometabolic regions that require other supporting information. For example, if the hypometabolic regions are in agreement with the sites indicated by MEG or VBM, then the regions are responsible for the seizure. Functional brain imaging may be indispensable for the explanation of semiology.
6. *Strategies for dealing with inadequate localization information or contradicting localization information* For patients with inadequate localization information or contradicting localization information, intracranial EEG may be applied rationally by implanting intracranial electrodes for long-term monitoring of electrical activities. However, attention should be paid to the following points: ① All information of the patients should be analyzed comprehensively and one or two rational hypotheses on epileptic activities propagation network should be proposed for purposive design of intracranial electrode implantation scheme in order to reveal the process of the brain activities during epileptic seizures. However, purposelessly implanting of excessive intracranial electrodes should be avoided. ② The dominance of intracranial EEG lies in that it can identify the site that presents the earliest abnormal electrical activities of seizure. Obviously, the temporal priority principle should be paid adequate attention. In other words, the comparison of the electrical activity information of intracranial EEG in multiple spatial sites and the semiology information is very important. The site that presents the earliest abnormal activities that are earlier than the first symptom has the highest localization significance and the site is closest to the true epileptogenic focus. ③ The possibility that a deep cortical structure is involved in the epileptic seizure process should be attached much importance, such as seizures from insular lobe, fronto-orbital, medial frontal cortex, and medial parietal cortex. ④ Information from cortical electrical stimulation should be fully utilized to help the localization. Intracranial EEG, especially cerebral depth electrode stimulation, can induce after discharges or epileptic seizure. A comparison of this information with that of routine seizures should be made for identifying the similarity between them. Cortical stimulation results can be used to plot a seizure network connection map for facilitating the localization of epileptogenic focus.
7. *Strategies for comprehensive evaluation and logical reasoning* The localization of epileptogenic focus is a process of comprehensive analysis. It is usually impossible to get all information for localization in many patients. Brain anatomic, neurophysiological, and brain network knowledge should be used to explain the neural activity process of each seizure. For this purpose, logical reasoning is essential. The physicians and surgeons in an epilepsy center should carry out comprehensive discussion in order to make a surgical protocol.

Cases of Frontal Lobe Epilepsy

2

Du Wei, Piao Yuanyuan, Xu Cuiping, Lin Yicong, and Chen Jia

Overview of Frontal Lobe Epilepsy

Anatomy of Frontal Lobe

Frontal lobe is the largest lobe of the brain. Its volume and weight account for 1/3–1/2 of the whole brain. Frontal lobe epilepsy is the second most common drug-resistant epilepsy (also known as drug refractory epilepsy), second to temporal lobe epilepsy (TLE), and accounting for 20%–30% of drug refractory epilepsy patients that need surgical treatment. Knowledge on the functions and anatomy of frontal lobe is crucial for understanding of frontal lobe seizures. Conventionally, the frontal lobe is divided into lateral frontal lobe, medial frontal lobe, and orbitofrontal lobe according to the origin site of frontal lobe epileptic seizures. The lateral frontal lobe consists of motor cortex (MC), premotor cortex (PMC), prefrontal lobe; the medial frontal lobe consists of primary motor cortex area, supplementary motor area (SMA), anterior cingulate cortex (ACC), and prefrontal lobe. Primary motor cortical area and SMA are among the most widely researched in studies of medial frontal lobe epilepsy.

Located in gyrus precentralis and anterior lobulus paracentralis, motor cortex regulates the voluntary movement of the body. Premotor cortex (Brodmann Area 6) is located anterior to the gyrus precentralis. It sends neuro-projection to primary motor cortex area and spinal cord anterior horn and participates in the preparation and learning of exercises.

Consisting of Brodmann Areas 9, 10, 44, 45, and 46, the prefrontal lobe cortex is involved in emotional processing, moral behaviors, motor control, working memory, and behavioral learning.

Consisting of Brodmann Areas 24, 25, and 32, the anterior cingulate cortex mainly receives afferences from dorsolateral prefrontal cortex, orbitofrontal lobe, insular lobe, and thalamus and sends neurofibral projecting to pre-motor cortex, orbitofrontal zone, cortical zone of anterior insular lobe, amygdala, and brain stem structure. Electrical stimulation of anterior cingulate cortex would give rise to simple archeokinetic movements of fingers, hands, lips, and tongue (e.g., touching, scrubbing, sucking, and licking); generally, the contralateral side of the body is affected. These movements are generally accompanied with euphoric emotional changes and/or variance and autonomic symptoms, such as mydriasis, facial flushing, tachycardia, and hyperventilation.

Consisting of the entire or the majority of Brodmann Area 6, SMA can be divided into SMA proper (2/3) and anterior region of SMA (1/3). Both parts receive afferences from thalamus, basal ganglia, cerebellum, cingulate cortex, anterior region of motor cortex, and posterior central region. However, SMA proper also receives cortical projections from anterior central area. SMA proper sends information through the corticospinal tract; anterior region of SMA sends information through corticobulbar tract. SMA is mainly responsible for the preparation of spontaneous movement. The SMA has an anterior part that represents head and face and a posterior part that represents upper extremities and lower extremities. Electrical stimulation of SMA proper can give rise to slow tonic contraction of proximal limbs and torso; generally bilateral lower limbs respond to the stimuli simultaneously or even the ipsilateral limbs (ipsilateral upper extremity or ipsilateral upper and lower extremities) manifest movements: head and eyes deviate to the contralateral side; and contralateral limbs or bilateral lower limbs and head experience such symptoms as numbness or tingling sensation. Stimulating the anterior region of SMA could give rise to inhibition of intention movement, i.e., the negative movement symptoms.

Clinical Manifestations

The majority of previous observations and studies held that frontal lobe epilepsy has the following semiological features:

D. Wei · P. Yuanyuan · X. Cuiping (✉)
Department of Neurosurgery, Beijing, China

L. Yicong · C. Jia
Department of Neurology, Beijing, China

Y. Wang (ed.), *Electroencephalogram for Presurgical Epilepsy Evaluation*, https://doi.org/10.1007/978-981-95-8003-3_2

Table 2.1 Division of frontal lobe regions and the regions' corresponding seizure symptoms

Site of origin	Seizure semiology
Cingulate cortex	Hypermotor, emotional symptoms (fear, risus), autonomic symptoms, dialeptic seizures, urinary incontinence
Supplementary motor area (SMA)	Postural or tonic deviation, hypermotor, body rotation, dystonia, verbigeration, oropharyngeal automatism, negative motor symptoms (reduction in movements of limbs or pause in speech), piloerection in bilateral or unilateral limbs, emotional symptoms (risus)
Motor cortex	Focal tonic or clonic movements
Dorsolateral prefrontal cortex	Tonic deviation, clonic limbs, pause in speech
Frontopolar	Tonic deviation, hypermotor, dialeptic seizures, clonic limbs, autonomic symptoms
Orbitofrontal zone	Olfactory hallucination, hypermotor, autonomic symptoms, urinary incontinence
Operculum insulae	Somatic sensory symptoms (electric shock, warm, pain), visceromotor and viscerosensory symptoms (throat tightness, dyspnea, pressure sensation in retrosternal or abdominal part), emotional symptoms (fear), chewing, drooling, gustatory hallucination, olfactory hallucination, ipsilateral facial jerk, pause in speech

many nocturnal episodes, frequent seizures, sometimes in clusters, brief duration; the patient rapidly regains consciousness after the seizure or only suffers from minimal post-ictal conscious disturbance; frontal lobe epilepsy would soon give rise to secondary generalized tonic-clonic seizure(s); asymmetric postural seizure(s) (abrupt, bilateral asymmetric tonic postural symptoms that last dozens of seconds); hypermotor seizures, and generally accompanied with obvious emotions (agitation, grief and indignation, agony, happiness); and the patient may experience auras of topoparesthesia or dyskinesia, usually with vocal symptoms. Some patients may manifest diverse auras, most of which are nonspecific, including somatosensory auras such as numbness, tingling, tightness, and heaviness; head auras (e.g., dizziness), fear, gustatory, olfactory, and upper abdominal auras The frontal lobe seizures can be divided into seven groups according to the origin site and semiologic features of seizure; their corresponding seizure symptoms are presented in Table 2.1.

Furthermore, in the EEG of children experiencing focal motor seizures after sleeping, wide sharp waves (SW) in central temporal region can be identified; most of such children have Self-limited epilepsy with centrotemporal spikes (SeLECTS), a condition with generally good prognosis; surgical treatment is not considered for such children, who should be differentiated from other patients with epilepsy.

EEG Characteristics

It is very difficult to localize the origin site of frontal lobe seizures with interictal scalp EEGs. In about 40% of the frontal lobe epilepsy, interictal EEGs show no epileptiform discharge. Long-term EEG monitoring may improve the detection rate of interictal epileptiform discharges. The distribution of interictal epileptiform discharges is usually quite generalized and concurrent spikes in bilateral hemispheres are quite common. Generally regional persistent epileptiform discharges can be seen in patients with dorsolateral prefrontal epilepsy, the site of epileptiform discharge is the same as the onset zone. However, in most patients whose epileptogenic focus is located in medial frontal lobe, interictal epileptiform discharge is not easily recorded or, if recorded, is multi-regional. In such patients, the recorded interictal epileptiform discharges are commonly seen in EEGs from midline leads such as Fz, Cz or F3, F4, Fp1, and Fp2. Rhythmic θ activities are quite common in midline lead in about 50% of the patients with frontal lobe epilepsy in awake state.

Even during a frontal lobe epileptic seizure, sometimes it is still much difficult to localize the epileptogenic focus with patient's ictal EEGs; this is mainly because: ① the initial clinical manifestation of seizure is generally abrupt hypermotor and postural tonic and as a result the initially recorded electrical activities of the brain are blurred or completely contaminated by motor artifacts, making it hard to analyze; ② the electrical activities of frontal lobe epilepsy rapidly give rise to synchronous propagation in bilateral frontal lobe through extensive neuro-fiber connection; as a result, it is rather difficult to distinguish one lateral from the other side; ③ EEGs obtained during the onset of seizure usually contain frequent low-amplitude β rhythms or attenuated and propagated β rhythms, which are susceptible to artifact by myoelectrical signal or other artifacts; ④ when epileptogenic focus is located in deep structures such as medial frontal, orbitofrontal, and insular opercula regions, no definite ictal EEG change can be recorded in some patients; and ⑤ electrical activities of dorsolateral prefrontal cortex (DLPFC) origin can also rapidly propagate to temporal lobe; as a result, definite ictal electrical activities can be recorded in temporal region, resulting in false localization.

Ictal EEGs may present rhythmic δ, θ, α, β activities, repetitive spikes or spike-and-wave complexes, electrical activities that are extensively suppressed, and/or nonrhythmic activities that are different from the background. Focal rhythmic discharges in seizure onset EEGs are mostly seen in patients with dorsolateral prefrontal cortex epilepsy, while seizure onset without focal rhythmic discharges is mostly seen in medial frontal lobe epilepsy.

Cases of Motor Cortex Epilepsy

Case 2.1 Precentral Gyrus Epilepsy

[Abstract of Medical Records]
Female, 17 years old.

1. *Chief complaint* Paroxysmal loss of consciousness and convulsion for 9 years.
2. *History of present illness* The patient experienced paroxysmal loss of consciousness and convulsion once without apparent predisposition 9 years ago. The frequency of seizures was about once per week for the next 2 years, and then progressed to 2–9 times per month. The seizure, lasting for 30 s to 2 min, was characterized by sudden right hand uplift, fingers in a claw-like position, right mouth twitching, eyes deviated upward and to the left, and head turned to the right, sometimes without complete loss of consciousness. Over the recent 2 months, the patient had frequent seizures and developed status epilepticus. Various antiseizure medications turned out to be ineffective. The patient has more than 10 seizures per day and is taking oxcarbazepine at 1200 mg/d; due to non-response to prior treatment with levetiracetam, the drug has been discontinued.
3. *Imaging examination*
   (a) MRI showed no abnormal signals.
   (b) PET showed decreased glucose metabolism over the left frontal region.
4. *EEG* For details, see Figs. 2.1, 2.2, 2.3, 2.4, and 2.5.

[Case Review]

1. *Case Characteristics*
   (a) *Seizure characteristics* ① Clustered seizures (more than 10 times per day). ② Early occurrence of motor symptoms during seizures (right mouth twitching). The seizure characteristics were consistent with those of frontal lobe epilepsy.
   (b) *EEG characteristics* ① Spike-and-wave complexes were observed over the central and parietal areas of bilateral posterior frontal regions on the interictal EEG. ② The low amplitude fast activity was observed over the left central and posterior frontal regions.

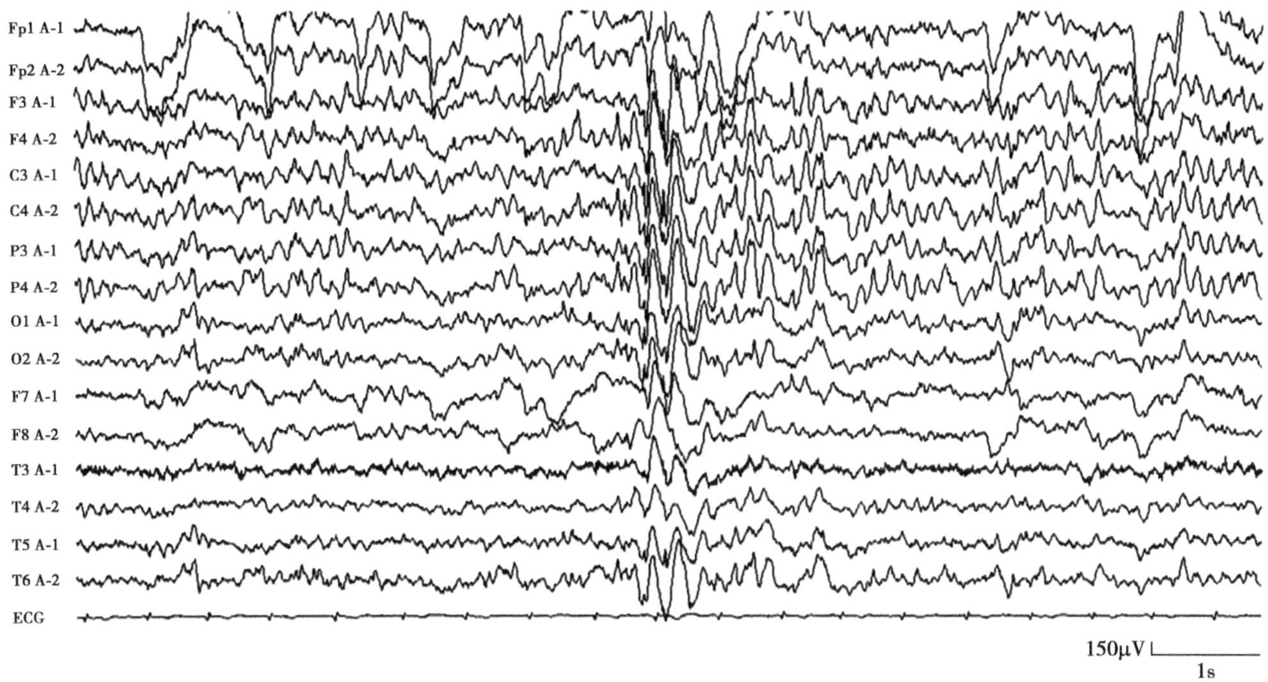

Fig. 2.1 Interictal scalp EEG
The basic rhythm was 8.0 Hz. Spike-and-wave complexes were observed over the bilateral posterior frontal (F3, F4) regions, central (C3, C4) region, and parietal (P3, P4) region

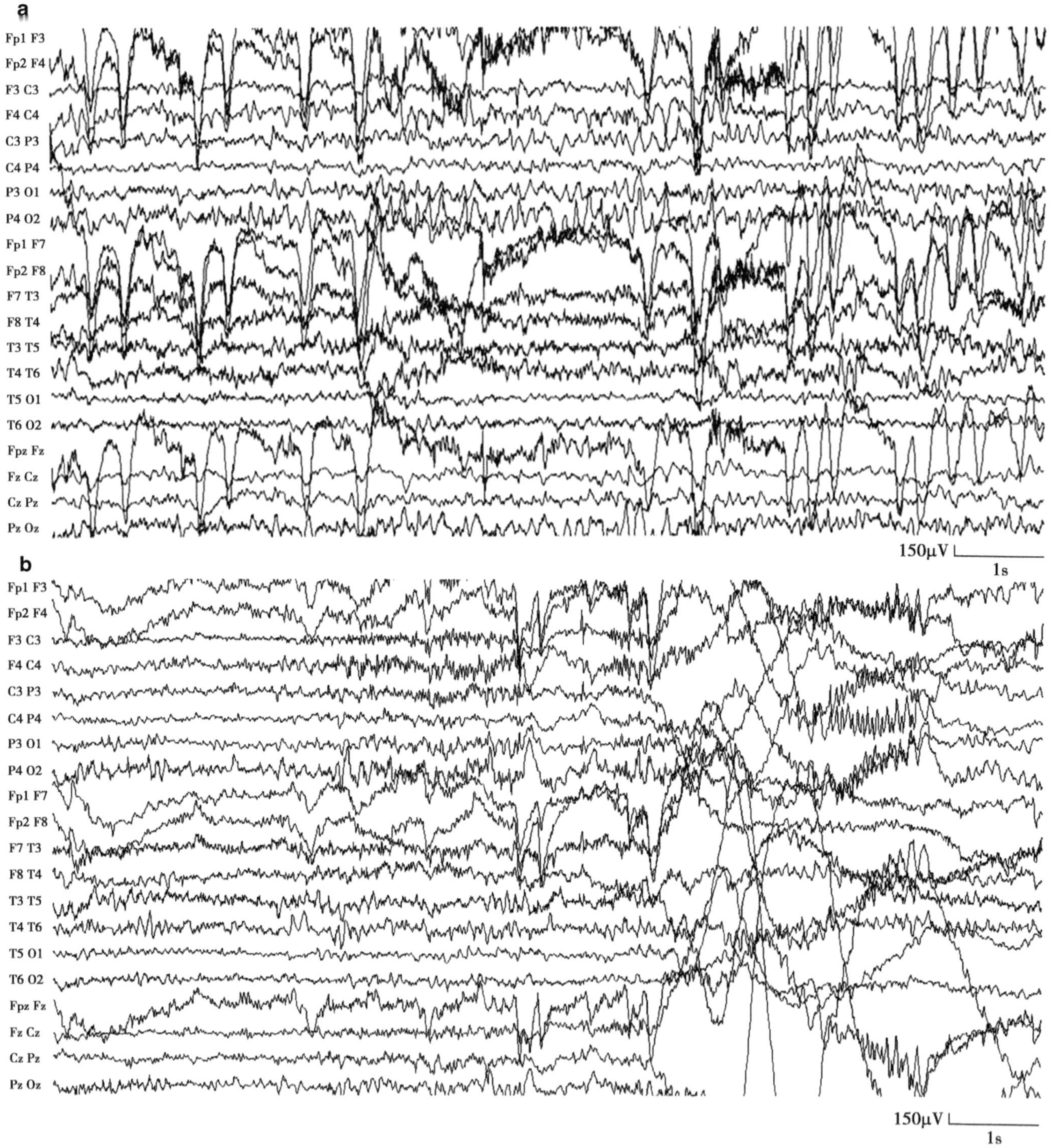

Fig. 2.2 Ictal scalp EEG. (**a**) The patient was sitting in bed and talking with her family members before the seizure. The EEG showed clear background, with multiple EMG artifacts in bilateral frontal regions (Fp1 F3, Fp2 F4, Fp1 F7, Fp2 F8, Fpz Fz). (**b**) At the time of seizure, the patient stopped talking and leaned back slowly, with her mouth deviated to the right, both upper limbs in flexion and obvious tonicity of the right upper limb, with slight trembling and loss of consciousness. EEG showed the low amplitude fast activity over the left posterior frontal (F3 C3) and central (C3 P3) regions, with amplitude increased and mixed with electrode artifacts. (**c**) At the end of the seizure, the patient sat up again and became conscious. The EEG recovered to the background

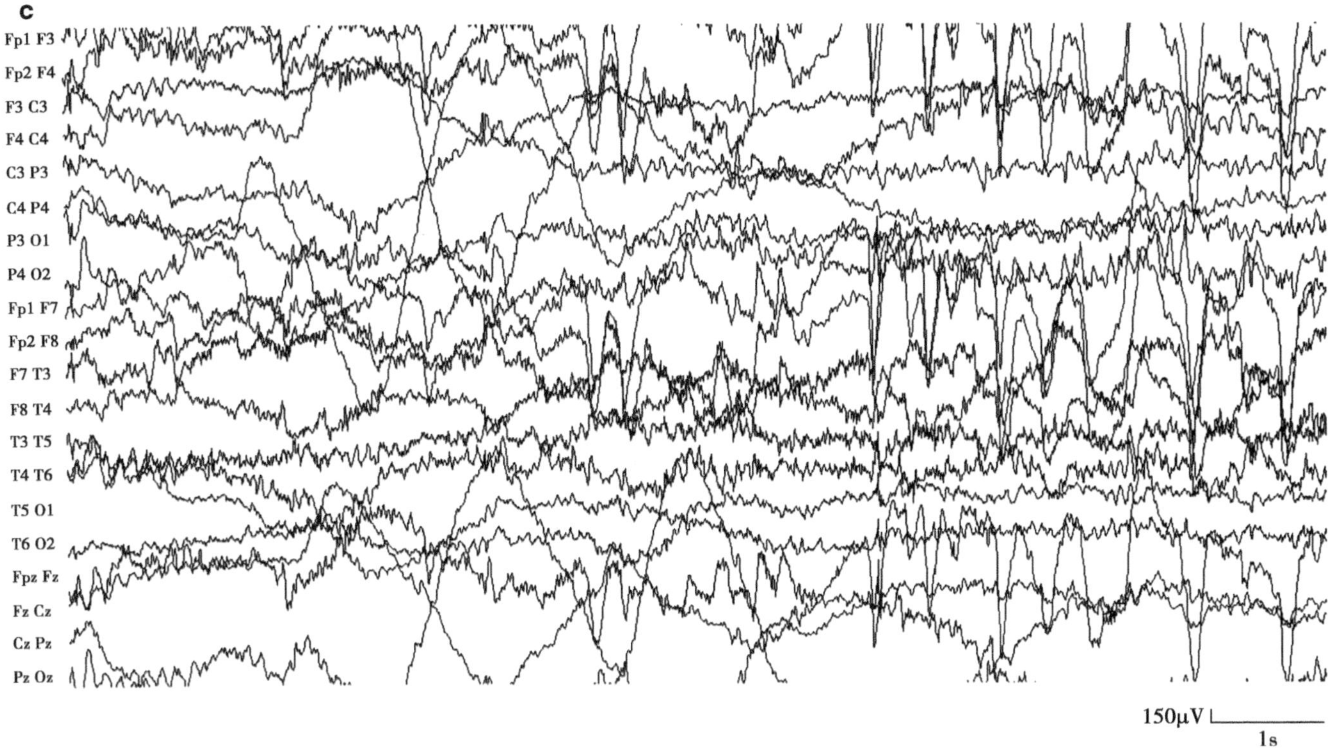

Fig. 2.2 (continued)

Fig. 2.3 Scheme of intracranial electrodes
Grid electrode 1: the upper part of the left central parietal region (the front of head) (32 contacts); Grid electrode 2: the lower part of the left posterior frontal central region (the back of head) (32 contacts)

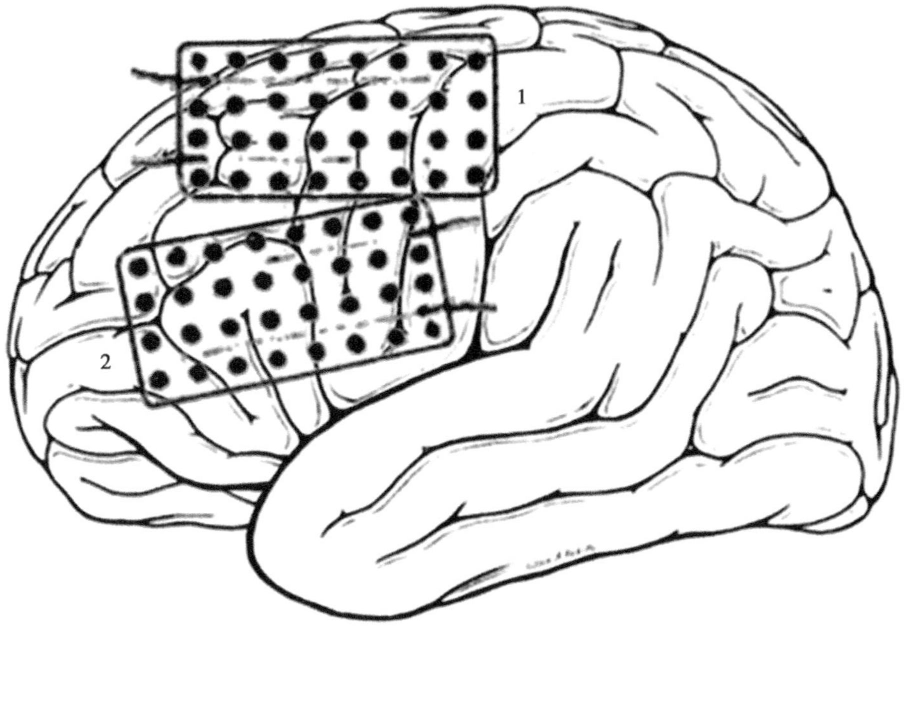

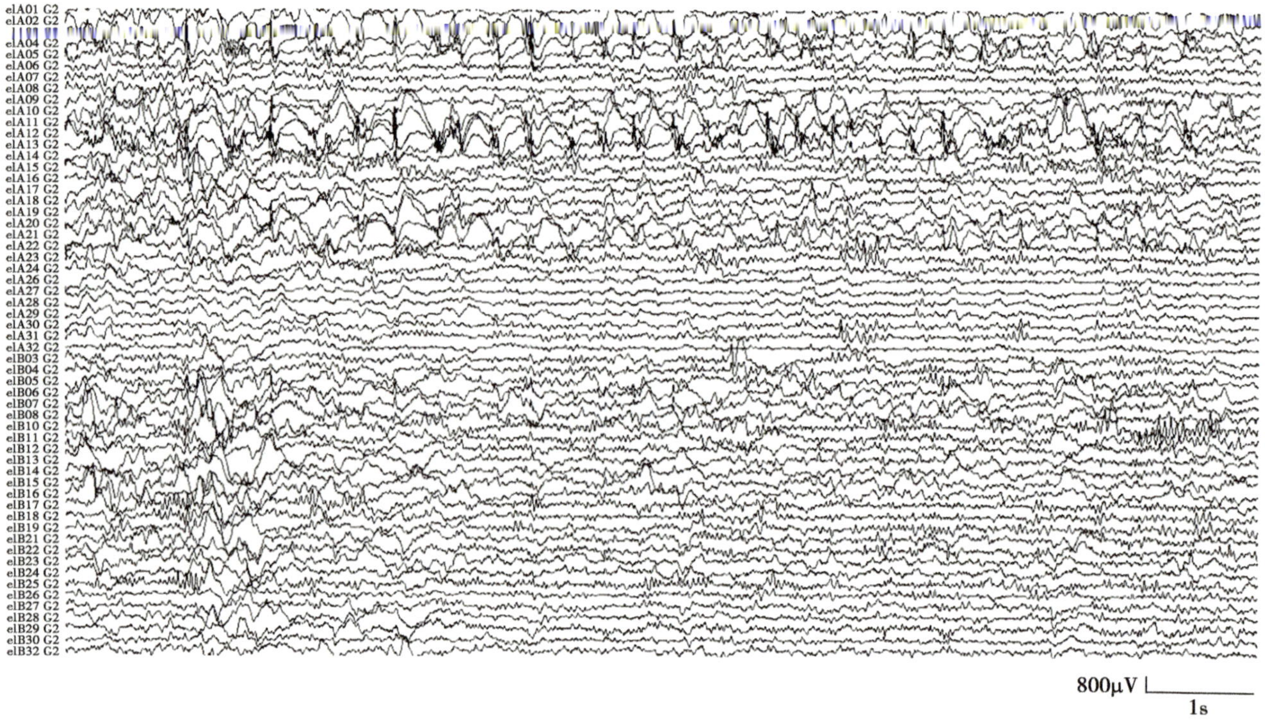

Fig. 2.4 Interictal intracranial EEG
The rhythms of limited spike-and-wave complexes and polyspikes were observed over the posterior part of left central region (contact numbers elA03, elA04, elA05, elA11, elA12, elA13, elA20, elA21)

2. *Diagnosis and treatment strategy and follow-up results*
The patient's seizure symptoms were consistent with the site of abnormal discharges on the EEG. It was hence considered that the seizure focus may be located over the left central and posterior frontal regions. In order to clarify the relationship of the epileptic focus with the sensorimotor and language cortices, a phase II evaluation was required. The intracranial electrodes should adequately cover the left central region and the posterior part of the left inferior frontal gyrus. The interictal IEEG showed significant abnormal discharges over the upper part of the left central cortex; the ictal IEEG showed the rhythm of spikes followed by the low amplitude fast activity over the upper part of left central cortex, indicating clear origin of seizures. The sensorimotor and language cortices were identified by cortical electrical stimulation. The origin of the seizure overlapped with the motor cortex of the right hand. To avoid postoperative right-hand motor dysfunction, limited focal resection of the left central region was performed. During the 1-year postoperative follow-up, the patient still had frequent seizures basically the same as that before operation. The main reason for the poor postoperative effect was believed due to the overlap between the seizure origin and the motor cortex of the right hand, and the epileptic focus was not completely resected.

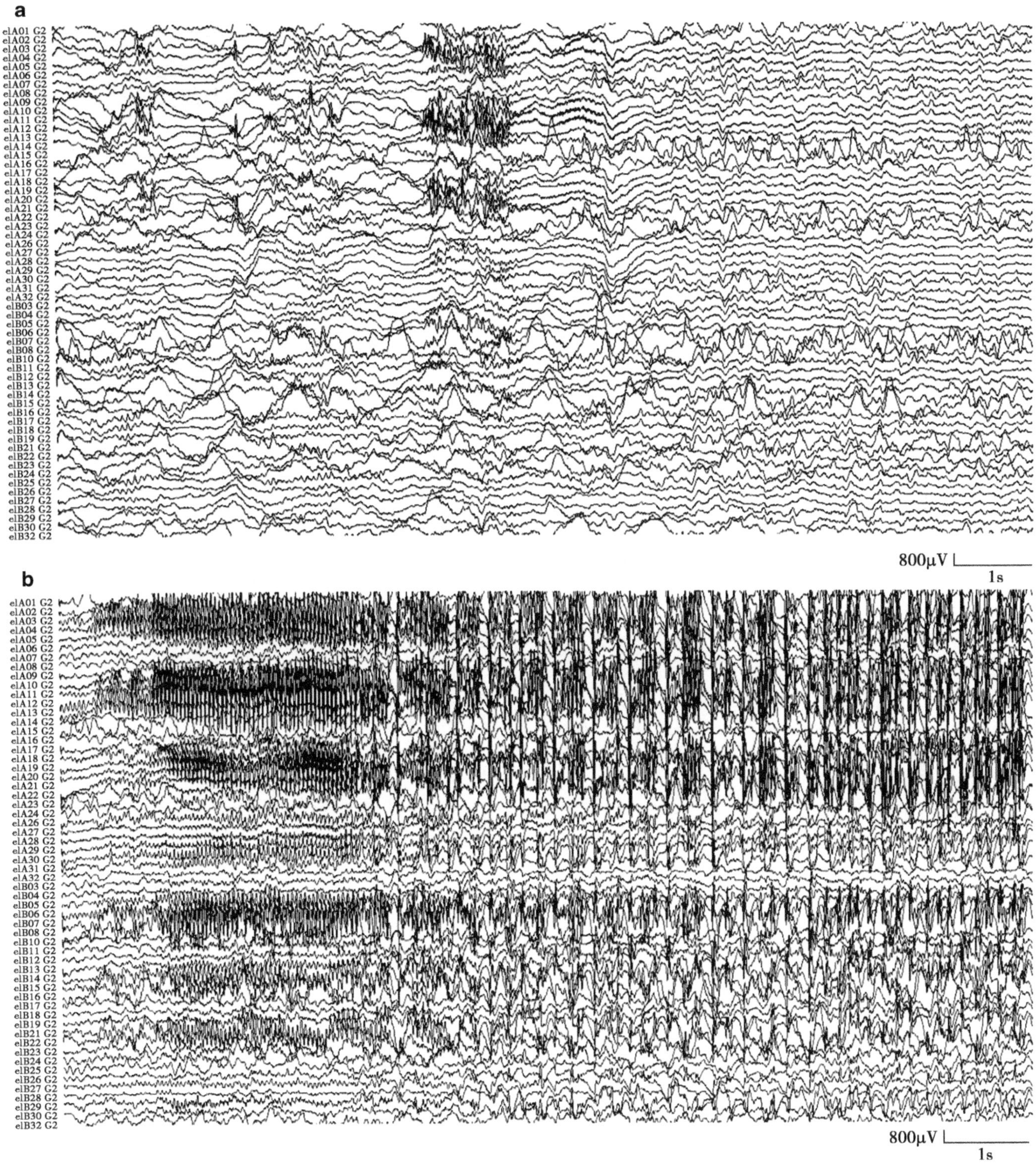

Fig. 2.5 Ictal EEG of intracranial electrodes. (**a**) Before the seizure, the patient was sleeping. The intracranial electroencepholography (IEEG) showed the rhythm of spikes and low amplitude fast activity in contact numbers over the upper part of left central parietal cortex (elA03, elA04, elA05, elA10, elA11, elA12, elA13, elA20, elA21). (**b**) During the seizure, the patient opened eyes and slowly looked to the left, with both upper limbs flexed. The IEEG showed the rhythm of spikes of high amplitude, over the anterior part of the central region (contact numbers elB06, elB07, elB08, elB14, elB15, elB16) and the posterior part of the central region (contact numbers elB21, elB22, elB29). (**c**) The patient experienced limb clonus, which slowly became tonic. The rhythm of spikes of high amplitude was observed on the IEEG. (**d**) The right upper limb of the patient was tonic and clonic. The rhythm of spike-and-wave complexes of high amplitude was observed. (**e**) The patient had flexed left upper limb and turned her head to the right, with limbs tonic and clonic in a decreasing frequency. The IEEG presentation was the same as **d**. (**f**) The patient's seizure ended. The IEEG was low amplitude activity

c

d

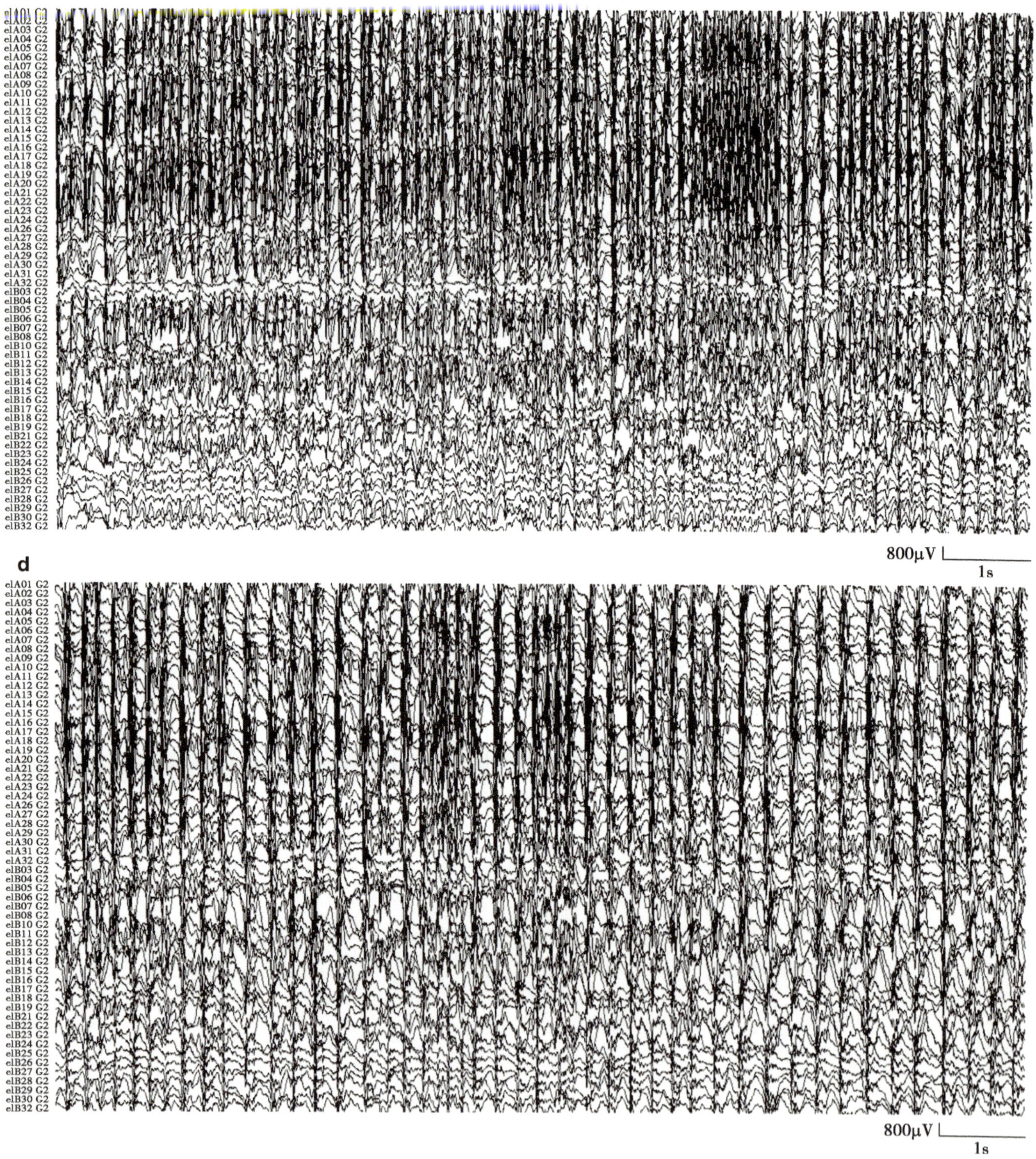

Fig. 2.5 (continued)

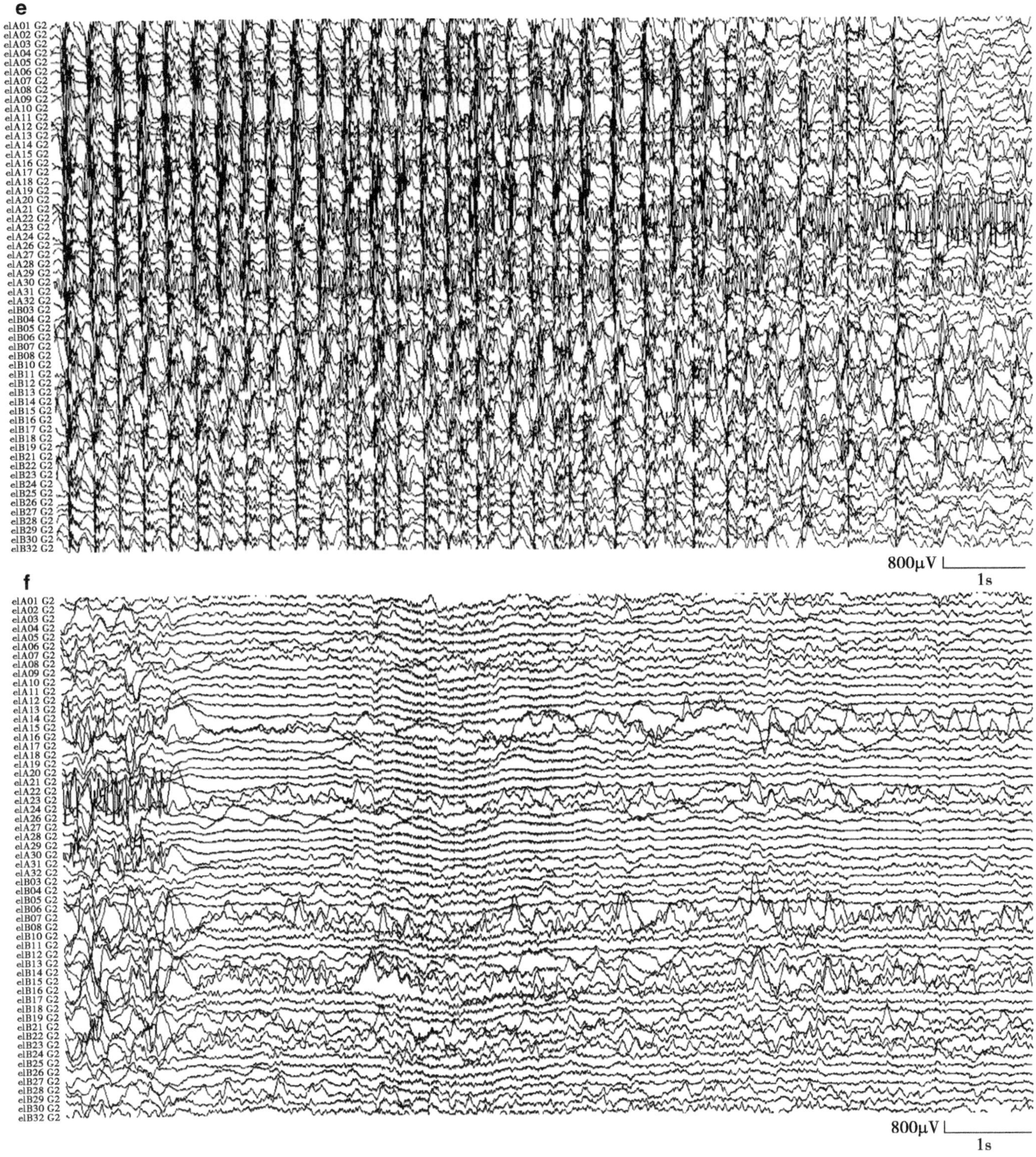

Fig. 2.5 (continued)

Case 2.2 Precentral Gyrus Epilepsy

[Abstract of Medical Records]
Male, 13 years old.

1. *Chief complaint* Paroxysmal loss of consciousness for 10 years.
2. *History of present illness* Loss of consciousness without predisposition 10 years ago, with left mouth twitching, which lasted about 1 min without limb convulsion. The antiseizure medications were ineffective. Over the past 10 years, the seizures were mainly characterized by loss of consciousness, left mouth twitching, flexion and tonic left upper limb, and synchronous tonicity of the right lower limb, which lasted 1–2 min. The seizures often occurred during the arousal from sleep. He is now orally taking carbamazepine 200 mg/dose t.i.d and sodium valproate 400 mg/dose t.i.d.

   Past history The patient was delivered at full term, with normal motor, language, and intellectual development.
3. *Physical examination* No neurological abnormalities were found.
4. *Imaging examination* MRI showed abnormal signals over the right frontal region.
5. *EEG* For details, see Figs. 2.6, 2.7, 2.8, and 2.9.

[Case Review]

1. *Case Characteristics*
   (a) *Seizure characteristics* ① The seizure was characterized by left mouth twitching, flexion and tonicity of the left upper limb, and synchronous tonicity of the right lower limb. ② Clustered seizures.
   (b) *EEG characteristics* Interictal EEG showed frequent spikes and spike-and-wave complexes over relevant leads over the right posterior frontal region.
   (c) *Imaging characteristics* MRI showed abnormal signals in right frontal region.
2. *Diagnosis and treatment strategy and follow-up results* The patient's semiology was consistent with the EEG and MRI. It was hence considered that the epileptic seizure focus may be located over the right central and posterior frontal region. In order to clarify the relationship between the epileptic focus and the sensorimotor cortex, intracranial electrodes were implanted over the right central and posterior frontal region. The interictal IEEG showed extensive epileptiform discharges; the ictal IEEG showed the extensive rhythm of spikes over the right central region. The relationship between motor cortex and epileptic foci was clarified by cortical electrical stimulation. The right posterior frontal region was surgically resected, and the central cortex was dissected. During the 1-year follow-up, there were few seizures, while the frequency of seizures was significantly less than that before surgery. The reason for the seizures post operation was believed to be the partial overlap between the epileptic focus and the motor cortex, as the epileptic focus was not completely resected by the surgery.

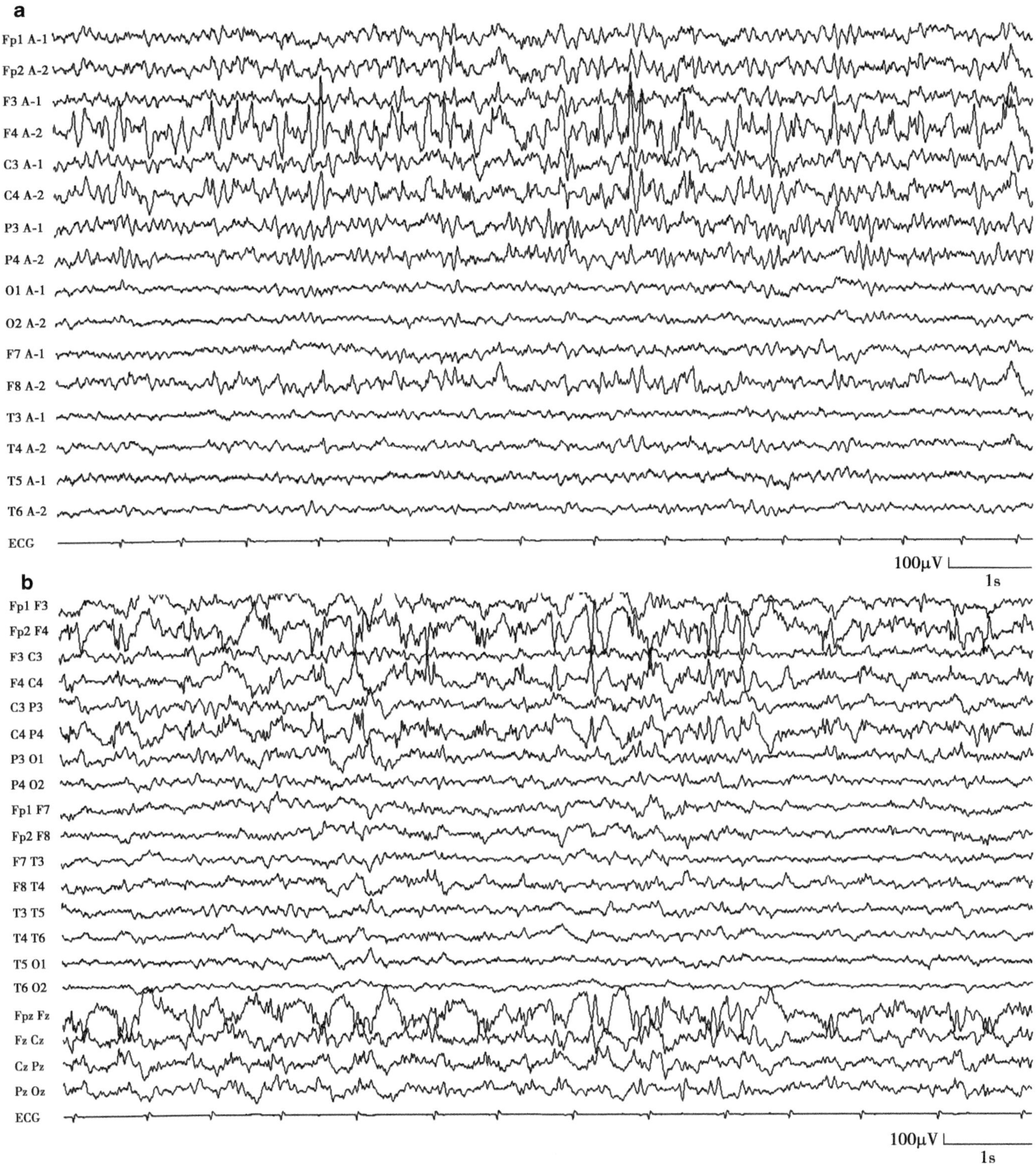

Fig. 2.6 Interictal scalp EEG. (**a**) The background occipital rhythm was 8.0–9.0 Hz, and rhythmic spike waves were observed over the right posterior frontal (F4) region. (**b**) The EEG showed the phase reversal of spikes over the right posterior frontal region (F4). No seizures were recorded

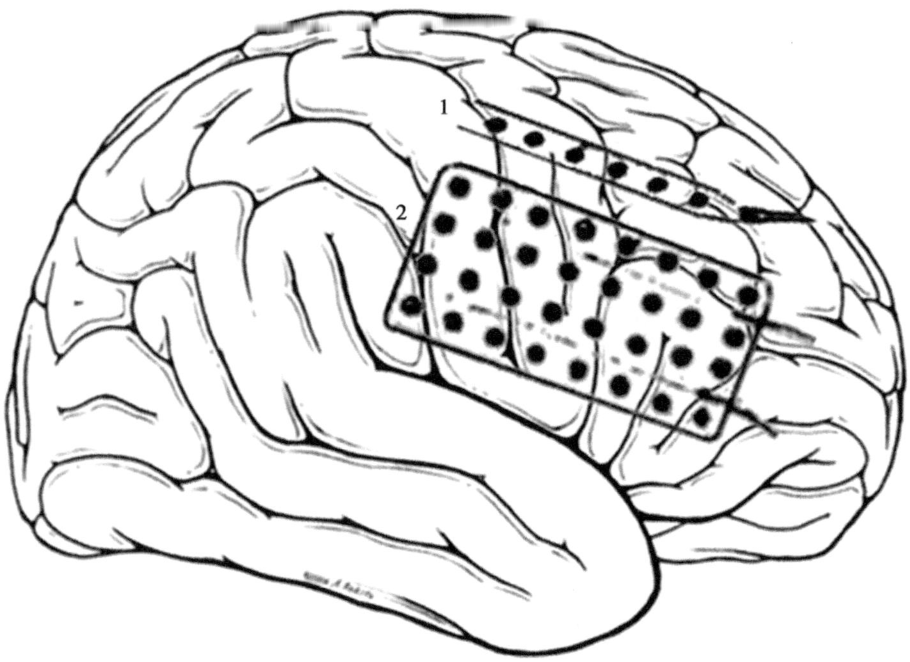

Fig. 2.7 Scheme of intracranial electrodes
Strip electrode 1: the upper part of right central region (6 contacts); Grid electrode 2: the middle of right central region (32 contacts)

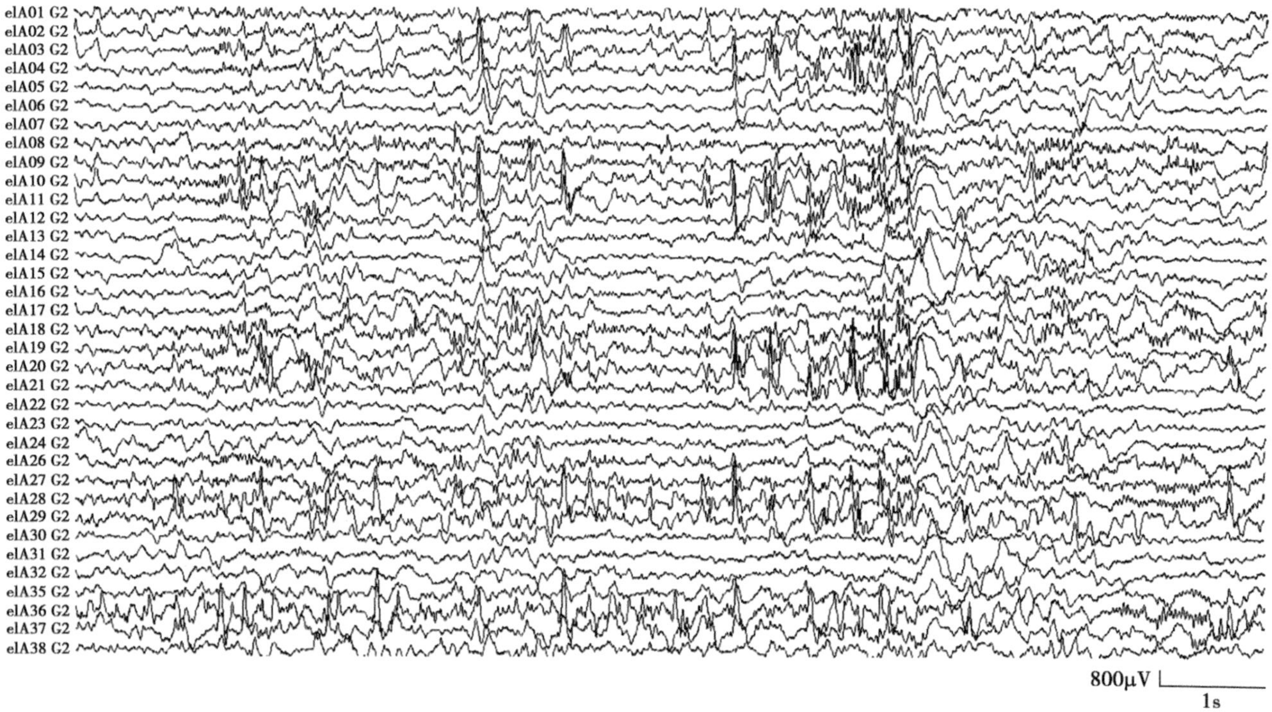

Fig. 2.8 Interictal intracranial EEG
Fast rhythms, spikes, and polyspike-and-wave complexes were observed over the upper part of right central region (contact numbers elA02, elA03, elA04) and the right middle central region (contact numbers elA09, elA10, elA11, elA12, elA17, elA18, elA19, elA20, elA21, elA27, elA28, elA29, elA36, elA37)

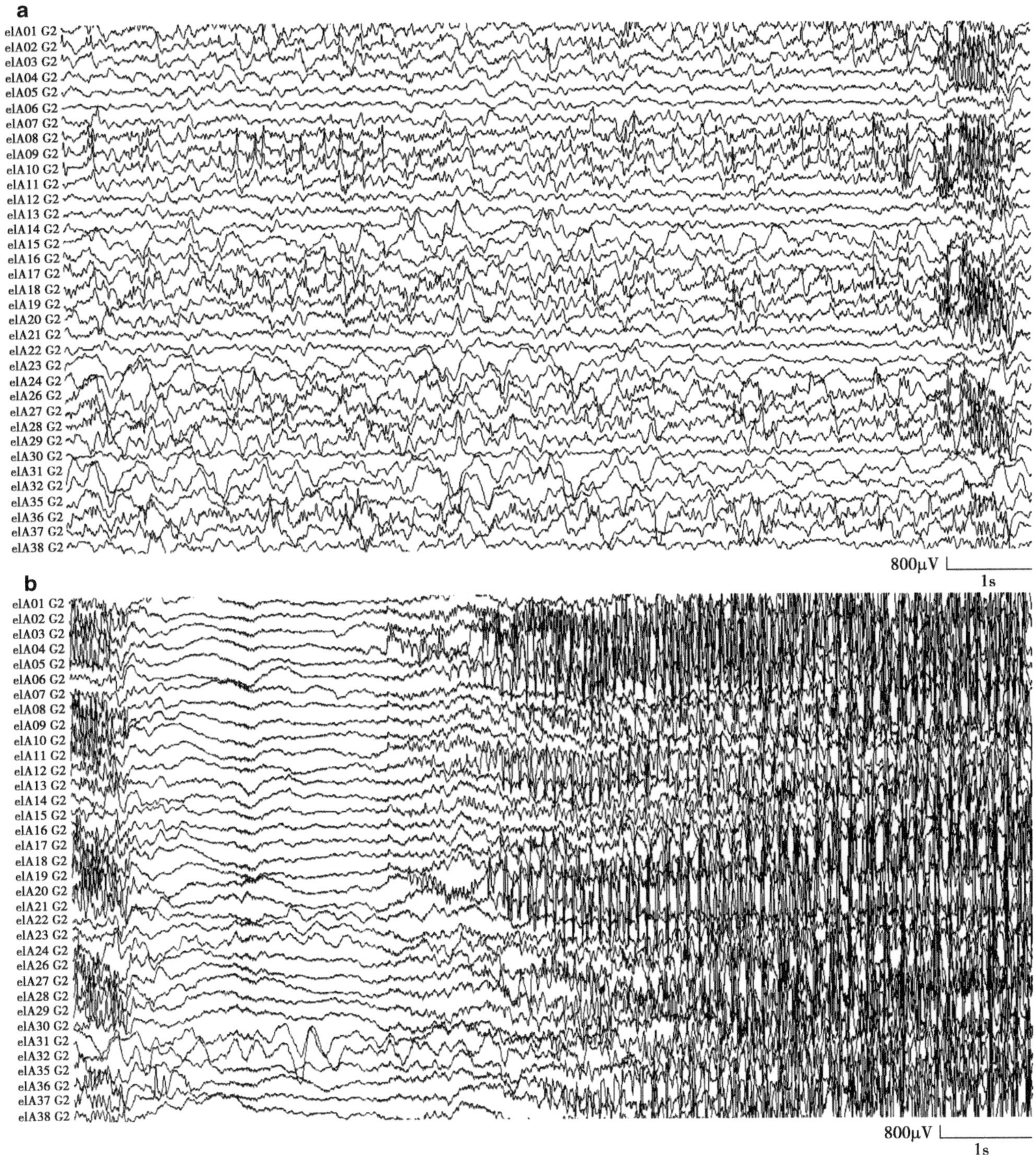

Fig. 2.9 Ictal EEG of intracranial electrodes. (**a**) The patient was supine with eyes closed before the seizure. The IEEG showed the rhythm of spikes of high amplitude over the upper part (contact numbers elA01, elA02, elA03, elA04) and the (contact numbers elA08, elA09, elA10, elA11, elA17, elA18, elA19, elA20, elA26, elA27, elA28, elA29, elA36, elA37) right middle central region. (**b**) During the seizure, the patient elevated his left upper limb and slowly extended it forward until it was tonic. His head was turned to the left; his right upper and lower limbs were flexed, and his left lower limb was tonic. After the amplitude was reduced, the IEEG showed the low amplitude fast activity over the upper part (contact numbers elA02, elA03, elA04) and the (contact numbers elA11, elA12, elA19, elA20) middle central region, followed by the rhythm of spikes of high amplitude that gradually generalized. (**c**, **d**) The patient had generalized tonic clonus. The rhythms of spike-and-wave complexes and polyspike-and-wave complexes were observed. (**e**, **f**) The patient had generalized tonic clonus. The rhythms of spike-and-wave complexes and polyspike-and-wave complexes were observed. (**g**) The patient had limb clonus in a decreasing frequency. The IEEG showed the rhythm of spikes of high amplitude, which gradually developed into the rhythms of spike-and-wave complexes and polyspike-and-wave complexes in a decreasing frequency until the end. (**h**) The patient's seizure ended. The IEEG showed extreme suppression and irregular slow waves over the right central region (contact numbers elA15, elA16, elA17, elA23, elA24, elA31, elA32) and spike-and-wave complexes at contact numbers elA28 and elA36

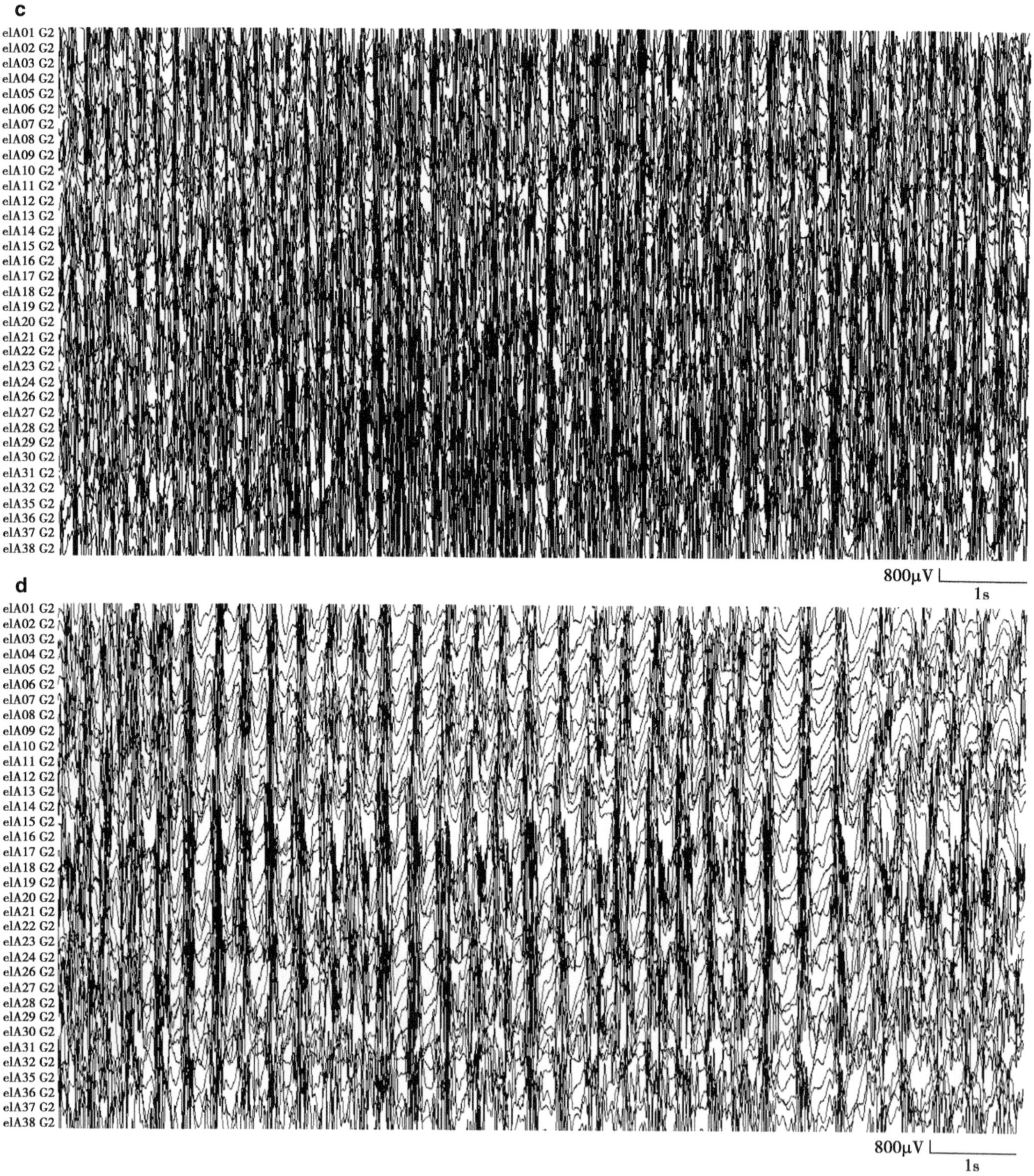

Fig. 2.9 (continued)

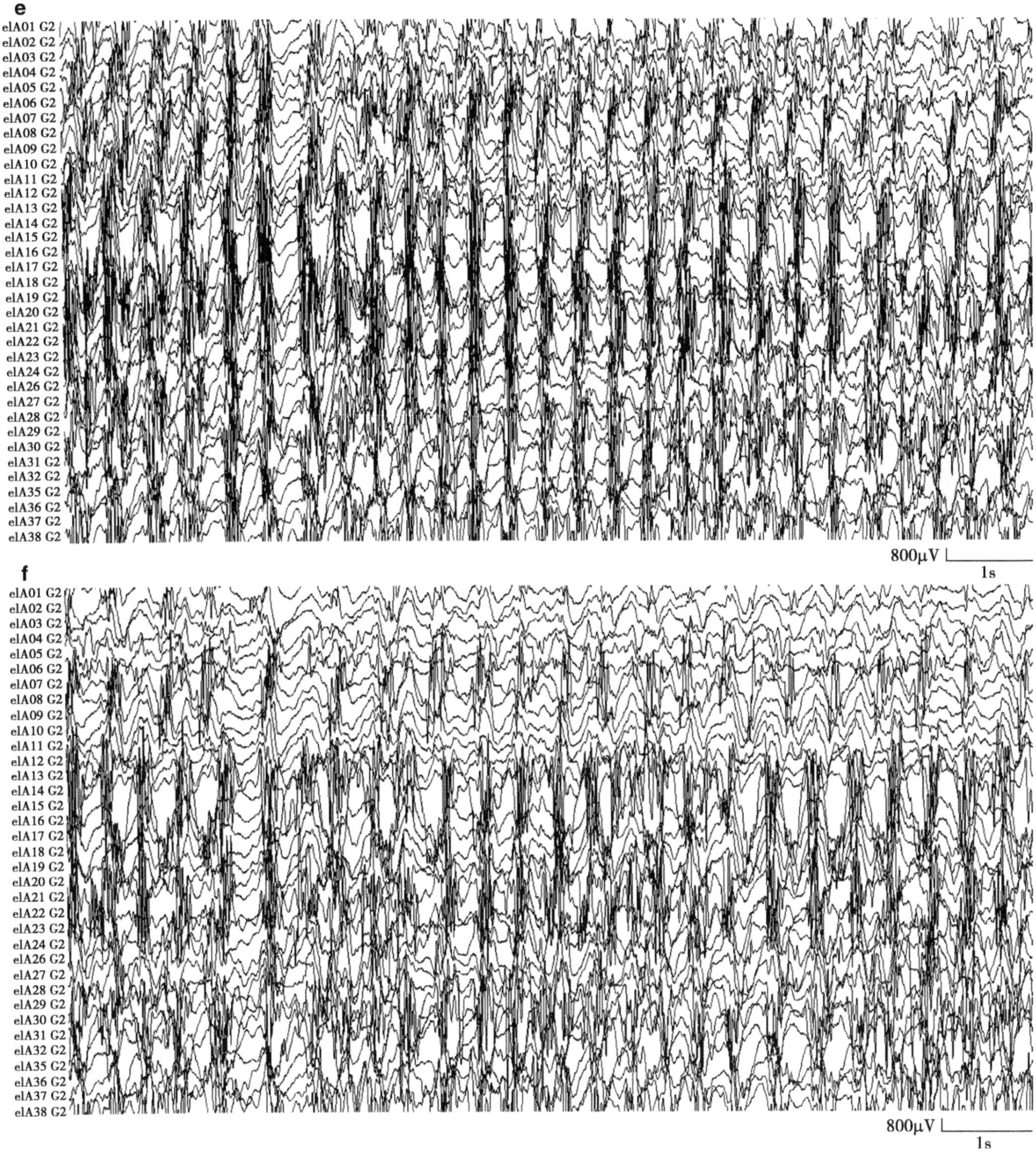

Fig. 2.9 (continued)

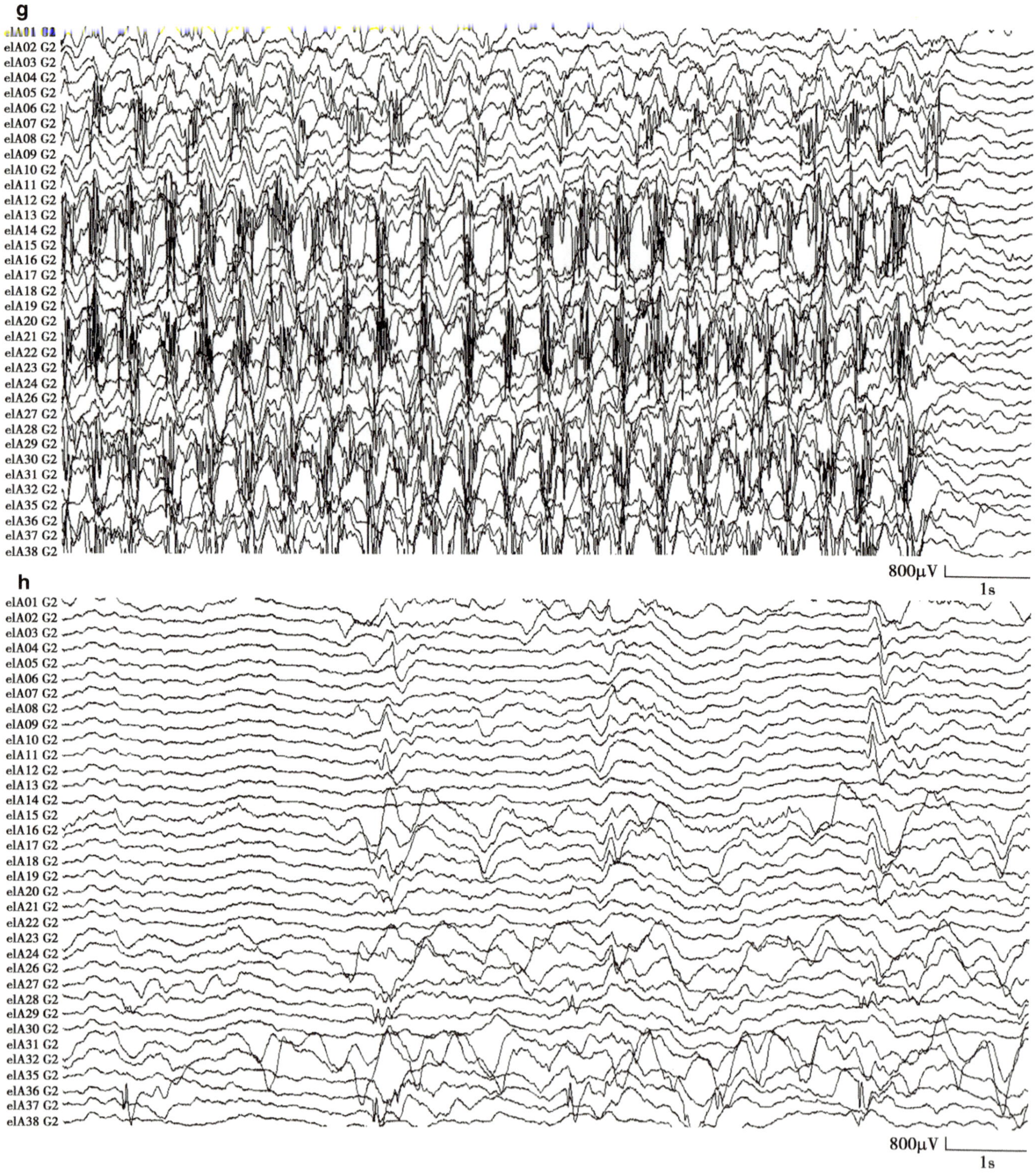

Fig. 2.9 (continued)

Case 2.3 Precentral Gyrus Epilepsy

[Abstract of Medical Records]
Female, 22 years old.

1. *Chief complaint* Paroxysmal limb convulsion for 13 years.
2. *History of present illness* The patient experienced a sudden generalized convulsion without any predisposition 13 years ago, with eyes gazing upward and loss of consciousness, which lasted 1–3 min. After the second seizure, she started to take medicine (name of which was unknown) and was seizure-free for 1 year. Two months after stopping medication, she started to have seizures again, which were characterized by twitching of the right lower limb, distortion of the mouth, and loss of consciousness. The treatment with medication and gamma knife was ineffective, and the seizures occurred 2–3 times a day. One year ago, the patient started taking topiramate (75 mg/dose b.i.d.) and carbamazepine (400 mg/dose b.i.d.), but still had seizures within 1 h after waking up every morning and noon. During the seizure, he felt tightness in the right lower limb, followed by two jerks. She then elevated the right upper limb and raised the left hand while fumbling, with her head turned to the left, which resolved after about 5 min. The patient was sometimes unconscious during the seizure.
3. *Personal and family history* No history of associated diseases.
4. *Physical examination* No neurological abnormalities were found.
5. *Imaging examination* MRI showed abnormal signals in left medial posterior frontal region.
6. *EEG* For details, see Figs. 2.10, 2.11, 2.12, 2.13, and 2.14.

[Case Review]

1. Case Characteristics
   (a) *Seizure characteristics* ① Twitching of right lower limb, followed by mouth distortion and loss of consciousness. ② The aura was clear: the tightness of right lower limb.
   (b) *EEG characteristics* ① Interictal EEG showed spikes over relevant leads over the bilateral frontal and the central regions, especially the left posterior frontal region. ② Ictal EEG showed EMG artifacts and electrode artifacts.
   (c) *Imaging characteristics* MRI showed abnormal signals in left medial posterior frontal region cortex.
2. *Diagnosis and treatment strategy and follow-up results* The patient's seizure symptoms were stereotyped, with clear aura. The MRI showed abnormal signals over the left posterior medial frontal cortex. According to the seizure aura and the results of MRI, it was considered that the epilepsy focus was located over the left central medial region. In order to clarify the relationship between the epileptic focus and the motor cortex, intracranial electrodes were implanted over the central area and left posterior frontal region and also over the area of abnormal MRI signals. The interictal IEEG showed the low amplitude fast activity and spikes over the leads over the left precentral gyrus and the middle upper part of the central and posterior frontal region; the ictal IEEG showed that the seizure origin was located over the medial central region, which soon spread to the upper part of the central and posterior frontal region. The left mesial precentral gyrus and posterior frontal region was resected. After the surgery, the patient was seizure-free during a 1-year follow-up. The seizure origin was clear, and the epileptic focus was completely resected, contributing to a satisfactory outcome of the operation.

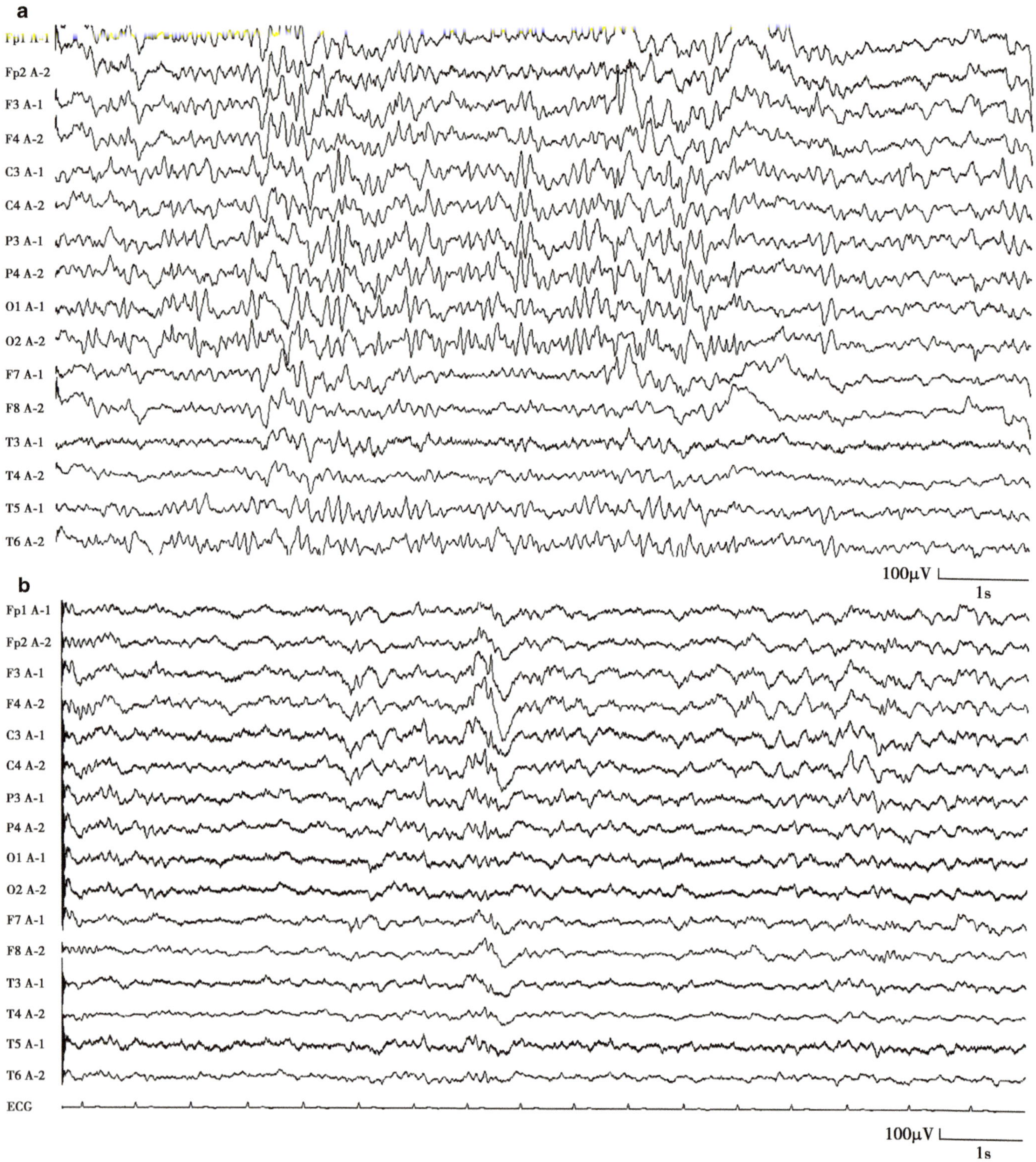

Fig. 2.10 Interictal scalp EEG. (**a**) The background occipital rhythm was 9.0 Hz. There were some medium-amplitude slow waves (5.0–6.0 Hz) mixed over the bilateral frontal and anterior temporal regions (Fp1, Fp2, F3, F4, F7, F8). In addition, spike-and-wave complexes were observed over the left posterior frontal region (F3). (**b**) The patient was asleep. Spikes were observed over the bilateral posterior frontal regions (F3 and F4), especially over the left side

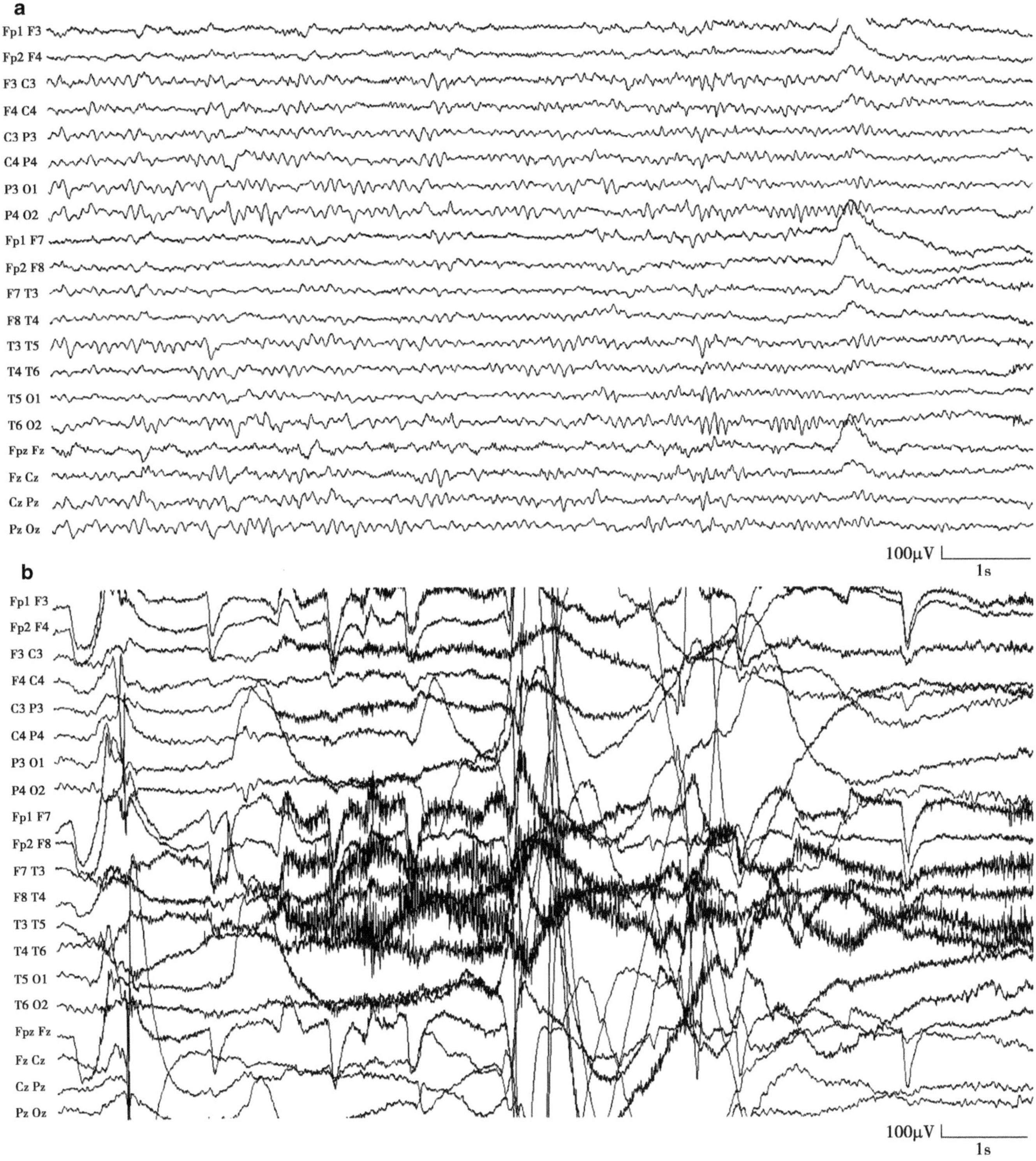

Fig. 2.11 Ictal scalp EEG. (**a**) The patient was conscious and supine with eyes closed before the seizure. The EEG was the awake background EEG. (**b**) The patient asked her family to mark when the seizure occurred. EEG showed some EMG artifacts and electrode artifacts. (**c**) The patient grasped the bed sheet and pillow with both hands, while involuntarily raising head. EEG showed some EMG artifacts and electrode artifacts. (**d**) At the end of the seizure, the EEG of the patient recovered to the background

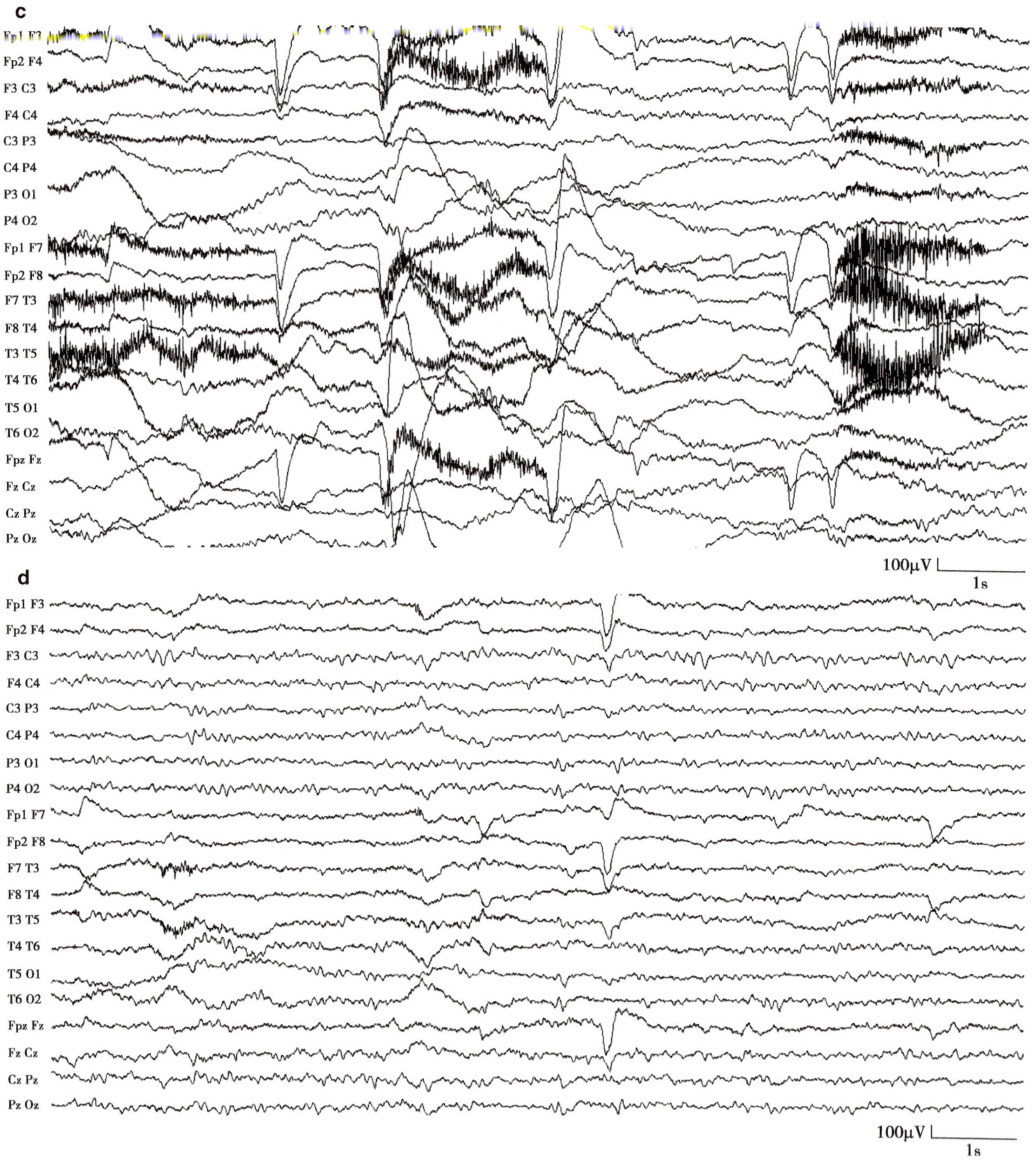

Fig. 2.11 (continued)

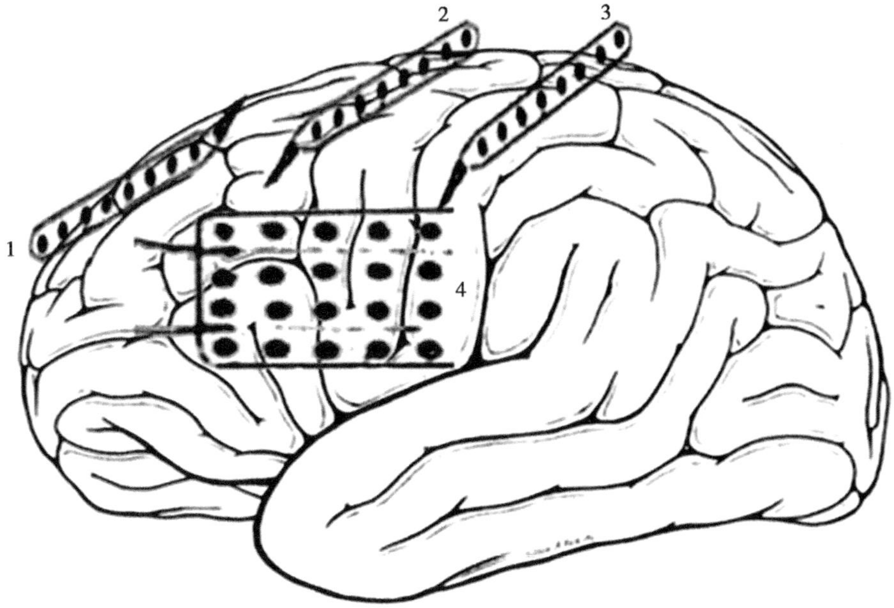

Fig. 2.12 Scheme of intracranial electrodes
Strip electrode 1: the left cingulate cortex (8 contacts); Strip electrode 2: the longitudinal fissure of the left precentral gyrus (8 contacts); Strip electrode 3: the longitudinal fissure of the left gyrus postcentralis (8 contacts); Grid electrode 4: the left central and posterior frontal region (20 contacts)

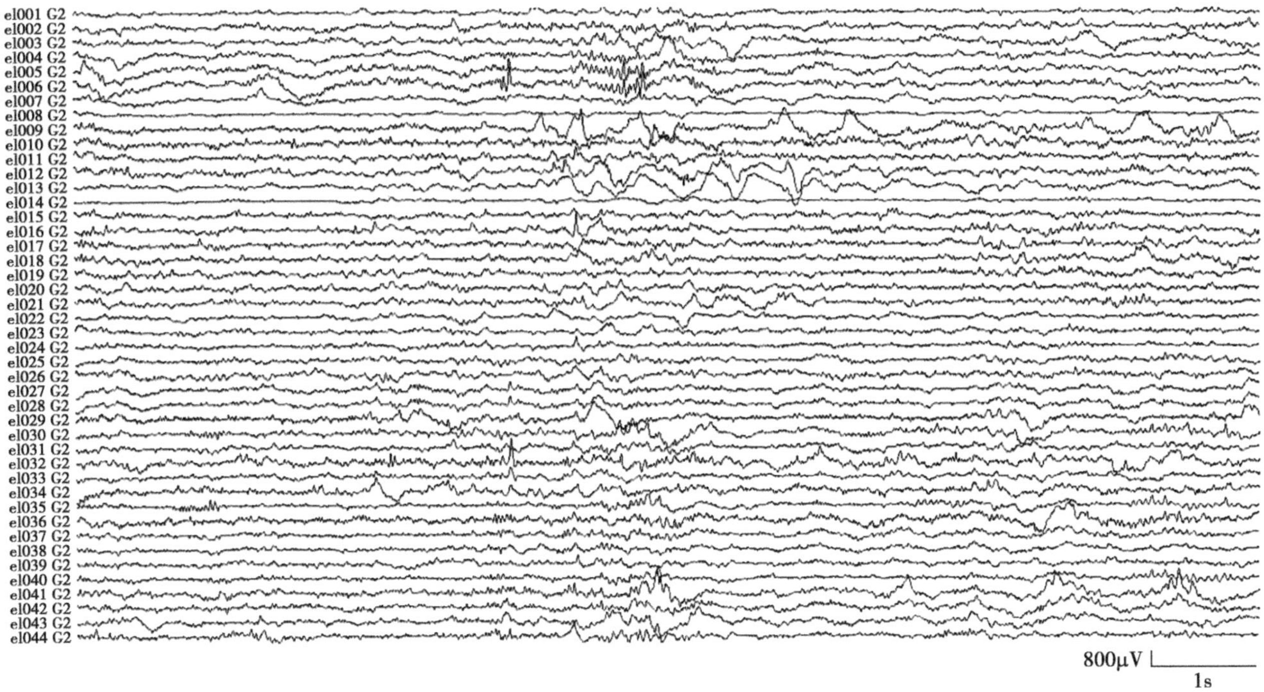

Fig. 2.13 Interictal intracranial EEG
The IEEG showed the low amplitude fast activity and slow waves over left precentral gyrus of the medial cortex (contact numbers el009, el010, el011, el012, el013), and the low amplitude paroxysmal fast activity and spike as well as waves over the middle upper part of the central and posterior frontal region (contact numbers el032 and el041), showing a rhythmical trend

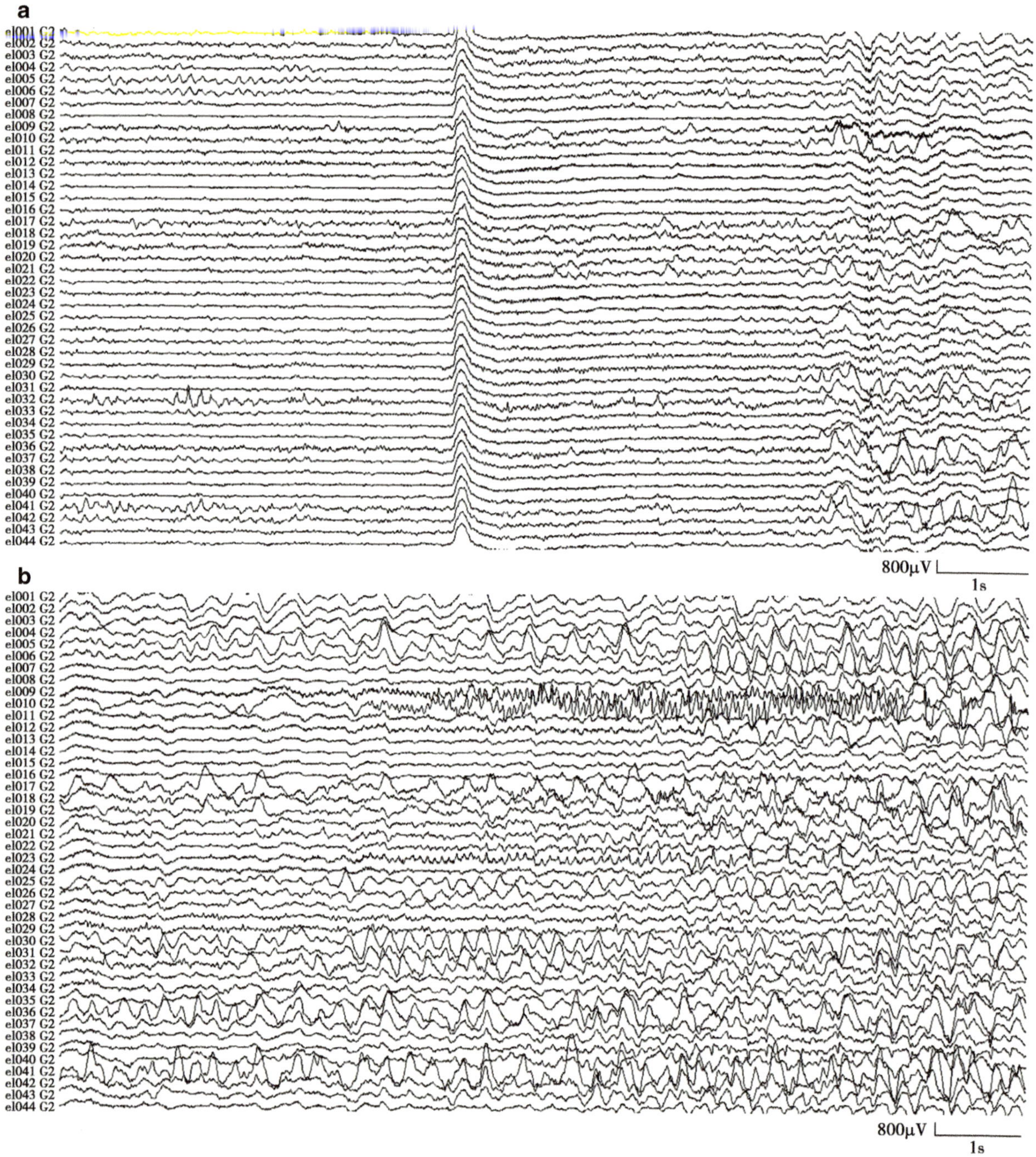

Fig. 2.14 Ictal EEG of intracranial electrodes. (**a**) The patient was conscious and supine with eyes closed before the seizure. The IEEG showed the low amplitude persistent fast activity over the left precentral gyrus (contact numbers el009, el010, el011, el012), the left gyrus postcentralis (contact numbers el022, el023, el024), and the middle upper part of the central and posterior frontal region (contact numbers el032, el036, el041), especially over the fissure of left precentral gyrus (contact number el009). (**b–d**) At the moment of seizure, the patient reported that she was experiencing a seizure. The right upper limb was slightly abducted and raised, and the left upper limb was raised and placed on the top of the head. About 2 s later, she lowered the left upper limb to the waist and fumbled, with her head and eyes slightly turned to the left. About 5 s later, her left hand stopped fumbling, while her eyes still gaze to the left. Her right upper limb was flexed and stiffened, with no response to any call. After about 15 s, she raised her left upper limb while fumbling with her left hand. The IEEG showed the low amplitude fast activity with increasing amplitude over the left central region (contact numbers el009, el010, el023); after about 5 s, the abovementioned rhythm of fast activity gradually developed into a rhythm of spikes with increasing amplitude, which lasted about 15 s. The rest of the leads developed a rhythm of slow waves. (**e, f**) After the seizure, the patient put her left upper limb on the chest, and rubbed a tissue with her left hand, and could answer questions. IEEG showed high-amplitude slow wave over the cingulate cortex (contact numbers el004, el005, el006), the longitudinal fissure (contact numbers el009, el010, el017), and the frontal region (contact numbers el025, el030, el035, el041), which recovered to background 20 s later

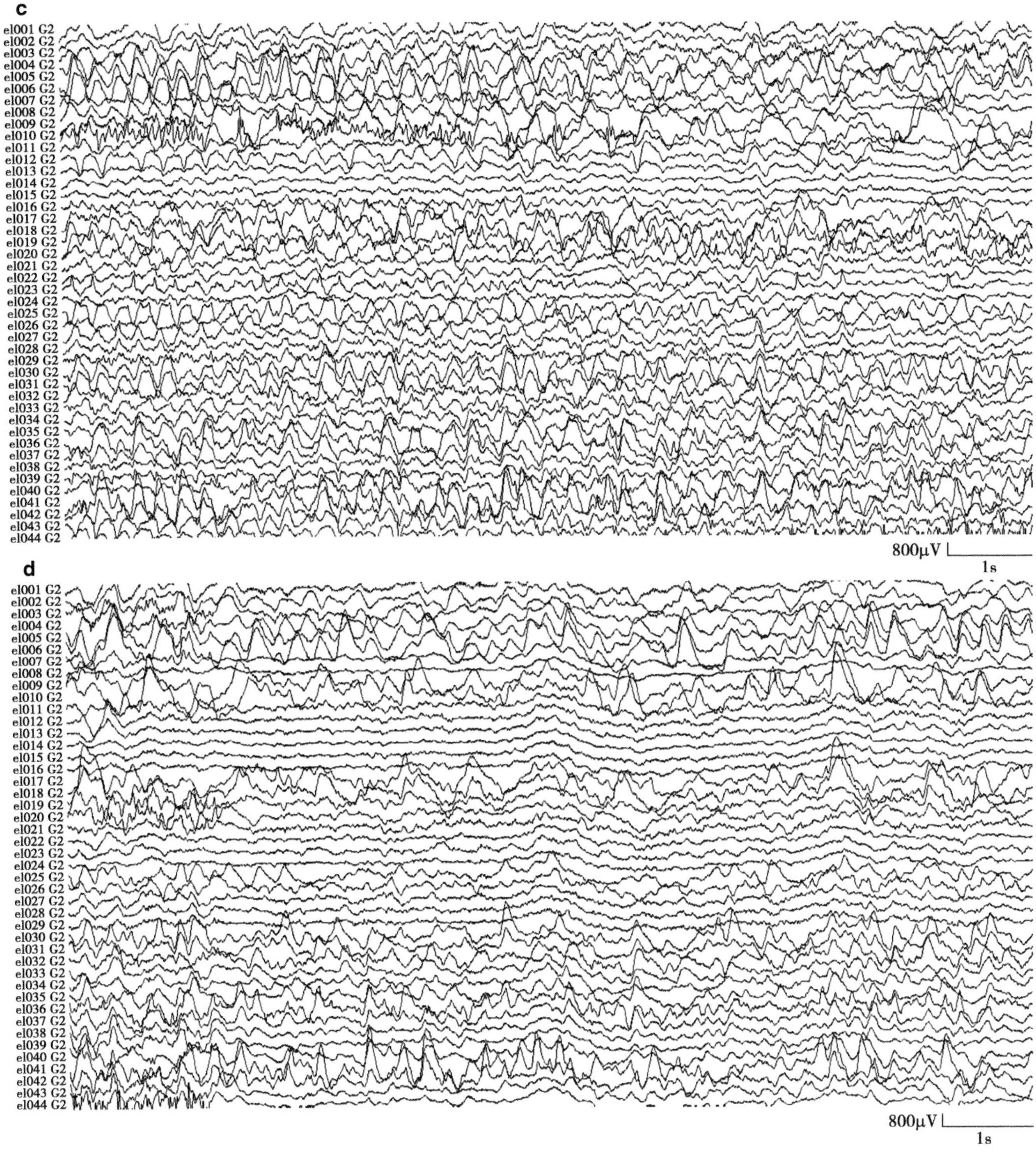

Fig. 2.14 (continued)

e

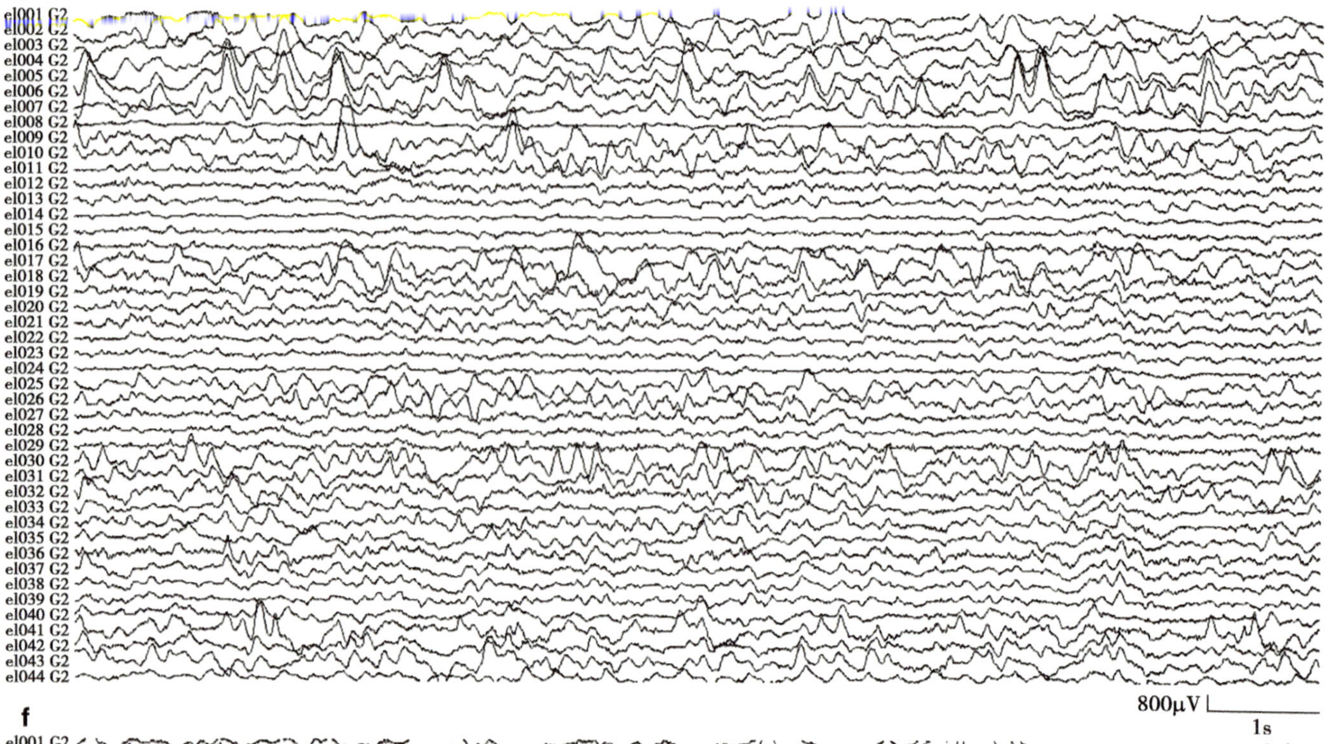

f

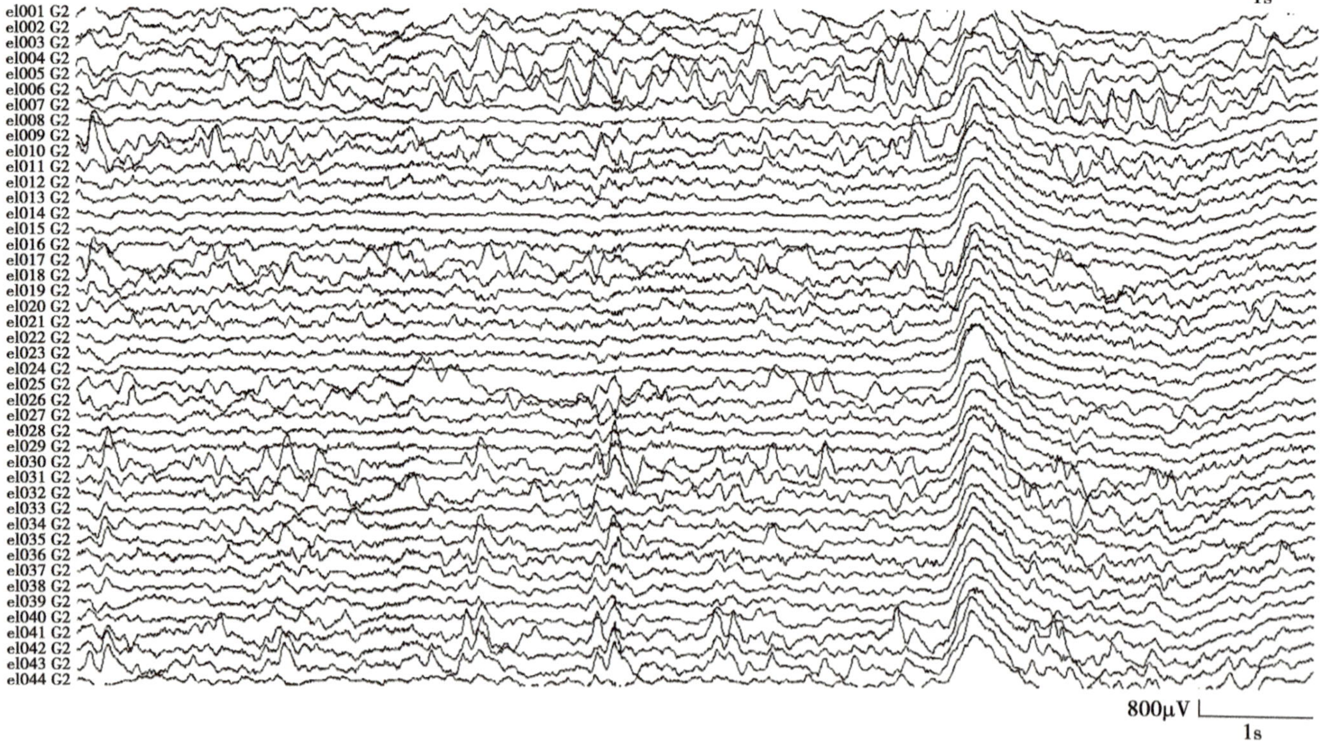

Fig. 2.14 (continued)

Case 2.4 Precentral Gyrus Epilepsy

[Abstract of Medical Records]
Female, 20 years old.

1. *Chief complaint* Paroxysmal limb convulsion for 20 years.
2. *History of present illness* At 2.5 months after birth, the patient had sudden onset of left limb convulsions with left facial twitching, and was diagnosed with "intracranial hemorrhage." At 4 years old, the patient had sudden onset of limb convulsions (unclear limb involvement). At 9 years old, the patient had another episode of unprovoked left limb twitching, eyes gazing to the upper left, and left facial twitching, which resolved after about 1 min. Since then, the patient has had multiple episodes at a frequency of 1–3 episodes per month, especially in the early morning (05:00–07:00), mostly peri-menstruation. The patient sometimes has warning signs (drowsiness, tiredness, or leg soreness). The patient had a similar manifestation in each episode: left limb convulsion, eyes gazing to the upper left, left facial twitching, and left facial numbness. The patient sometimes has systemic involvement during episodes, with twitching of the limbs, flexion of the upper limbs, and tonicity of lower limbs, which resolve after the symptoms last for tens of seconds to 2 min, at a frequency of about 2 episodes per year. Since the onset of the disease, the patient has been treated with traditional Chinese medicines (unknown), topiramate, and carbamazepine, with poor responses. The patient is currently receiving daily oral carbamazepine: 175 mg in the morning, 175 mg in the afternoon, and 250 mg in the evening. The patient had irregular menstrual cycle in the past more than 2 years, with prolonged menstruation (7–15 days) and increased menstrual blood volume.
3. *Past history* The patient was delivered at full term, with normal motor, language, and intellectual development.
4. *Personal and family history* No history of associated diseases.
5. *Physical examination* No neurological abnormalities were found.
6. *Neuropsychological examination* Moderate intelligence; verbal intelligence quotient (VIQ) = 103; performance intelligence quotient (PIQ) = 101, and full intelligence quotient (FIQ) = 102.
7. *Imaging examination*
   (a) MRI showed abnormal signals over the right temporoparietal cortex, which was considered as encephalomalacia (ischemia and sequelae of necrotic changes).
   (b) fMRI showed motor center located anteromedially to the encephalomalacia and compensation activation over the contralateral motor center.
8. *EEG* For details, see Figs. 2.15, 2.16, 2.17, 2.18, and 2.19.

[Case Review]

1. *Case Characteristics*
   (a) *Seizure characteristics* ① Left limb and mouth twitching. ② Aura of numbness in the left cheek.
   (b) *EEG characteristics* ① Interictal EEG showed sharp waves over the right frontal and anterior temporal regions. ② Ictal EEG showed spike-and-wave complexes over the bilateral frontal regions, the frontal midline, and the anterior temporal region, especially on the right.
   (c) *Imaging characteristics* MRI showed encephalomalacia over the right frontal, temporal, and parietal regions.
2. *Diagnosis and treatment strategy and follow-up results* The patient's semiology was consistent with the EEG and MRI. It was hence considered that the epileptic focus was located over the central area of right posterior frontal region. In order to clarify the relationship between the epileptic focus and the sensorimotor cortex, intracranial electrodes were implanted over the right central and posterior frontal region. The postoperative interictal IEEG showed scattered spikes and spike-and-wave complexes over the central area of right posterior frontal region; the ictal IEEG showed that the seizure origin was located over the right posterior frontal region and the lower part of the central region. The relationship between motor cortex and epileptic foci was clarified by cortical electrical stimulation. The right posterior frontal region and the lower part of the central region were surgically resected. After the surgery, the patient was seizure-free in a 1-year follow-up. The foci and lesions were completely resected, contributing to a satisfactory outcome of the operation.

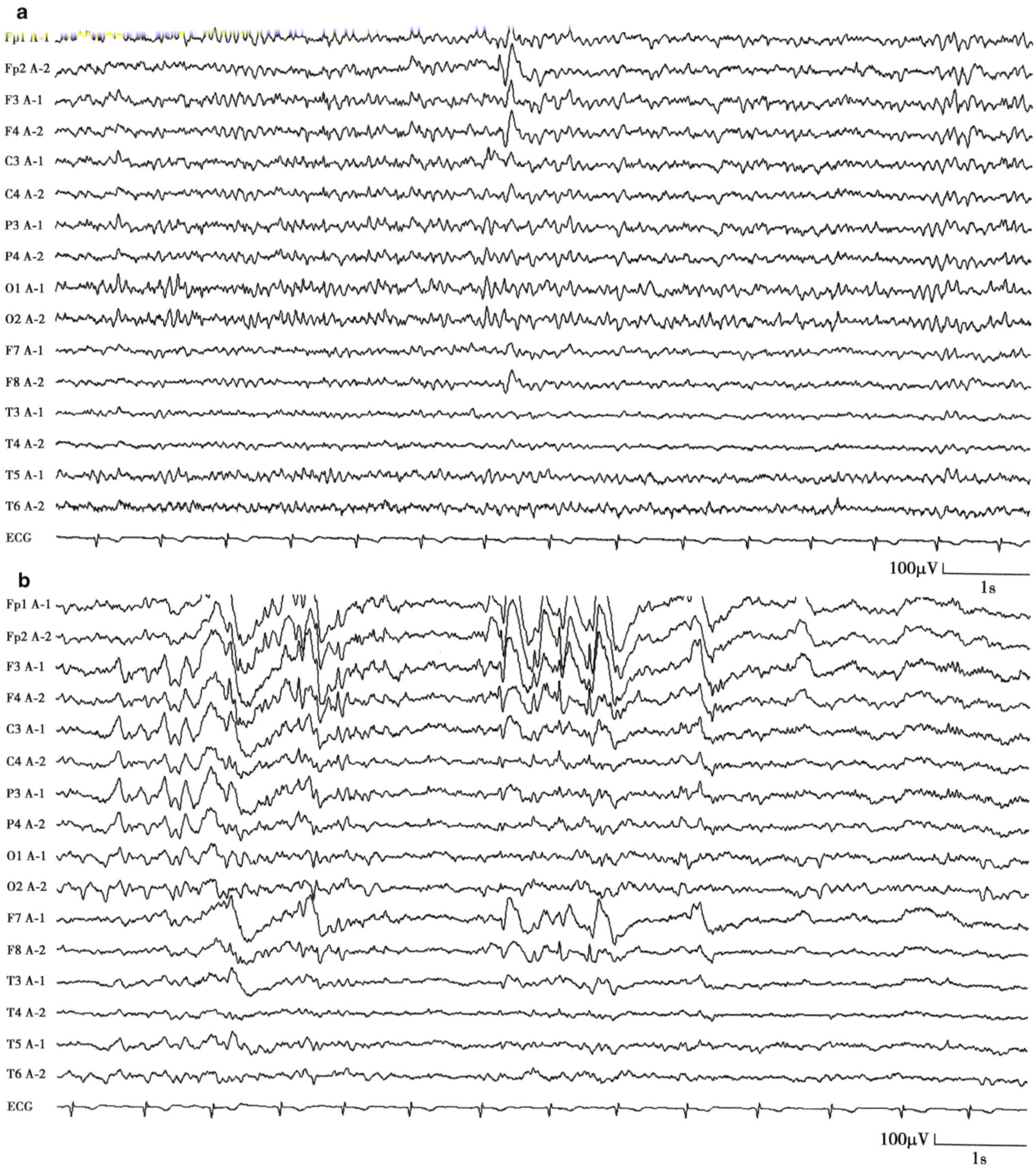

Fig. 2.15 Interictal scalp EEG. (**a**) The patient was awake. The EEG showed a background occipital rhythm of 10.0 Hz with a few scattered sharp waves over the right frontal polar (Fp2), frontal (F4), and anterior temporal regions (F8). (**b**) The patient was asleep. The EEG showed spike-and-wave complexes over bilateral frontal polar (Fp1, Fp2), posterior frontal (F3, F4), and anterior temporal regions (F7, F8), especially on the right

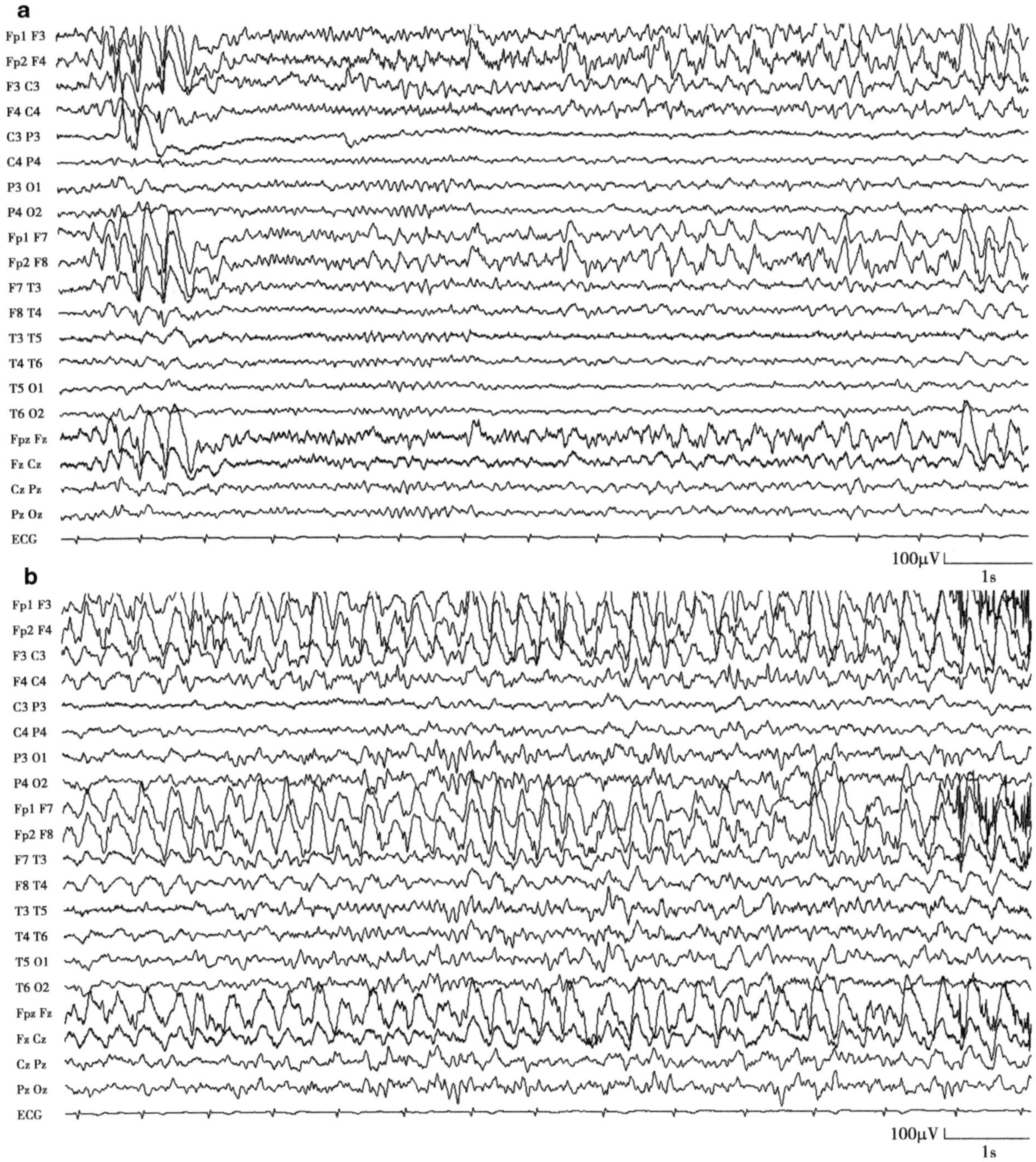

Fig. 2.16 Ictal scalp EEG. (**a**) About 13 s before the seizure, the patient was supine with eyes closed. The EEG showed the rhythm of spike-and-wave complexes over the bilateral frontal regions (Fp1 F3, Fp2 F4, Fp1 F7, Fp2 F8) and frontal midline (Fpz Fz, Fz Cz), especially the right, which lasted about 2 s. It was followed by the low amplitude fast activity over the bilateral frontal regions (Fp1 F3, Fp2 F4, Fp1 F7, Fp2 F8), especially over the right frontal region, which lasted about 4 s. The amplitude increased and the frequency decreased. (**b**) The patient remained supine with eyes closed. The EEG showed the rhythms of waves and spike-and-wave complexes of high amplitude over the bilateral frontal regions (Fp1 F3, Fp2 F4, Fp1 F7, Fp2 F8) and frontal midline (Fpz Fz, Fz Cz). (**c**) The patient gazed to the upper left with both eyes and turned head and body to the left. EEG showed numerous EMG artifacts. (**d**) The patient still turned head to the left, with both upper limbs flexed and both lower limbs flexed and raised, while making "ah" sounds. Mixed EMG artifacts were seen. (**e**) The patient's limbs were abducted while been tonic and clonic. EMG artifacts were seen. (**f**) The patient's limbs were tonic and clonic. EMG artifacts were seen. (**g**) The patient had clonus in a decreasing frequency. Numerous EMG artifacts were observed. (**h**) The patient had clonus in a decreasing frequency. Numerous EMG artifacts were observed. (**i**) The patient's seizure ended, and the movements stopped. The EEG showed polyspike-and-wave complexes over the bilateral frontal regions (Fp1 F3, Fp2 F4, Fp1 F7, Fp2 F8), the left temporoparietal regions (F7 T3, T3 T5, T5 O1, P3 O1), and the frontoparietal midline (Fpz Fz, Pz Oz), mixed with some irregular slow waves of medium and high amplitude. Flat waves with low amplitude were observed over the remaining leads. (**j, k**) The patient's seizure ended, and the movements stopped. The EEG showed polyspike-and-wave complexes over the bilateral frontal regions (Fp1 F3, Fp2 F4, Fp1 F7, Fp2 F8), the left temporoparietal regions (F7 T3, T3 T5, T5 O1, P3 O1) and the frontoparietal midline (Fpz Fz, Pz Oz), mixed with some irregular slow waves of medium and high amplitude. Flat activity with low amplitude was observed over the remaining leads. (**l**) The patient was wheezing heavily and was still unconscious. The EEG showed flat waves of low amplitude, mixed with some EMG artifacts

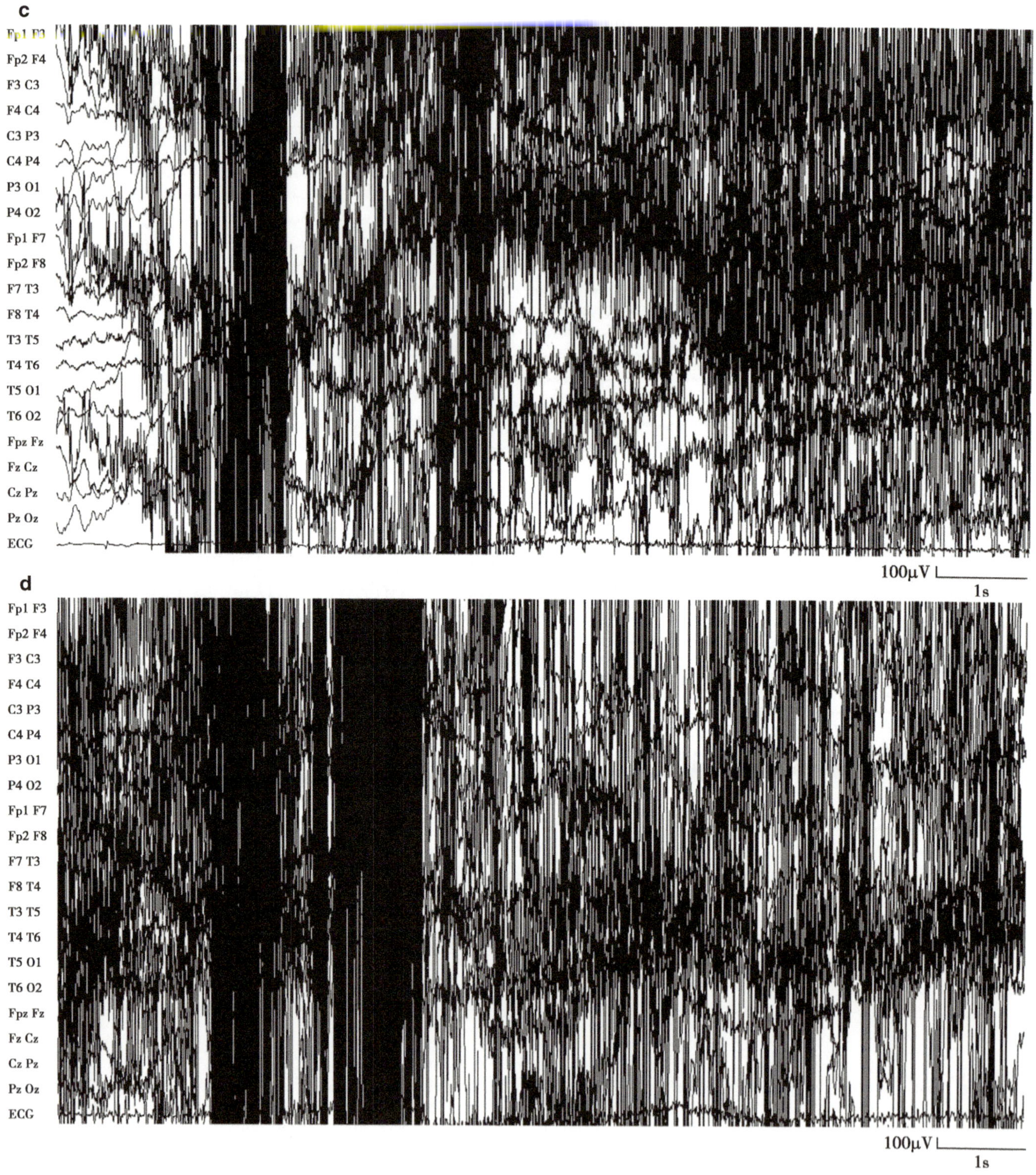

Fig. 2.16 (continued)

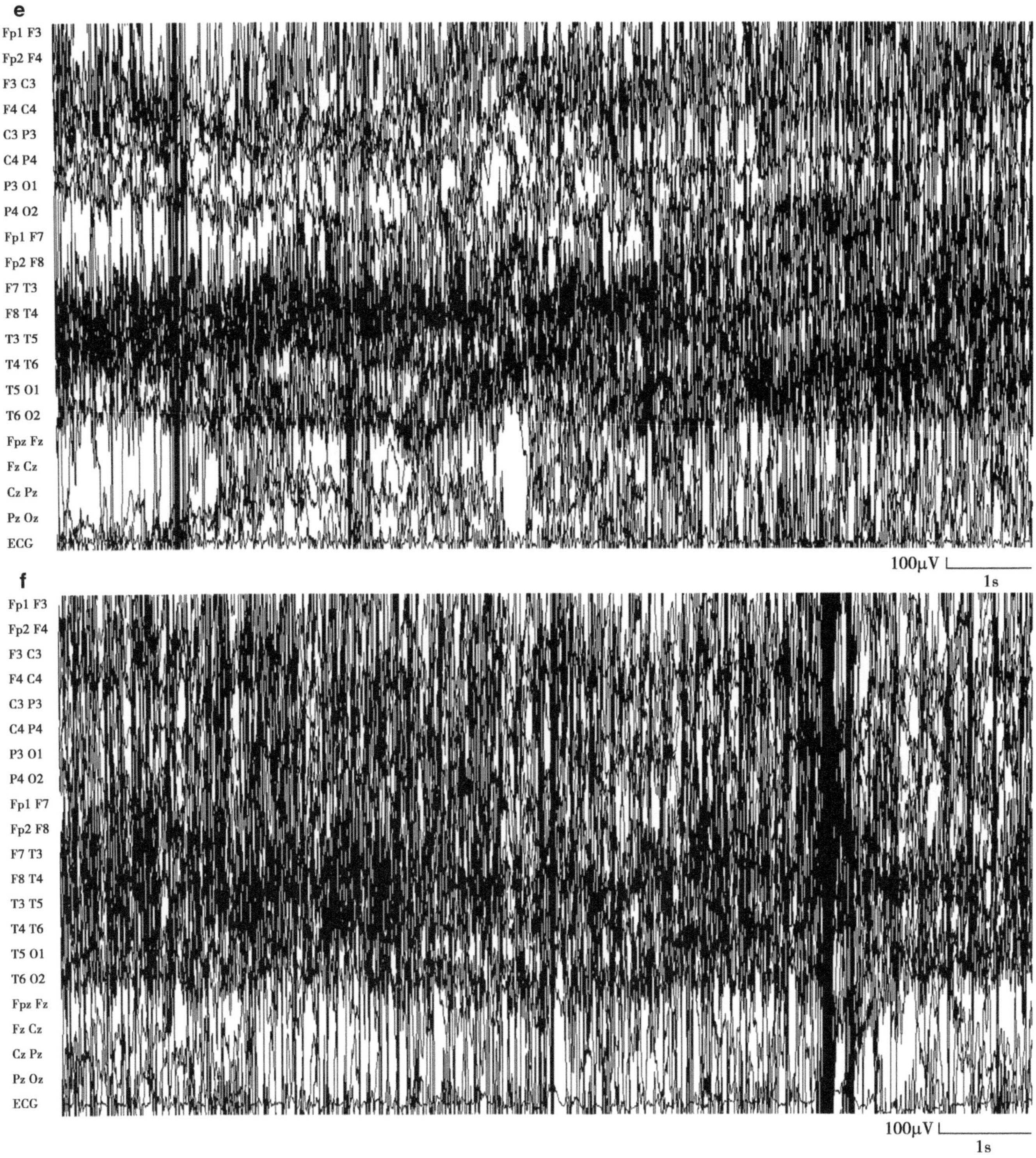

Fig. 2.16 (continued)

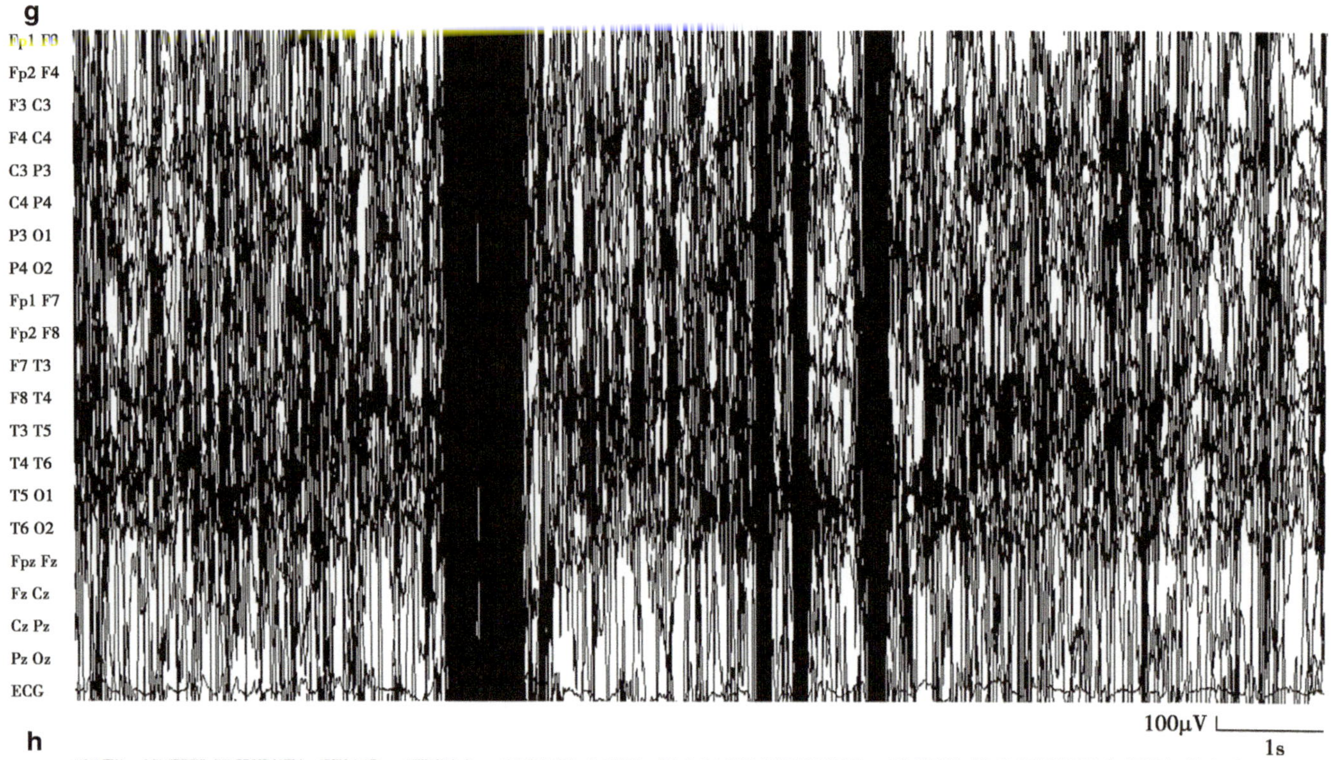

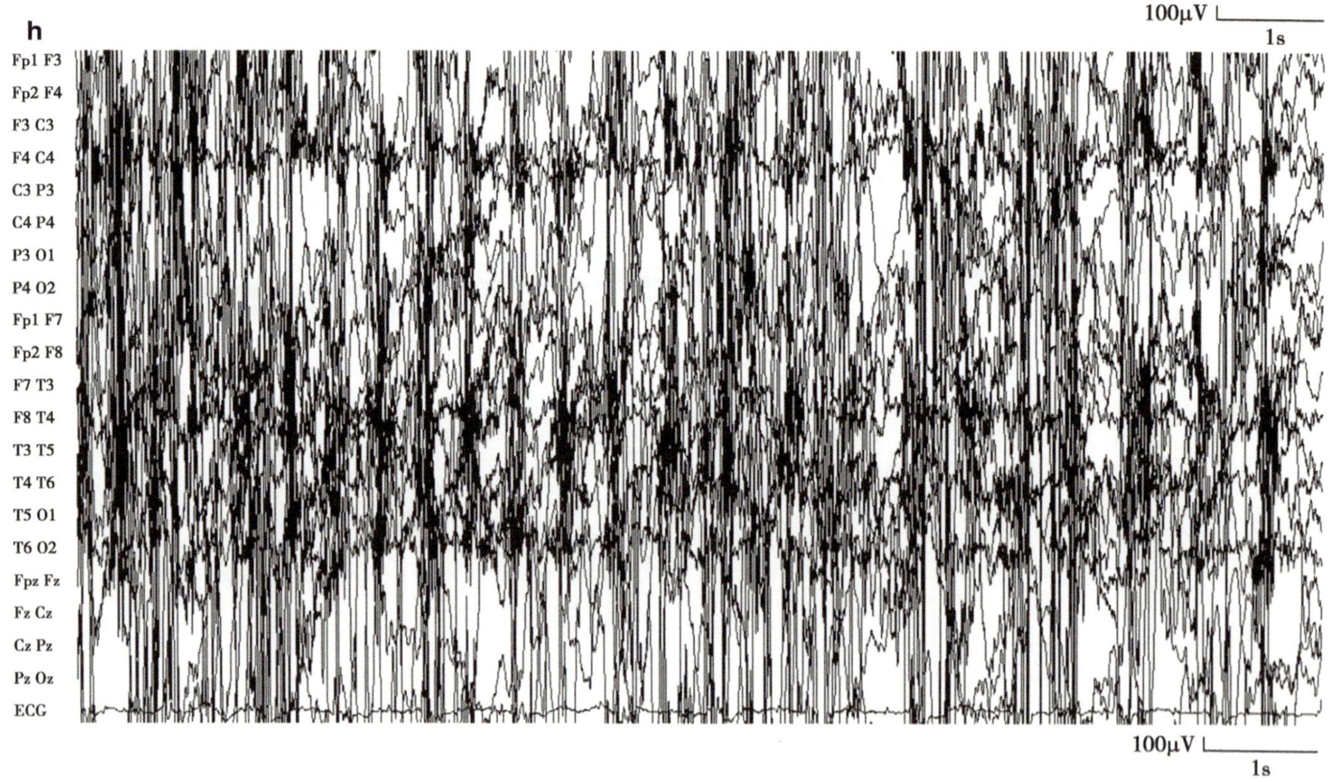

Fig. 2.16 (continued)

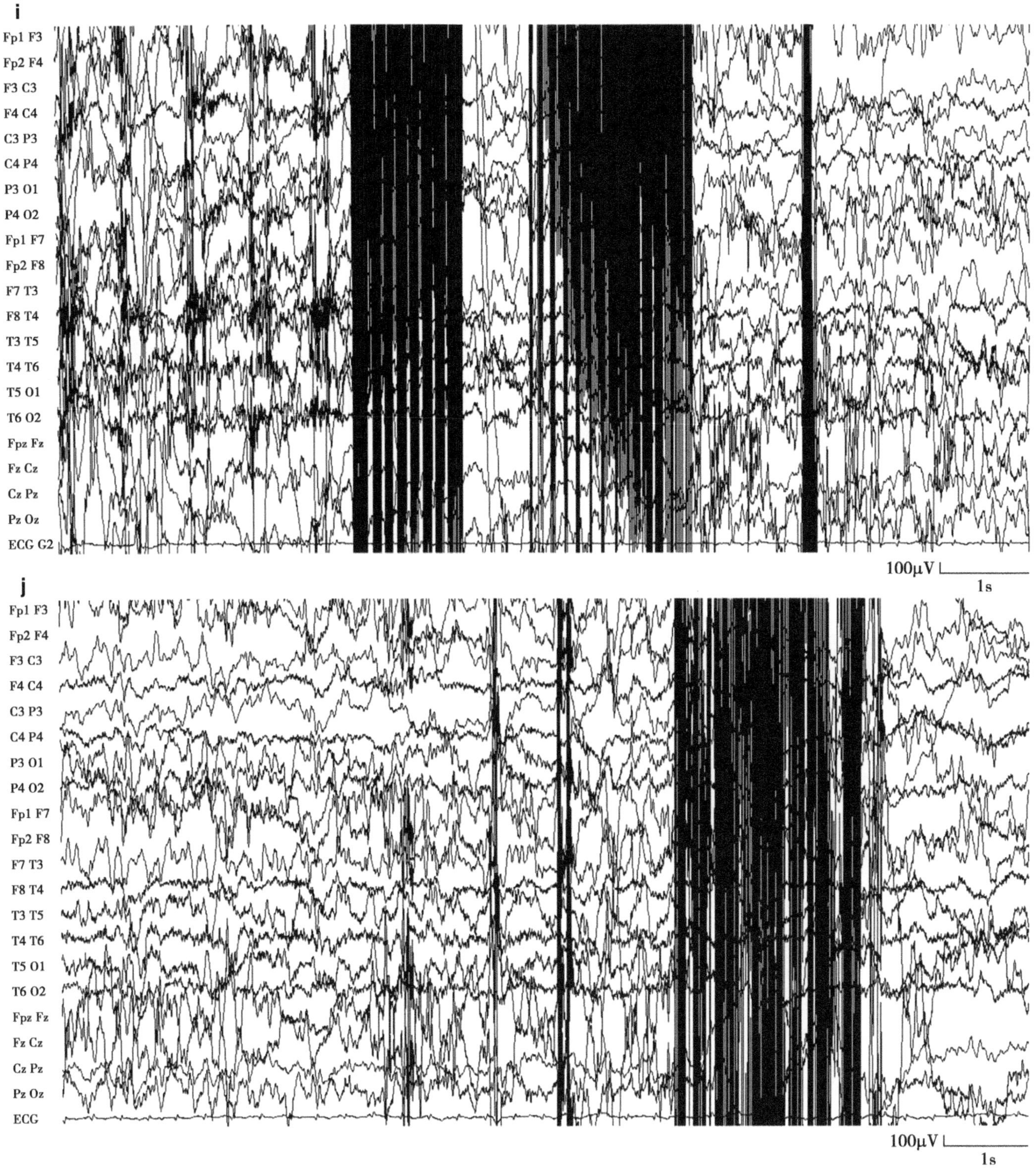

Fig. 2.16 (continued)

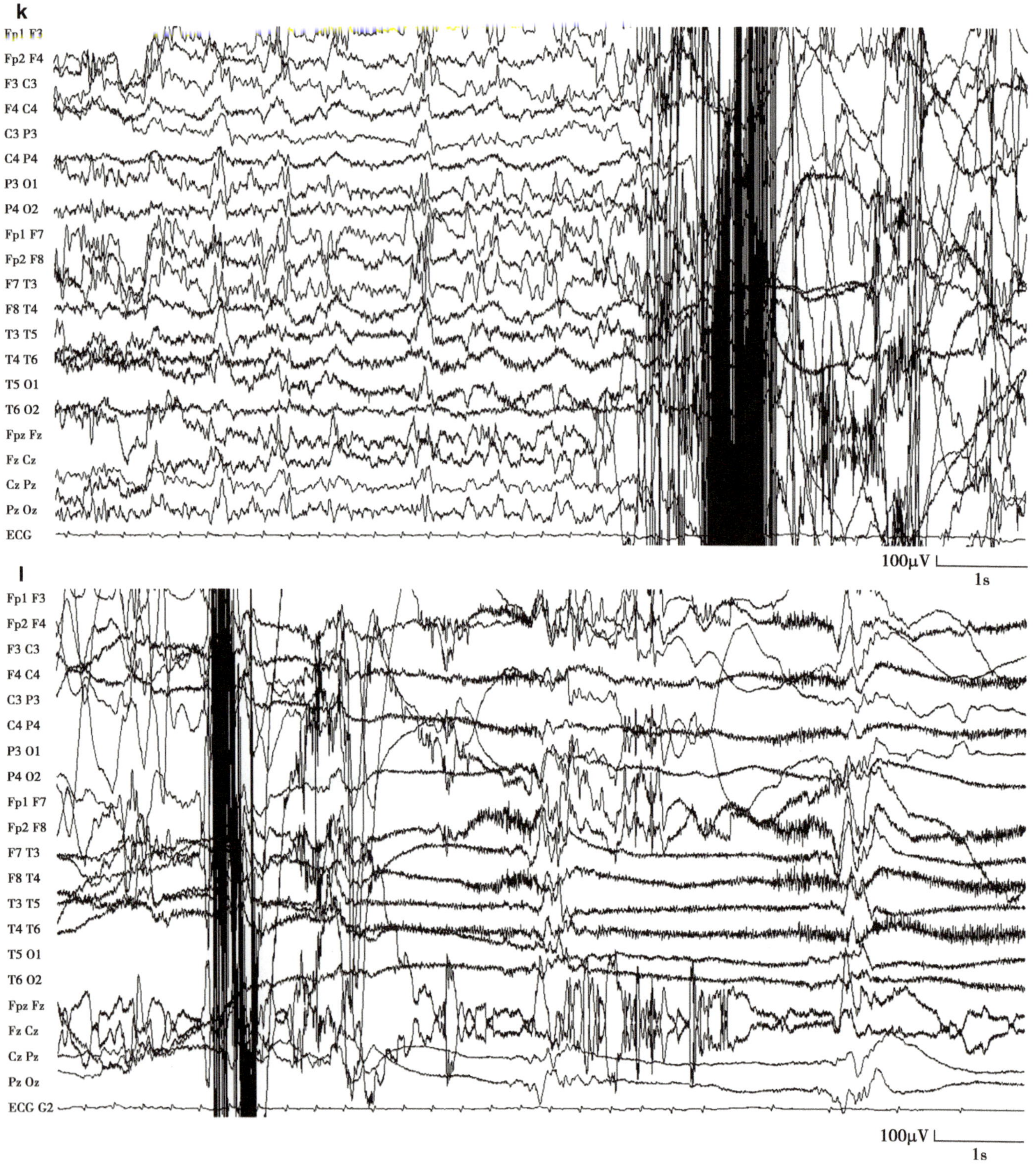

Fig. 2.16 (continued)

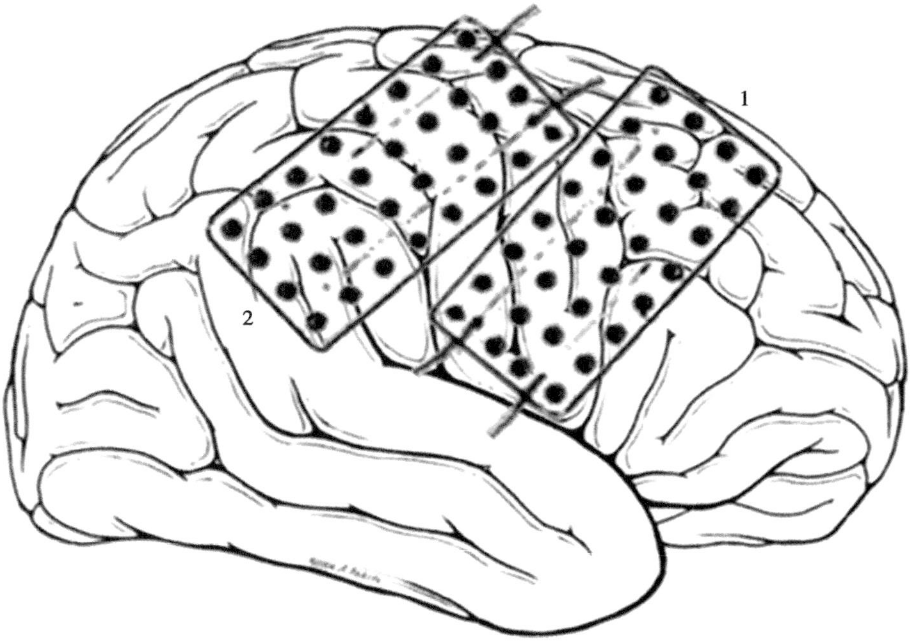

Fig. 2.17 Scheme of intracranial electrodes
Grid electrode 1: the right central and posterior frontal region (32 contacts); Grid electrode 2: the right central parietal region (32 contacts)

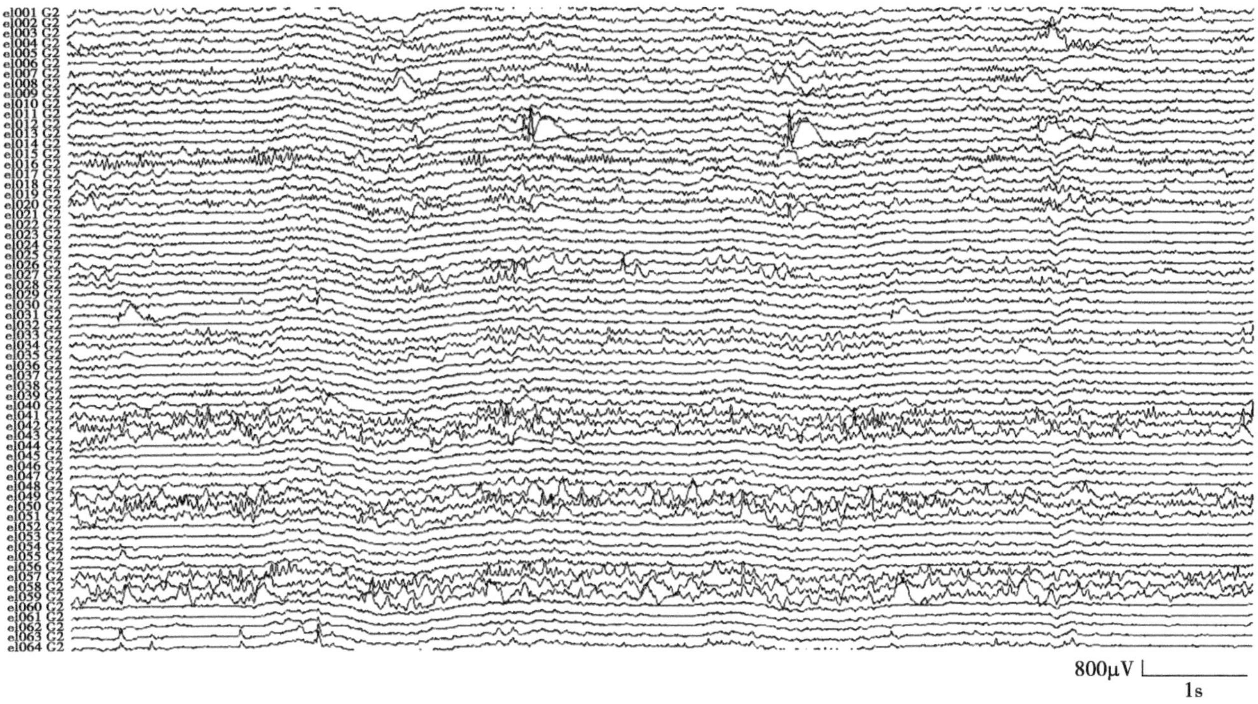

Fig. 2.18 Interictal intracranial EEG
IEEG showed scattered spike-and-wave complexes over the right posterior frontal (contact numbers el004, el007, el008, el013, el014, el031) and central regions (contact numbers el063 and el064), especially over the posterior frontal region (contact number el013)

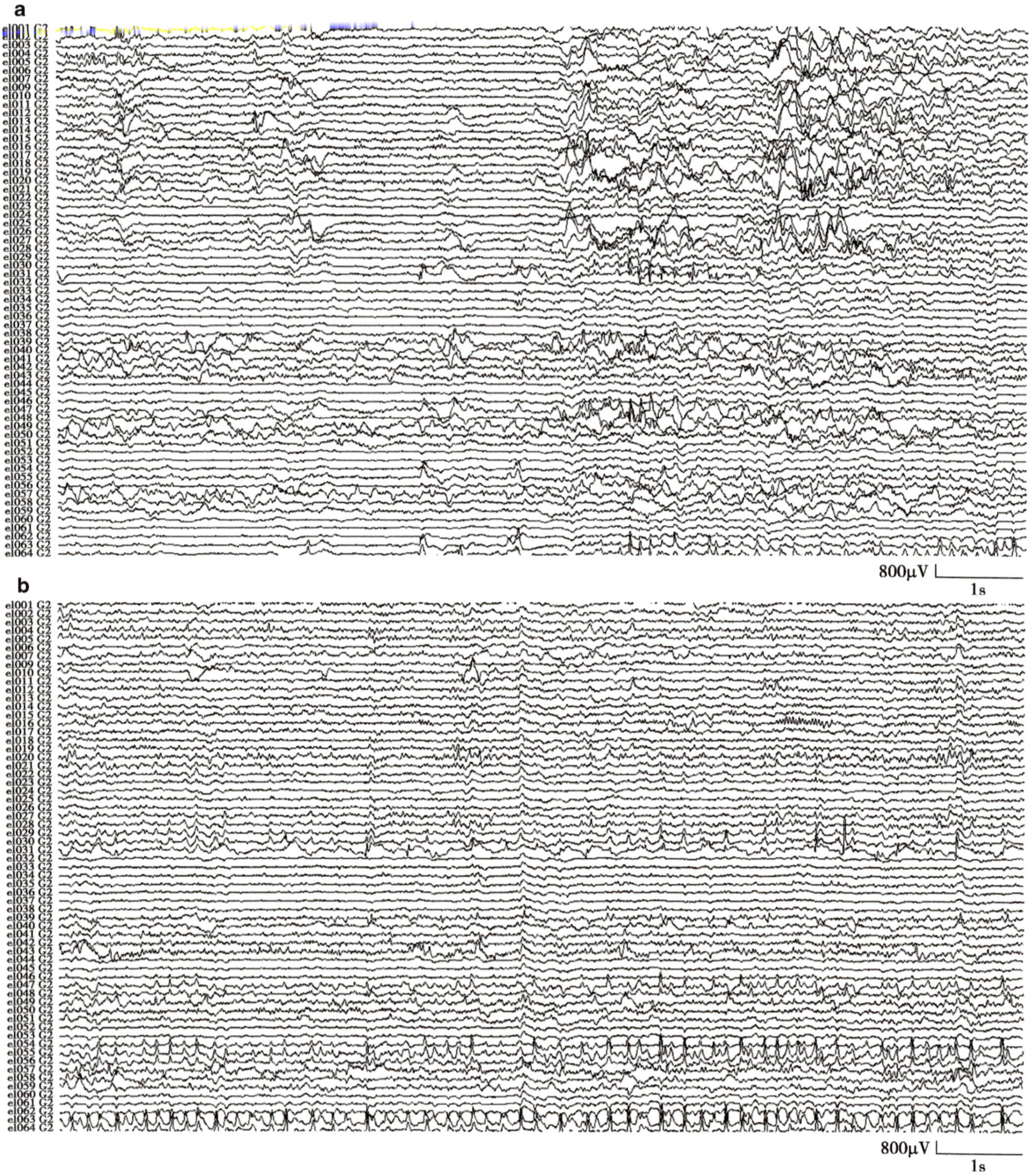

Fig. 2.19 Ictal intracranial EEG. (**a**) The patient was in left-sided decubitus position before the seizure. The IEEG showed sharp waves over the right posterior frontal region (contact numbers el030 and el031) and central region (contact numbers el039, el040, el047, el048, el054, el055, el056, el063, el064), which were gradually rhythmic, especially over the central region (contact numbers el063, el064), which lasted about 6 s. (**b, c**) During the seizure, the patient reported a seizure sensation to his family and then turned the body slightly to the right, followed by flexion and slight elevation of the two upper limbs. The IEEG showed sustained rhythmic sharp waves over the right posterior frontal region (contact numbers el030 and el031) and central region (contact numbers el047, el048, el055, el056, el062, el063, el064) with increasing amplitude, which gradually extended to the central and parietal regions, especially over the middle upper part of the central region (contact numbers el055, el056, el063, el064). (**d**) The patient had mild clonus in both upper limbs. The patient's IEEG manifestations were the same as shown in **c**. (**e**) At the end of the seizure, the patient changed to a supine position, and the IEEG recovered to the background

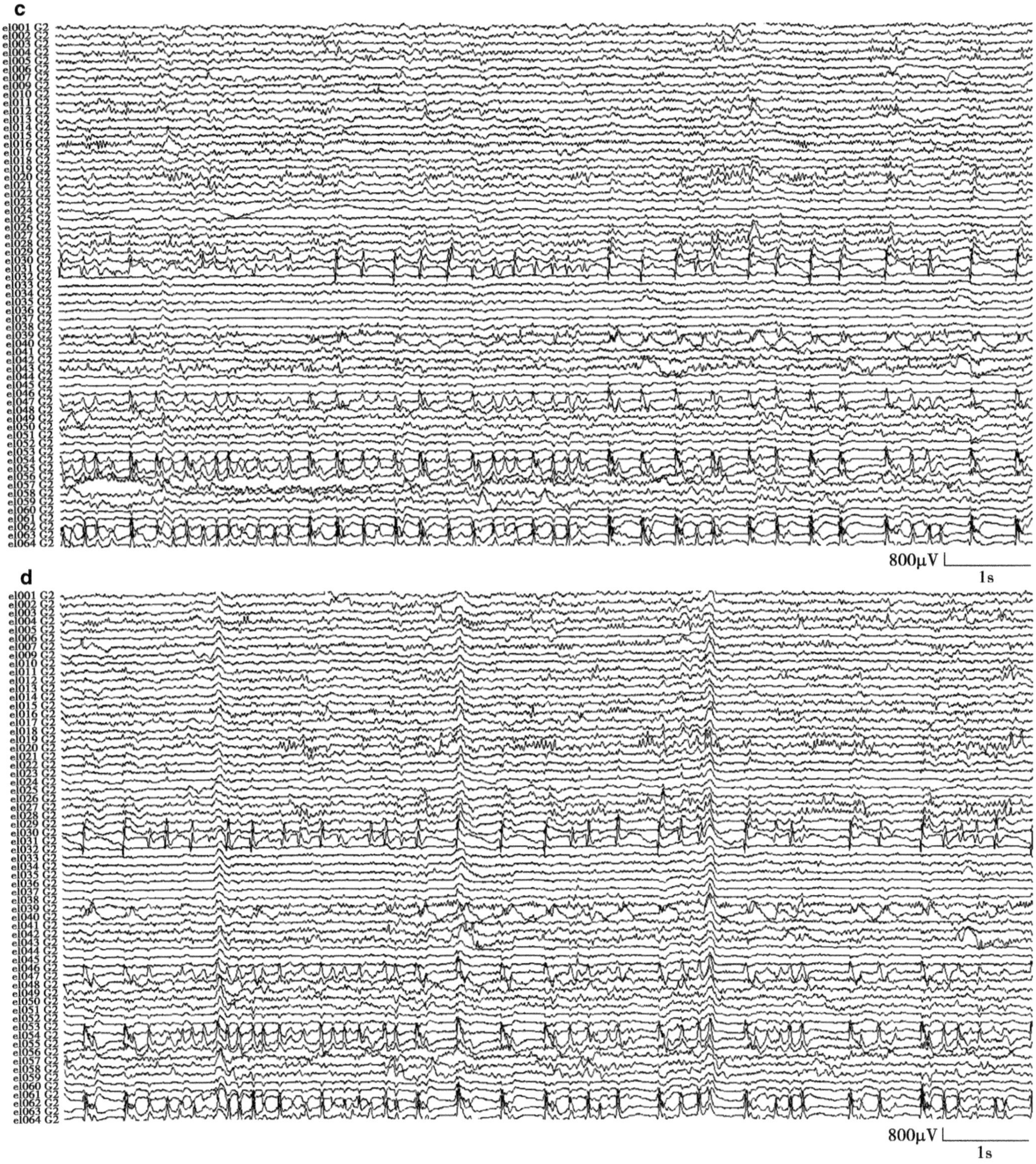

Fig. 2.19 (continued)

e

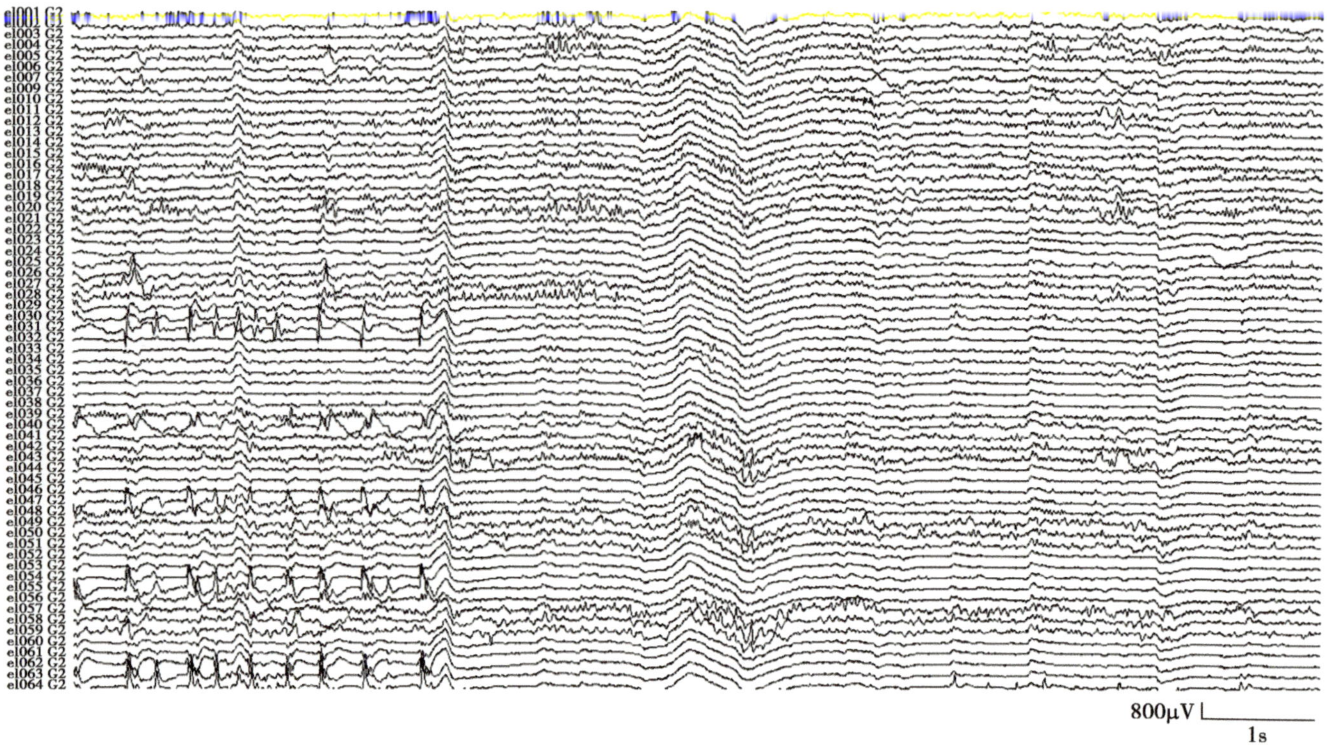

Fig. 2.19 (continued)

Cases of Dorsolateral Prefrontal Cortex Epilepsy

Case 2.5 Premotor Cortex Epilepsy

[Abstract of Medical Records]
Male, 26 years old.

1. *Chief complaint* Recurrent episodic twitching for 10 years, worsening for more than 1 month.
2. *History of present illness* The patient suffered from a sudden onset of tachypnea 10 years ago, with eyes turning upward and failure to answer questions. Seizure type 1: His two upper limbs were flexed, two lower limbs were tonic, with tongue biting and urinary incontinence, which lasted for about 2 min and then resolved. There was no aura. After the seizure, the patient fumbled and then got fully awake after 5–10 min. On average, 1 seizure occurred every 2 days. Seizure type 2: sometimes, it was only manifested by turning the head aimlessly and looking from side to side, with 2–3 jerks of both upper limbs. Both kinds of seizures occurred at night. He has been treated with multiple drugs including carbamazepine, sodium valproate, and traditional Chinese medicine. During the recent 1 month, the seizures have become frequent and occur every night, often type 2. Now the patient is taking sodium valproate orally.
3. *Personal and family history* No history of associated diseases.
4. *Physical examination* The patient was poorly articulate and had nothing else special. Psychological assessment: VIQ = 128, PIQ = 105, FIQ = 120.
5. *Imaging examination*
   (a) MRI showed abnormal signals over the right frontal region.
   (b) MRS showed that the NAA concentration over the left hippocampus was lower than that in the right corresponding area.
   (c) SPECT showed decreased blood perfusion over the posterior part of the right basal ganglia and the temporal lobe.
6. *EEG* For details, see Figs. 2.20, 2.21, 2.22, 2.23, and 2.24.

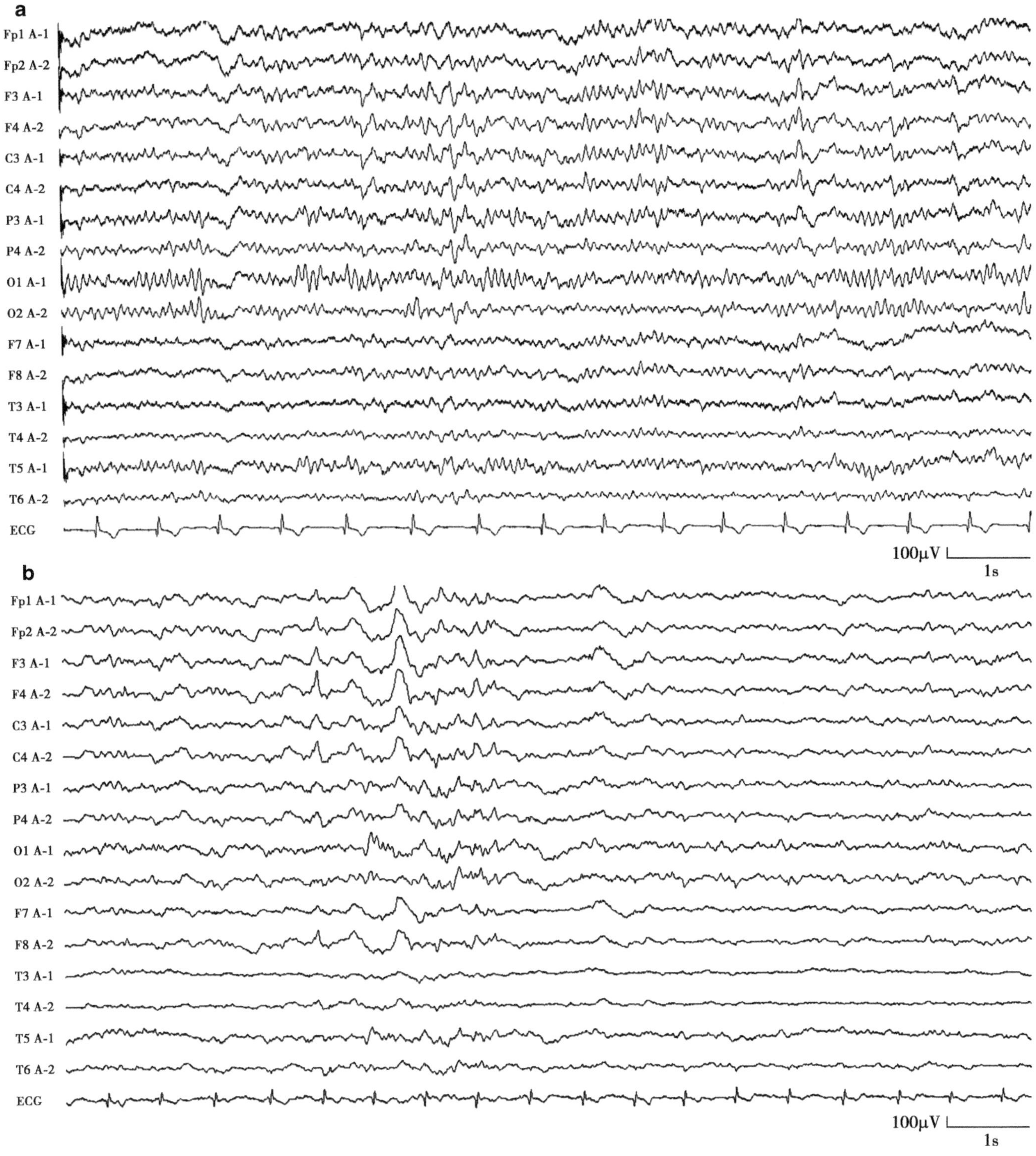

Fig. 2.20 Interictal scalp EEG. (**a**) The EEG showed a background occipital rhythm of 9.0 Hz mixed with some slow of 5.0–7.0 Hz of low and medium amplitude. (**b**) The EEG showed stage II of sleep, and scattered sharp waves over the right frontal region (F4) and the anterior temporal region (F8), which spread to the left central region (C4)

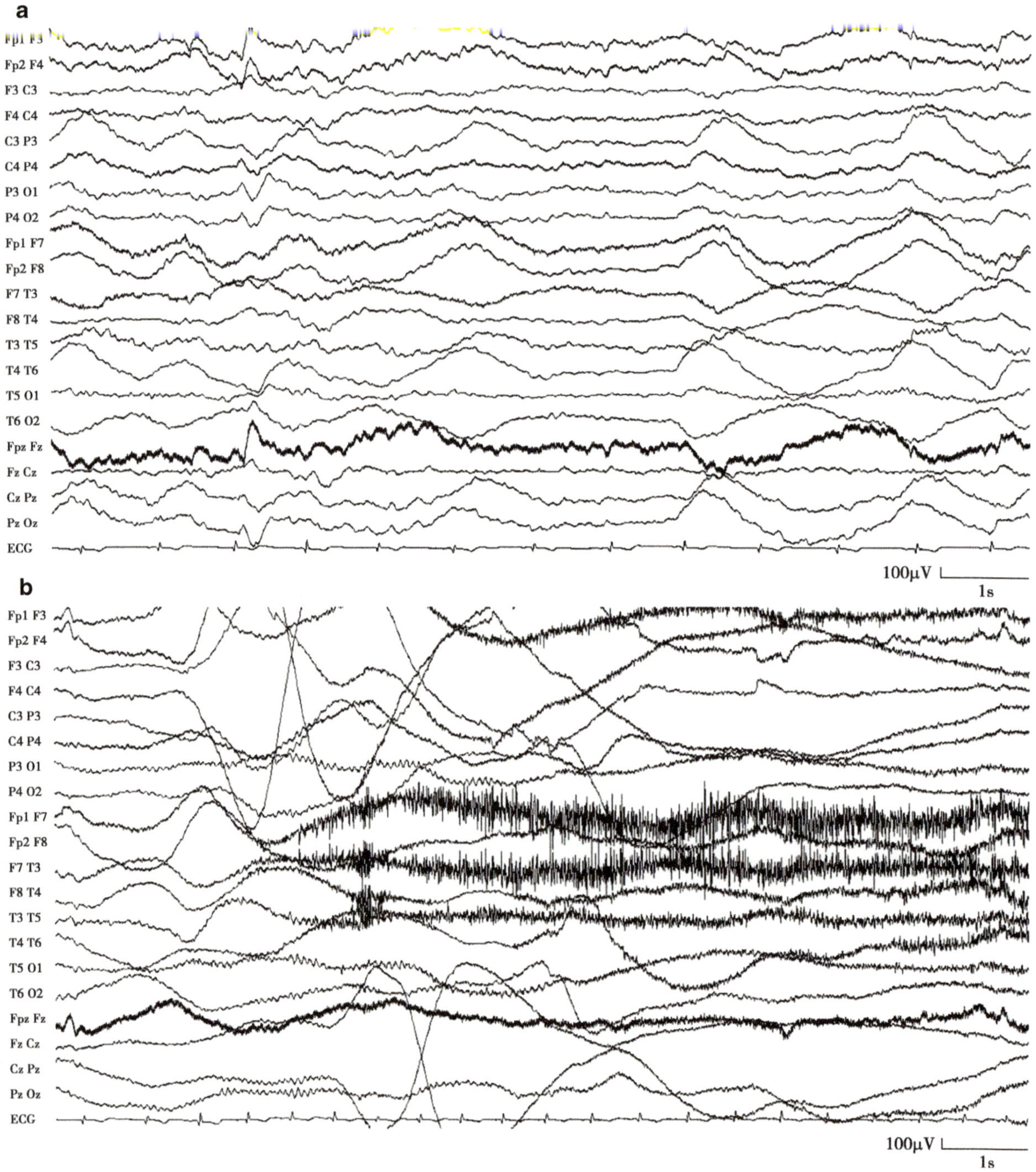

Fig. 2.21 Ictal scalp EEG. (**a**) Sixteen second before the seizure, the patient was asleep in a right-sided decubitus position, with the upper limbs crossed on the chest. The EEG showed the stage II of sleep, and artifacts caused by poor contact of electrodes over the midline (Fpz Fz). (**b**) The patient opened his eyes and gazed forward during the seizure, then sat up slowly with the right upper limb slightly abducted and tonic. The EEG showed flat waves of low amplitude and many electrode artifacts over all leads; the low amplitude fast activity were observed over the bilateral parieto-occipital (P3 O1, P4 O2), posterior temporo-occipital (T5 O1, T6 O2), and midline regions (Cz Pz, Pz Oz); and EMG artifacts can be seen over the bilateral fronto-temporal regions, especially on the left. (**c**) The patient's upper limbs were tonic and slightly abducted, and the lower limbs were flexed and raised. The patient lay down with the help of his family. The EEG showed the rhythm of sharp waves of low amplitude over the bilateral frontal (F3 C3, F4 C4) and frontal midline regions (Fz Cz) with increasing amplitude, especially on the right (F4 C4). (**d**) The patient vocalized with tonic limbs. EMG and electrode artifacts were observed. (**e, f**) The patient had tonic and clonic limbs. Numerous EMG artifacts were observed. (**g**) The patient had tonic and clonic limbs. Numerous EMG artifacts were observed. (**h**) The patient's limbs were still having clonic jerks in a decreasing frequency, with salivating. The EEG showed irregular 3.0–5.0 Hz slowing of high amplitude and the rhythm of spike-and-wave complexes over the bilateral middle frontal regions (Fp1 F3, Fp2 F4, F3 C3, F4 C4), and EMG artifacts were showed over the bilateral temporal regions. (**i**) The seizure ended, while his wheezing was heavy. EEG showed oculomotor artifacts over the bilateral frontal poles (Fp1 F3, Fp2 F4, Fpz Fz, Fz Cz) and EMG artifacts over the bilateral temporal regions. (**j**) The seizure ended. The EEG showed reduced amplitude, mixed with electrode artifacts and artifacts over the bilateral temporal regions

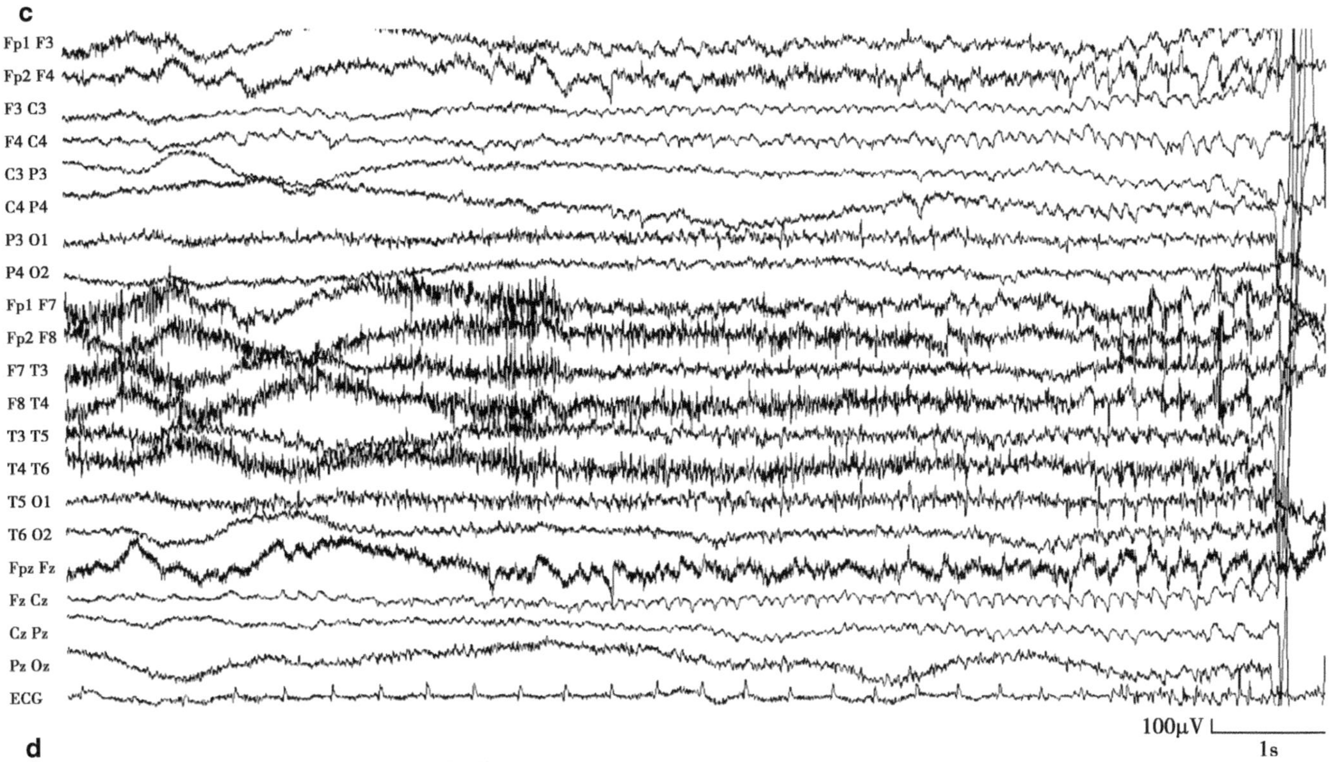

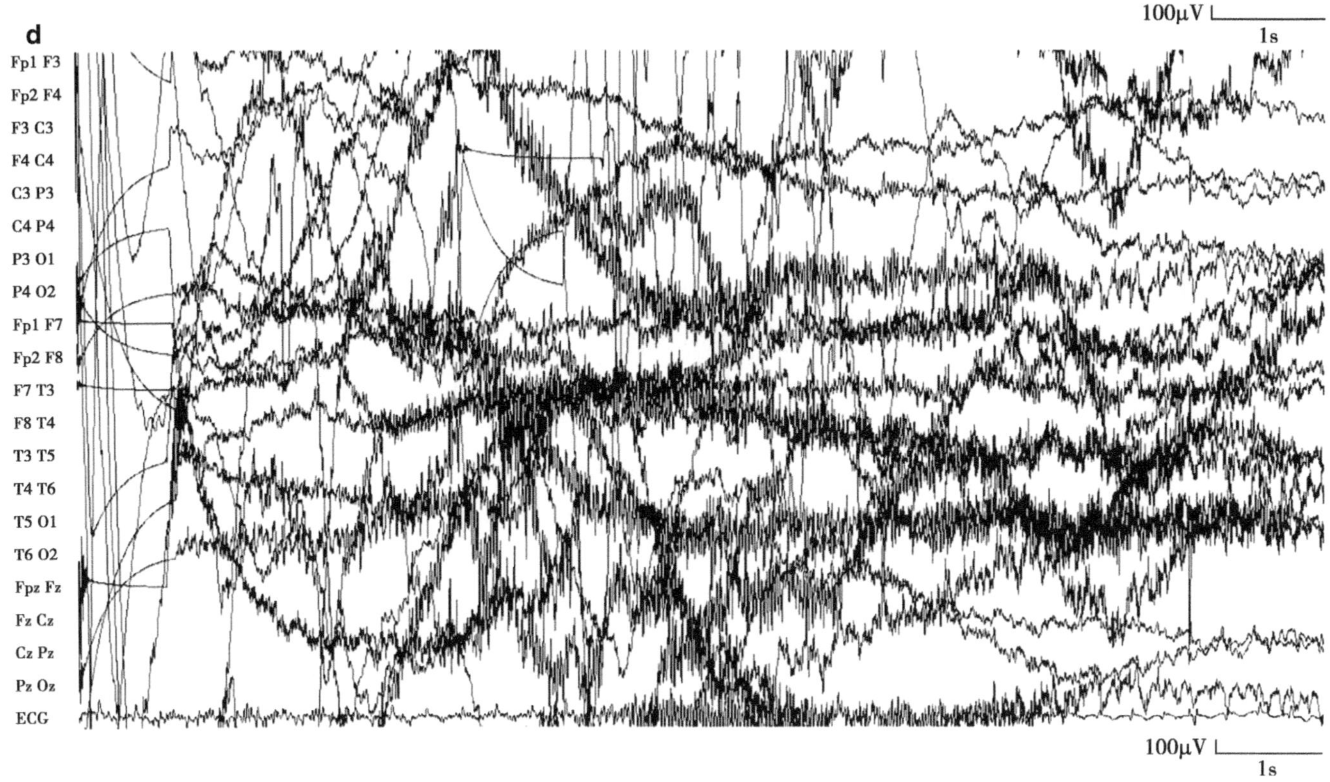

Fig. 2.21 (continued)

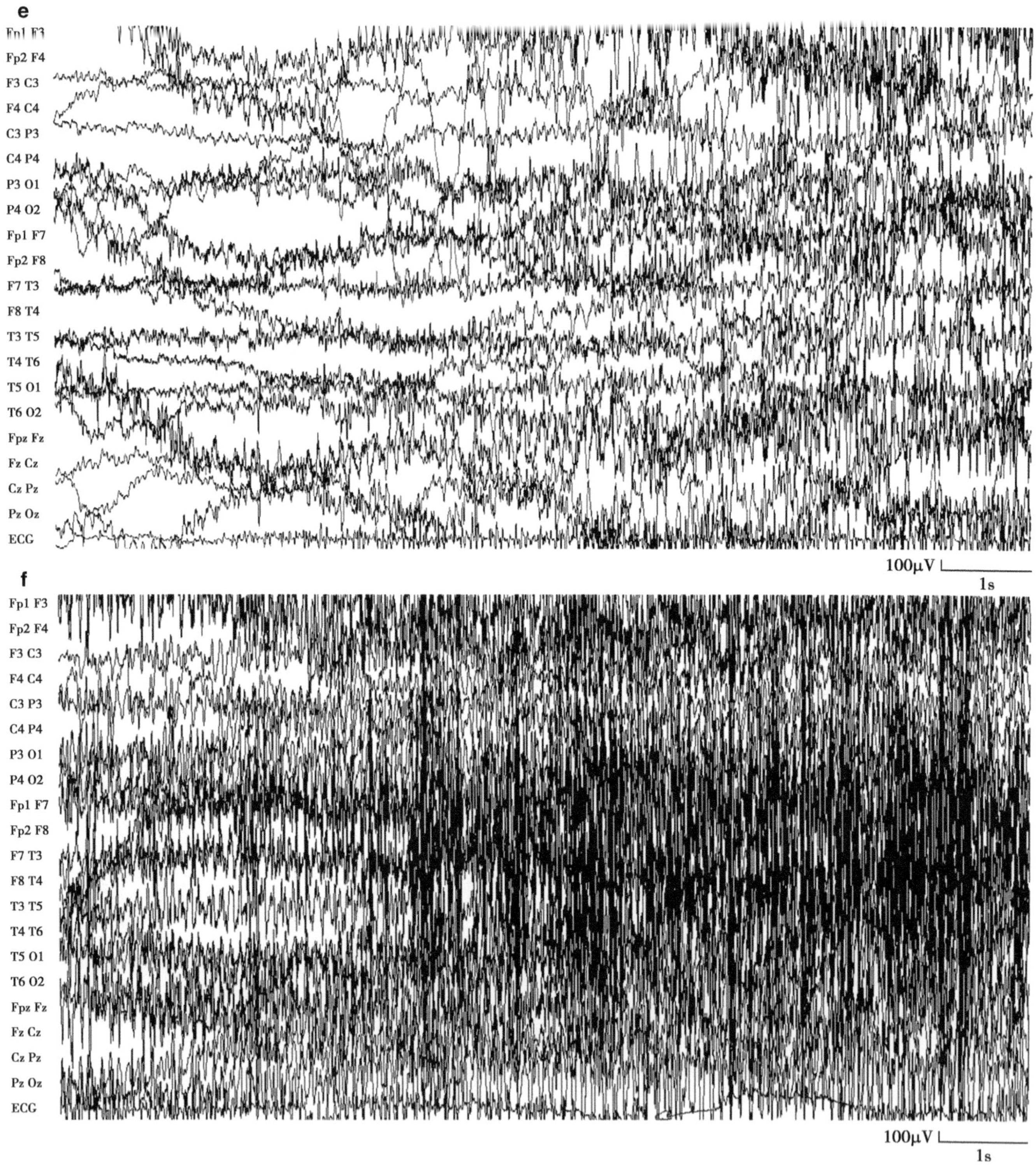

Fig. 2.21 (continued)

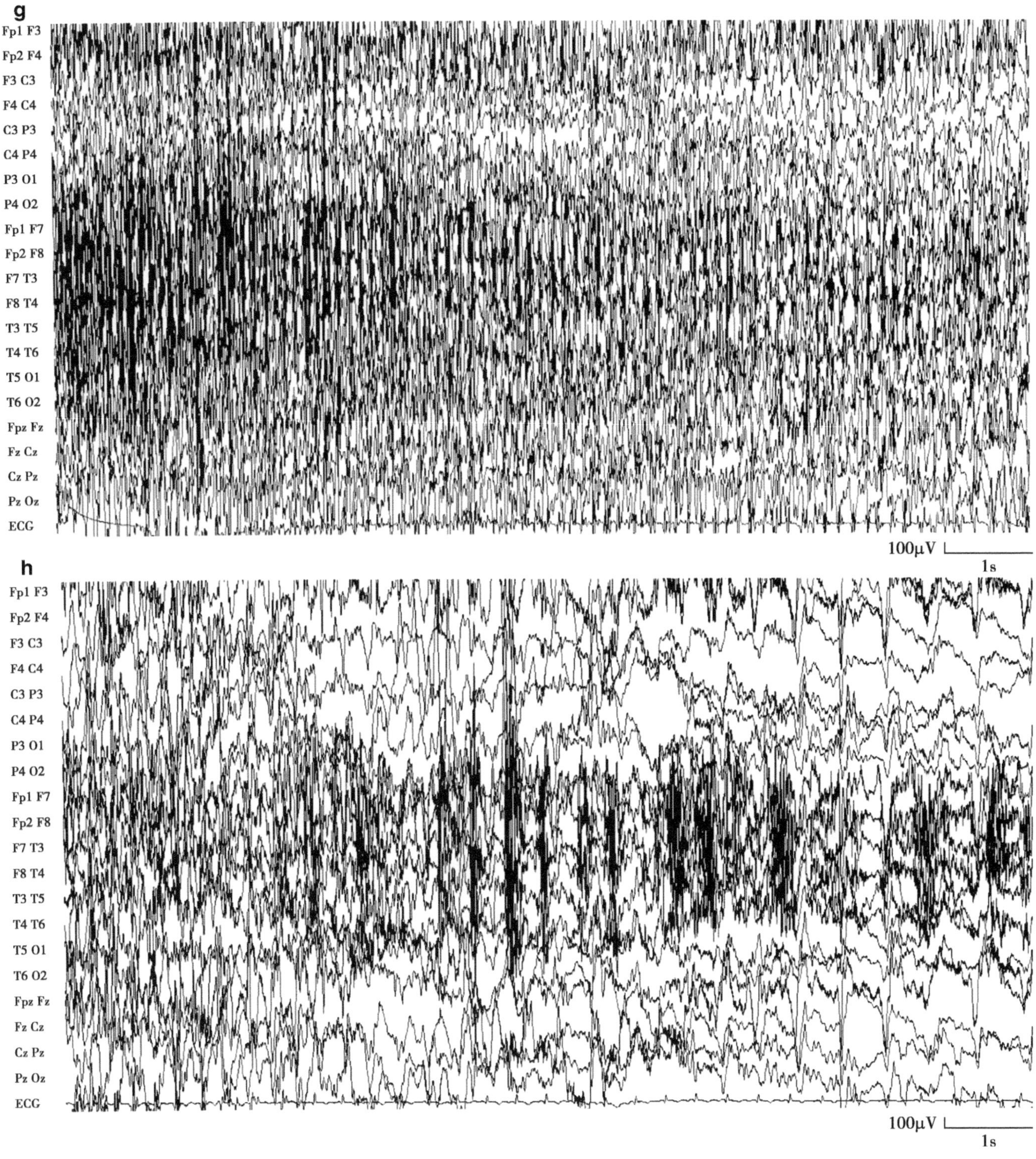

Fig. 2.21 (continued)

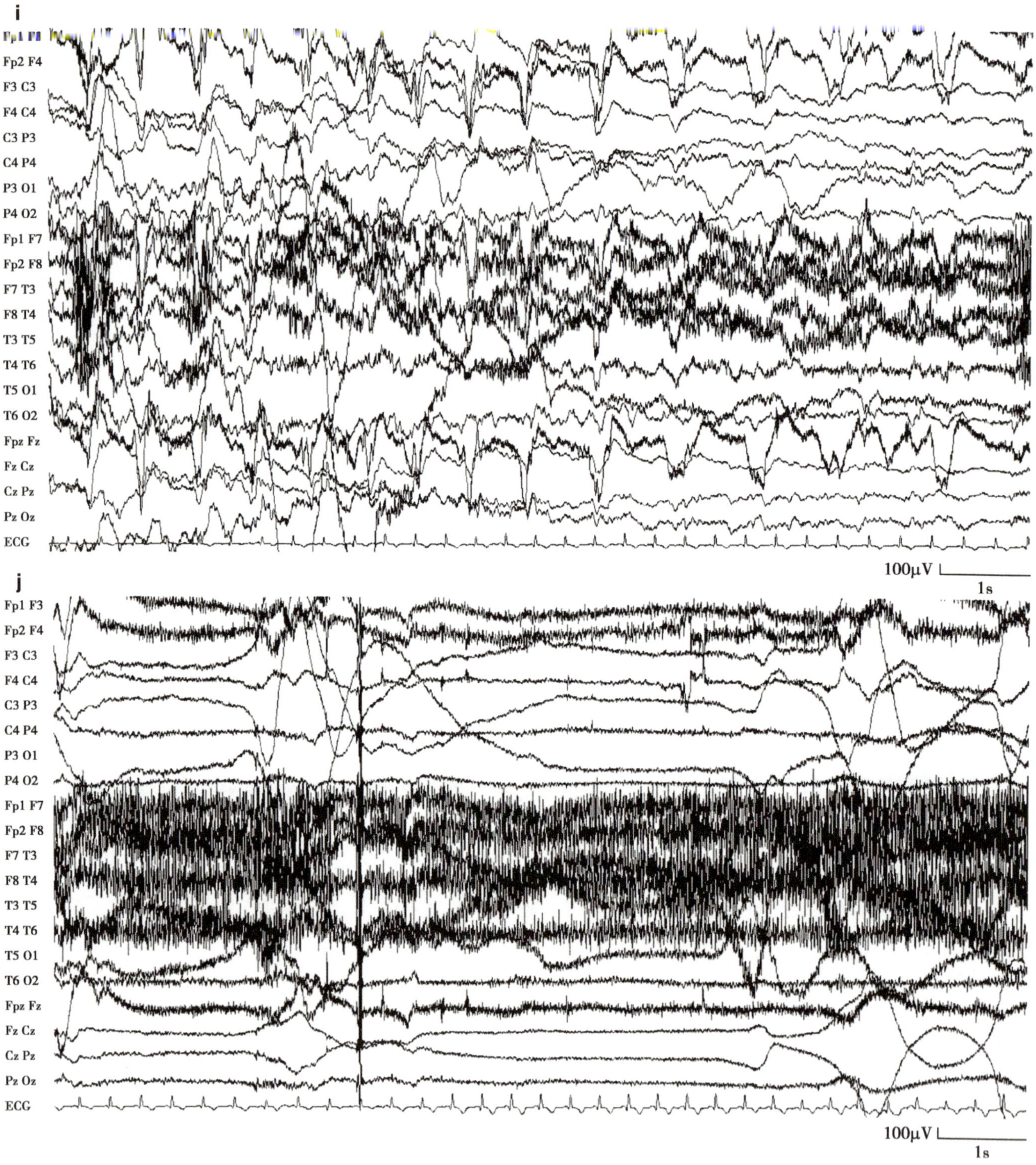

Fig. 2.21 (continued)

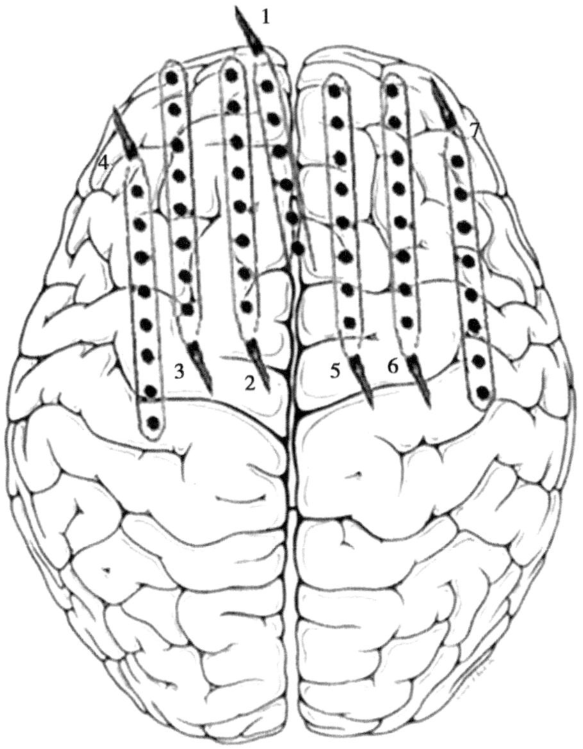

Fig. 2.22 Scheme of intracranial electrodes
Strip electrode 1: the left medial frontal cortex (6 contacts); Strip electrode 2: the left superior frontal gyrus (8 contacts); Strip electrode 3: the left middle frontal gyrus (8 contacts); Strip electrode 4: the left frontal central region (8 contacts); Strip electrode 5: the right superior frontal gyrus (8 contacts); Strip electrode 6: the right middle frontal gyrus (8 contacts); Strip electrode 7: over the right frontal central region (8 contacts)

[Case Review]

1. *Case Characteristics*
   (a) *Seizure characteristics* ① Sudden shortness of breath during sleep, failure to answer questions. ② No aura. ③ Seizures occurred at night.
   (b) *EEG characteristics* ① Interictal EEG showed sharp waves over the right frontal and anterior temporal region, which spread to the right central region. ② Ictal EEG showed the low amplitude fast activity over the bilateral parieto-occipital and posterior temporal-occipital cortices.
   (c) *Imaging characteristics* Suspicious abnormal signals were observed over the right frontal region.
2. *Diagnosis and treatment strategy and follow-up results* The seizure focus was to be located in the frontal lobe based on the characteristics of the patient's semiology, while the side could not be clarified noninvasively. Therefore, intracranial electrodes were implanted over the bilateral frontal regions, involving the central area of the posterior frontal region. The interictal IEEG showed extensive epileptiform discharges, the rhythms of spike wave complex, spikes and low amplitude fast activity over the left frontal fissure and the central region, and repetitive spikes and the rhythm of spikes over the right frontal region; the ictal IEEG showed that the seizure origin was located over the right frontal region. The right frontal region was surgically resected. After the surgery, the patient was seizure-free during a 1-year follow-up. The seizure origin was clear, and the epileptic focus was completely resected, contributing to a satisfactory outcome of the operation.

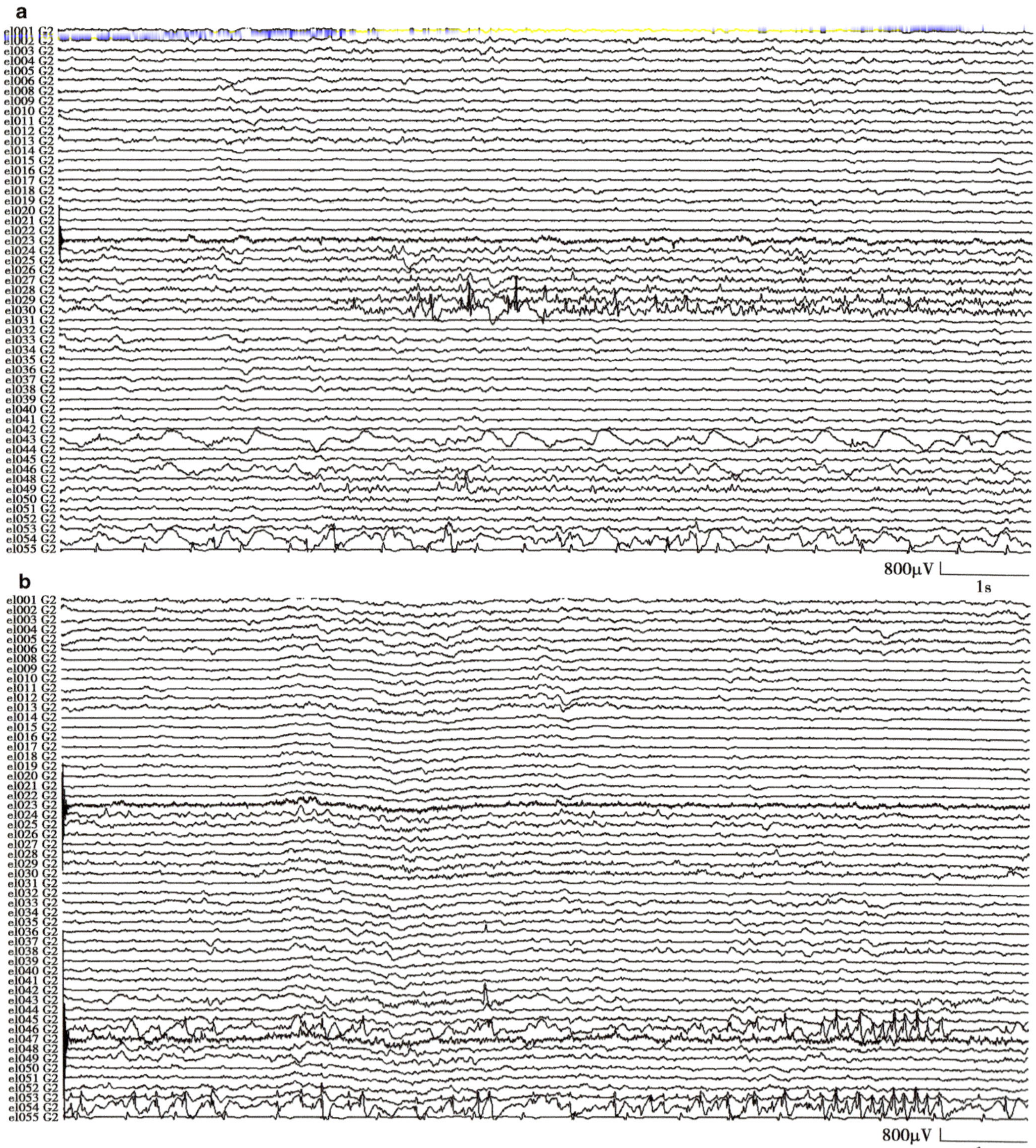

Fig. 2.23 Interictal intracranial EEG. (**a**) The IEEG showed focal spikes and the low amplitude fast activity over the left frontal central region (contact numbers el029 and el030). (**b**) The IEEG showed repetitive spikes and paroxysmal spike rhythms of high amplitude over the right frontal and central regions (contact numbers el046, el053, el054). (**c**) The IEEG showed spike-and-wave complexes over the left medial frontal cortex (contact numbers el02, el03, el04, el05) and the central region (contact numbers el028, el029, el030); it also showed the rhythm of spike-and-wave complexes over the right frontal region (contact numbers el046, el053, el054)

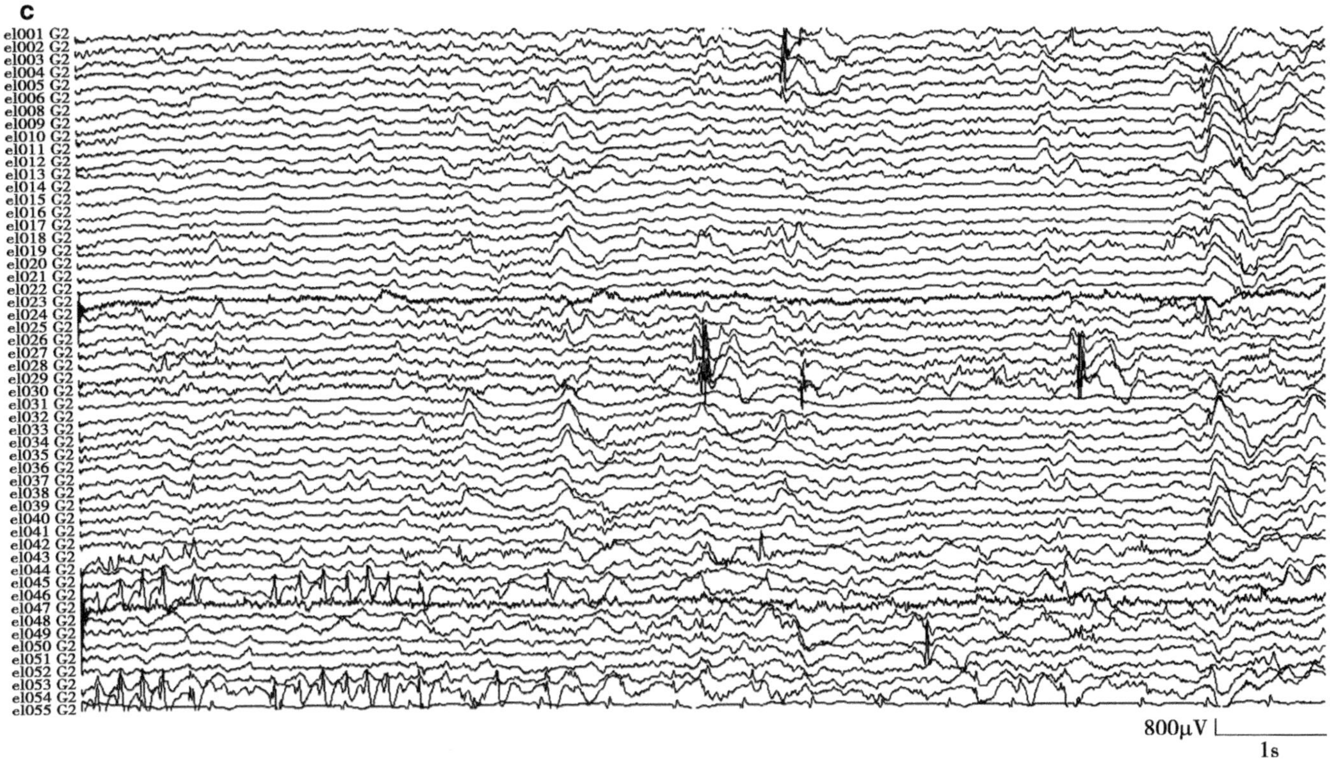

Fig. 2.23 (continued)

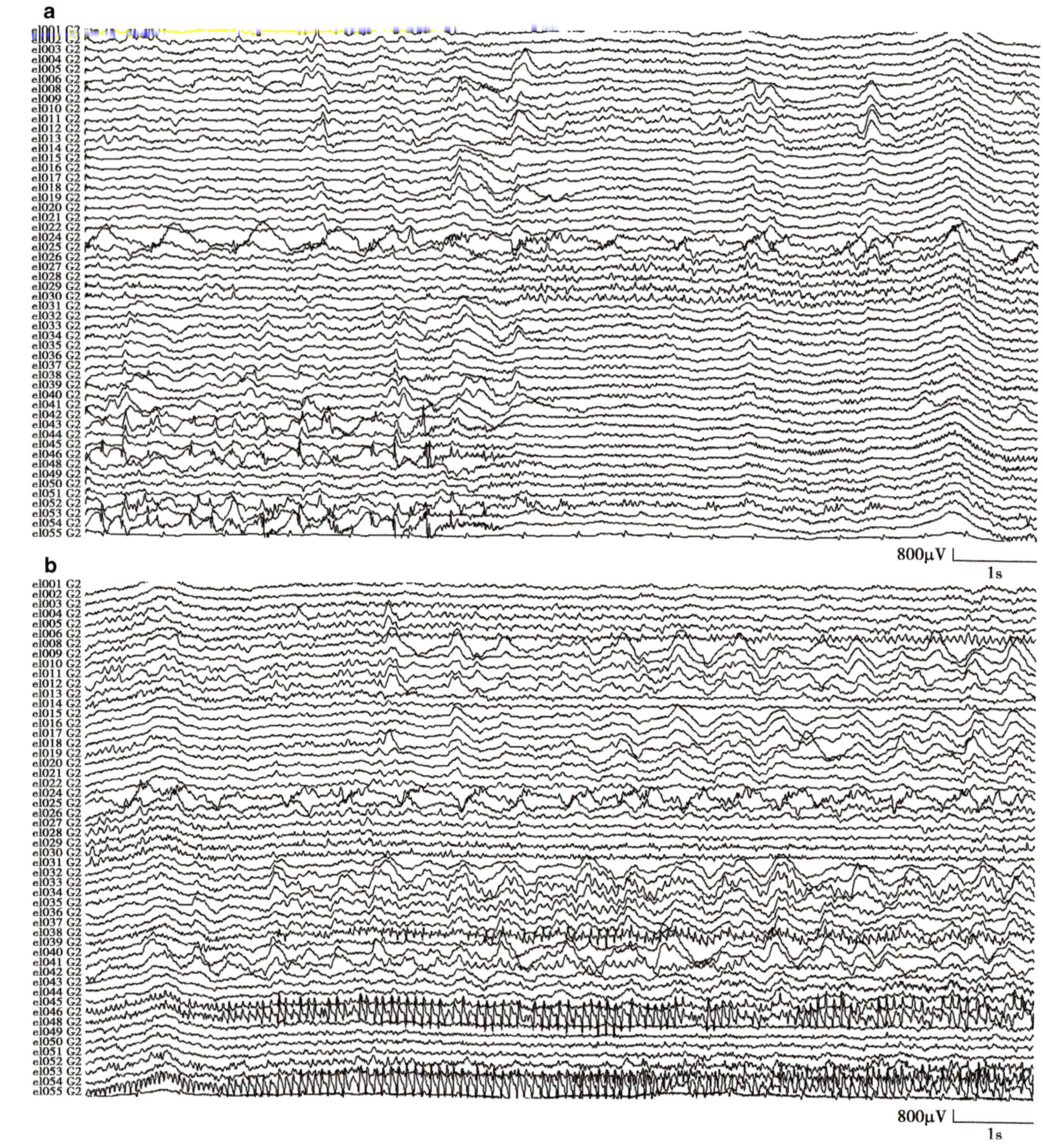

Fig. 2.24 Ictal EEG of intracranial electrodes. (**a**) The patient was asleep before the seizure. Five second before the seizure, the IEEG showed wave amplitude decreasing, rhythmic spikes, and the low amplitude fast activity over the right frontal region (contact numbers el043, el044, el045, el046, el052, el053, el054), and the low amplitude fast activity waves over the left frontal region (contact numbers el024, el025, el027, el028, el029, el030). (**b**) During the seizure, the patient opened eyes and stared, and was slightly short of breath. The IEEG showed increasing rhythm, and the rhythm of spikes over the right frontal region (contact numbers el038, el045, el046, el053, el054). (**c**) The patient's right upper limb was flexed and stiff, and his head was raised slowly, and failed to answer questions. The IEEG showed that the rhythm of sharp waves over the right frontal region, which gradually spread to the left frontal fissure (contact number el06) and the frontal central region (contact numbers el024, el025, el030). (**d**) The patient's upper limbs were flexed and shaken, and his lower limbs were flexed and raised slowly, with the eyes gazing to the left. The rhythms of spike-and-wave complexes and spikes of high amplitude were observed. (**e, f**) The patient had tonic and clonic limbs and vocalized. The IEEG showed the rhythm of spikes with increasing amplitude, especially over the left frontal central region (contact numbers el024, el025, el029, el030). (**g, h**) The patient had tonic-clonic limbs. The IEEG presentation was the same as **f**. (**i, j**) The patient had tonic-clonic limbs. The IEEG presentation was the same as **f**. (**k**) The patient had tonic-clonic. The IEEG showed the rhythm of spikes over the right frontal region. (**l**) The seizure stopped, while his wheezing was heavy. The rhythm of spike wave complexes of high amplitude was observed

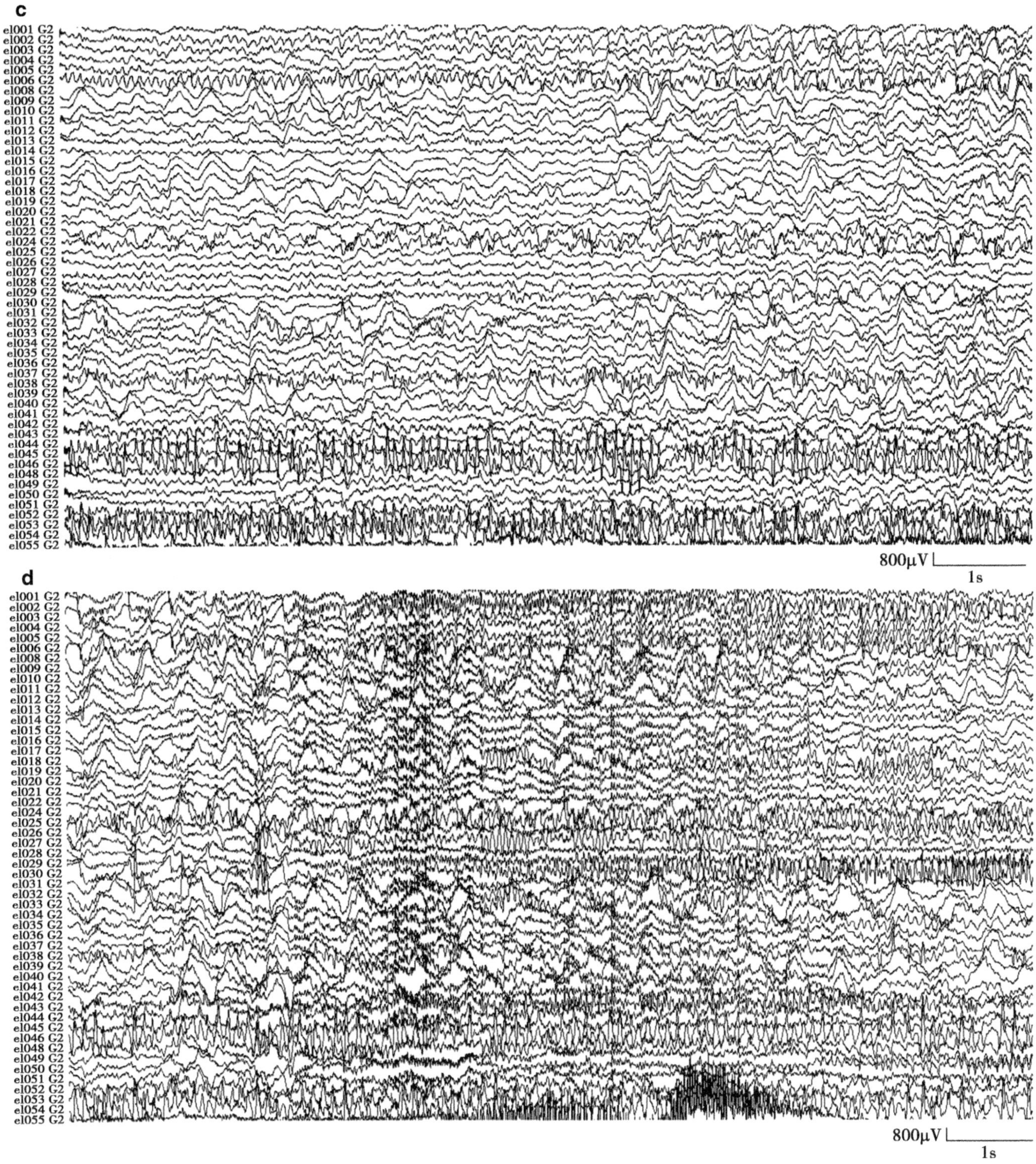

el001 G2
el002 G2
el003 G2
el004 G2
el005 G2
el006 G2
el008 G2
el009 G2
el010 G2
el011 G2
el012 G2
el013 G2
el014 G2
el015 G2
el016 G2
el017 G2
el018 G2
el019 G2
el020 G2
el021 G2
el022 G2
el024 G2
el025 G2
el026 G2
el027 G2
el028 G2
el029 G2
el030 G2
el031 G2
el032 G2
el033 G2
el034 G2
el035 G2
el036 G2
el037 G2
el038 G2
el039 G2
el040 G2
el041 G2
el042 G2
el043 G2
el044 G2
el045 G2
el046 G2
el048 G2
el049 G2
el050 G2
el051 G2
el052 G2
el053 G2
el054 G2
el055 G2

Fig. 2.24 (continued)

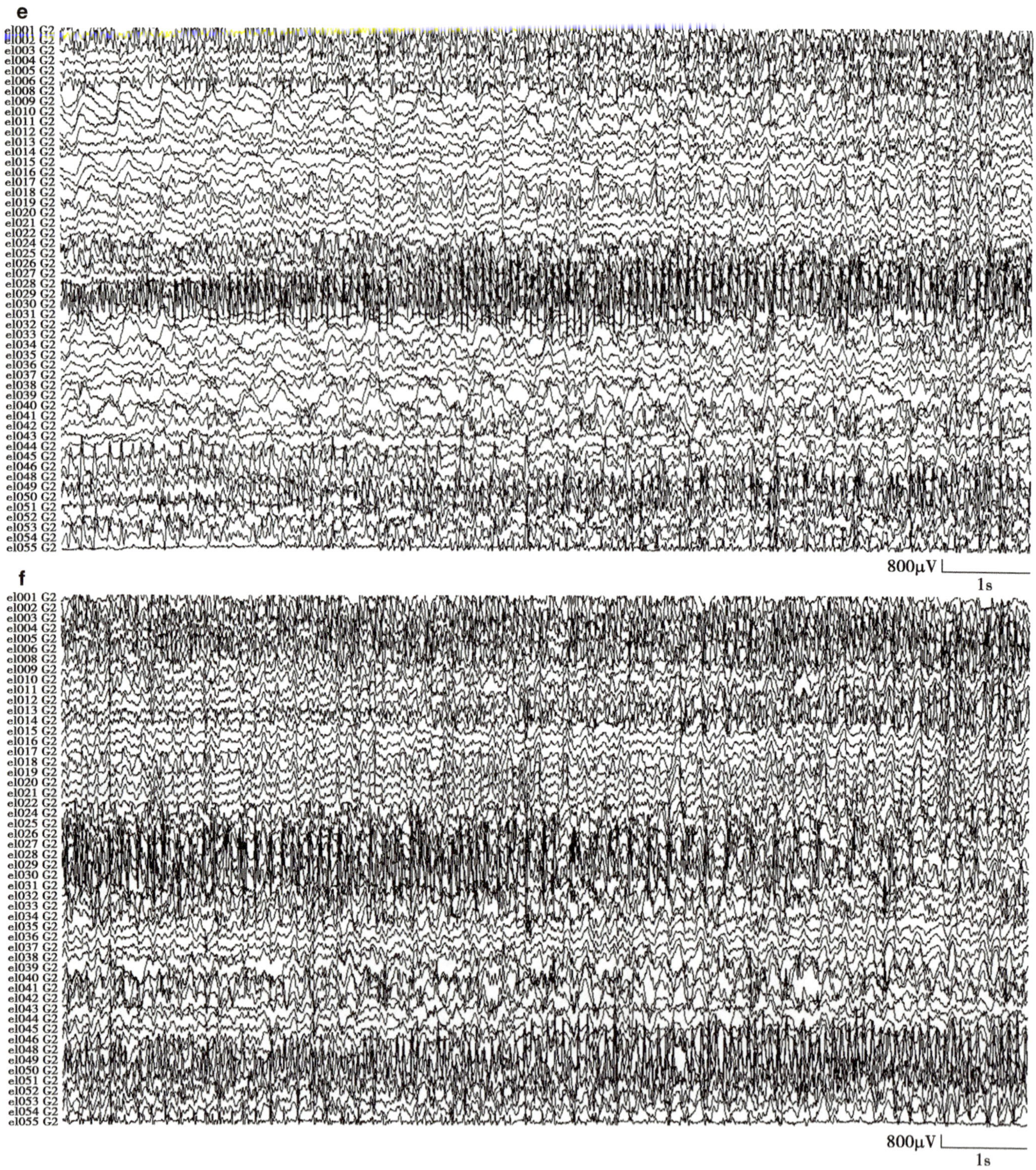

Fig. 2.24 (continued)

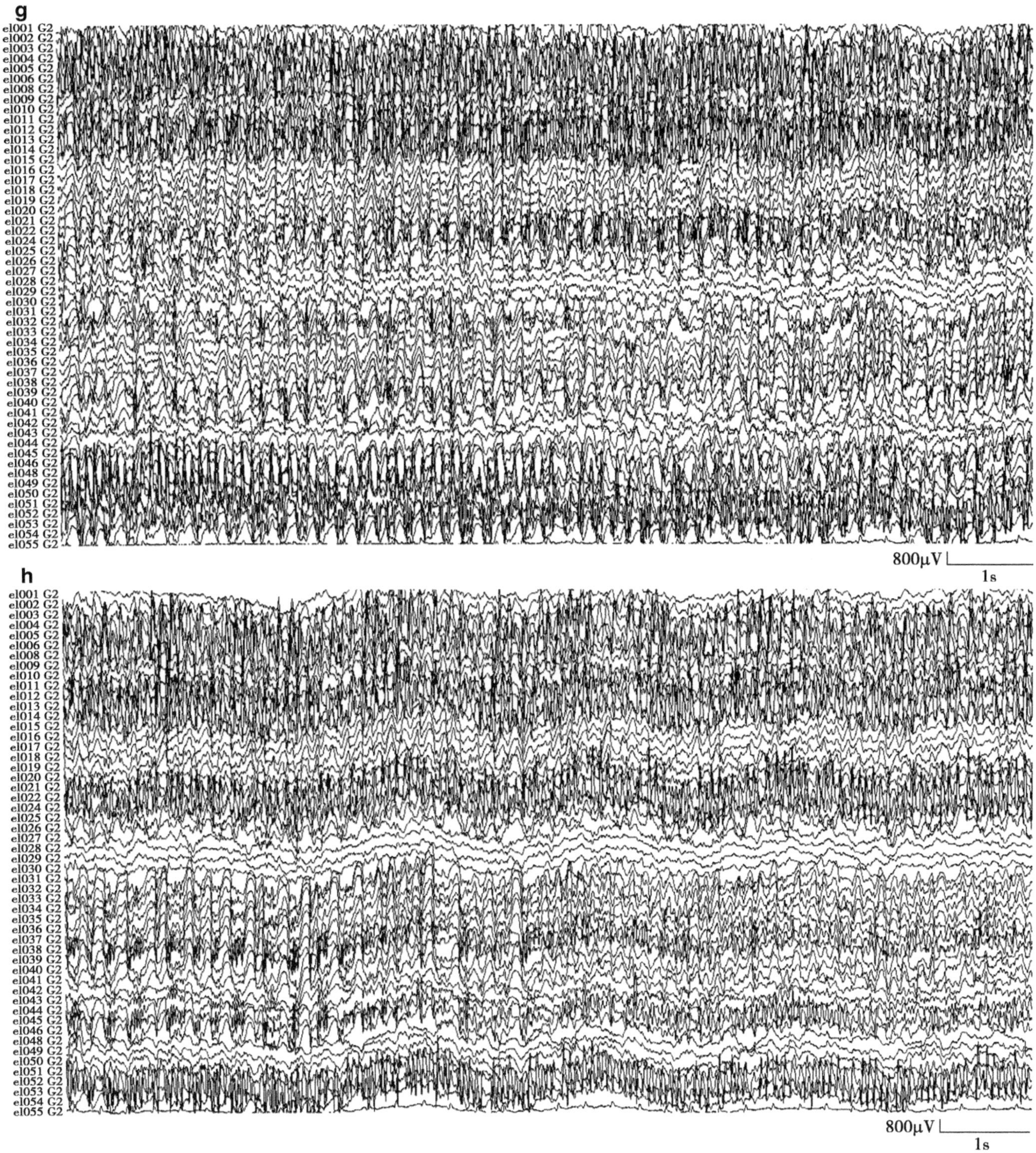

Fig. 2.24 (continued)

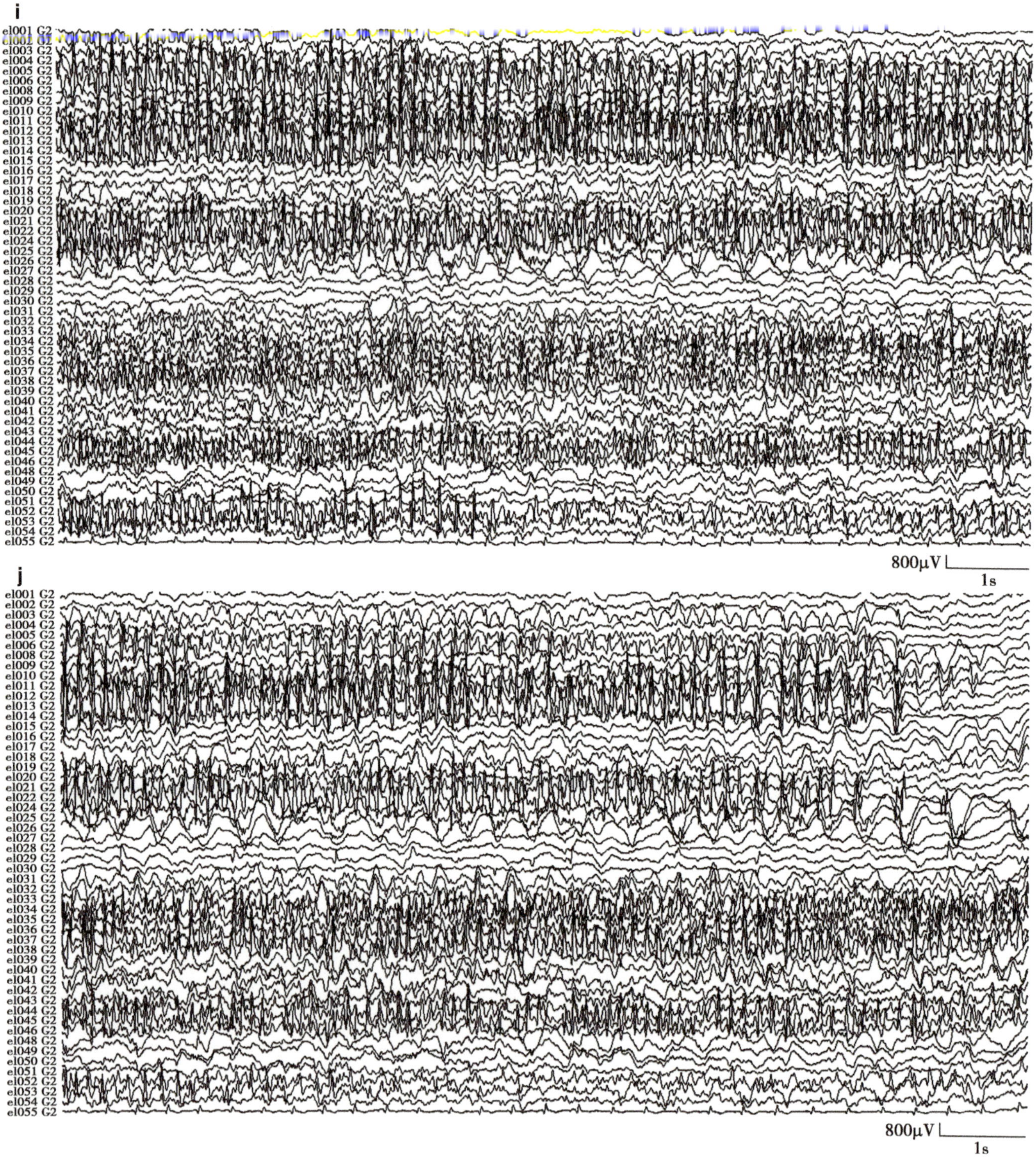

Fig. 2.24 (continued)

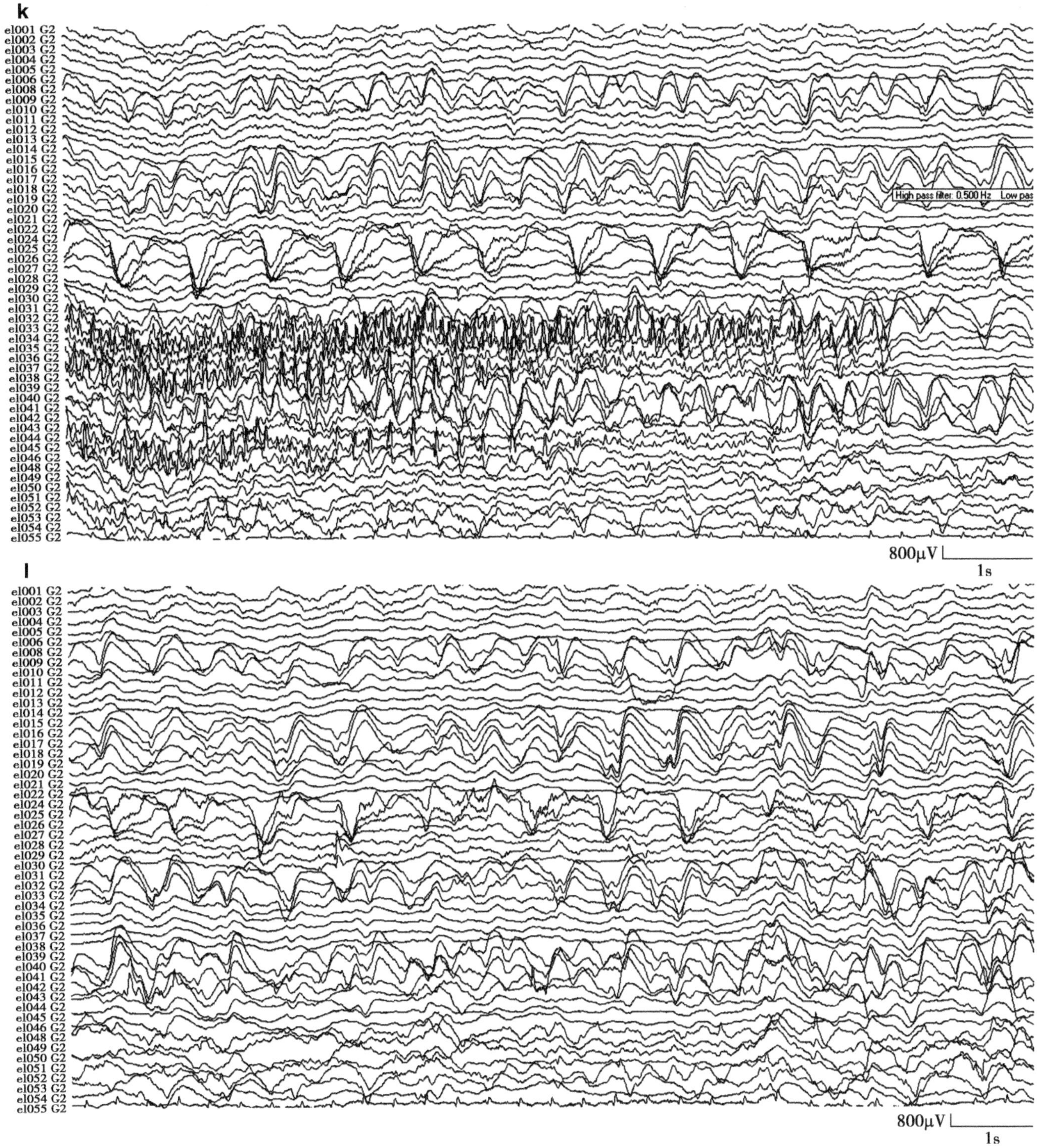

Fig. 2.24 (continued)

Case 2.6 Middle Frontal Gyrus Epilepsy

[Abstract of Medical Records]
Male, 33 years old.

1. *Chief complaint* Paroxysmal convulsion for 23 years.
2. *History of present illness* The patient was diagnosed with epilepsy 23 years ago when he started having episodic loss of consciousness and limb twitching with 3–5 seizures per month. After starting treatment with medications such as carbamazepine, his seizures were essentially under control, and he was basically seizure-free after 1 year. Ten years ago, the patient had seizures again, which was characterized by loss of consciousness, aimless wandering, and sometimes generalized twitching. He was successively given phenytoin sodium, carbamazepine, the effects of which were unsatisfactory. There were various seizure types, including the following: ① discomfort, chest tightness, followed by loss of consciousness, tonic-clonic limbs, with or without involuntary fumbling of limbs, lasting 3–5 min and then resolved, sometimes wandering and jumping aimlessly after waking up; ② sudden panting, with or without loss of consciousness or generalized convulsions, for a short duration; and ③ sudden stupor, ending with chewing for a few seconds. The seizures occurred 2–3 times or 8–9 times a month when the patient took medicines. When the seizures were frequent, the patient behaved abnormally, such as hitting and hurting others. He has been admitted twice into psychiatric hospitals. Since the onset of the disease, the patient suffered from memory loss, unresponsiveness, irritability, and a tendency to strike others.
3. *Past history* The patient was delivered in obstructed labor, and suffered from loss of consciousness and generalized tonic-clonic seizure when he had a fever within 6 months after birth.
4. *Personal and family history* No history of associated diseases.
5. *Physical examination* With clear consciousness but memory impairment; with no abnormalities in the heart, lungs, and abdomen.
6. *Imaging examination* MRI showed no abnormalities.
7. *EEG* For details, see Figs. 2.25, 2.26, 2.27, 2.28, and 2.29.

[Case Review]

1. *Case Characteristics*
   (a) *Seizure characteristics* ① There were two seizure types: one was Focal to bilateral tonic-clonic seizure; the other was loss of consciousness. ② The aura was feeling uncomfortable in the heart and chest tightness.
   (b) *EEG characteristics* ① Interictal EEG showed sharp waves over the right sphenoidal electrode. ② Ictal EEG showed numerous EMG artifacts.
   (c) *Imaging characteristics* MRI showed no abnormalities.
2. *Diagnosis and treatment strategy and follow-up results* The side and specific location of the seizure focus could not be clarified based on the patient's semiology, EEG, and MRI. The electrodes should cover the medial frontal cortex, orbitofrontal region, dorsolateral frontal cortex, and temporal region based on the semiology. Therefore, intracranial electrodes were implanted over the bilateral frontal and temporal regions. The interictal IEEG showed extensive epileptiform discharges, and slow waves over the bilateral medial frontal cortex, spike wave complexes over the right temporal region, sharp waves over the left temporal region, and the low amplitude fast activity, sharp waves, and slow waves over the right frontal region. The ictal IEEG revealed that the seizure origin was located over the right frontal region and showed the low amplitude fast activity over the right medial frontal cortex, orbitofrontal region, and dorsolateral frontal region, especially the dorsolateral frontal region. The right frontal region was surgically resected, and the patient was seizure-free during a 1-year postoperative follow-up. The seizure origin was clear, and the epileptic focus was completely resected, contributing to a satisfactory outcome of the operation. Some of the manifestations in this patient were similar to temporal lobe epilepsy, which may be caused by epileptiform discharges involving the temporal lobe during seizures.

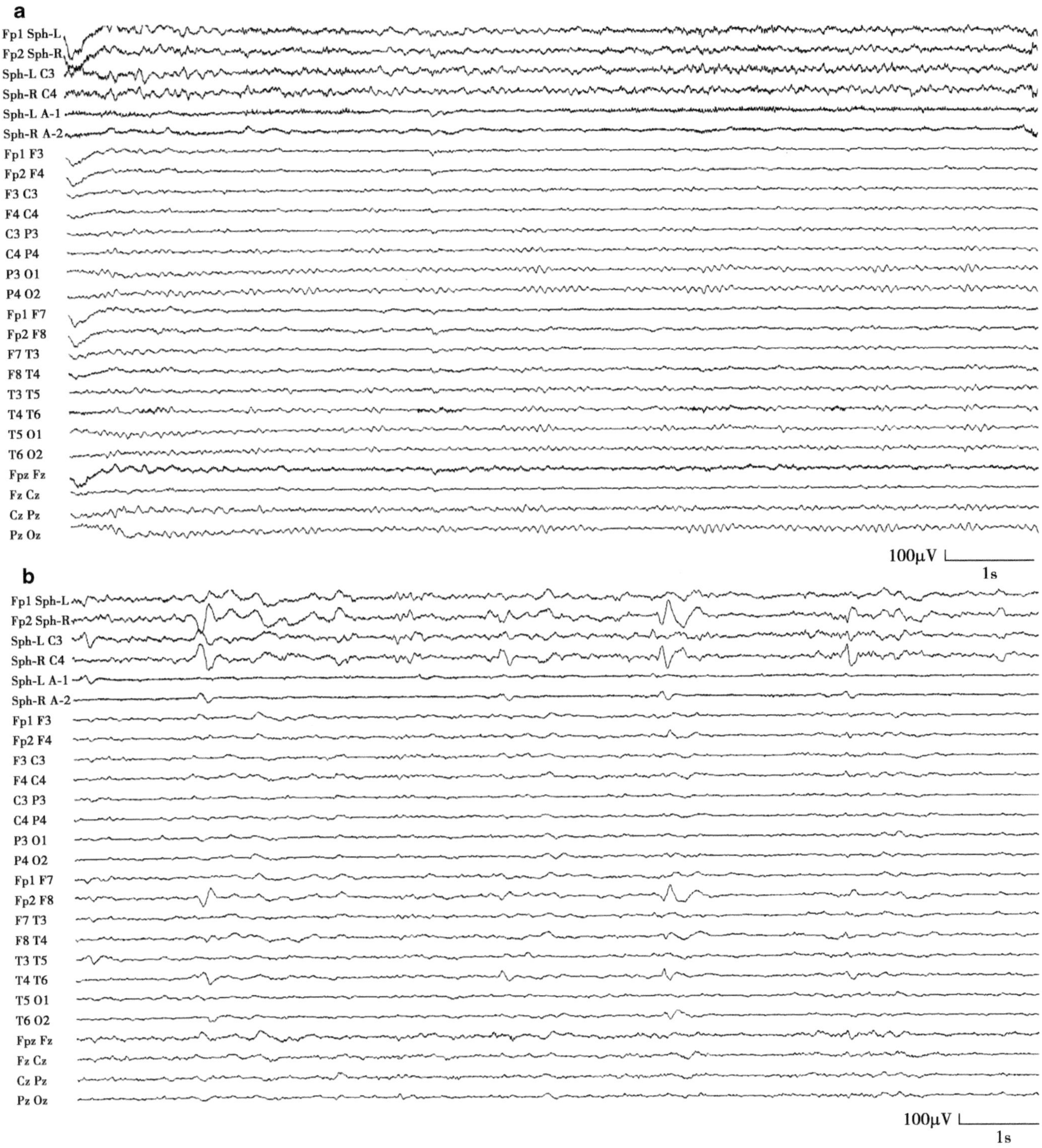

Fig. 2.25 Interictal scalp EEG. (**a**) The EEG had a background occipital rhythm of 9.0 Hz and showed some 4.0–5.0 Hz slowing of medium and high amplitude mixed over the bilateral frontal regions. (**b**) The EEG of stage II of sleep showed the scattered sharp waves over the right sphenoidal electrode, and sharp-and-wave complexes of low amplitude were seen over the right temporal region

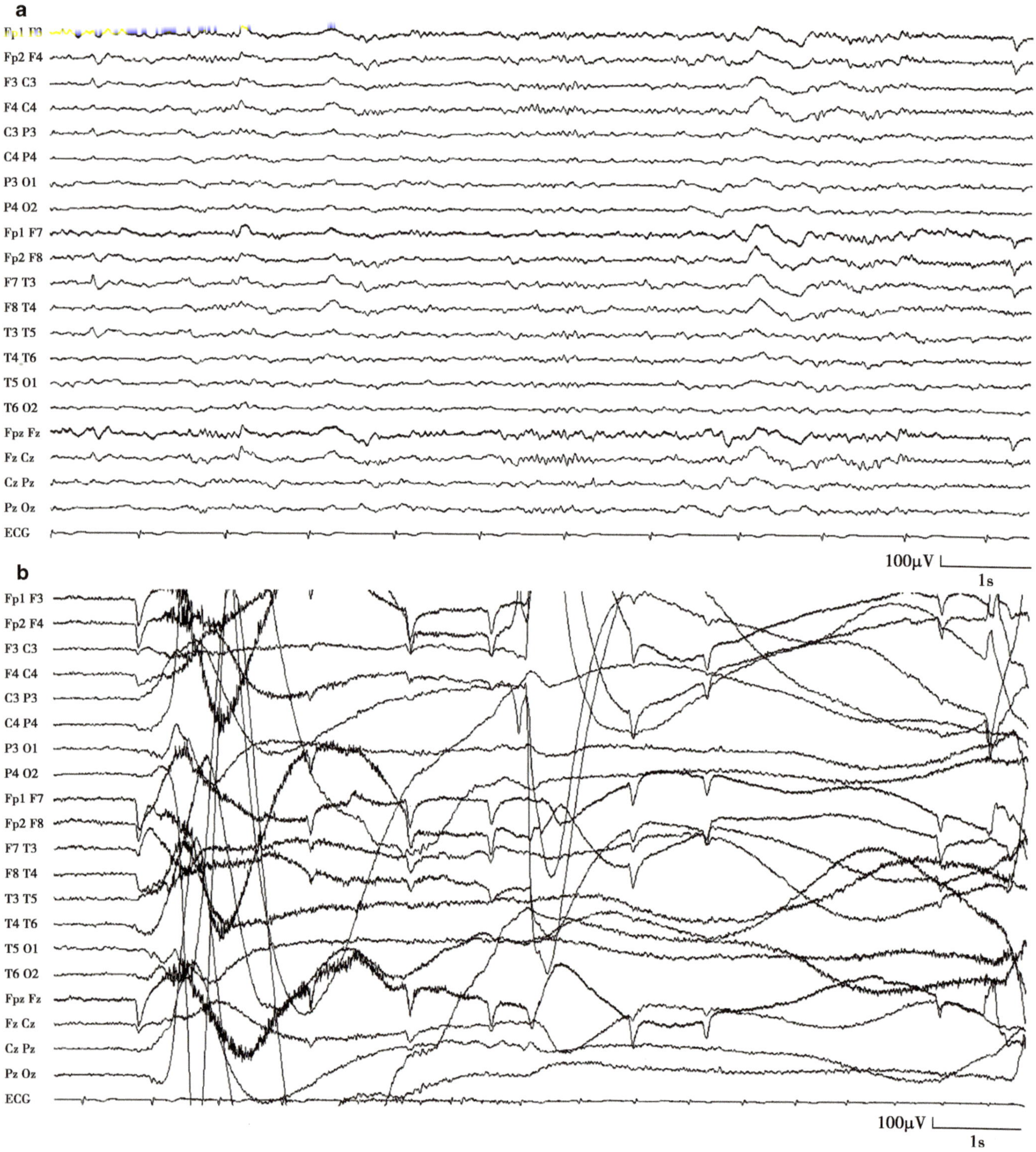

Fig. 2.26 Ictal scalp EEG. (**a**) The patient was asleep before the seizure. The EEG was presented the background of stage II of sleep. (**b**) The patient opened his eyes after awaking. The EEG showed α suppression when the patient was awake. (**c**) During the seizure, the patient placed his hands on his forehead, held his breath, and made a forceful "um" sound in his throat for about 8 s, then sat up from the bed, chewed, pulled the electrode wire with his right hand, and looked backward with his head turned to the right for about 10 s. Numerous EMG artifacts were mixed. (**d**) During the seizure, the patient placed his hands on the upper part of the orbits, held his breath, and made a forceful "um" sound in his throat for about 8 s, then sat up from the bed, chewed, pulled the electrode wire with his right hand, and looked backward with his head turned to the right for about 10 s. Numerous EMG artifacts could be found. (**e**) At the end of the seizure, the patient lay down again. The EEG showed that each lead had low amplitude activity with EMG and electrode artifacts, which lasted about 15 s before the background was recovered

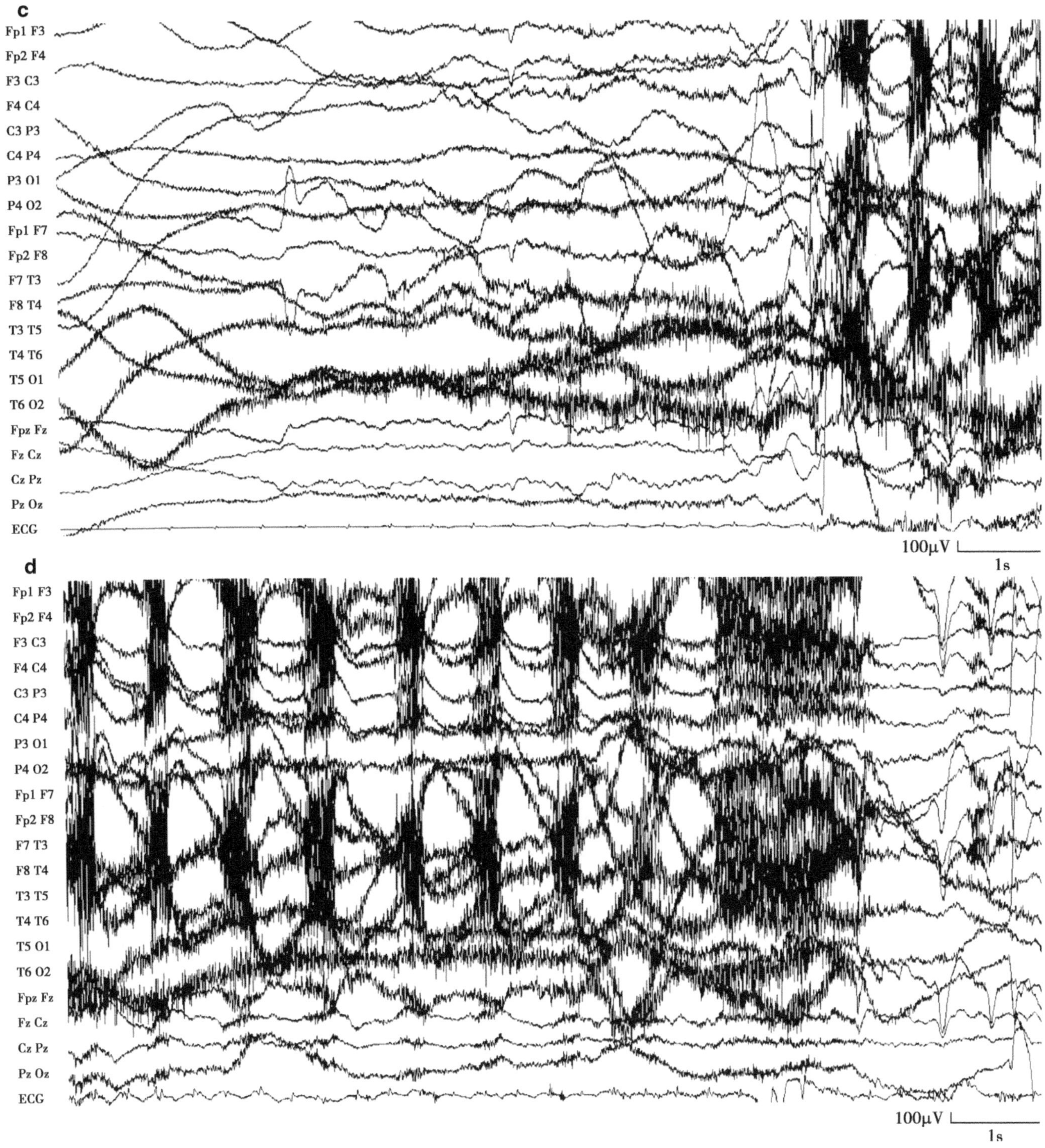

Fig. 2.26 (continued)

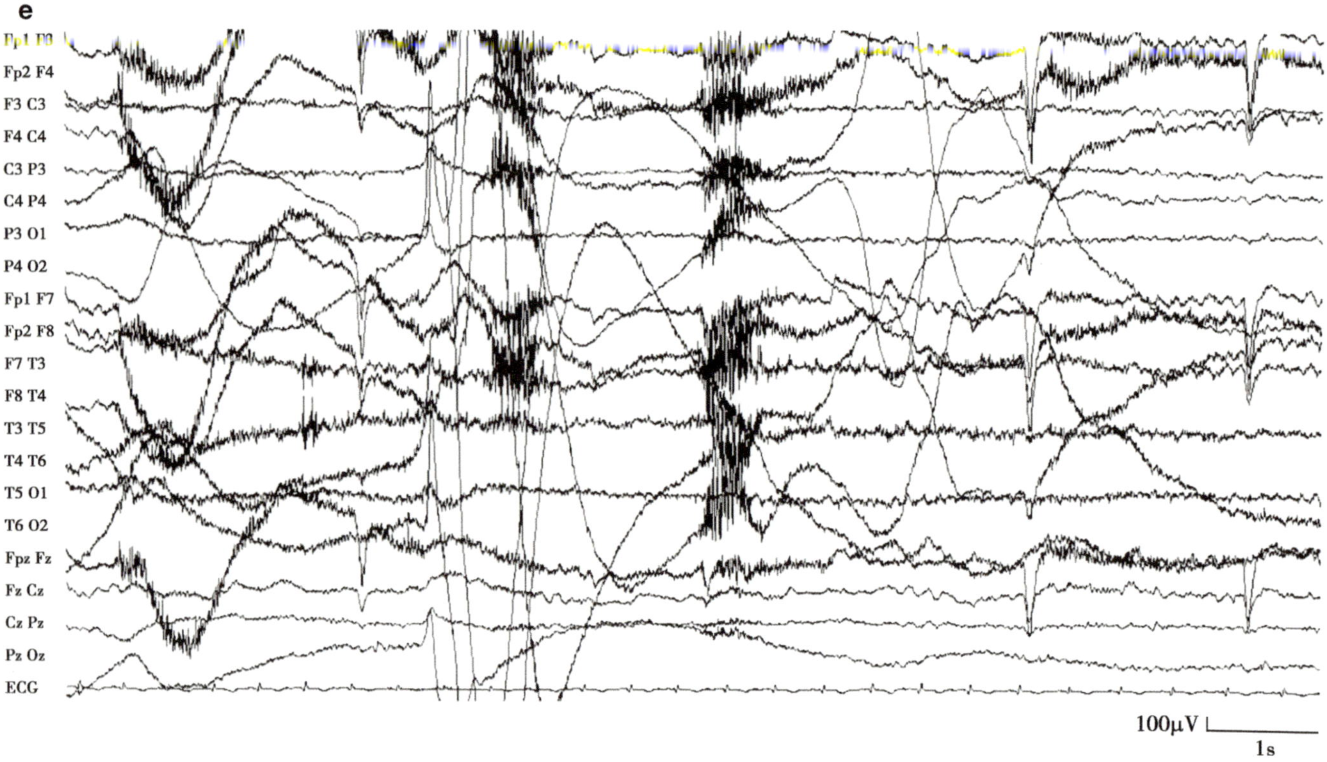

Fig. 2.26 (continued)

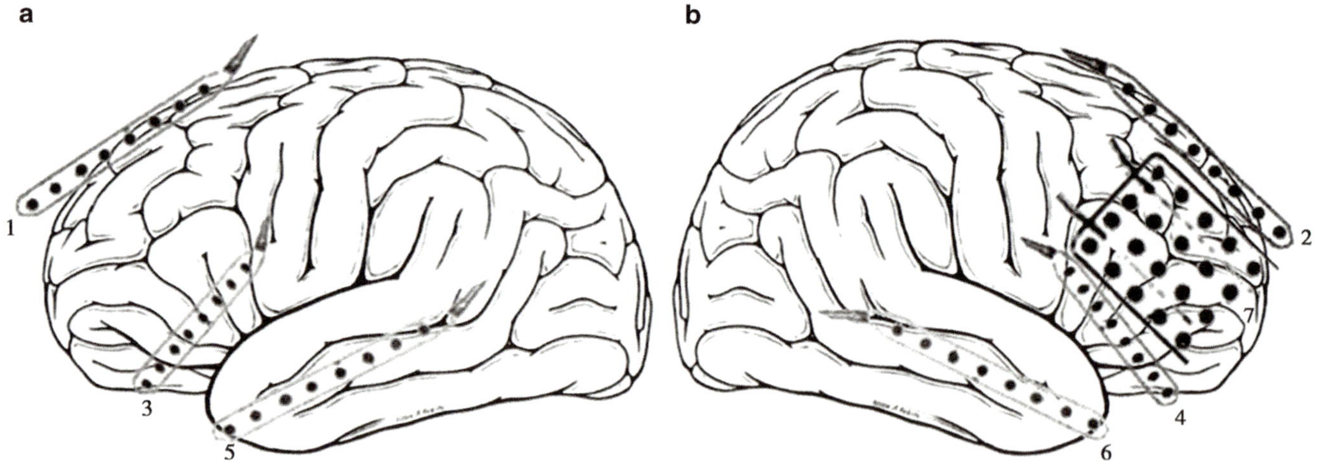

Fig. 2.27 Scheme of intracranial electrodes. (**a**) Strip electrode 1: the left medial frontal cortex (8 contacts). Strip electrode 3: the left orbitofrontal region (8 contacts); Strip electrode 5: the left temporal pole (8 contacts). (**b**) Strip electrode 2: the right medial frontal fissure (8 contacts); Strip electrode 4: the right orbitofrontal region (8 contacts); Strip electrode 6: the right temporal pole (8 contacts); Grid electrode 7: the right frontal convex (20 contacts)

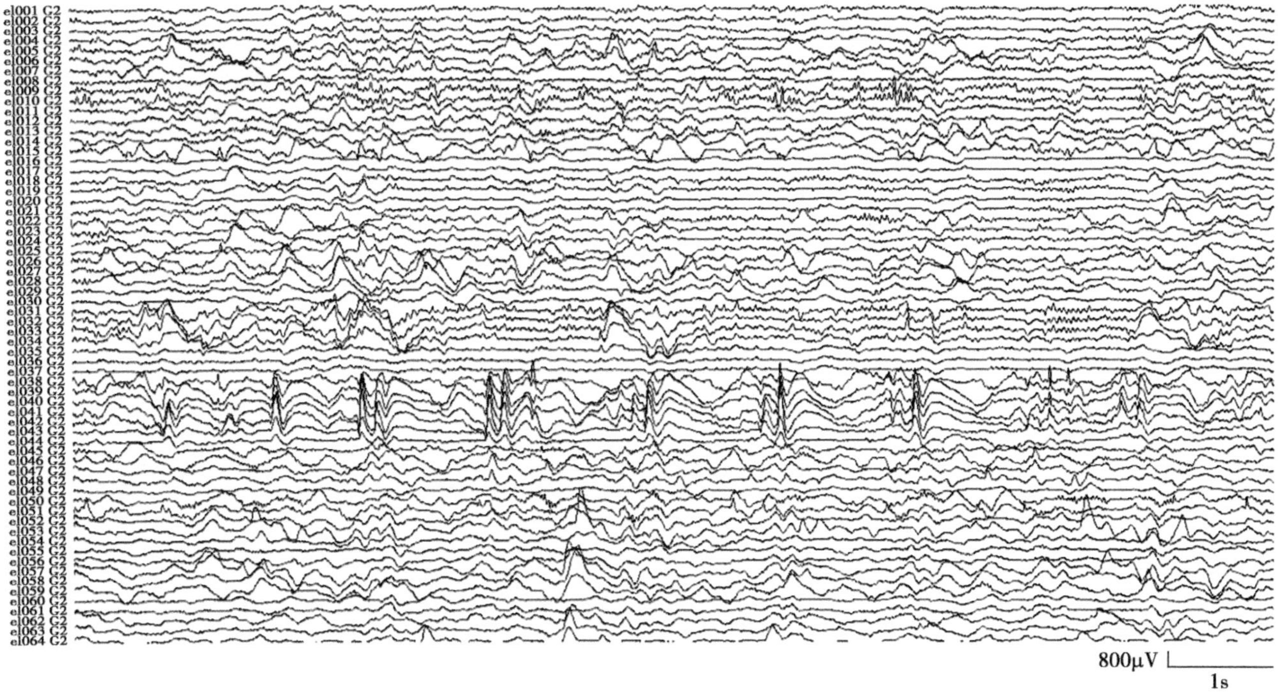

Fig. 2.28 Interictal intracranial EEG
The sleep EEG showed many rhythmic slow waves of medium amplitude over the bilateral medial frontal cortex (contact numbers el05, el06, el07, el013, el014, el015, el018, el022, el026, el027, el028) and the orbitofrontal region (contact numbers el018, el022, el026, el027, el028), among which the electrode of the right medial cortex (contact number el015) was mixed with a few sharp waves of low and medium amplitude; showed paroxysmal spikes of extremely high amplitude over the right temporal region (contact numbers el038, el039, el040, el041, el042, el043), and the synchronous sharp waves of medium and high amplitude over the left temporal region (contact numbers el031, el032, el033, el034); showed low amplitude fast activity over the right middle and inferior frontal gyrus (contact numbers el045, el046, el050, el051), among which sharp waves were emitted over the middle frontal gyrus (contact numbers el050 and el051); and showed slow waves of medium and high amplitude over the middle and posterior part of the frontal region (contact numbers el047, el048, el049, el052, el053, el054, el057, el058, el059, el062, el063, el064)

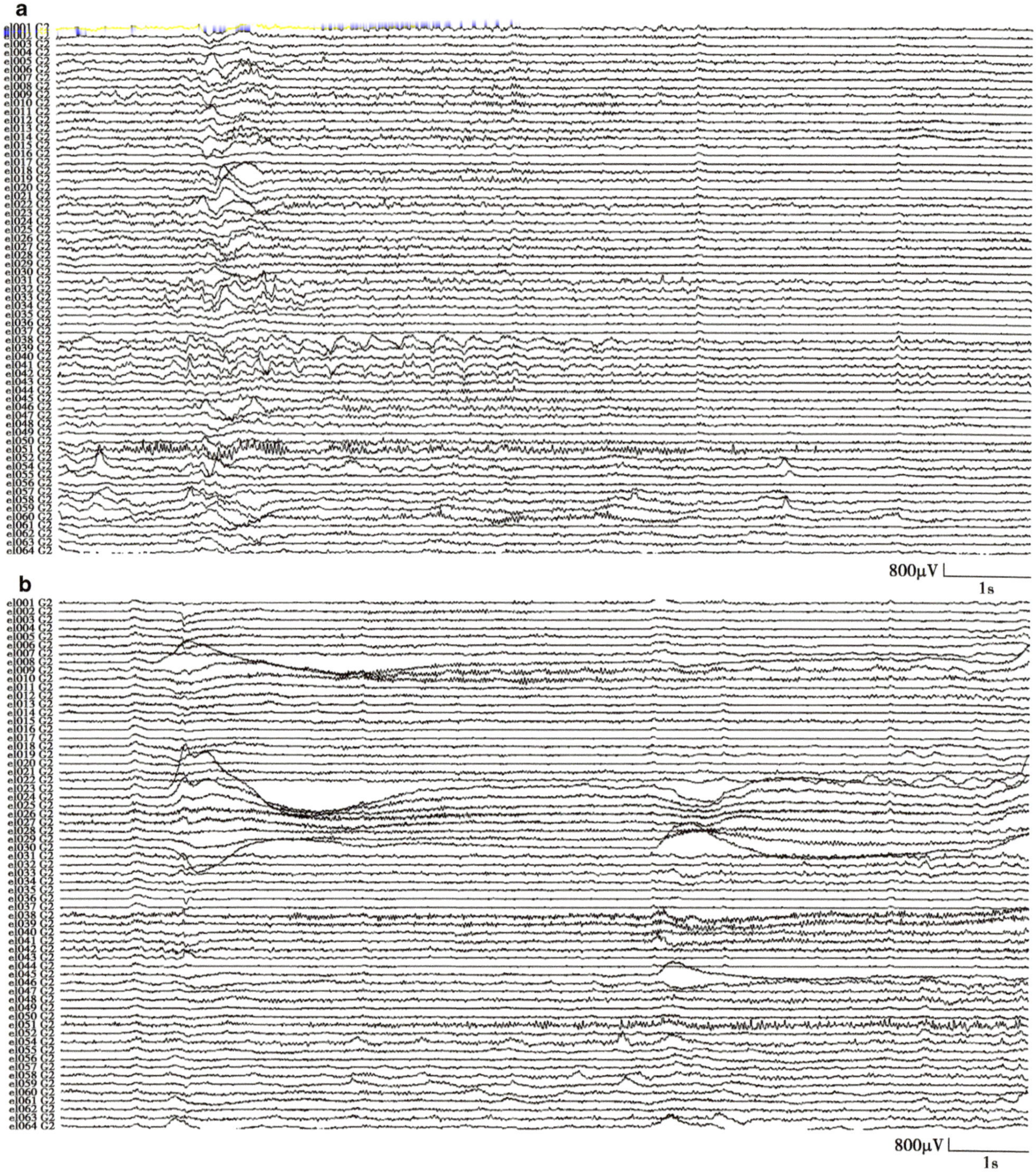

Fig. 2.29 Ictal intracranial EEG. (**a**) The patient was asleep before the seizure. The IEEG showed the low amplitude fast activity over the right medial frontal cortex (contact numbers el012, el013, el014), the right orbitofrontal region (contact numbers el026 and el027), and the mid-anterior part of the right frontal convex (contact numbers el045, el046, el050, el051, el058, el059, el060), especially at the electrode over the middle and superior frontal gyrus (contact number el051), manifested as abnormally early appearance of waves of high amplitude; it also showed the low amplitude fast activity following the rhythm of slowing over the right temporal pole (contact numbers el038, el039, el040, el041, el042). (**b**) During the seizure, the patient opened eyes and stared, pursing his lips while making an "um" sound in his throat forcefully. The IEEG showed the low amplitude persistent fast activity over the right electrodes, especially over the right medial frontal cortex (contact numbers el08, el09, el010), the right orbitofrontal region (contact numbers el025, el026, el027, el028), the right temporal pole (contact numbers el038, el039), and the right middle and inferior frontal gyrus (contact number el051). (**c**) The patient still vocalized and sighed after about 10 s, then chewed, kicked with both lower limbs, and grasped the quilt with both hands. IEEG still showed the low amplitude persistent fast activity over the bilateral medial frontal cortex (contact numbers el03, el04, el05, el09, el010, el011), the right orbitofrontal region (contact numbers el025, el026, el027, el028), the right temporal pole (contact numbers el038, el039, el040, el041, el042) and right frontal region (contact numbers el046, el047, el048, el052, el053, el058, el059, el062, el063), and showed rhythmic spikes of high amplitude over the anterior part of the right middle and inferior frontal gyrus (contact numbers el046 and el051). (**d**) The patient's seizure ended. The IEEG recovered the background

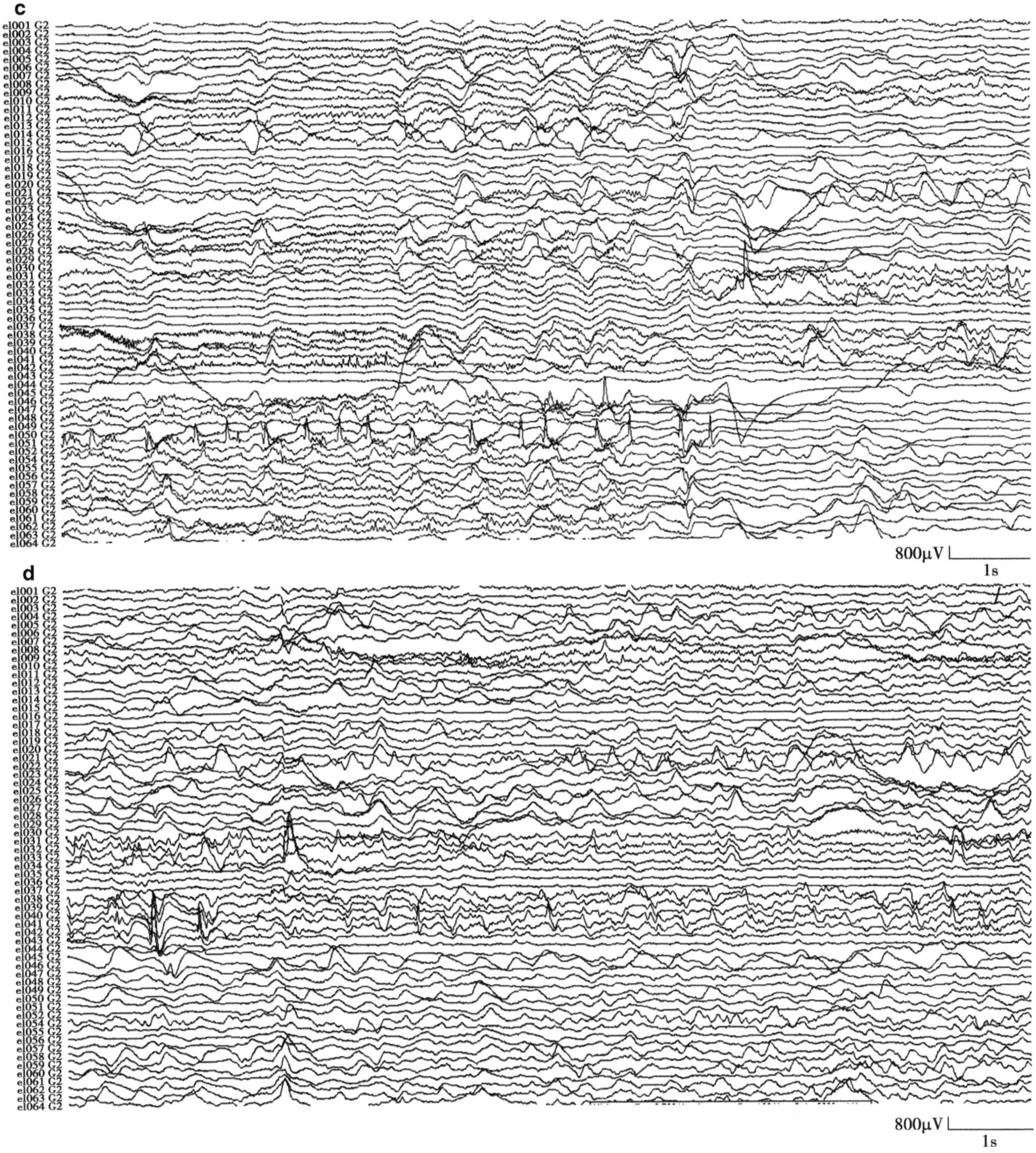

Fig. 2.29 (continued)

Case 2.7 Middle and Inferior Frontal Gyrus Epilepsy

[Abstract of Medical Records]
Male, 9 years old.

1. *Chief complaint* Episodic impairment of consciousness with limb twitching for 7 months.
2. *History of present illness* The patient started showing the absence of mind and giggles 7 months ago out of no apparent predisposition, with his right upper limb twitching. Since then the seizures repeated in the pattern of absence of mind, giggles, and twitching of the right upper and lower limbs and even the four limbs. Sometimes he would shout with panic and fumble with both upper limbs, which resolved in less than 1 min. There was no apparent aura. The seizures usually occurred during the day and night up to 20 times a day. He is now orally taking carbamazepine 400 mg/dose b.i.d, lamotrigine 25 mg/dose b.i.d, and topiramate 25 mg/dose b.i.d. The effect was poor.
3. *Past history* The patient was delivered at full term, with normal motor, language, and intellectual development.
4. *Personal and family history* No history of associated diseases.
5. *Physical examination* No neurological abnormalities were found.
6. *Imaging examination* MRI showed no specific abnormal changes.
7. *EEG* For details, see Figs. 2.30, 2.31, 2.32, 2.33, and 2.34.

[Case Review]

1. Case Characteristics
   (a) Seizure characteristics ① The seizure was manifested by absence of mind, giggles, and twitching of the right upper and lower limbs. ② There was no aura. ③ The patient sometimes shouted with panic and fumbled with both upper limbs. ④ The seizures occurred during the day and night. ⑤ Clustered seizures (up to more than 20 times a day). The seizure characteristics above were consistent with those of frontal lobe epilepsy.
   (b) *EEG characteristics* ① Interictal EEG showed spikes over the left frontal region. ② Ictal EEG showed the rhythm of spikes over the left frontal region, frontal midline, and left anterior temporal region, and showed the phase reversal at F7.
   (c) *Imaging characteristics* MRI showed no specific abnormal changes.

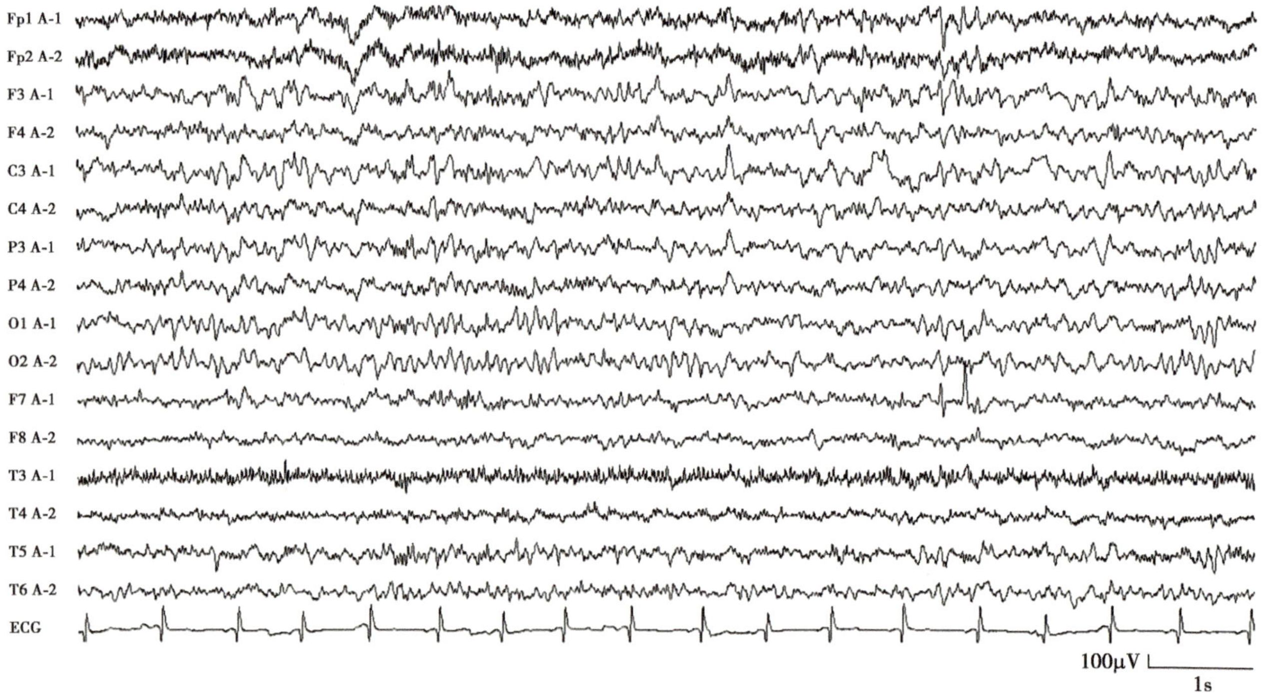

Fig. 2.30 Interictal scalp EEG
The EEG had a background occipital rhythm of 10.0 Hz and showed a few 4.0–5.0 Hz slow waves of medium and high amplitude mixed over the left frontal region (F3) and the central region (C3), and the of scattered spikes was seen over the left frontal region (F3) and anterior temporal region (F7)

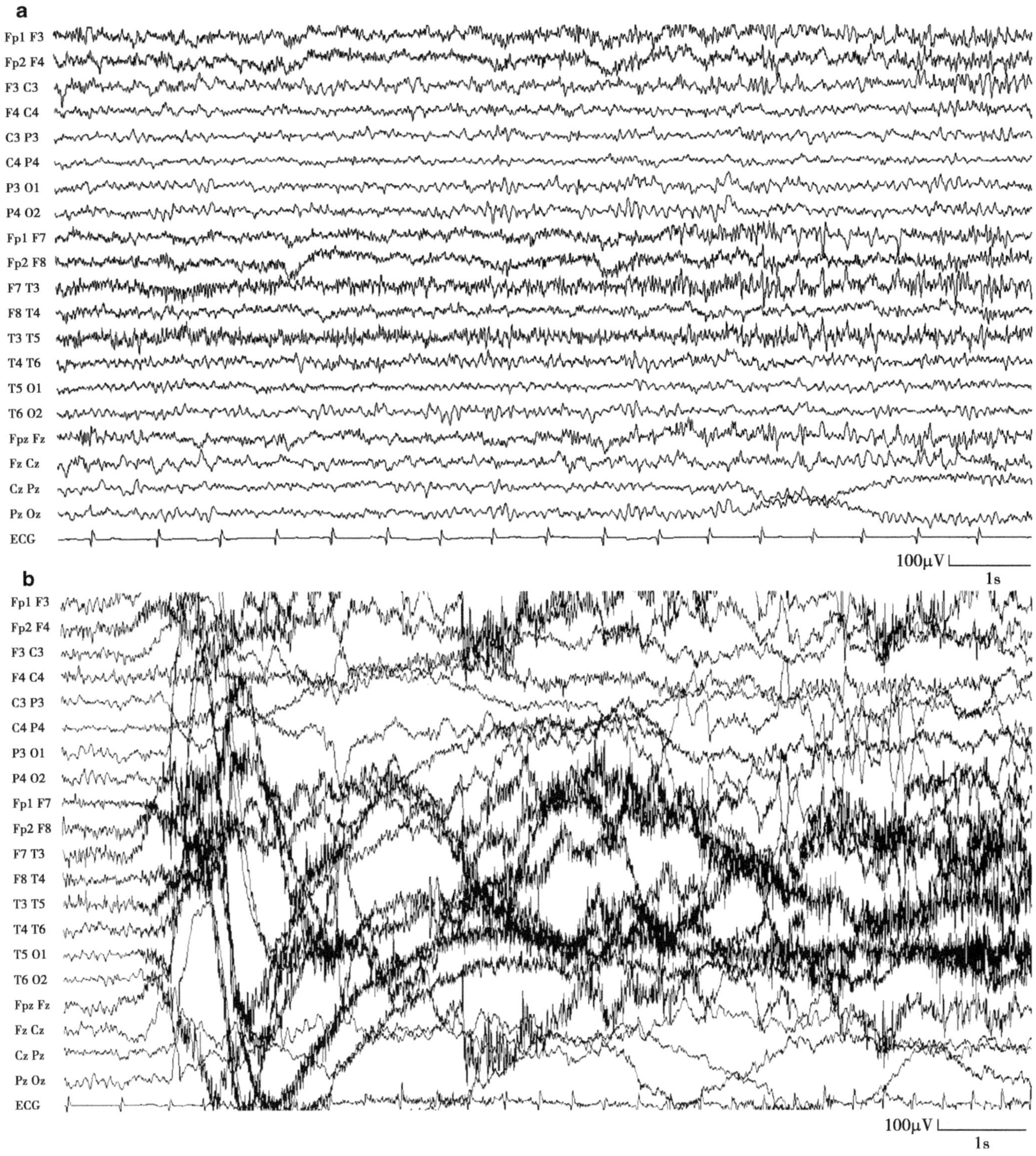

Fig. 2.31 Ictal scalp EEG. (**a**) The patient was awake and supine with eyes closed before the seizure. Three second before the seizure, in addition to the waves shown on the EEG when the patient was awake, the EEG showed the short-term rhythm of spikes over the left frontal region (Fp1 F3, F3 C3), frontal midline (Fpz Fz), left frontal region, anterior temporal region (Fp1 F7, F7 T3), and showed phase reversal over left anterior temporal region (F7). (**b**) During the seizure, the patient suddenly opened his eyes, raised his head and tried to sit up, while patting his abdomen with both hands for several times and then grasping his clothes. Electrode and EMG artifacts were observed. (**c**) The patient tried to sit up by raising his head. The EEG was the same as **b**. (**d**) At the end of the seizure, the patient lay down again. The EEG showed sharply contoured slow waves of high amplitude over the bilateral frontal regions (Fp1 F3, Fp2 F4, Fp1 F7, Fp2 F8) and frontal midline (Fpz Fz, Fz Cz)

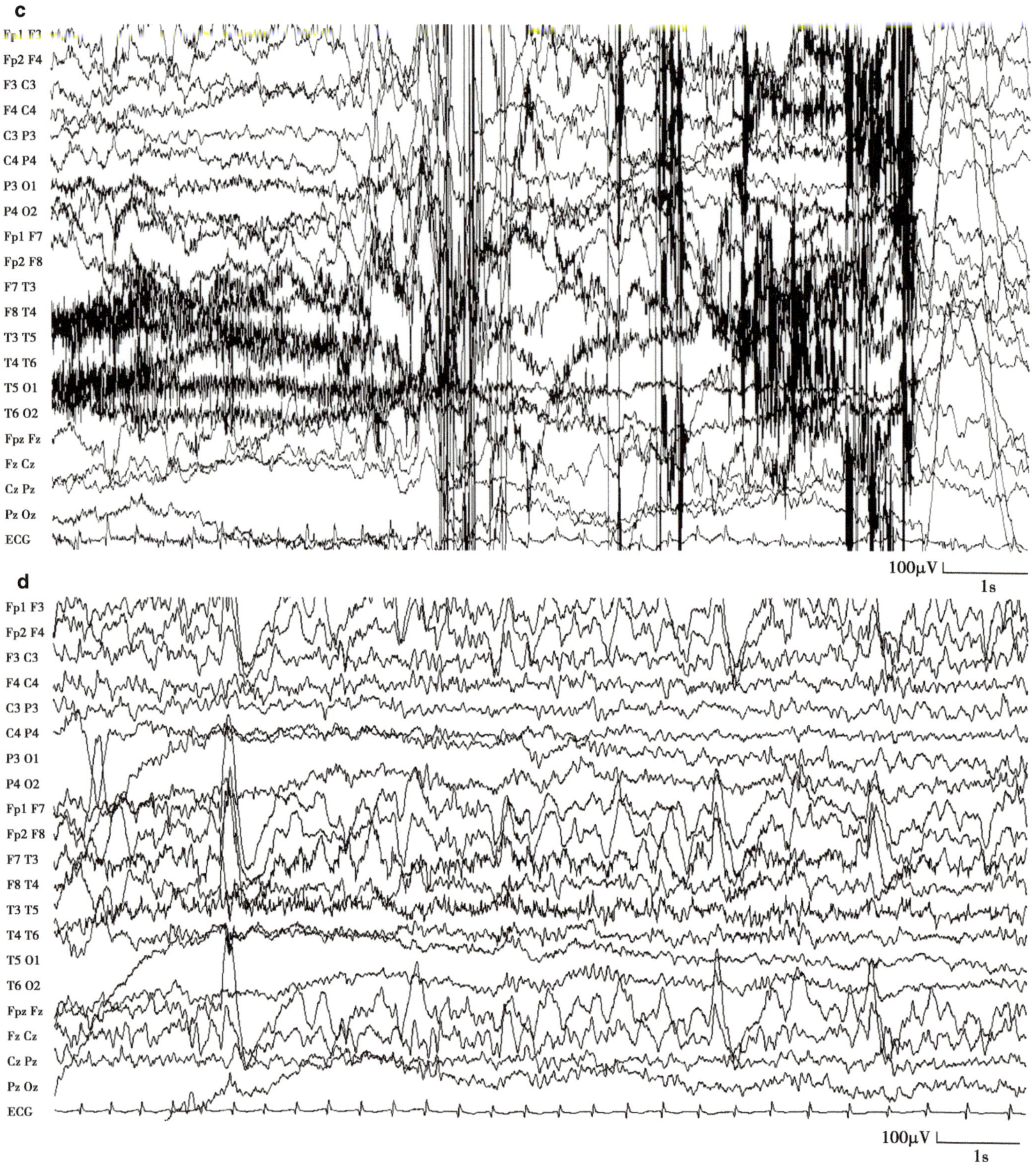

Fig. 2.31 (continued)

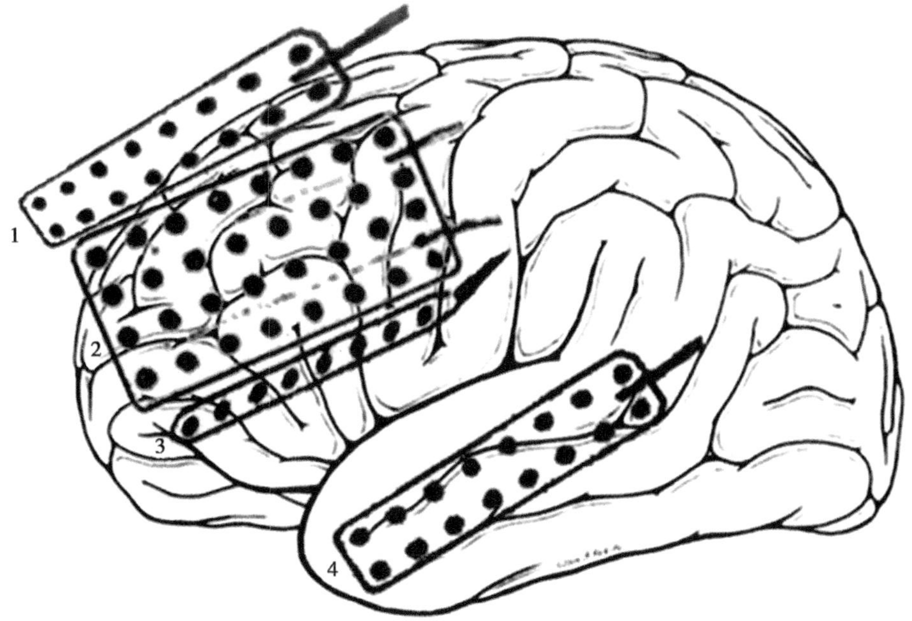

Fig. 2.32 Scheme of intracranial electrodes Grid electrode 1: the left superior frontal gyrus to medial frontal cortex (16 contacts); Grid electrode 2: the left middle and inferior frontal gyrus (32 contacts); Strip electrode 3: the left orbitofrontal region (8 contacts); Grid electrode 4: the left temporal region (16 contacts)

2. *Diagnosis and treatment strategy and follow-up results*
   The patient's semiology included the twitching of right upper and lower limbs with panic, sometimes with shouting and fumbling of both upper limbs. The ictal EEG showed the rhythm of spikes over the left frontal region, frontal midline, and left anterior temporal region. The MRI showed no suggestive information. In combination with the information, the focus was located at the left side. In addition, the seizure origin was considered to be located over the frontal lobe based on the semiology, especially over the medial frontal cortex or orbitofrontal region. However, the left temporal region could not be completely excluded. Intracranial electrodes were hence implanted over the left frontal and temporal regions. The interictal IEEG showed significantly abnormal discharges over the left middle and inferior frontal gyrus and the orbitofrontal region; the ictal IEEG examination confirmed that the origin was located over the left middle and inferior frontal gyrus and the orbitofrontal region. The left middle and inferior frontal gyrus were resected surgically. After the surgery, the patient was seizure-free during a 4-year follow-up. The sites of epileptic foci of the patient were identified, and the epileptic foci were completely resected surgically, contributing to a satisfactory postoperative outcome.

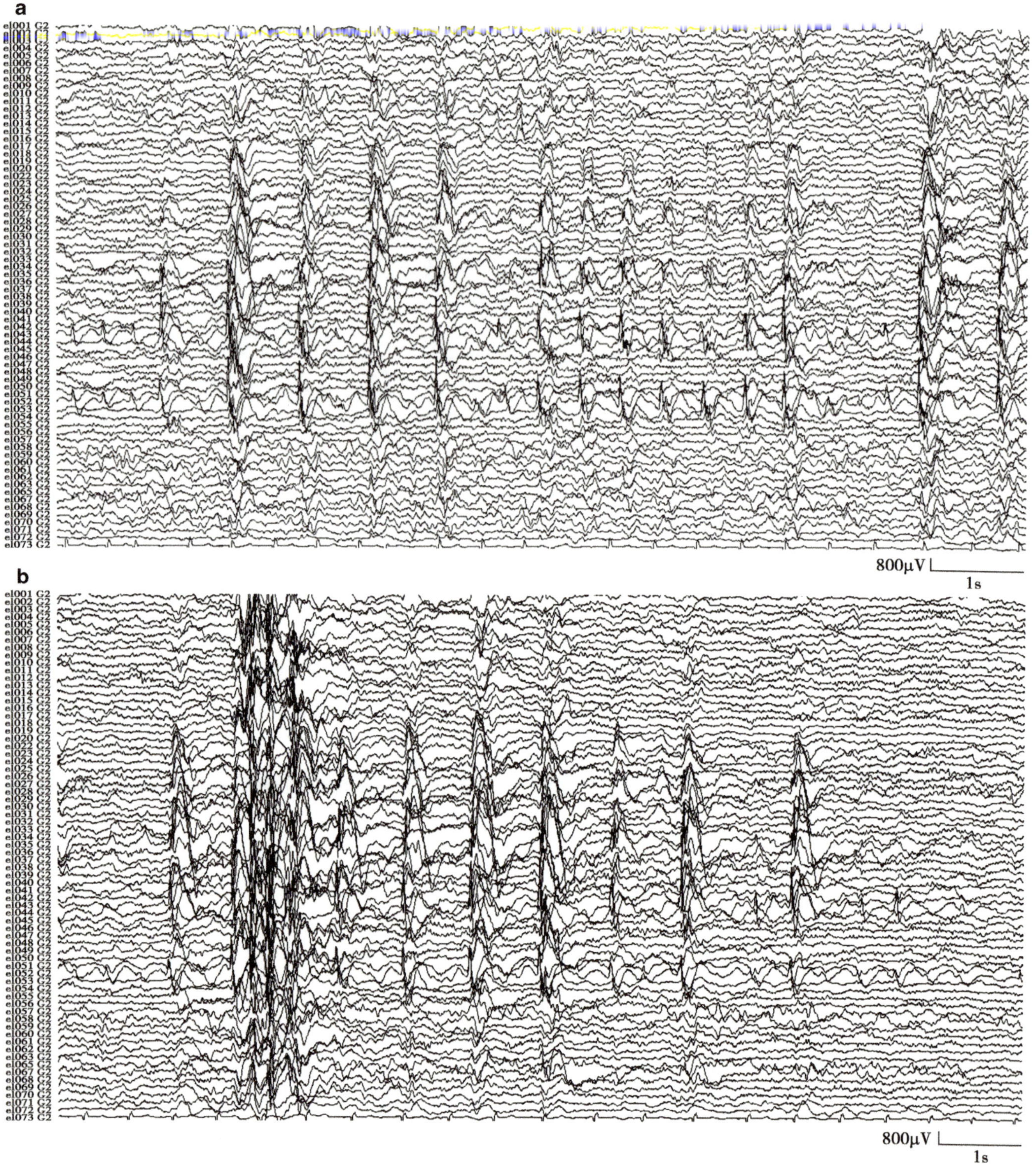

Fig. 2.33 Interictal intracranial EEG. (**a**) The EEG showed rhythmic spike-and-wave complexes over the left middle and inferior frontal gyrus (contact numbers el017, el018, el019, el020, el025, el026, el027, el034, el035, el042, el043, el044) and over the orbitofrontal region (contact numbers el051, el052, el053). (**b**) The EEG showed polyspike-and-wave complexes and spike-and-wave complexes extensively over the left frontal and temporal regions, sometimes bursting, especially over the left middle and inferior frontal gyrus (contact numbers el020, el022, el023, el033, el034, el035, el036, el041, el042, el043, el044) and the orbitofrontal region (contact numbers el051, el052). The discharges spread to the left temporal region (contact numbers el057, el058, el059, el060, el061, el062, el063, el067, el068, el069)

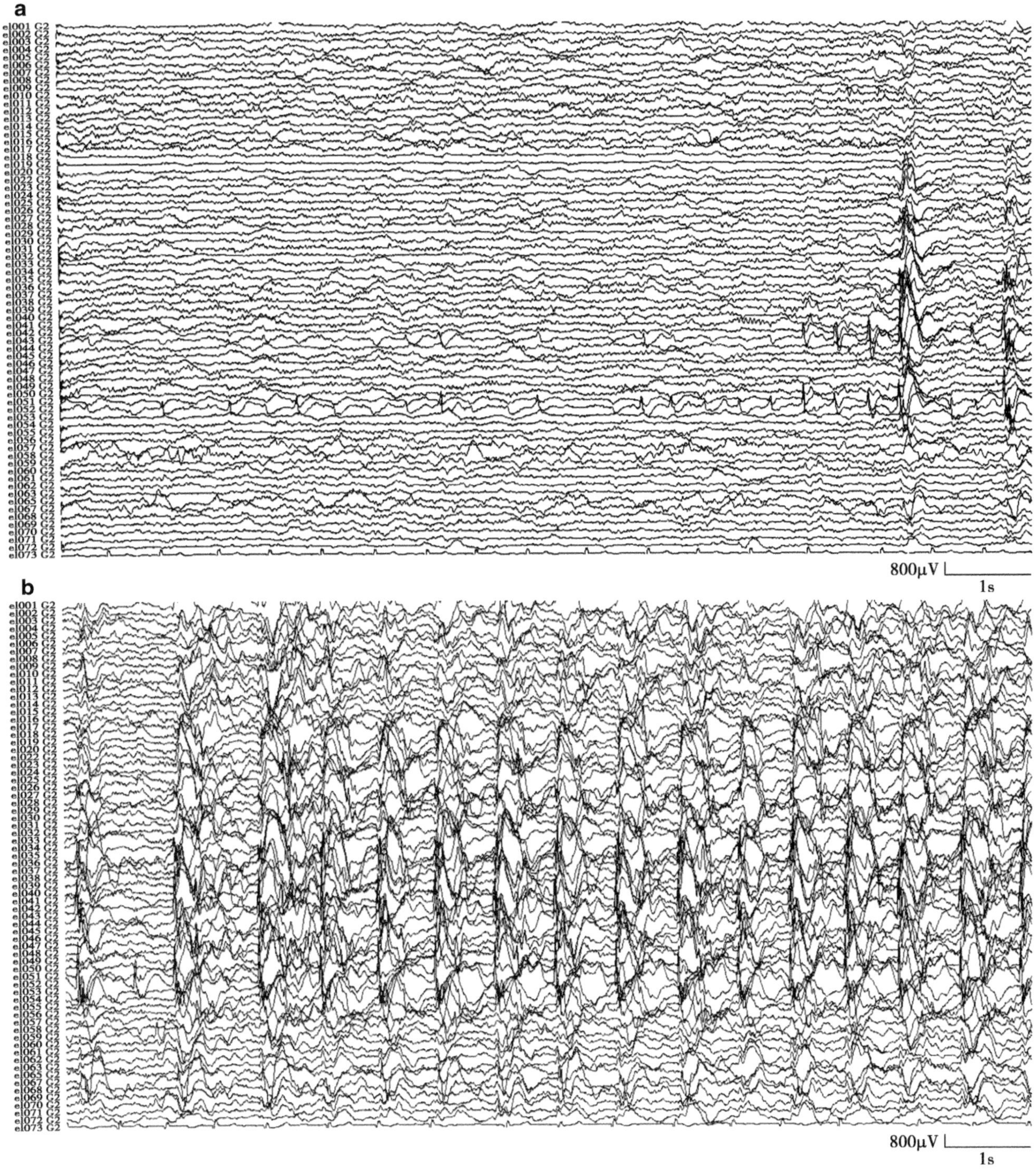

Fig. 2.34 Ictal EEG of intracranial electrodes. (**a**) The patient was conscious and supine with eyes closed before the seizure. The IEEG showed rhythmic spikes over the left orbitofrontal region (contact numbers el051 and el052) and inferior frontal gyrus (contact number el043), followed by the extensive rhythm of spike-and-wave complexes over the left frontal region. (**b**, **c**) The patient was conscious and supine with eyes closed before the seizure. The IEEG showed rhythmic spikes over the left orbitofrontal region (contact numbers el051 and el052) and inferior frontal gyrus (contact number el043), followed by the extensive rhythm of spike-and-wave complexes over the left frontal region. (**d**) The patient suddenly sat up during the seizure, grunted in his mouth, and started to fumbling for the sheet after tapping his hands several times. The IEEG showed the rhythm of spikes over the left orbitofrontal region (contact numbers el050, el051, el052), inferior frontal gyrus (contact numbers el042, el043), and temporal region (contact number el067), with the amplitude gradually increasing and discharges extending to the middle and superior frontal gyrus (contact numbers el011, el025, el026, el027, el033, el034, el035, el036). (**e**) The patient stopped fumbling with both hands, turned his head to the left side from time to time, and failed to answer questions. The IEEG showed the rhythm of spike-and-wave complexes of extremely high amplitude over the left frontal region. (**f**) The patient's seizure ended. The rhythm of slow waves was observed on the IEEG, which lasted relatively longer

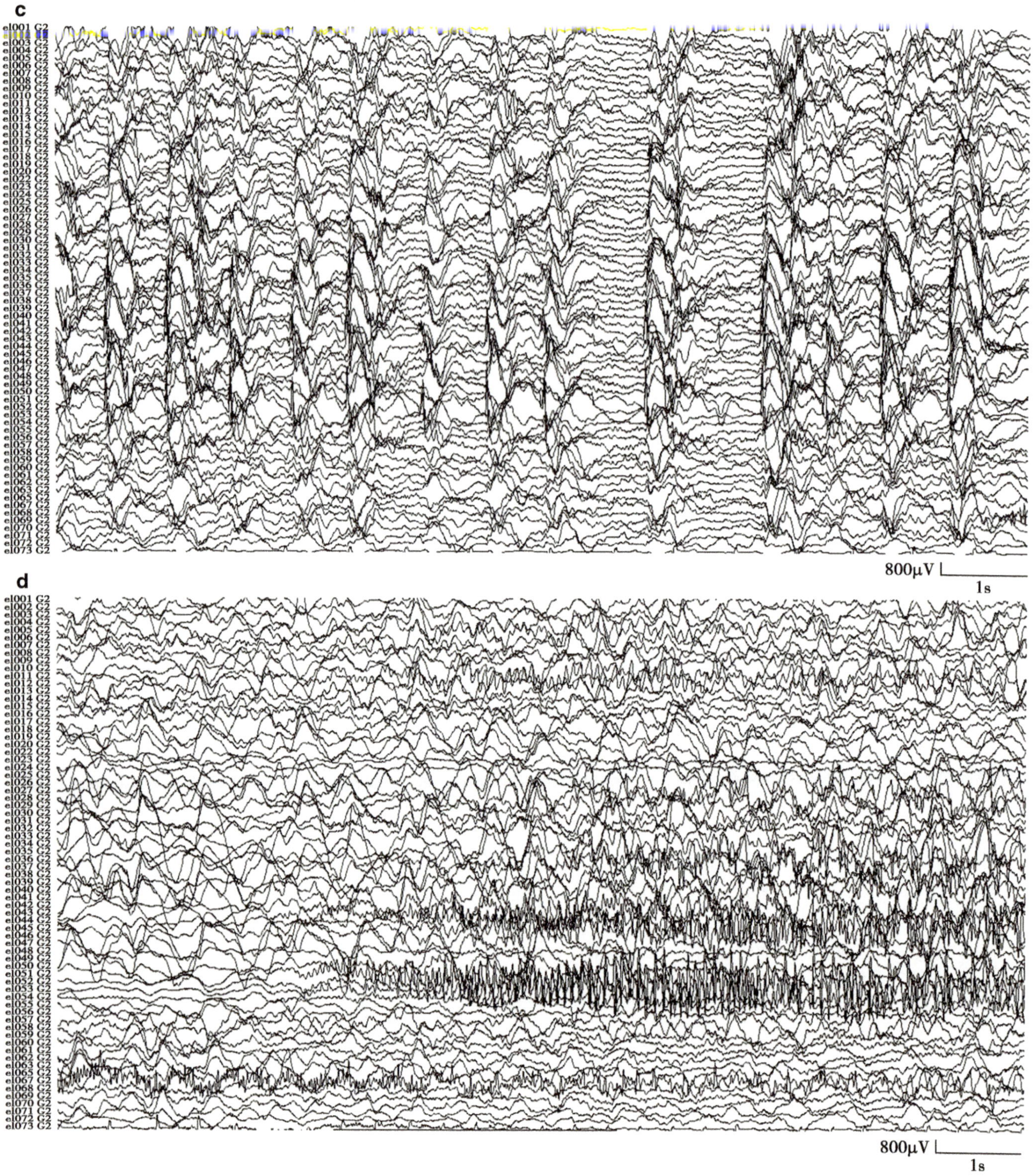

Fig. 2.34 (continued)

e

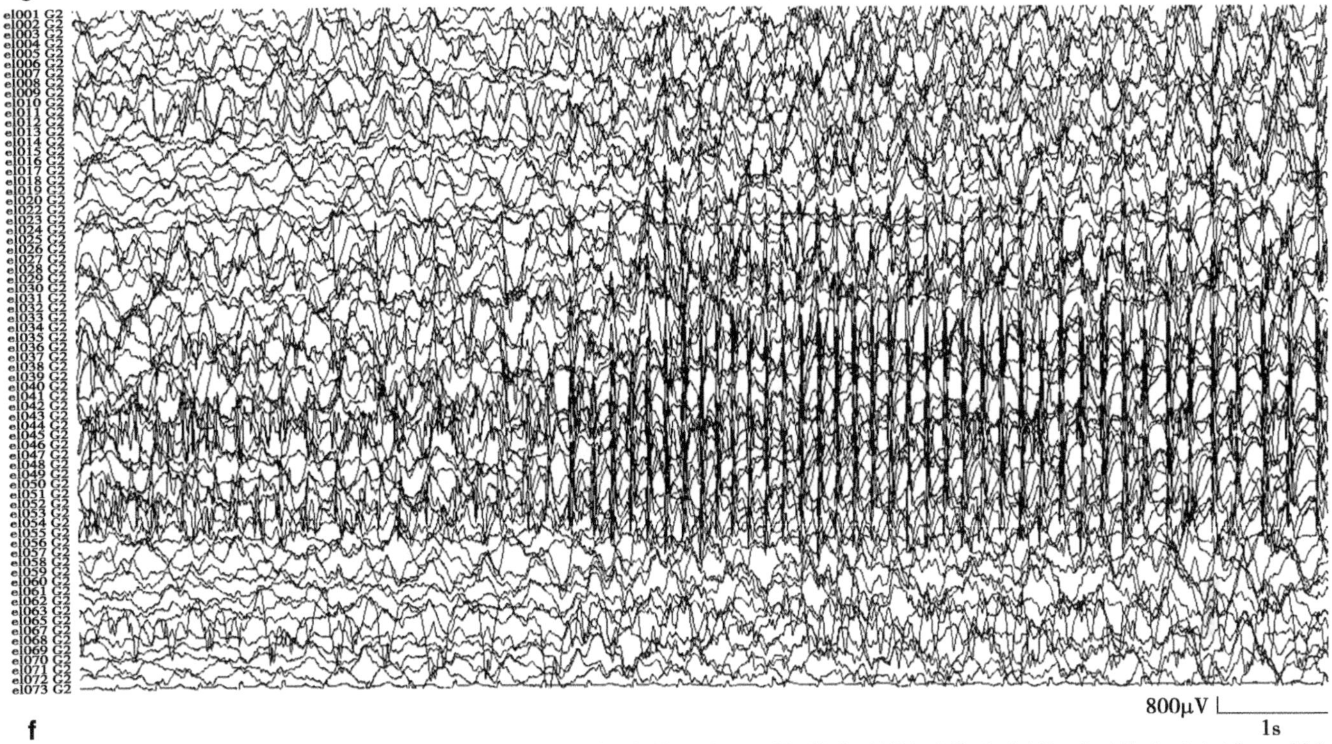

f

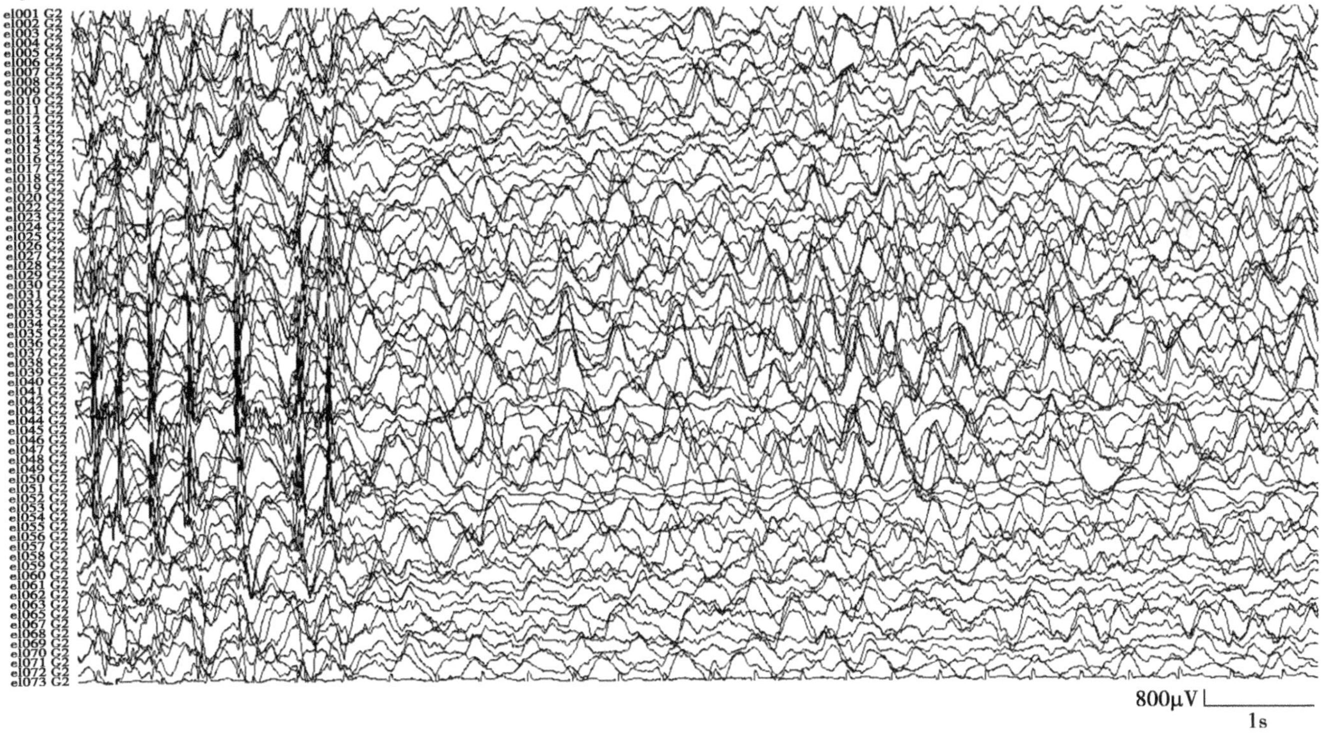

Fig. 2.34 (continued)

Case 2.8 Posterior Inferior Frontal Gyrus Epilepsy

[Abstract of Medical Records]
Female, 6 years old.

1. *Chief complaint* Paroxysmal left eyelid twitching for 3 years.
2. *History of present illness* The patient developed involuntary left eyelid twitching and clonus when playing 3 years ago without obvious predisposition, which resolved after tens of seconds. Since then the seizures repeated every day, and the symptoms gradually developed into the simultaneous twitching of left eyelid and mouth. Before the seizure, there was an aura of pain of left eye. After the seizure, she could recall the whole process, but failed to answer questions during the seizure, which lasted for more than 10 s to tens of seconds and occurred during the day and night. She experienced "grand mal" twice due to fever, which were characterized by tonic twitching of the limbs and resolved after about 2 min, the details of which are not known. No similar seizures occurred afterward. She was diagnosed as epilepsy. The treatment with carbamazepine, sodium valproate, and topiramate failed to completely control the seizures. She is now regularly taking 375 mg of oxcarbazepine in the morning and 450 mg in the evening, levetiracetam 500 mg/dose b.i.d., and lamotrigine 100 mg/dose b.i.d. orally. The seizures still occur daily.
3. *Past history* The patient was delivered at full term and had a history of two febrile convulsions.
4. *Personal history* Her development was normal for her age, with fair intelligence. She is now in pre-school.
5. *Physical examination* The movement of finger-to-nose with left hand was less stable and accurate than the opposite side.
6. *Imaging examination* MRI showed no obvious abnormalities.
7. *EEG* For details, see Figs. 2.35, 2.36, 2.37, 2.38, and 2.39.

[Case Review]

1. *Case Characteristics*
   (a) *Seizure characteristics* ① Left eyelid and mouth twitching. ② Aura of left eye pain. ③ No definite loss of consciousness during the seizure.
   (b) *EEG characteristics* ① Interictal EEG showed the scattered spikes of extremely high amplitude over the leads over the right posterior frontal and central cortices. ② Ictal EEG showed irregular θ waves mixed with the low amplitude fast activities over the right parietal, occipital, and posterior temporal regions.
   (c) *Imaging characteristics* MRI showed no obvious abnormal changes.
2. *Diagnosis and treatment strategy and follow-up results* The patient's seizure symptoms were consistent with the suggestive information of the EEG. It was hence considered that the epileptic focus was located over the central area as well as right posterior frontal region. In order to clarify the relationship between the epileptic focus and the sensorimotor cortex, intracranial electrodes were implanted over the central area of right posterior frontal region. The interictal IEEG showed significantly abnormal discharges over the central area and the right posterior frontal region; the ictal IEEG clarified the site of origin. The relationship between motor cortex and epileptic foci was clarified by cortical electrical stimulation. The lower middle part of the central area and the right posterior inferior frontal region were resected surgically. During a 6-month postoperative follow-up, the patient still had seizures, the reason for which was analyzed to be the partial overlap of the epileptic focus with the motor cortex, and the incomplete removal of the epileptic focus by surgery.

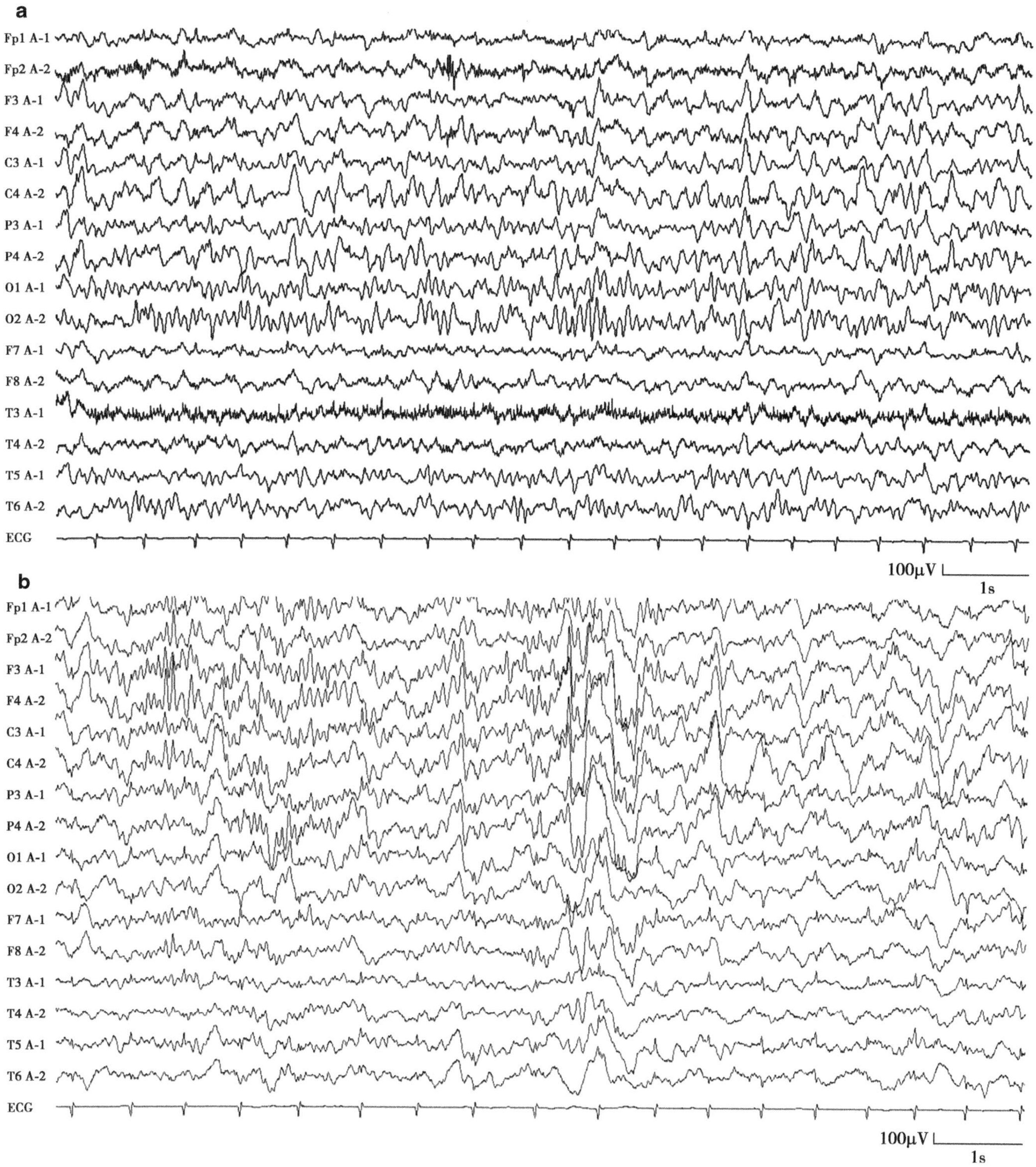

Fig. 2.35 Interictal scalp EEG. (**a**) The EEG had a background occipital rhythm of 9.0 Hz and showed some 4.0–5.0 Hz slow waves of medium and high amplitude mixed over the bilateral posterior frontal regions (F3, F4), the right central region (C4), the parietal region (P4), and the anterior temporal region (F8). (**b**) The EEG was presented as stage II of sleep and showed basically symmetrical bilateral vertex and spindles, and the spikes of extremely high amplitude over the right posterior frontal region (F4), the anterior temporal region (F8), and the central region (C4), which spread to the left parietal region (P4)

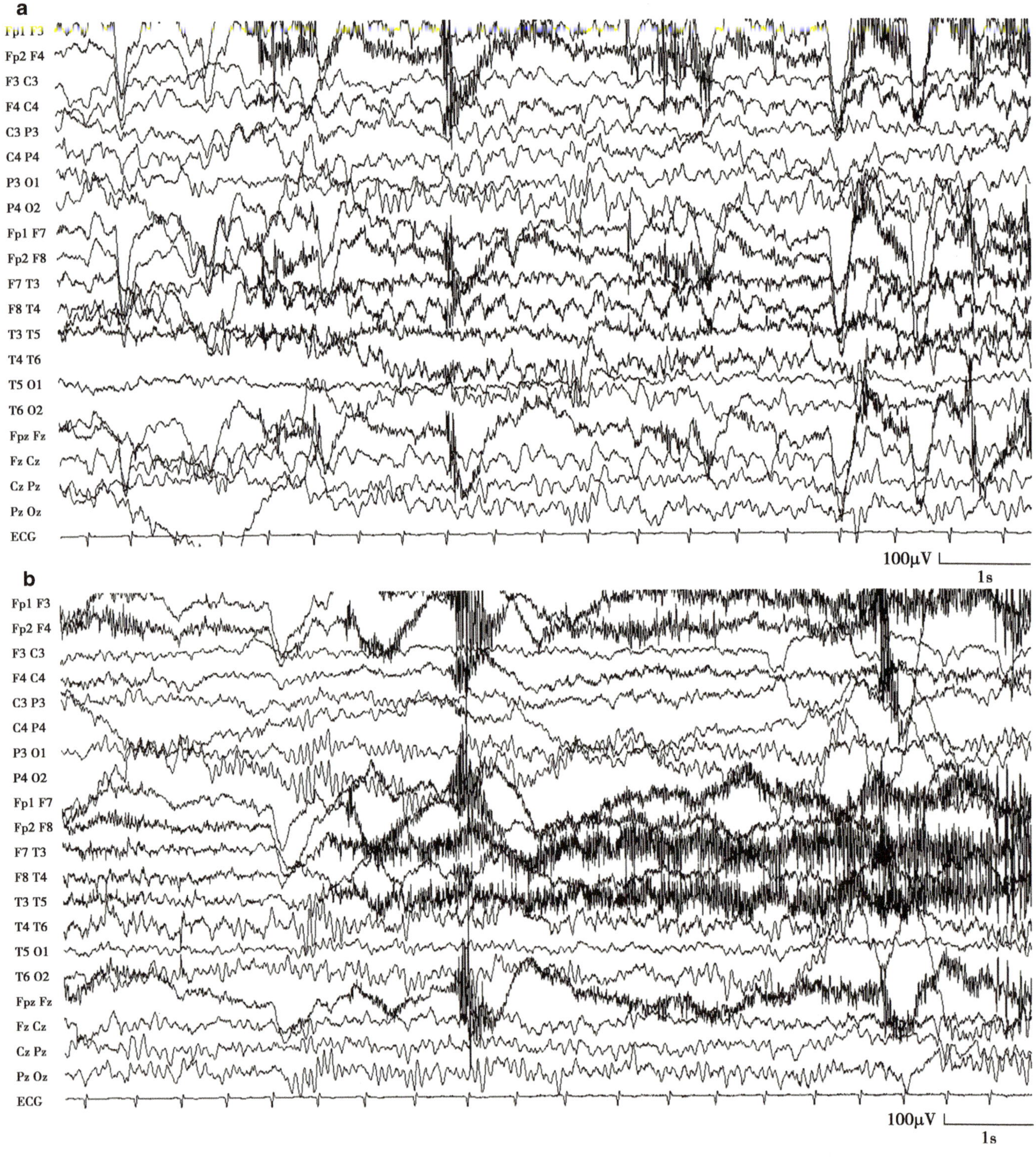

Fig. 2.36 Ictal scalp EEG. (**a**) The patient was lying supine and awake 10 s before the seizure. The EEG had a background occipital rhythm of 8.0 Hz, and showed some EMG artifacts over the bilateral frontal regions (Fp1 F3, Fp2 F4, Fp1 F7, Fp2 F8, Fpz Fz), and many 3.0–4.0 Hz slow waves of medium and high amplitude over the bilateral posterior frontal regions (F3 C3, F4 C4), the central region (C3 P3, C4 P4), and the right temporal region (F8 T4, T4 T6). (**b**) The patient had eyes closed and left mouth twitching during the seizure. The EEG showed irregular θ waves mixed with fast of low amplitude especially over the right parietal and occipital regions (P4 O2) and the posterior temporal region (T4 T6, T6 O2), the frequency and amplitude of which gradually decreased. It also showed numerous EMG artifacts over the bilateral frontal regions (Fp1 F3, Fp2 F4, Fp1 F7, Fp2 F8, Fpz Fz) and the temporal region (F7 T3, F8 T4). (**c**) The patient had persistent left mouth twitching. The EEG showed numerous artifacts over the bilateral frontal regions (Fp1 F3, Fp2 F4, Fp1 F7, Fp2 F8, Fpz Fz) and the temporal region (F7 T3, F8 T4, T3 T5, T4 T6). (**d**) The patient had intermittent left mouth twitching, and the limbs remained over the pre-ictal position. The EEG presentation was the basically same as **c**. (**e**) When the twitching gradually stopped, the patient opened her eyes. The EEG recovered to the background EEG with a few electrode wobble artifacts and EMG artifacts. (**f**) At the end of the seizure, the patient's limbs resumed locomotor. The EEG presentation was the same as **e**

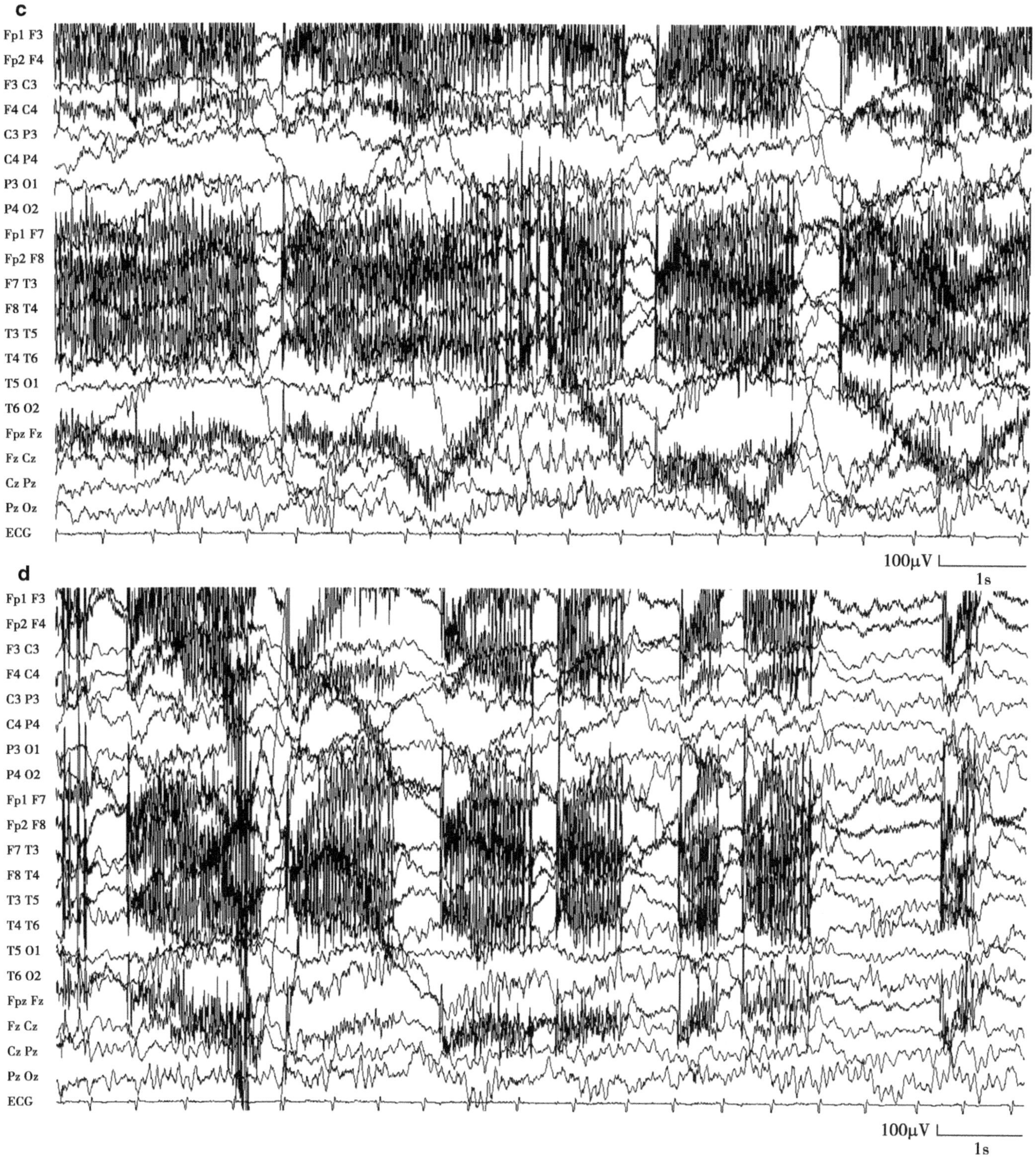

Fig. 2.36 (continued)

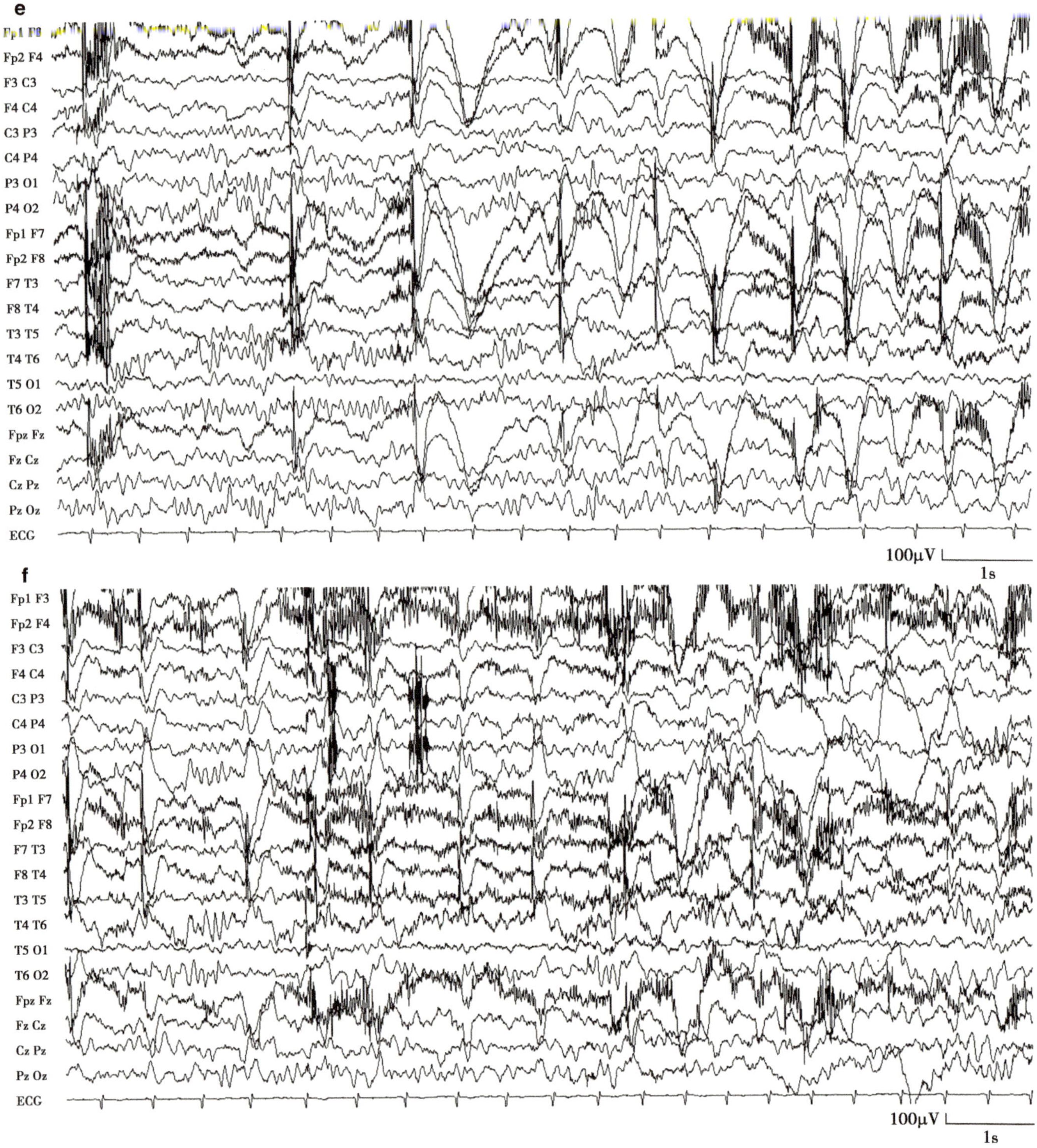

Fig. 2.36 (continued)

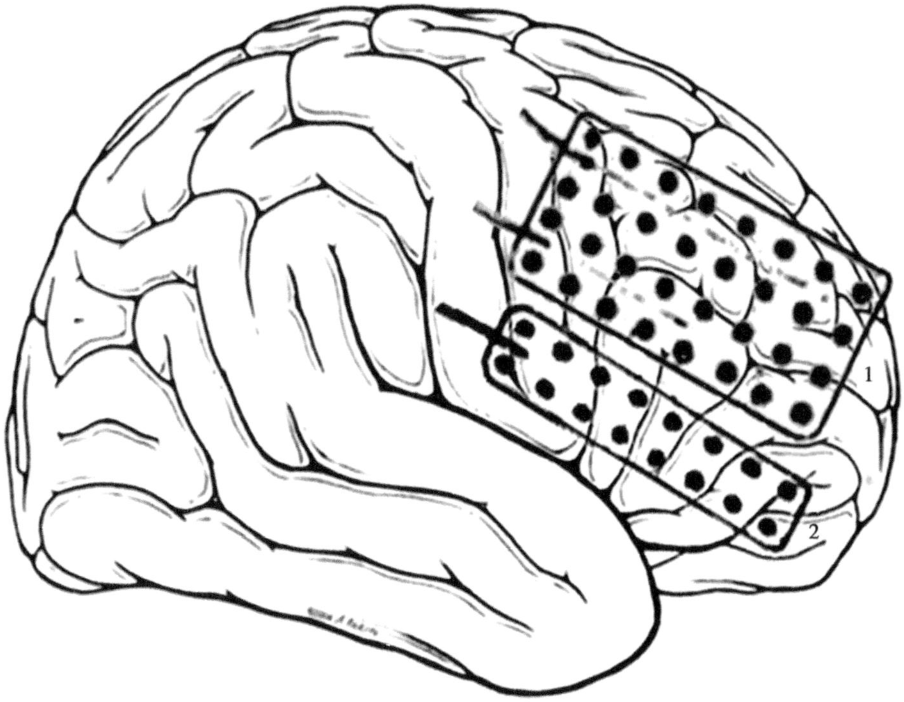

Fig. 2.37 Scheme of intracranial electrodes
Grid electrode 1: the middle upper part of the central area of the right posterior frontal region (32 contacts); Grid electrode 2: the lower part of the central area as well as the right posterior frontal region (16 contacts)

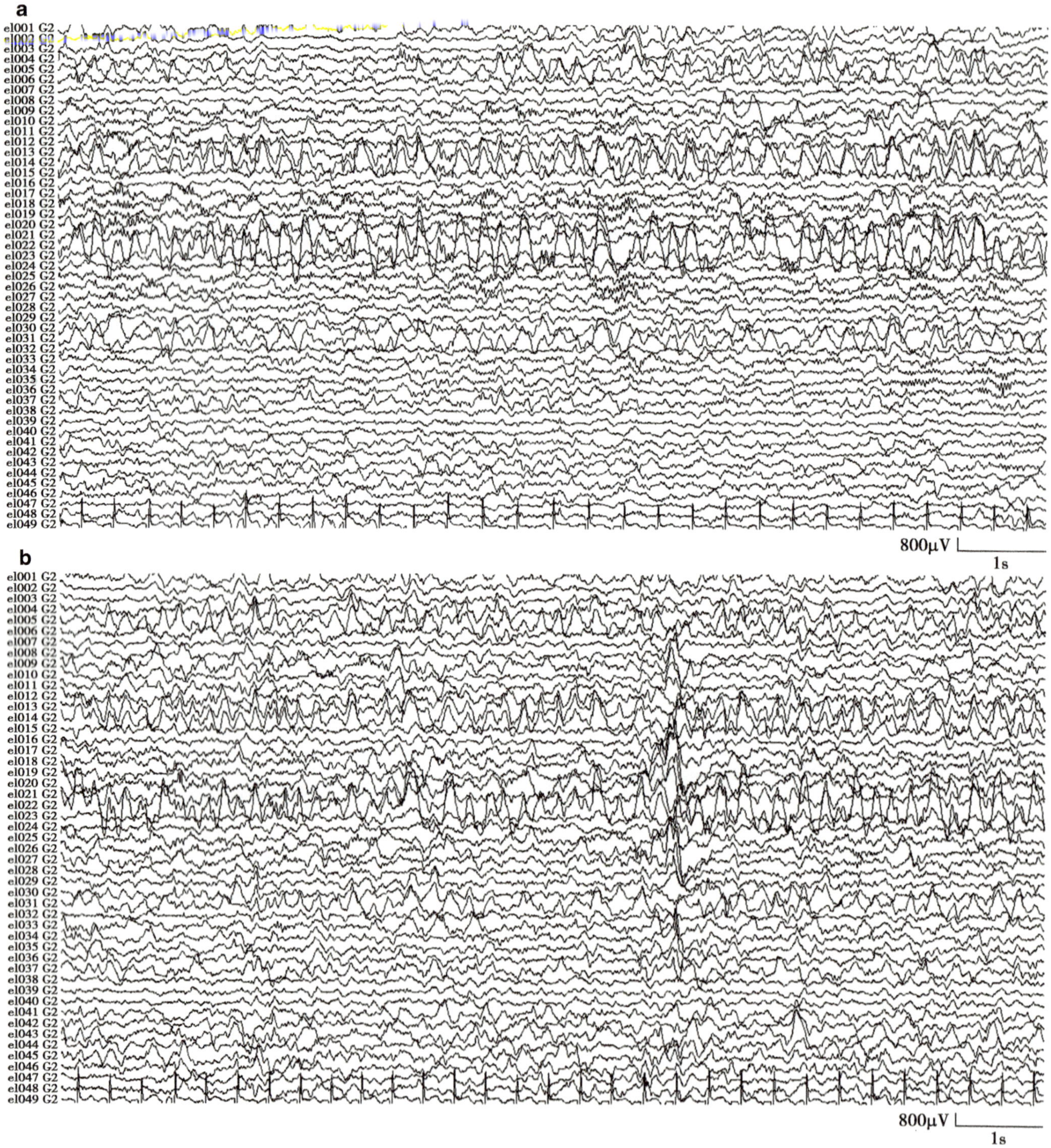

Fig. 2.38 Interictal intracranial EEG. (**a**) The IEEG showed the rhythms of persistent slow waves of high amplitude and sharpened slow waves over the middle upper part of the central area of the right posterior frontal region (contact numbers el04, el05, el013, el014, el022, el030, el031). (**b**) The IEEG showed spikes of high amplitude over the middle upper part of the central area of the right posterior frontal region (contact numbers el017, el018, el025, el026, el027, el033, el034, el035)

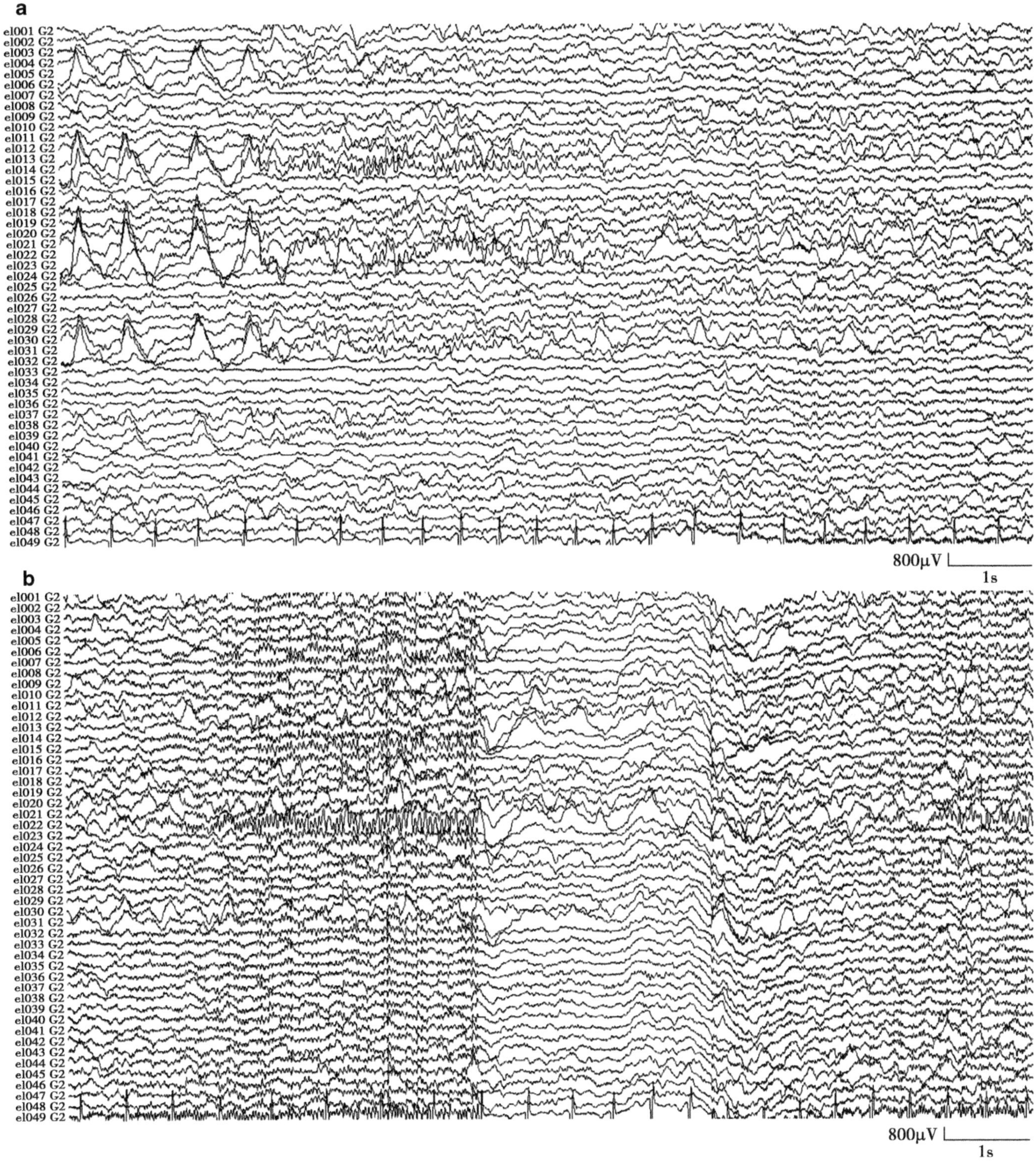

Fig. 2.39 Ictal EEG of intracranial electrodes. (**a**) The patient was asleep 2 s before the seizure. The IEEG showed a decrease in wave amplitude, and the low amplitude fast activity over the middle upper part of the central area of the right posterior frontal region (contact numbers el013, el014, el021, el022, el030, el031). (**b**) During the seizure, the patient's mouth was distorted to the left, and her lower limbs were slightly shaken, with a slight twitching of the left hand. The IEEG showed that the spike-and-wave complexes rhythm gradually became stronger over the middle upper part of the central region of the right posterior frontal cortex (contact numbers el06, el07, el014, el015, el016, el022), with increased amplitude, lasting 4–5 s. (**c**) The seizure ended. The IEEG recovered to the background EEG

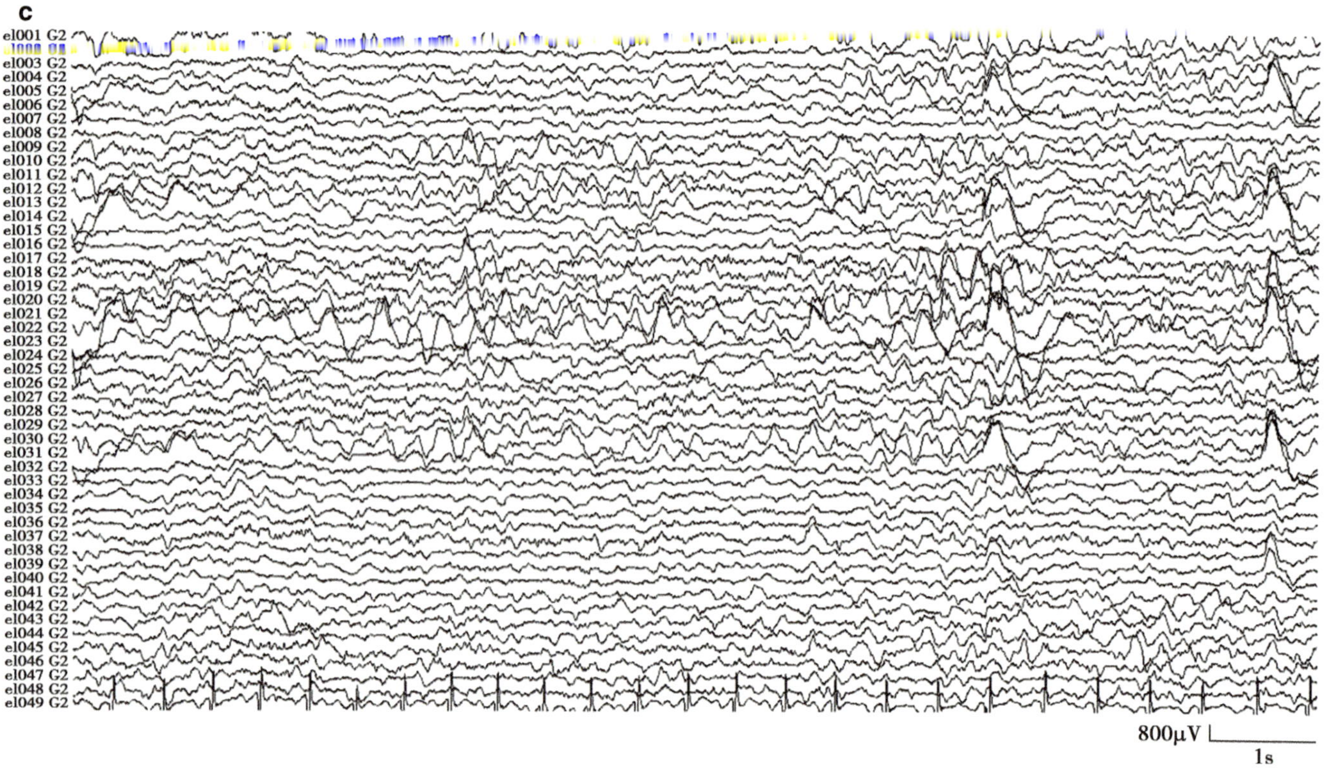

Fig. 2.39 (continued)

Case 2.9 Posterior Inferior Frontal Gyrus Epilepsy

[Abstract of Medical Records]
Male, 17 years old.

1. *Chief complaint* Episodic loss of consciousness and twitching for 6 years.
2. *History of present illness* The patient had a sudden onset of shouting, loss of consciousness, and tonic clonus of the limbs during sleep without any cause 6 years ago, which lasted for several minutes and then resolved. At present, there are two types of seizures: One is episodic absence of mind, with chewing and fumbling, which lasts for dozens of seconds and resolves. There is no aura before the seizure, and the patient cannot recall after the seizure. The other is manifested as sudden screaming during sleep and loss of consciousness, with twitching of the limbs, which resolves after 2–3 min and occurs 1–2 times/day on average. Antiseizure medications failed to control the seizure, the patient is now taking traditional Chinese medicines such as Kexianling, with poor effect.
3. *Past history* The patient had noticeable jaundice when he was a neonate and was diagnosed with right cerebral arteritis at the age of 11 months.
4. *Physical examination* He was conscious. Grade 5 muscle strength of the right limb, Grade 5 proximal muscle strength of the left upper limb, Grade 4 distal muscle strength, flexion contracture, Grade 4 muscle strength of the left lower limb, hypermyotonia of the left lower limb, tendon reflex (+++) of the left lower limb, left Babinski sign (positive), and Babinski sign (negative) on the right.
5. *Imaging examination* MRI showed no obvious abnormalities.
6. *EEG* For details, see Figs. 2.40, 2.41, 2.42, 2.43, and 2.44.

[Case Review]

1. *Case Characteristics*
   (a) *Seizure characteristics* ① Two seizure types. ② No aura before seizure.

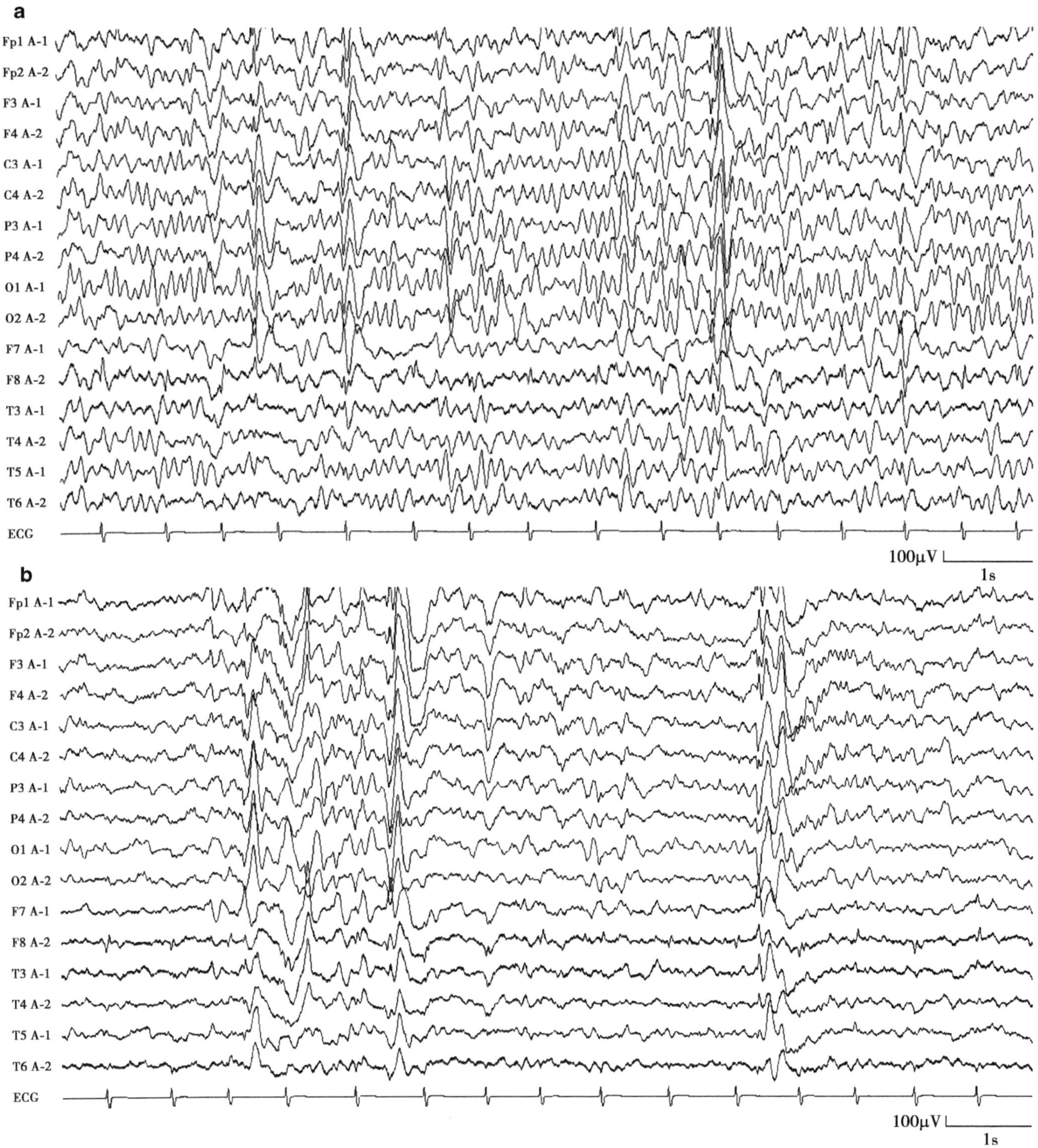

Fig. 2.40 Interictal scalp EEG. (**a**) The EEG had a basic rhythm of 8.0 Hz and was mixed with many 5.0–7.0 Hz slow waves of medium and high amplitude. A few spikes of high amplitude and spike-and-wave complexes were observed over the bilateral frontal regions (Fp1, Fp2, F3, F4), and anterior temporal region (F7, F8). (**b**) The abnormal waves during sleeping were the same as that shown by **a**, and spread to all leads

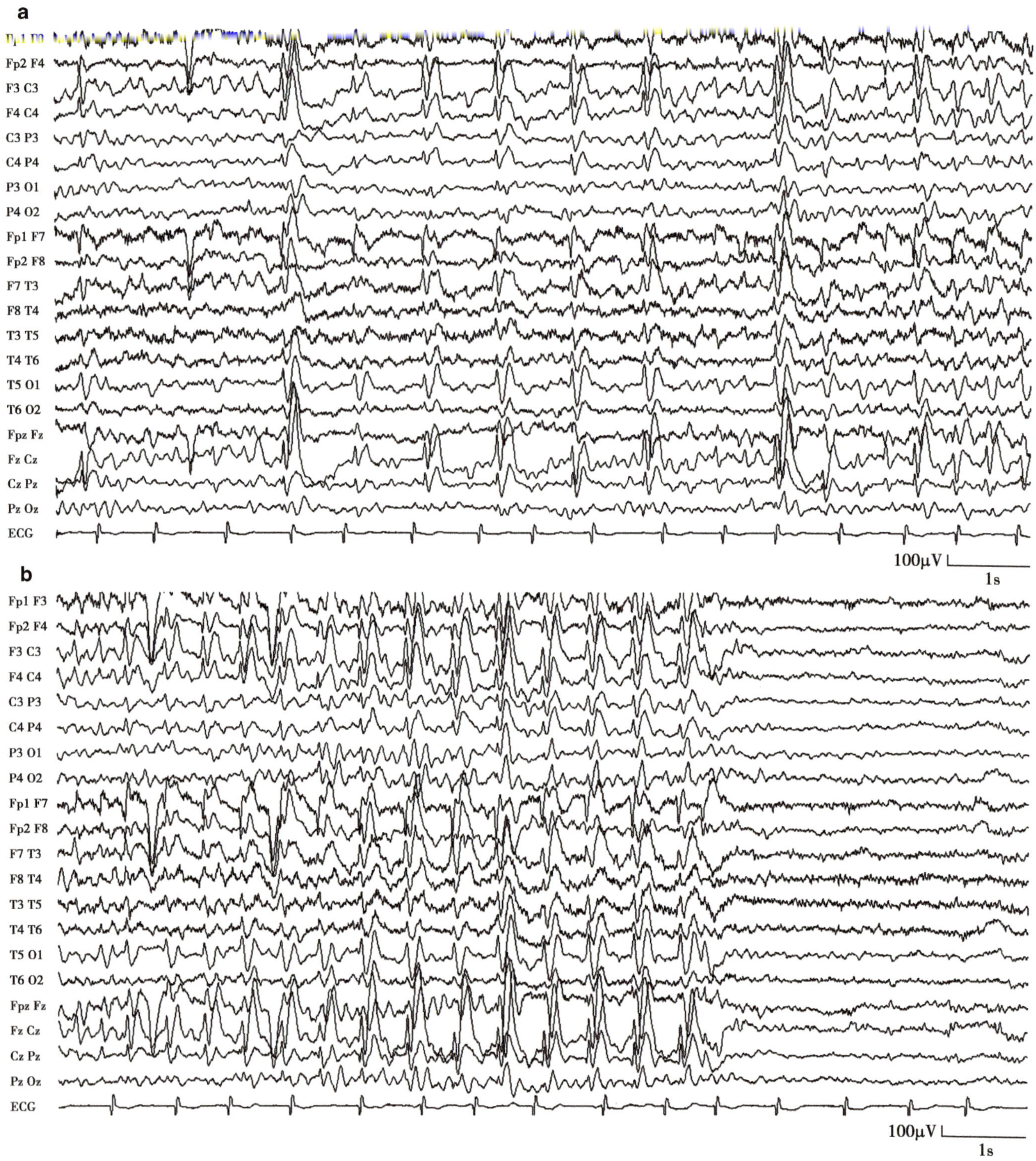

Fig. 2.41 Ictal scalp EEG. (**a**) 32 s before the seizure, the patient was lying and reading a book with both lower limbs flexed. The EEG showed rhythmic spike-and-wave complexes of high amplitude in frontal central region (Fp1 F3, Fp2 F4, F3 C3, F4 C4, C3 P3, C4 P4) and the midline (Fpz Fz, Fz Cz, Cz Pz), left temporal region (F7 T3, T3 T5, T5 O1), and showed phase inversion over the lead F7. (**b**) The patient remained the above position 24 s before the seizure. The EEG showed rhythmic spike-and-wave complexes with a gradual increase in frequency, and a low amplitude activity after about 9 s. (**c**) The patient's left foot trembled slightly. The EEG showed the low amplitude fast activity over the bilateral frontal central region (Fp1 F3, Fp2 F4, F3 C3, F4 C4, C3 P3, C4 P4), the midline (Fpz Fz, Fz Cz, Cz Pz), the bilateral frontal and temporal regions (Fp1 F7, Fp2 F8, F7 T3, F8 T4), and the left posterior temporal region (T3 T5, T5 O1), among which the wave rhythm was lower and the frequency was higher over the bilateral frontal regions (Fp1 F3, Fp2 F4, Fpz Fz). (**d**) During the seizure, the patient's limbs were moving like riding a bike. EEG showed many EMG artifacts and electrode wobble artifacts mixed. (**e**) The patient sat up and still held the book with both hands. The EEG was the same as **d**. (**f**) The patient lay down with the help of his family members, and the seizure ended. The EEG recovered to the background EEG

c

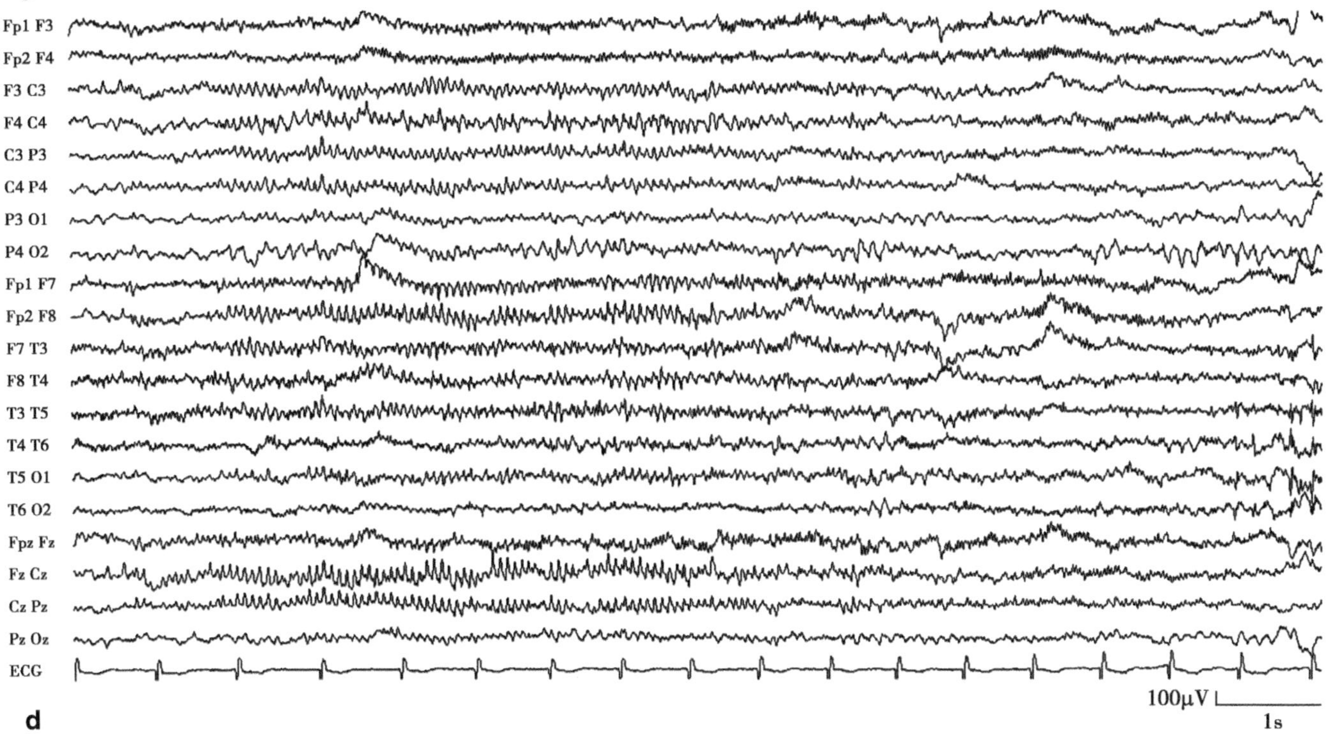

d

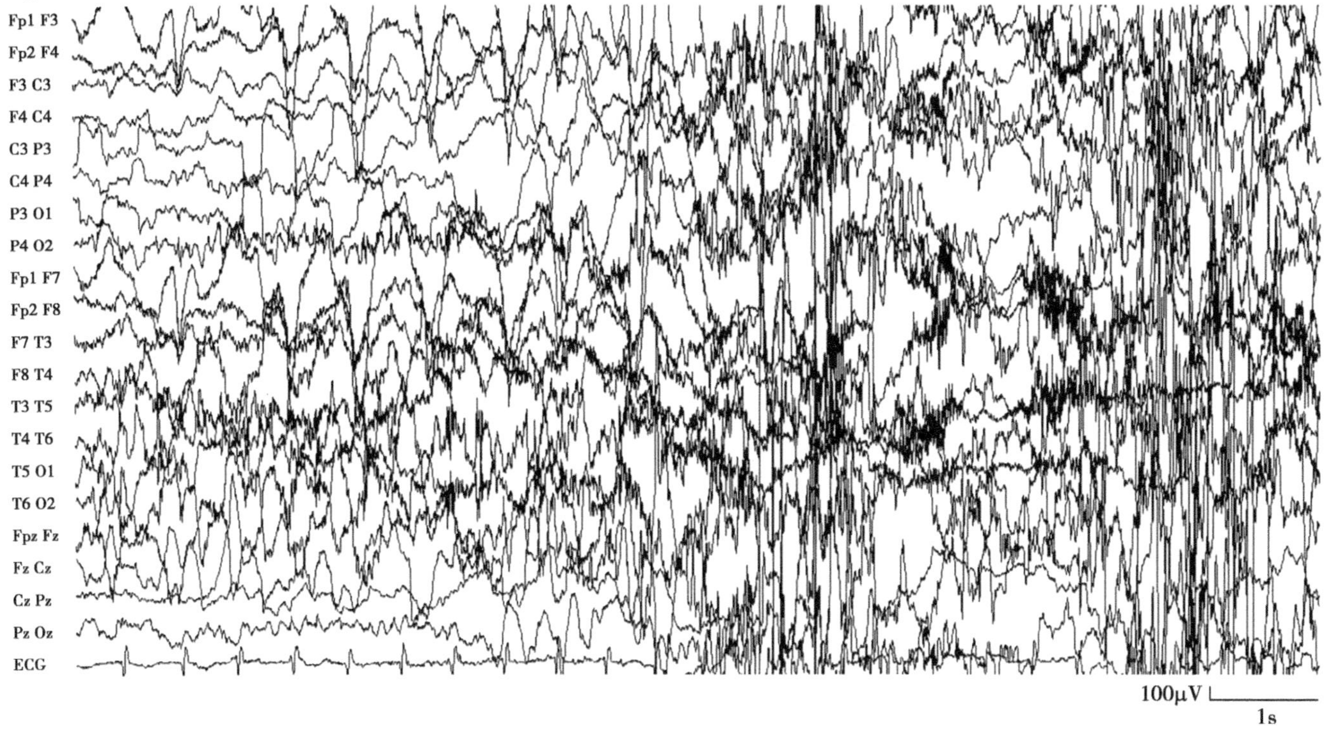

Fig. 2.41 (continued)

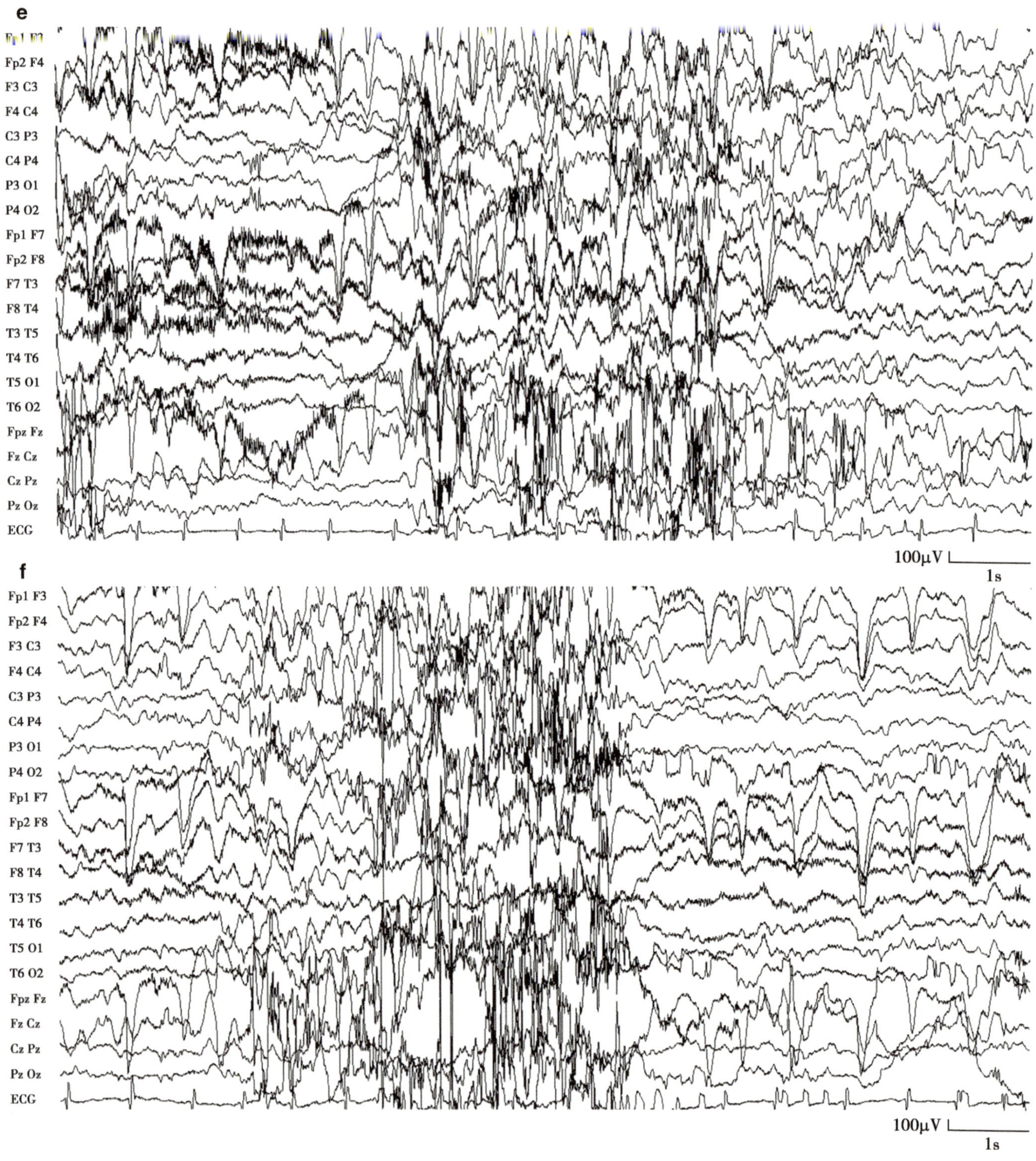

Fig. 2.41 (continued)

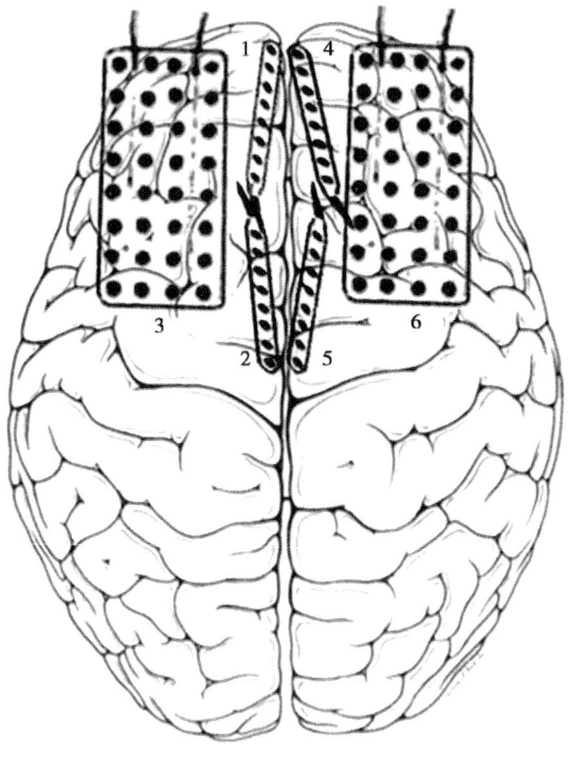

Fig. 2.42 Scheme of intracranial electrodes
Strip electrode 1: the left medial prefrontal cortex (8 contacts); Strip electrode 2: the left posterior medial frontal cortex (8 contacts); Grid electrode 3: the left dorsolateral prefrontal cortex (32 contacts); Strip electrode 4: the right anterior medial frontal cortex (8 contacts); Strip electrode 5: the right posterior medial frontal cortex (8 contacts); Grid electrode 6: the right dorsolateral prefrontal cortex (32 contacts)

(b) *EEG characteristics* ① Interictal EEG showed extensive abnormal discharges, and spikes and spike-and-wave complexes over the bilateral frontal and anterior temporal regions. ② Ictal EEG showed simultaneous rhythmic spike-and-wave complexes over the anterior part of the scalp bilaterally, especially on the left.

(c) *Imaging characteristics* MRI showed no obvious abnormalities.

2. *Diagnosis and treatment strategy and follow-up results* The patient's MRI was negative; occasional right-sided jerking symptoms were observed during seizures; interictal and ictal EEGs showed that the information was insufficient for determining the side (more possibly on the left). According to the seizure symptoms and EEG features, the frontal region was considered as the epileptic focus. Therefore, intracranial electrodes were implanted over the bilateral frontal regions. The interictal IEEG showed extensive discharges, and the ictal IEEG showed a clear origin located over the posterior part of left middle and inferior frontal gyrus. The left middle and inferior frontal gyrus were resected surgically. After the surgery, the patient was seizure-free during a 4-year follow-up. The reasons for the success of the treatment were identified in the analysis as follows: the epileptic focus was accurately positioned and completely resected, contributing to a satisfactory outcome.

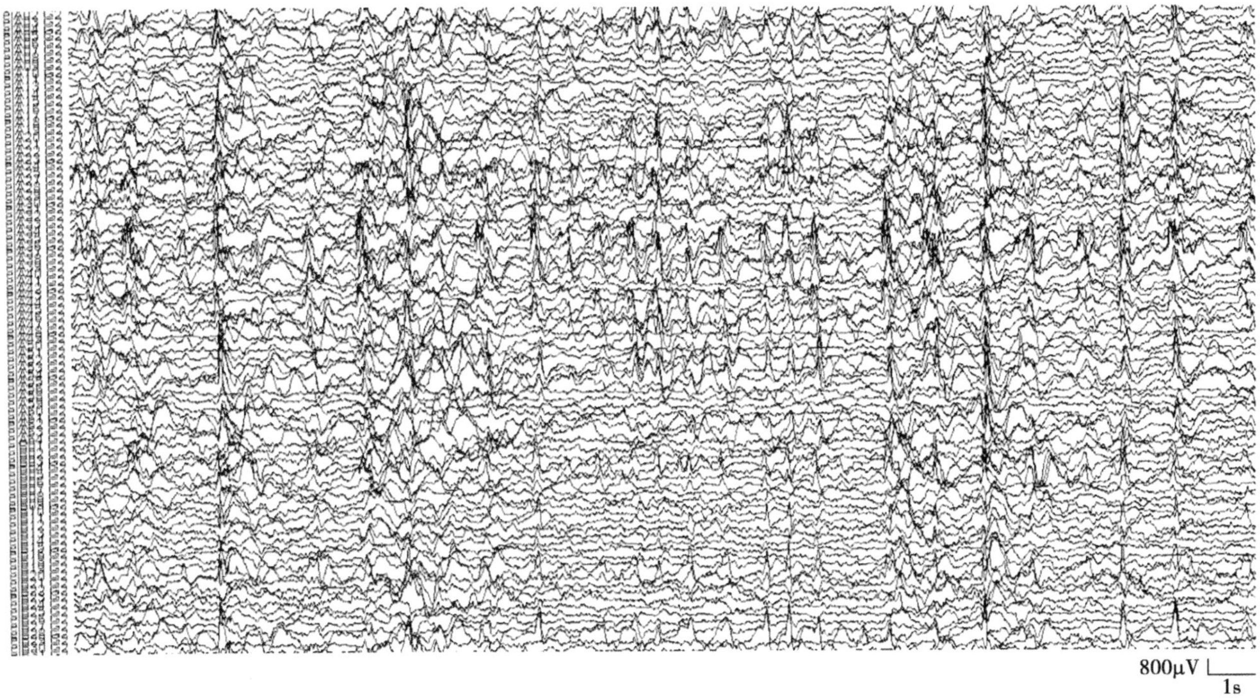

Fig. 2.43 Interictal intracranial EEG
The background IEEG showed extensive spikes, and rhythmic sharp waves over the left medial prefrontal area (contact numbers elA02, elA03, elA04, elA05), posterior medial frontal area (contact numbers elA53, elA54, elA55), left dorsolateral prefrontal cortex (contact numbers elA27, elA28, elA29, elA36, elA37, elA38, elA39, elA40, elA44, elA45, elA46, elA47, elA48), which spread to the right dorsolateral prefrontal cortex (contact numbers elB20, elB21, elB28, elB29)

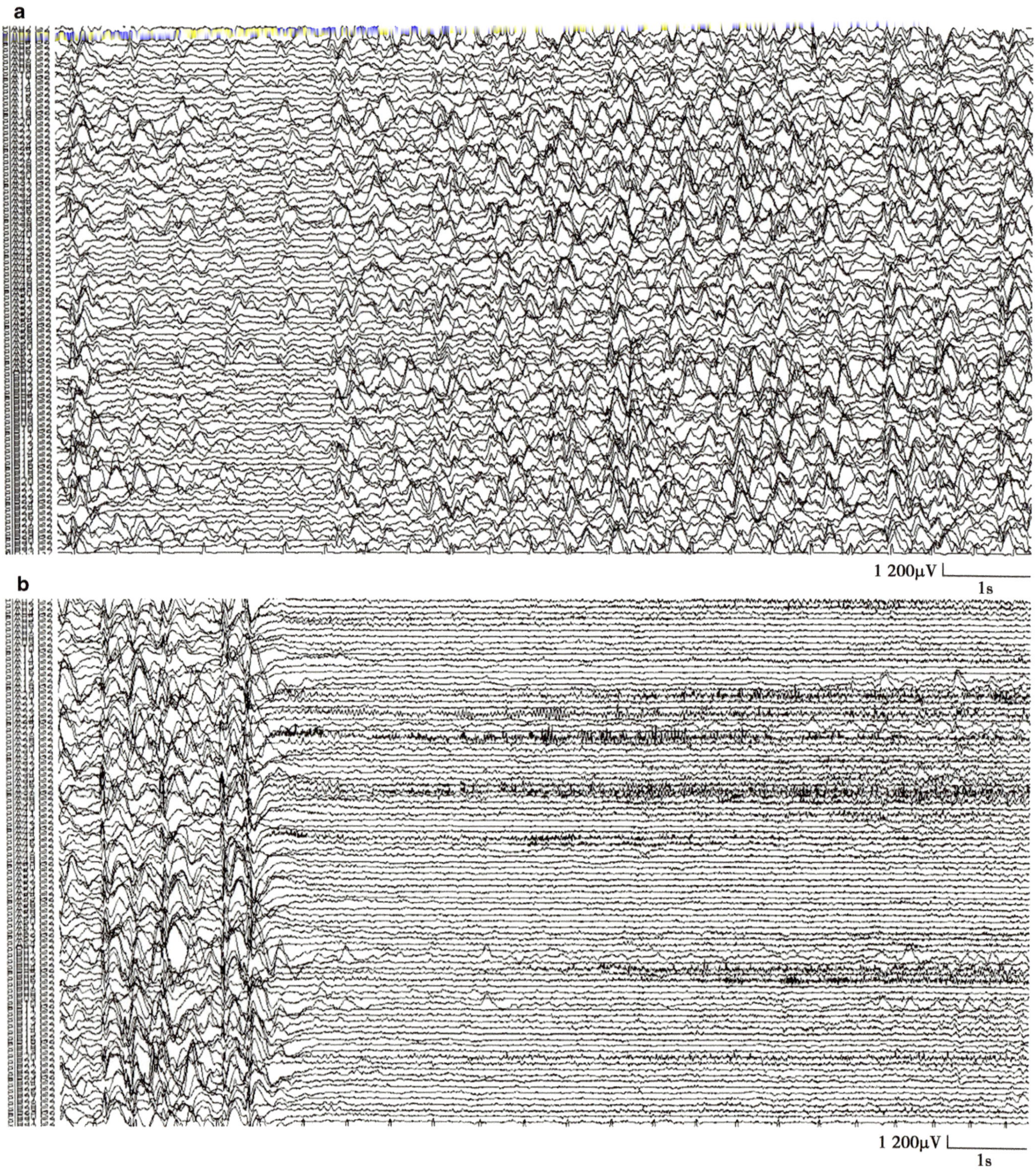

Fig. 2.44 Ictal intracranial EEG. (**a**) The patient was sleeping before the seizure, and was slightly short of breath after waking. The IEEG showed increased wave amplitude of abnormal electrical activities. (**b**) The patient had several slight left mouth twitches, a movement of the right lower limb, flexion of the right upper limb, and eyes closed. The IEEG showed wave amplitude decrease at the beginning of the seizure, and the low amplitude fast activity over the left dorsolateral prefrontal cortex (contact numbers elA20, elA23, elA28, elA36, elA37, elA45), which lasted for 3 s and then spread to the left medial prefrontal cortex (contact numbers elA02, elA03) and the right dorsolateral prefrontal cortex (contact numbers elB03, elB04, elB05, elB20). (**c**) The seizure ended. The IEEG recovered to the original background EEG

c

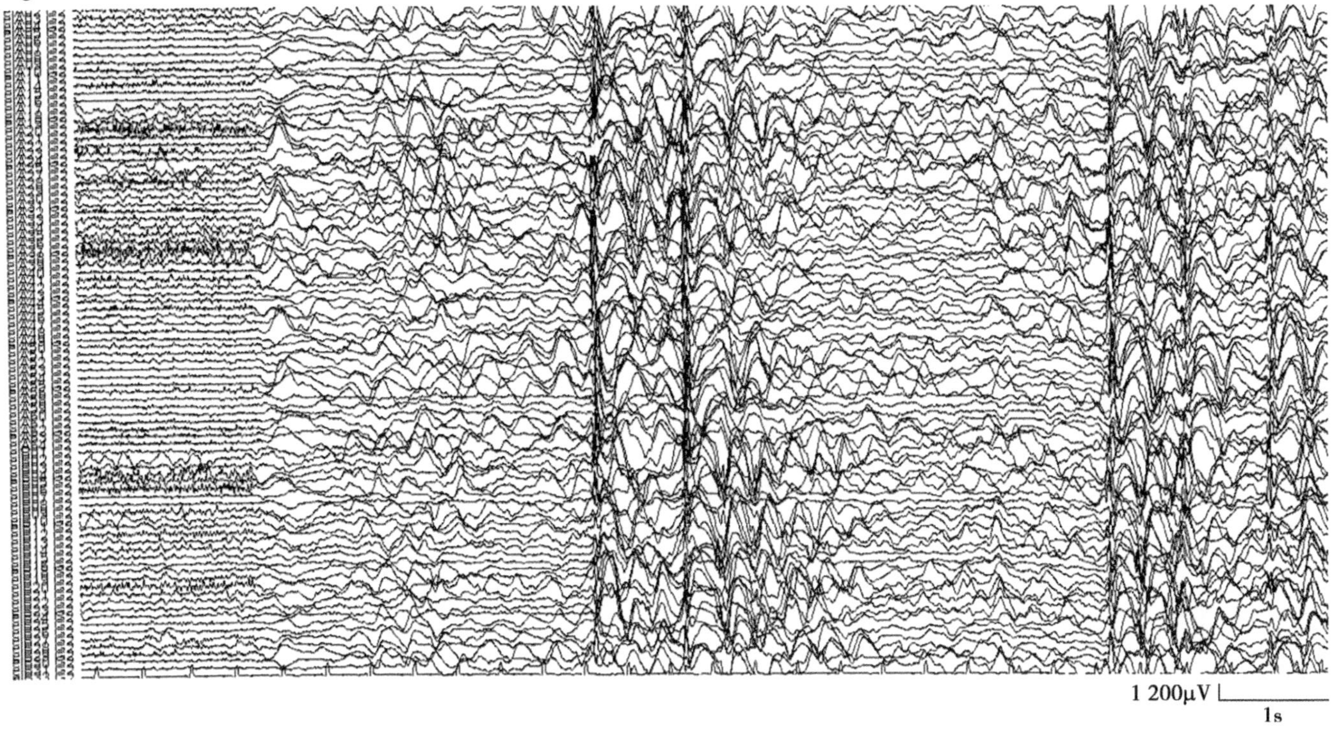

Fig. 2.44 (continued)

Cases of Medial Frontal Lobe Epilepsy

Case 2.10 Medial Frontal Lobe Epilepsy (Superior Frontal Gyrus)

[Abstract of Medical Records]
Male, 23 years old.

1. *Chief complaint* Paroxysmal limb convulsion for 20 years.
2. *History of present illness* The patient suddenly experienced twitching of the limbs, foamed at the mouth, and lost consciousness during sleep 20 years ago, which ended in 2–3 min. Since then, the seizures have been recurrent at a frequency of 1 time every 2–3 days. After treatment with phenobarbital and carbamazepine, the seizure type changed to sudden absence of mind and dropping objects to the ground, which lasted for a few seconds or tens of seconds, occasionally with twitching of the limbs, mostly at night. Seven years ago, the frequency of seizures increased, and the drug treatment regimen was adjusted. The treatment with carbamazepine, phenytoin sodium, and clonazepam was not effective. At the time of admission, he had 1–2 seizures per day, which were characterized by rigidity of the limbs and loss of consciousness.
3. *Past history* The patient was delivered at full term, with normal motor, language, and intellectual development.
4. *Imaging examination* MRI showed no obvious abnormal changes.
5. *EEG* For details, see Figs. 2.45, 2.46, 2.47, 2.48, and 2.49.

[Case Review]

1. *Case Characteristics*
   (a) *Seizure characteristics* ① Nocturnal seizures, 1–2 times per day. ② Short duration of seizures, with slightly asymmetric postural tonicity.
   (b) *EEG characteristics* ① Interictal EEG showed the rhythm of paroxysmal 2.5–3.0 Hz spike-and-wave complexes of high amplitude, especially over the anterior head bilaterally. ② Ictal EEG showed irregular fast activity of low amplitude over the frontal midline.
   (c) *Imaging characteristics* MRI showed no obvious abnormal changes.

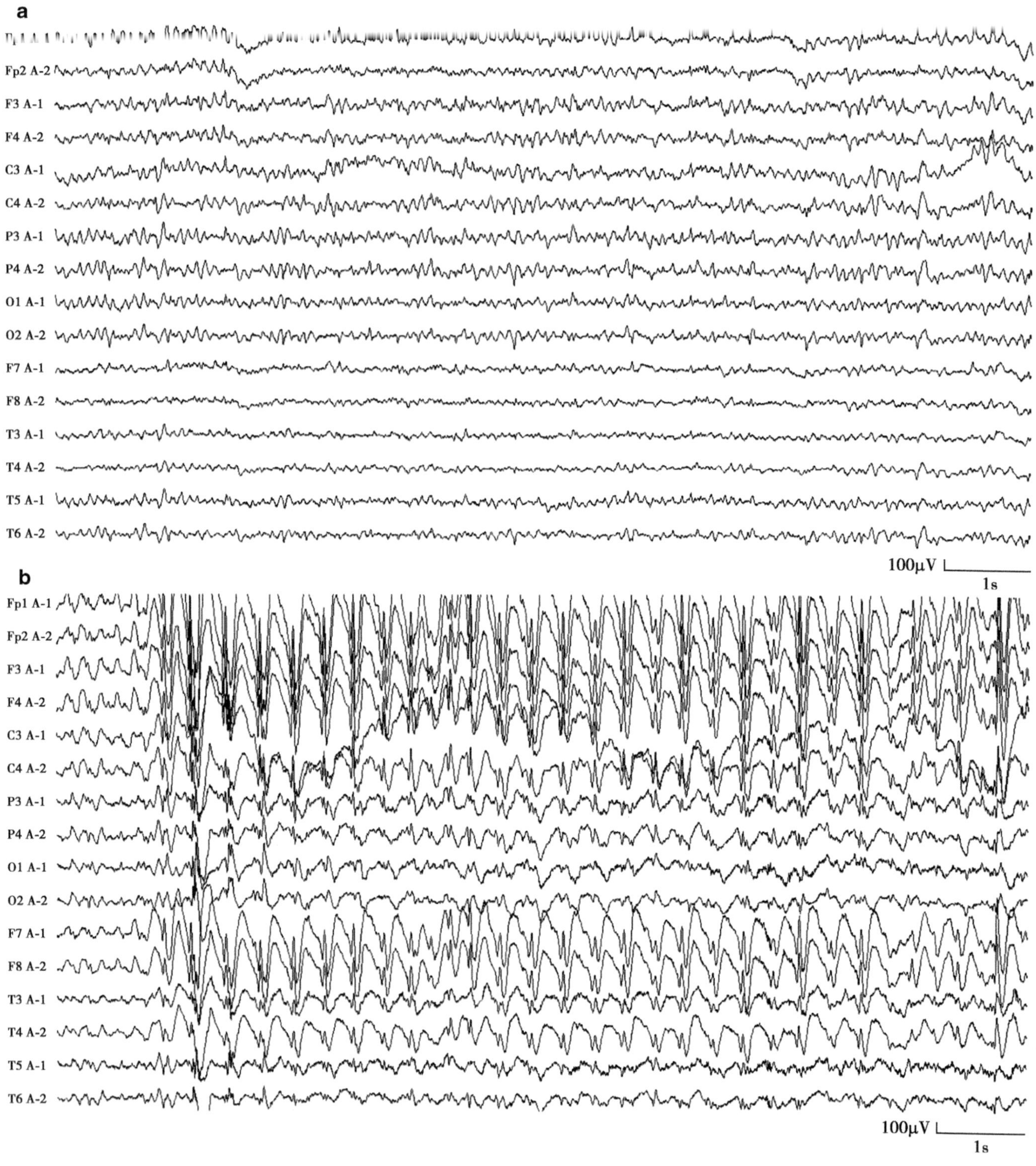

Fig. 2.45 Interictal scalp EEG. (**a**) The EEG showed a basic rhythm of 8.0 Hz and a few 5.0–7.0 Hz slow waves of low and medium amplitude. (**b**) The EEG showed the rhythm of paroxysmal 2.5–3.0 Hz spike-and-wave complex of high amplitude, especially over the anterior head bilaterally (Fp1, Fp2, F3, F4, F7, F8)

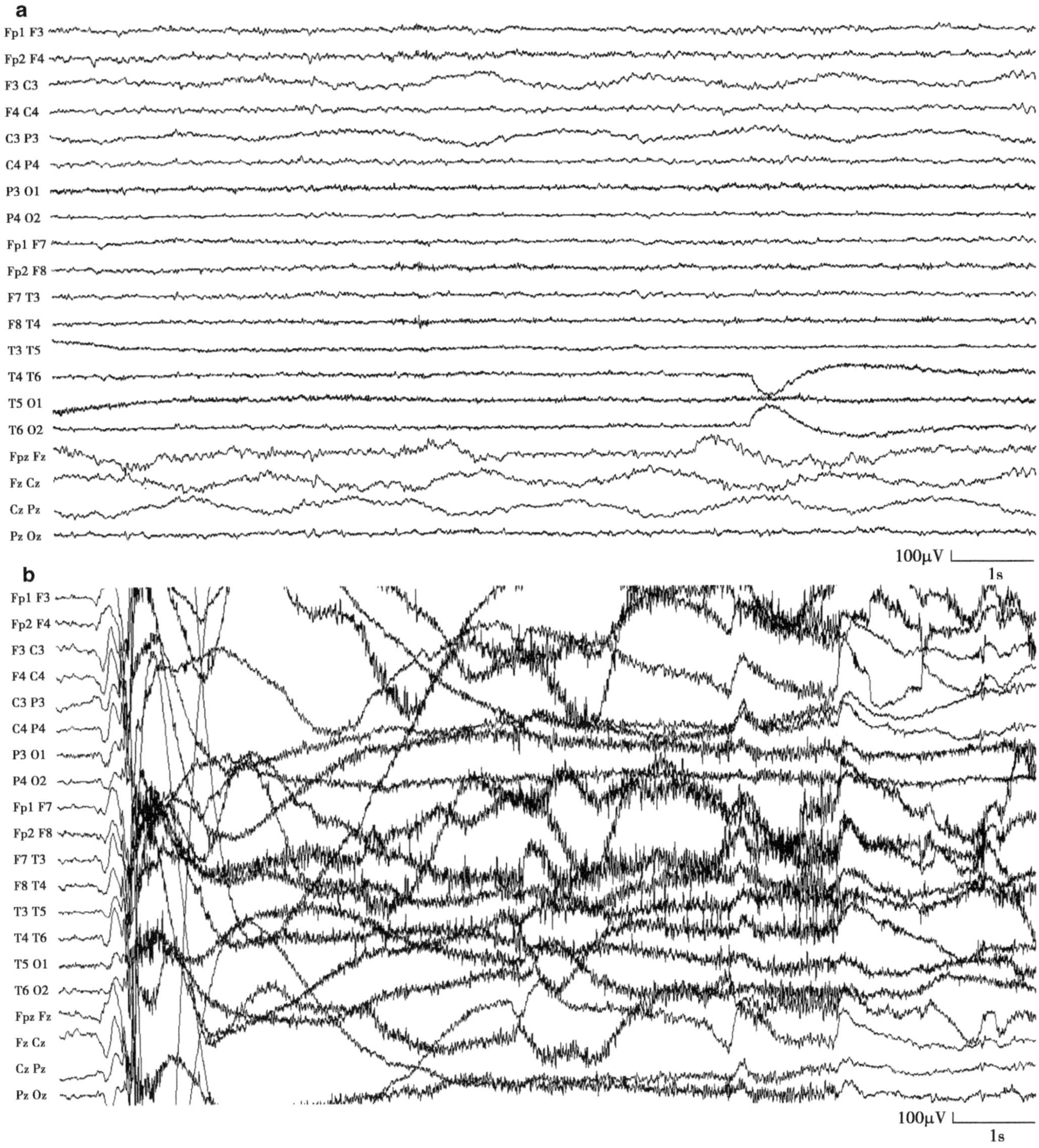

Fig. 2.46 Ictal scalp EEG. (**a**) The patient was asleep before the seizure. The EEG was the background EEG of stage I of sleep, and showed fast activity of low amplitude over the leads over the frontal midline (Fpz Fz, Fz Cz). (**b**) The patient suddenly turned his eyes upward, slightly raised his head, raised his left upper limb, and slightly raised his right hand in a tonic state for about 15 s. The EEG showed slow waves of high amplitude followed by EMG artifacts. (**c**) The patient lowered his upper limbs while chewing in his mouth. The EEG showed many electrode wobble artifacts and EMG artifacts. (**d**) The seizure ended. The EEG showed the rhythm of spike-and-wave complexes of high amplitude, especially over the anterior head bilaterally (Fp1 F3, Fp2 F4, F3 C3, F4 C4, Fp1 F7, Fp2 F8, F7 T3, F8 T4, Fpz Fz, Fz Cz). (**e**) The seizure ended. The EEG showed the rhythm of spike-and-wave complexes of high amplitude, especially over the anterior head bilaterally (Fp1 F3, Fp2 F4, F3 C3, F4 C4, Fp1 F7, Fp2 F8, F7 T3, F8 T4, Fpz Fz, Fz Cz)

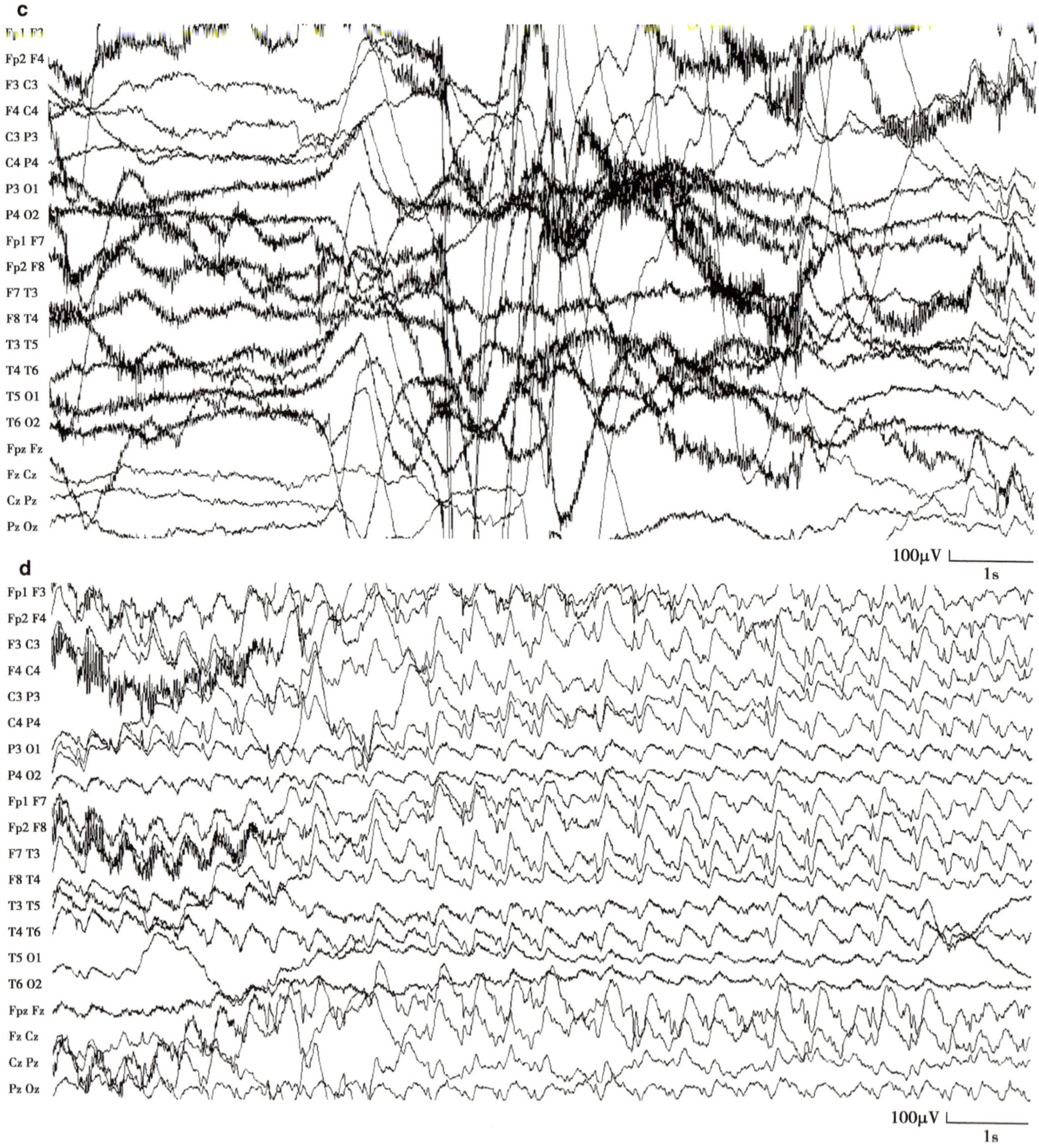

Fig. 2.46 (continued)

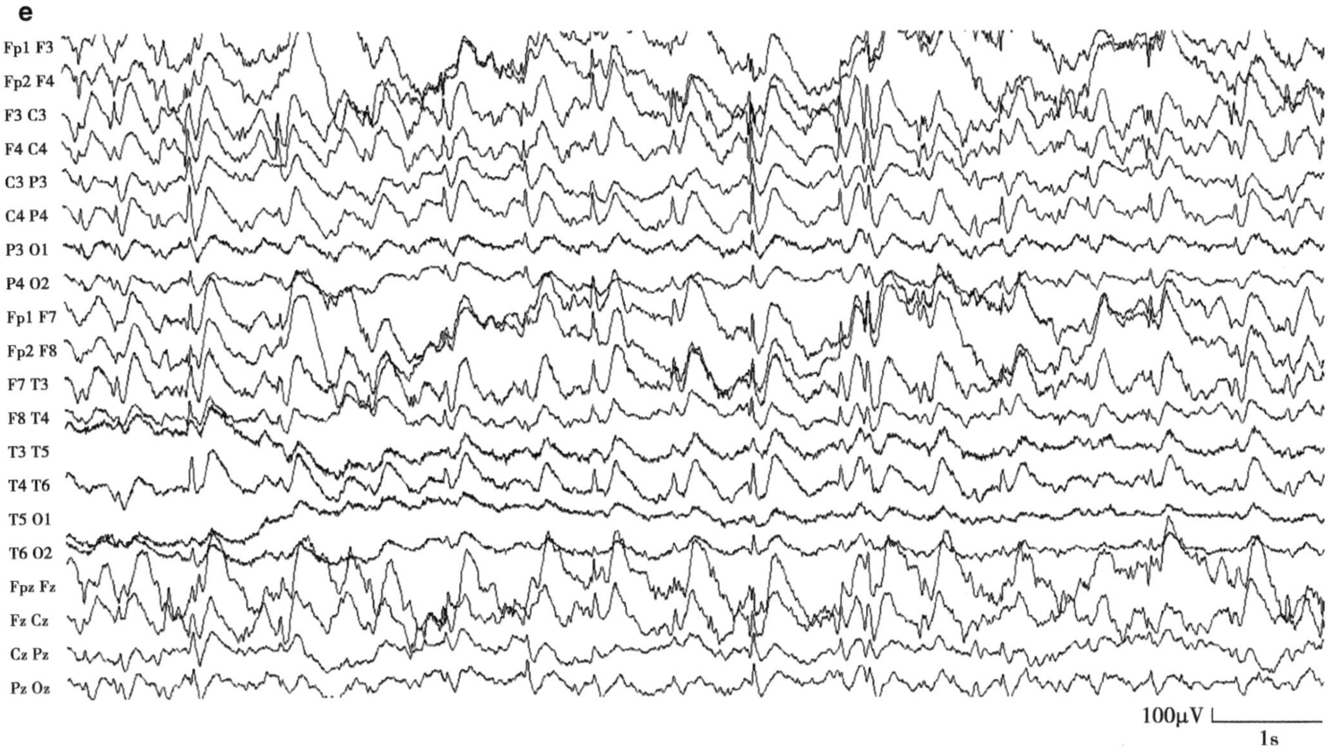

Fig. 2.46 (continued)

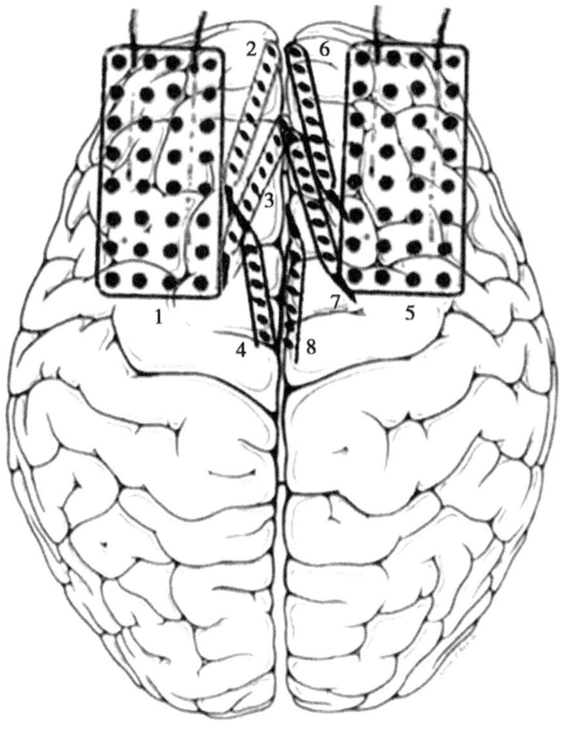

Fig. 2.47 Scheme of intracranial electrodes
Grid electrode 1: the left dorsolateral prefrontal cortex (32 contacts); Strip electrode 2: the left medial prefrontal cortex (8 contacts); Strip electrode 3: the left medial frontal cortex (8 contacts); Strip electrode 4: the left posterior medial frontal cortex (6 contacts); Grid electrode 5: the right dorsolateral prefrontal cortex (32 contacts); Strip electrode 6: the right medial prefrontal cortex (8 contacts); Strip electrode 7: the right medial frontal cortex (8 contacts); Strip electrode 8: the right posterior medial frontal cortex (6 contacts)

2. *Diagnosis and treatment strategy and follow-up results*
   There was insufficient information for determination of the side of seizure symptoms, but the motor symptoms during seizure were characterized by slightly tonicity over the left upper limb, suggesting that the epileptic focus might be located on the right side. The interictal EEG showed fast activities of low amplitude and rhythmic sharp waves over the anterior head bilaterally, while the ictal EEG showed the same over the frontal midline; MRI showed no significant abnormal changes. According to the above information, it was considered that the epileptic focus was located over the frontal lobe, while the side of the focus was unclear. Intracranial electrodes were hence implanted over the frontal lobes bilaterally. The interictal IEEG showed extensive abnormal discharges, and the ictal IEEG showed that the origin site was not restricted. The right middle and superior frontal gyrus including medial cortex and frontal pole were resected, and the corpus callosum was incised. After 2 years of postoperative follow-up, there were still a few seizures. The reason for this was considered to be the extensive range of the interictal EEG and the ictal IEEG of the patient, and the cortical excitability was high. Although the epileptic focus was resected, the peripheral cortices with high excitability may become secondary epileptic foci. Therefore, there were still a few seizures after surgery.

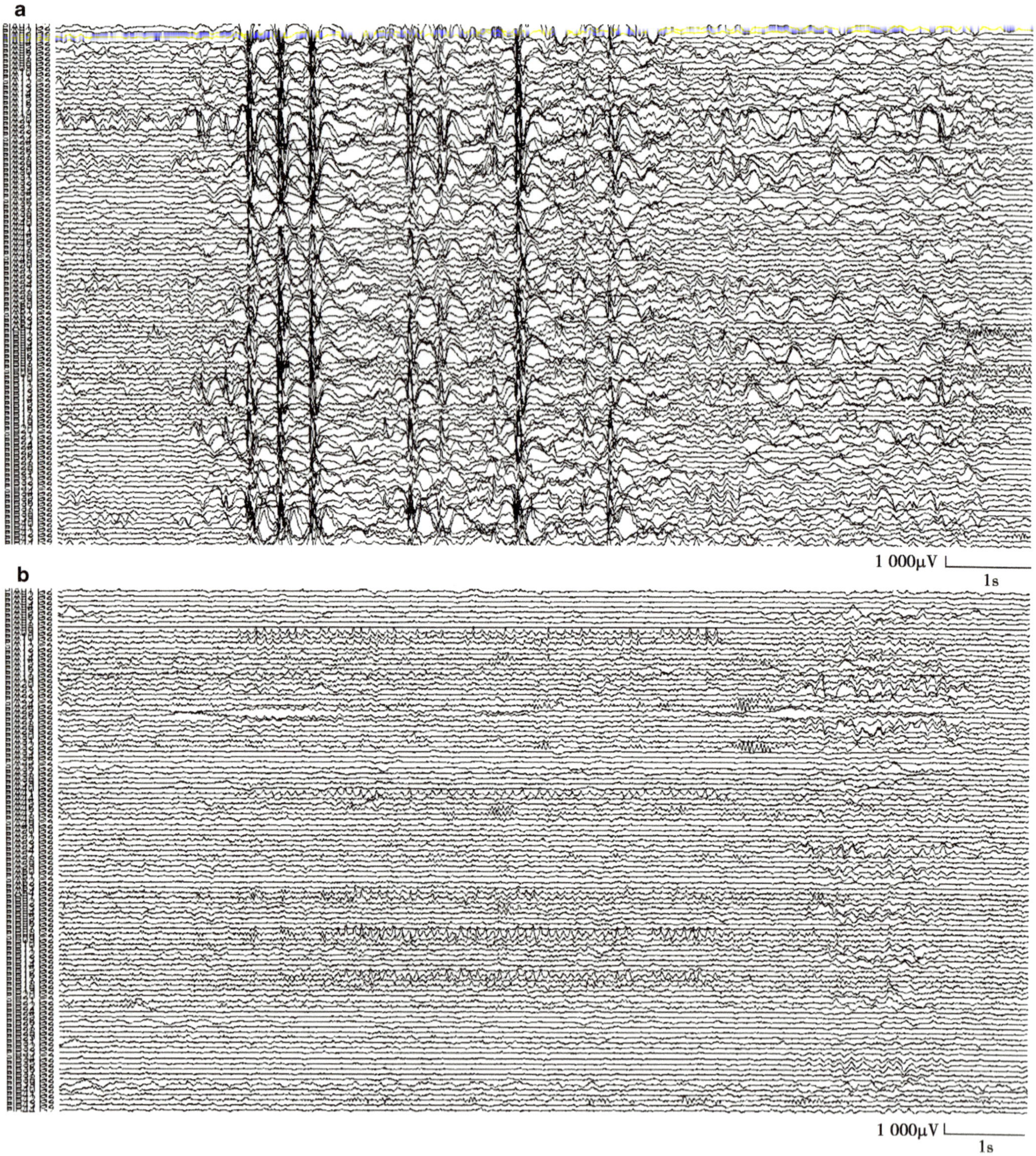

Fig. 2.48 Interictal intracranial EEG. (**a**) The IEEG showed the burst of the rhythm of spike-and-wave complexes of high amplitude and multi-spike-and-wave complexes, especially over the bilateral dorsolateral frontal cortices (contact numbers elA06, elA12, elA20, elA21, elA28, elA29, elA58, elA59, elA60, elB04, elB05, elB06, elB11, elB12, elB13, elB20, elB21). (**b**) The IEEG showed the rhythm of paroxysmal sharp waves over the bilateral dorsolateral frontal cortices, especially on the right (contact numbers elA64, elB01, elB08, elB09, elB16, elB17, elB18)

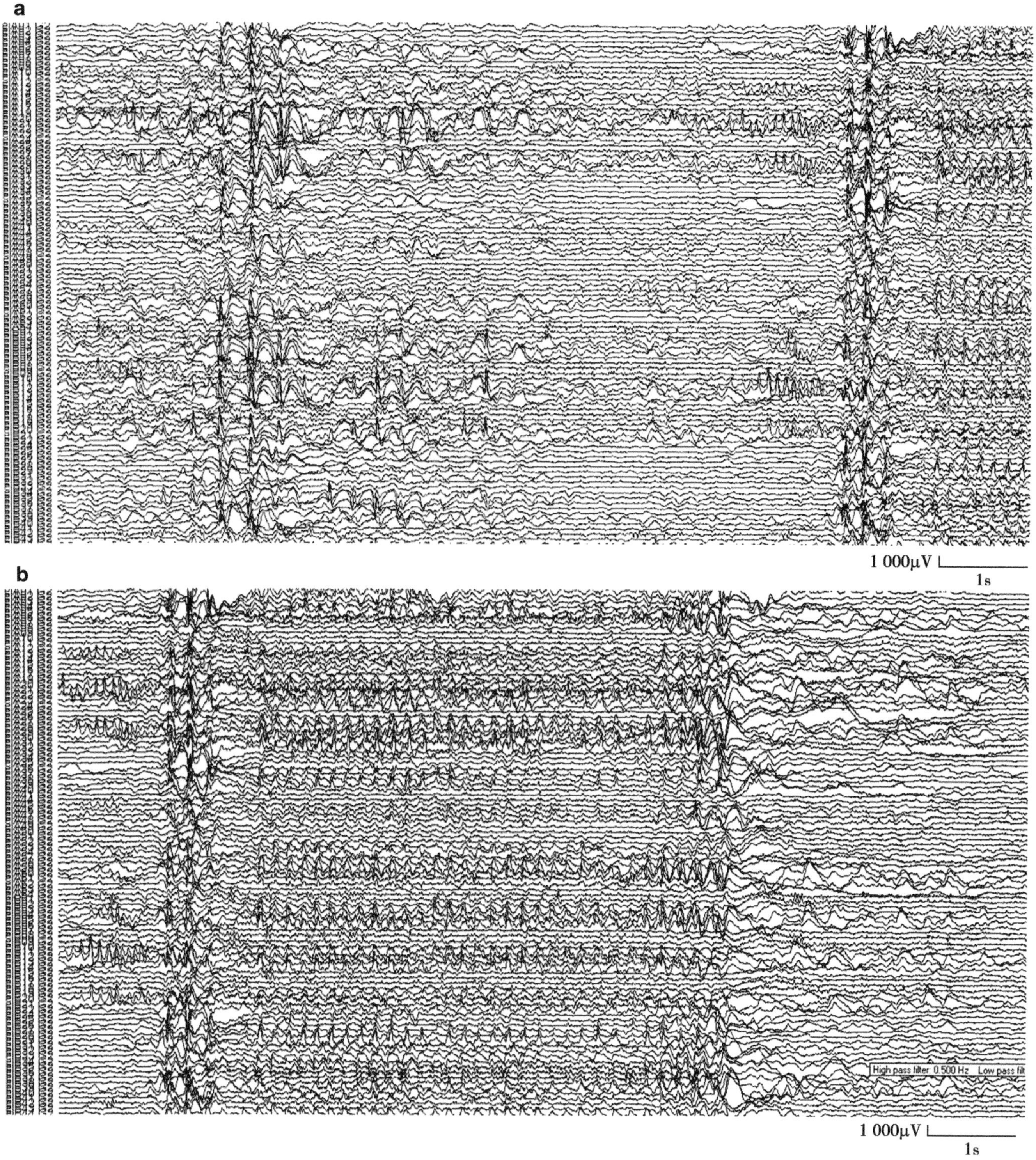

Fig. 2.49 Ictal EEG of intracranial electrodes. (**a**) The patient was asleep before the seizure. The IEEG showed rhythmic spike-and-wave complexes on the bilateral dorsolateral frontal cortices (contact numbers elA13, elA14, elA21, elA22, elA28, elA29, elB03, elB04, elB05, elB11, elB12, elB19, elB20). (**b**) During the seizure, the patient raised the left upper limb, slightly raised the right upper limb, turned the body to the right, and buried the head between both upper limbs, which lasted 8–9 s. The IEEG showed the low amplitude fast activity and spikes of high amplitude over the bilateral dorsolateral frontal cortices (contact numbers elA13, elA14, elA21, elA22, elA28, elA29, elB03, elB04, elB05, elB11, elB12, elB19, elB20) and the right medial frontal cortex (contact numbers elB29, elB30, elB34, elB35, elB36, elB37, elB44). (**c**) After the seizure, the patient's body still maintained the position of right lateral decubitus and fell asleep again. The IEEG gradually recovered to the background EEG

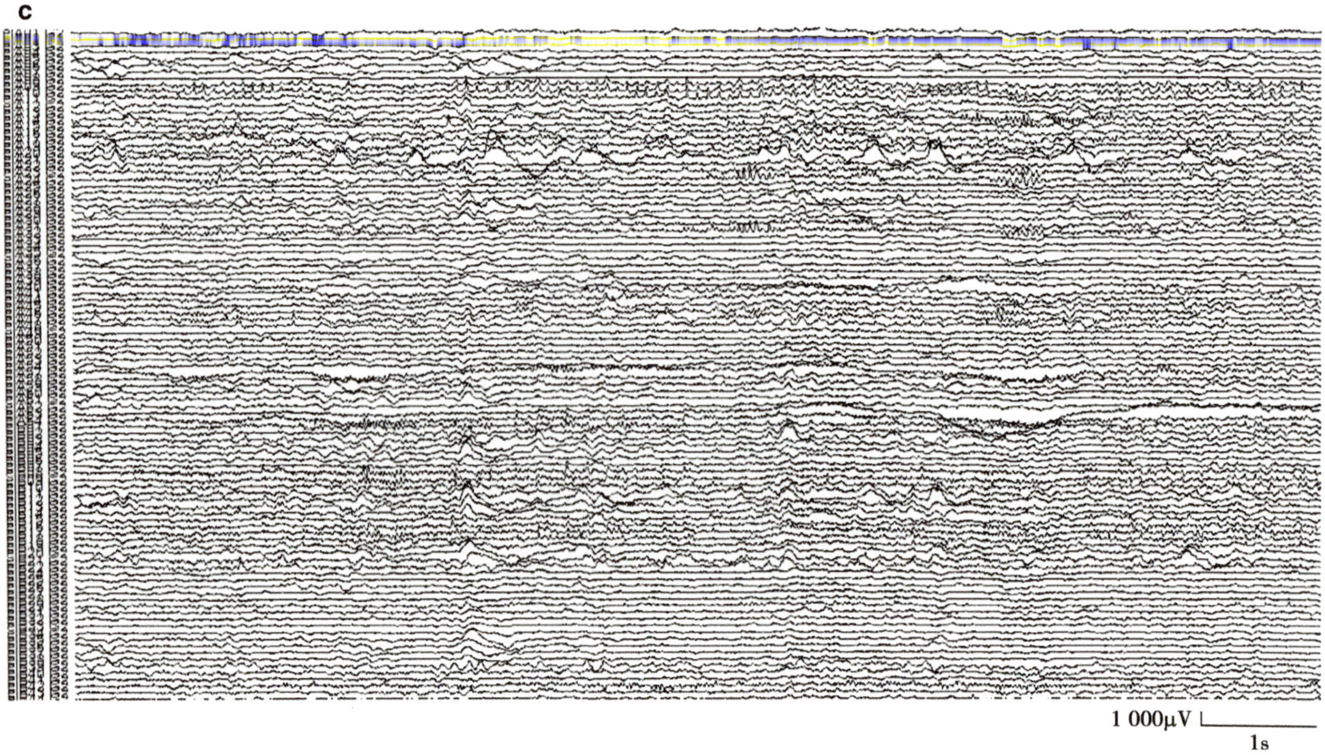

Fig. 2.49 (continued)

Case 2.11 Medial Frontal Lobe Epilepsy (Cingulate Cortex)

[Abstract of Medical Records]
Male, 21 years old.

1. *Chief complaint* Paroxysmal limb convulsion with loss of consciousness for 15 years.
2. *History of present illness* The patient has had unexplained right mouth and eyelid twitching since 15 years ago; an episode occurs every 2–3 months, lasting approximately 30 s for each episode. He was diagnosed with epilepsy at a children's hospital. The patient started on oral medication. He was treated with phenytoin sodium, carbamazepine, sodium valproate, phenobarbital, and traditional Chinese medicines, while the disease was not well controlled. Later the seizure type changed slightly and was manifested as eyes staring, head turned to the right, right mouth twitching, tonic limbs, and vocalization, with loss of consciousness.

   The patient had a seizure every 2–3 months, each lasting 1–2 min. The seizures usually occurred at night during sleep. One and a half years ago, the patient was hospitalized for carbon monoxide poisoning and was in a coma for 20 h. In the past 8 months, the patient had frequent seizures, which were mainly manifested as the raising of the right upper limb, the turning of head to the right, and right mouth twitching, with loss of consciousness, which lasted about 1 min and occurred 1–2 times a day; another seizure type was manifested as staring at both eyes, lowering the head, and straightening both upper limbs, which lasted for a few seconds and occurred 3–20 times a day. Before the seizure, the patient felt a sense of "swelling" of the right upper limb. The seizures occurred during both wakefulness and sleep. The patient was treated with zonisamide while orally taking sodium valproate (200 mg/dose t.i.d.) 6 months ago, but the seizures were still frequent, more than 10 times a day.
3. *Personal history* The patient was delivered at term without any history of birth injury or asphyxia.
4. *Family history* His mother had a history of epilepsy.
5. *Physical examination* No neurological abnormalities were found.
6. *Imaging examination*
   (a) MRI showed that the right hippocampus was slightly smaller than the contralateral one.
   (b) MRS showed that the NAA concentration over the left hippocampus (NAA/Cr: 1.53) was slightly lower than the corresponding part on the right (NAA/Cr: 1.62). The CHO concentration over the left hippo-

campus (CHO/Cr: 1.32) was slightly higher than the corresponding part on the right (CHO/Cr: 1.62).

7. *EEG* For details, see Figs. 2.50, 2.51, 2.52, 2.53, and 2.54.

[Case Review]

1. Case Characteristics
   (a) *Seizure characteristics* ① The patient raised the right upper limb, turned his head to the right, and had right mouth twitching during the seizure, with loss of consciousness. ② Cluster seizures (about 10 or more seizures per day). ③ The patient felt swelling of the right upper limb before the seizure.
   (b) *EEG characteristics* ① Interictal EEG showed the rhythm of 4.0–5.0 Hz slow waves of low and medium amplitude over the leads over the left central and temporal regions. ② Ictal EEG showed sharp waves of low amplitude over the leads over the midline.
   (c) *Imaging characteristics* MRI examinations showed that the right hippocampus was slightly smaller than the contralateral one.
2. *Diagnosis and treatment strategy and follow-up results* The patient had a clear aura of seizure (feeling "swelling" over the right upper limb). The interictal EEG showed the rhythm of slow waves over the left central and temporal regions, and the ictal EEG showed sharp waves of low amplitude over the leads over the midline (Cz). Based on the seizure symptoms and the EEG information, intracranial electrodes were implanted over the central area of the left posterior frontal region. As the Cz sharp wave was obvious during the seizure, the electrodes needed to cover the medial frontal cortex. The interictal IEEG showed that the abnormal discharges were mainly over the left medial frontal cortex, orbitofrontal region, and the central area as well as the posterior frontal region; the ictal IEEG showed that the site seizure zone was located over the left medial frontal cortex and the middle upper part of the central area as well as the posterior frontal region. After the sensorimotor cortex was identified by cortical electrical stimulation, the left middle and superior frontal gyrus, medial frontal gyrus, and posterior frontal region were resected. The postoperative effects were good. The MRI changes in this patient were irrelevant to localization.

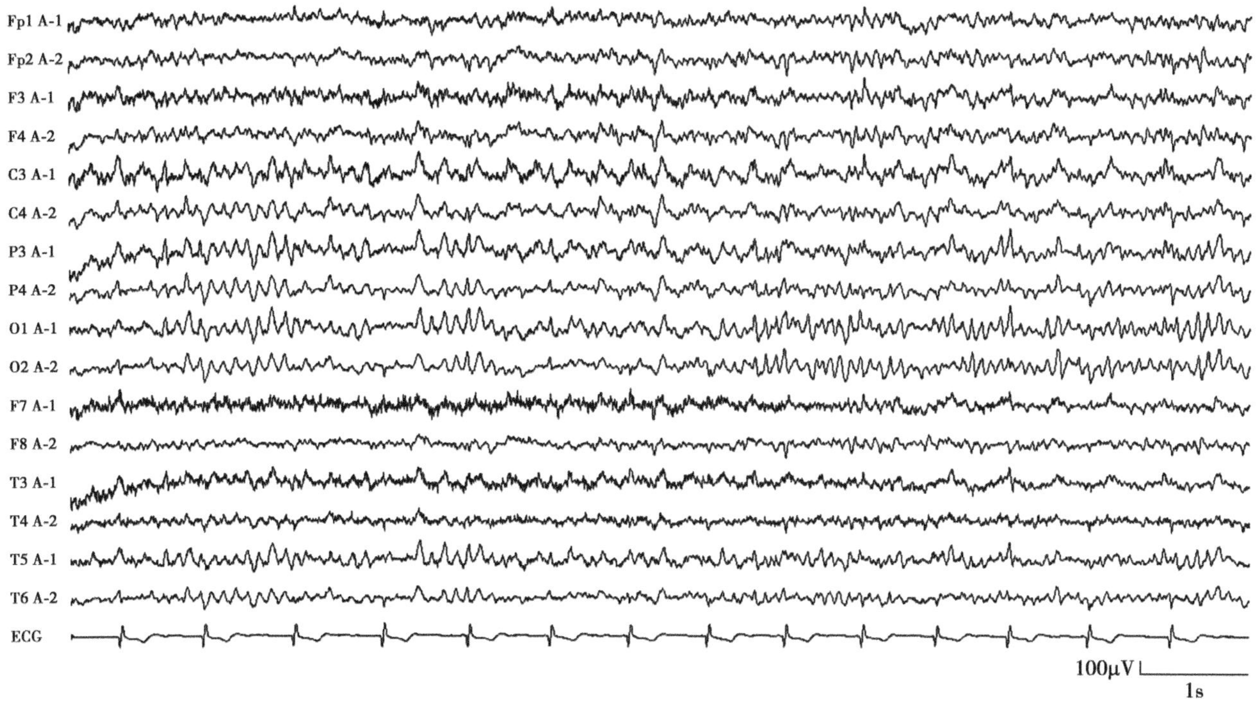

Fig. 2.50 Interictal scalp EEG
It had a basic rhythm of 9.0 Hz, and showed the rhythm of 4.0–5.0 Hz slow waves of low and medium amplitude over the left central region (C3) and the temporal region (T3)

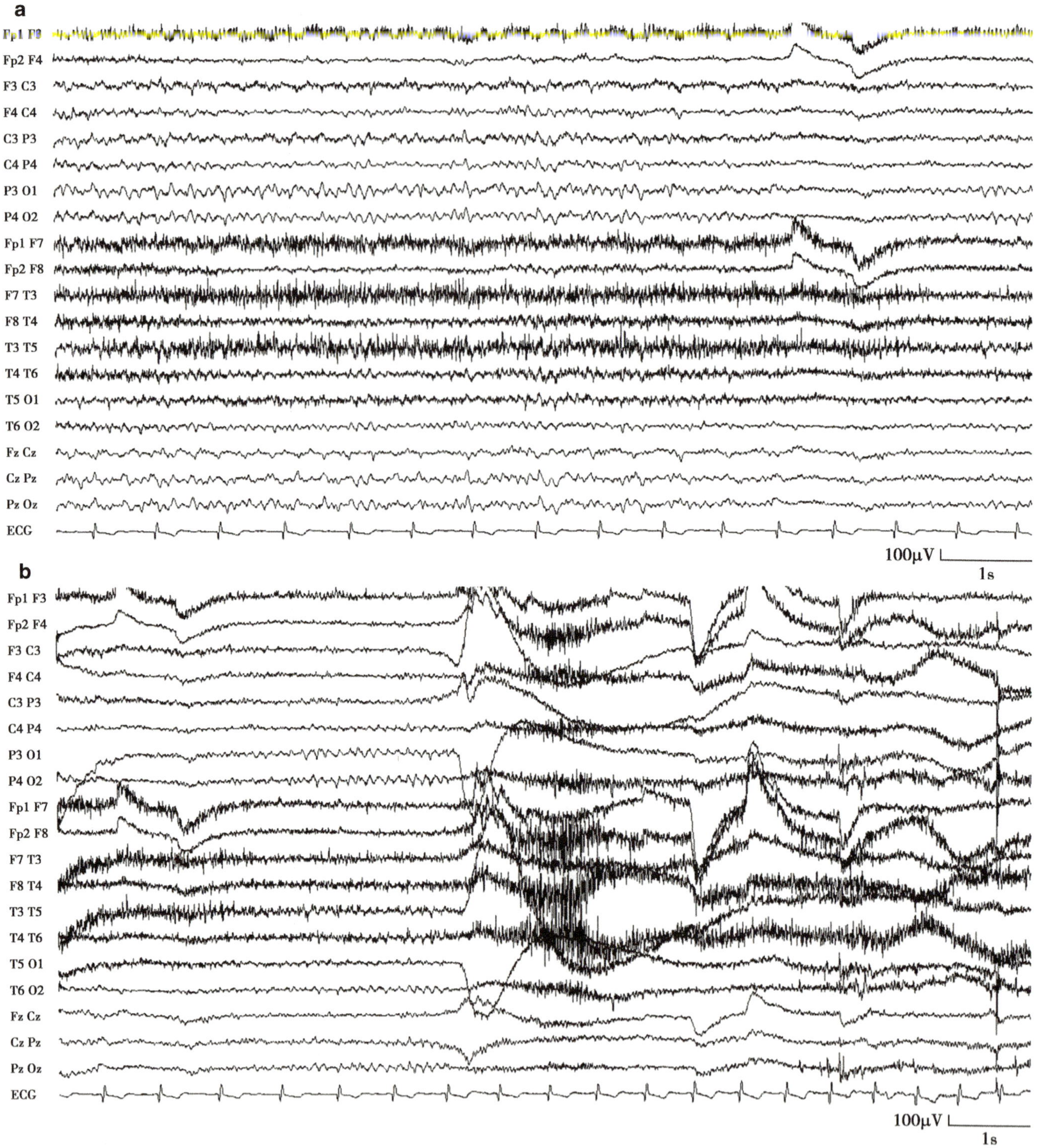

Fig. 2.51 Ictal scalp EEG. (**a**) The patient was conscious and supine with eyes closed before the seizure. The EEG was the background EEG when the patient was awake, and showed sharp waves of low amplitude over the midline (Cz) and EMG artifacts over the bilateral temporal regions. (**b**) During the seizure, the patient opened his eyes, raised his upper body, and tried to sit up from bed. The EEG showed α wave suppression with the patient eyes open, and obvious EMG artifacts in each lead. (**c**) The patient's lower limbs were slightly flexed and the body was moved from side to side in bed. The EEG showed obvious EMG artifacts. (**d**) At the end of the seizure, the patient lay down with his eyes closed. The EEG showed periodic-like spikes of medium to high amplitude over the midline (Cz, Pz)

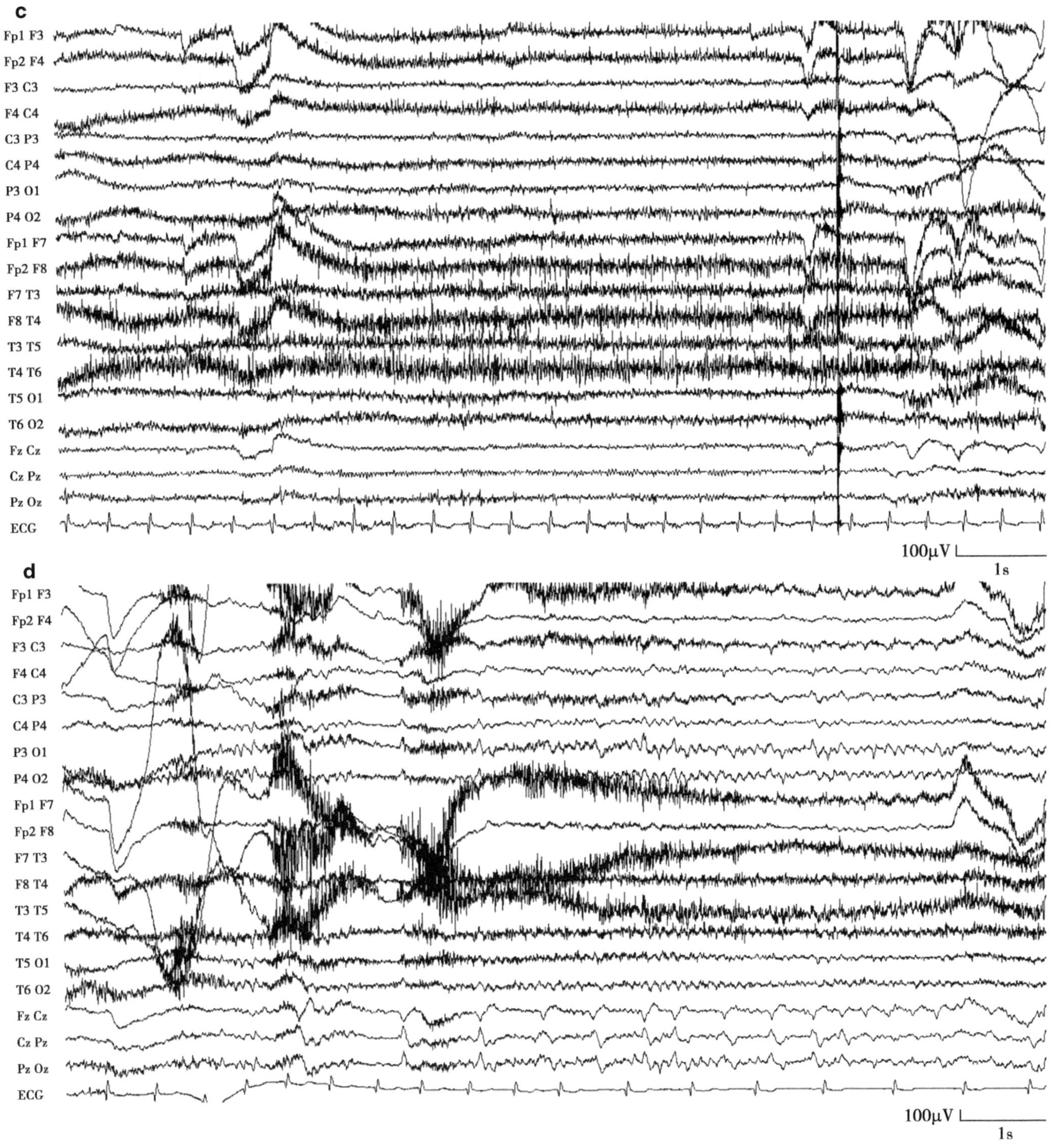

Fig. 2.51 (continued)

Fig. 2.52 Scheme of intracranial electrodes
Grid electrode 1: the left frontal fissure (16 contacts); Grid electrode 2: the left orbitofrontal region (16 contacts); Grid electrode 3: central area and the posterior areas of the left superior frontal gyrus (32 contacts); Strip electrode 4: the right medial prefrontal cortex (8 contacts); Strip electrode 5: the right posterior medial frontal cortex (8 contacts)

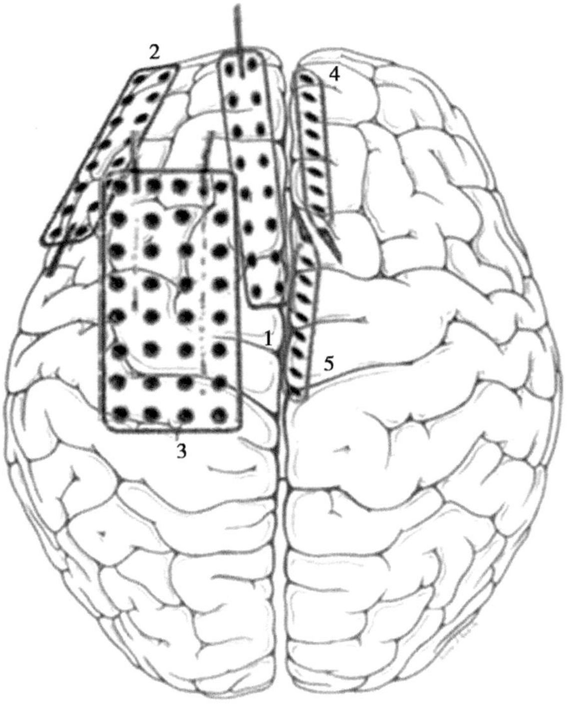

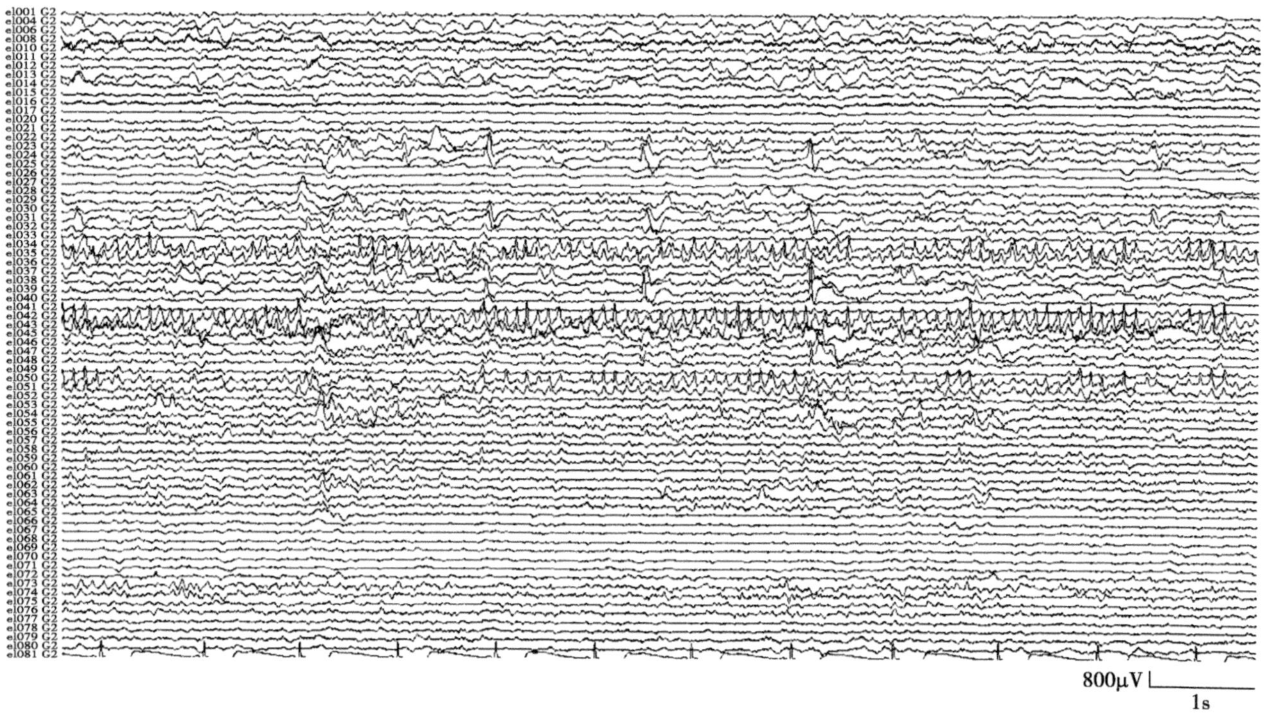

Fig. 2.53 Interictal intracranial EEG
Sharp waves were observed over the left orbitofrontal region (contact numbers el022, el023, el024, el030, el031) and the left posterior frontal region (contact numbers el038, el039, el047, el053, el054, el064)

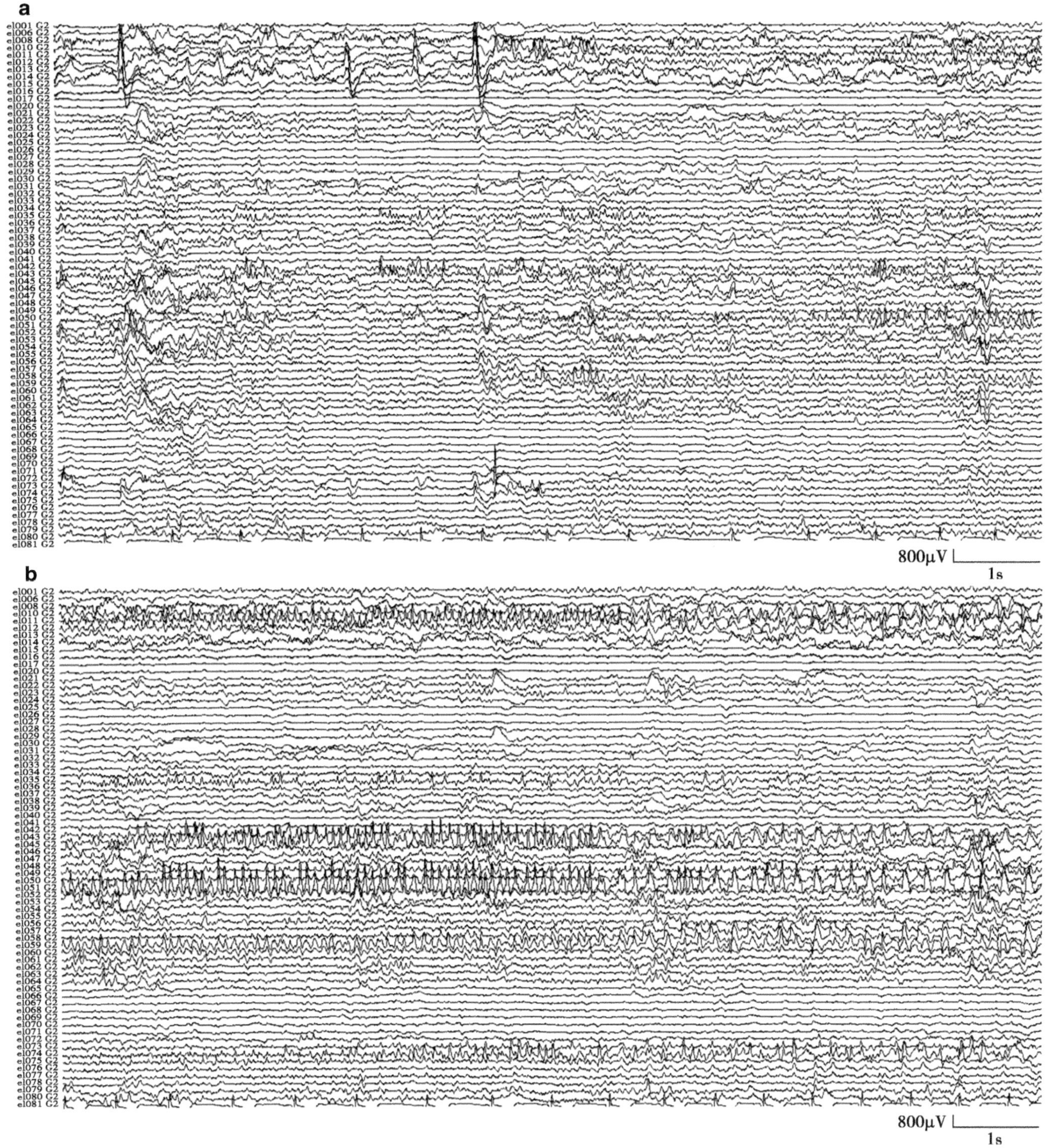

Fig. 2.54 Ictal intracranial EEG. (**a**) The patient was supine with eyes closed before the seizure. The IEEG showed the rhythms of spikes of high amplitude and low amplitude fast activity over the left medial frontal cortex (contact numbers el008, el010, el011, el012, el013, el014); sharp waves of low and medium amplitude over the left inferior frontal gyrus (contact numbers el024, el030, el031, el032); and the low amplitude fast activity over the central area and the left posterior medial frontal region (contact numbers el035, el036, el042, el043, el050, el051, el059, el060). (**b**) The patient remained supine with eyes closed. The IEEG showed the rhythm of spikes over the left medial frontal cortex (contact numbers el010, el011, el012) and over the central area and the left posterior frontal region (contact numbers el035, el042, el043, el051, el059, el060); and the synchronous spike rhythm over the right posterior medial frontal cortex (contact number el074). (**c**) During the seizure, the patient opened his eyes and looked from side to side aimlessly. The IEEG showed amplitude reduction, mixed with wobble artifacts. (**d**) The patient closed eyes and grasped the sheet slightly with both hands later when the seizure occurred. The IEEG recovered to the background EEG. (**e**) The patient raised his head after the seizure and tried to sit up. The IEEG was the same as **d**. (**f**) At the end of the seizure, the patient lay down again with eyes closed while keeping quiet. The IEEG was the same as **d**

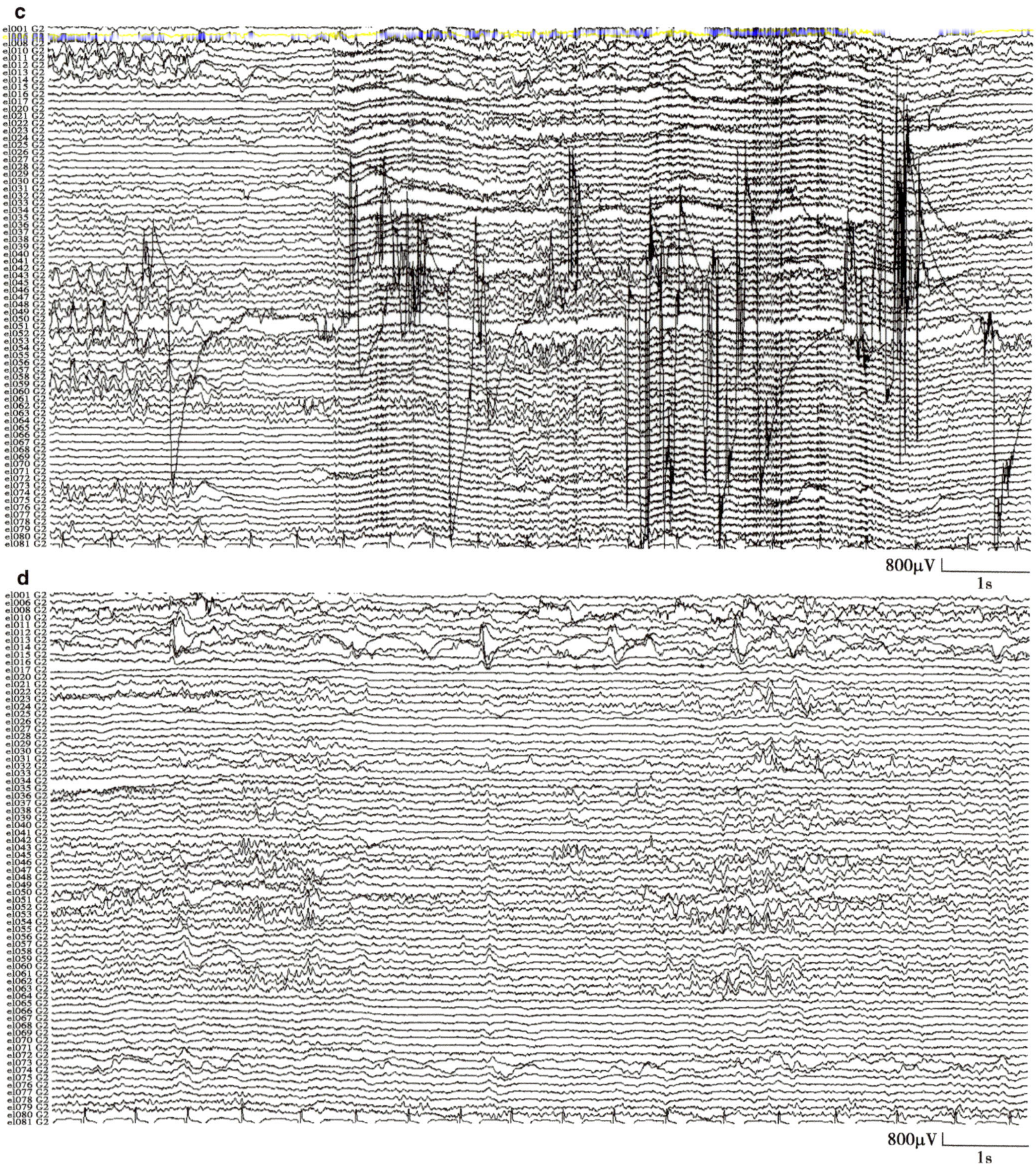

Fig. 2.54 (continued)

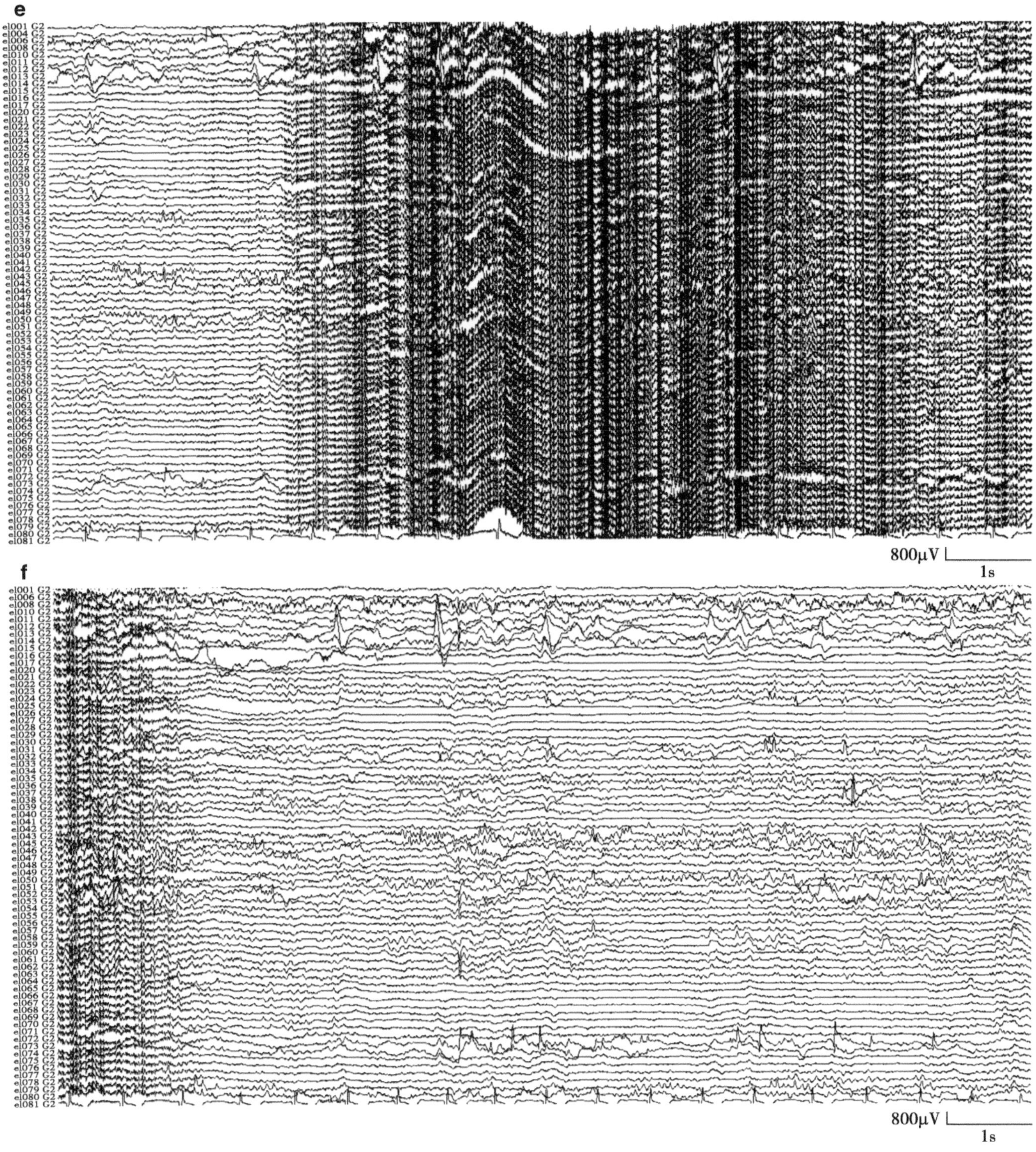

Fig. 2.54 (continued)

Cases of Basis Frontalis Epilepsy

Case 2.12 Orbitofrontal Epilepsy

[Abstract of Medical Records]
Female, 8 years old.

1. *Chief complaint* Episodic loss of consciousness for 7 years.
2. *History of present illness* The patient had episodic loss of consciousness with the movements of tonic limb 7 years ago. The patient felt discomfort in abdomen and felt suffocated for a few seconds to 1 min before the seizure, and failed to answer questions in most cases during the seizure, with the flexion of both upper limbs. One or both of her lower limbs sometimes were abducted or flexed without clonus. The patient often felt tired after the seizure occurred, which resolved in about 10 min. Sometimes the patient smack lips after the seizure. In the early stage of the disease, the patient had one seizure per day; in the past 1 year, the patient had frequent seizures, with about 10 seizures per day. Since the onset of the disease, the patient has been taking various drugs such as sodium valproate, lamotrigine, and topiramate successively. In the past year, she has been treated with sodium valproate at a dose of 200 mg/dose b.i.d. and oxcarbazepine at a dose of 150 mg b.i.d., with unfavorable response. At present, she has poorer intelligence than her peers, a good appetite, and normal bladder and bowel function.
3. *Past history* The patient was delivered at full term, with normal motor, language, and intellectual development.
4. *Personal and family history* No history of associated diseases.
5. *Physical examination* The patient was conscious and had poor cortical functions, especially in terms of computing power. No other positive neurological signs were observed. Psychological assessment: VIQ = 55, PIQ = 35, FIQ = 39
6. *Imaging examination*
   (a) MRI showed abnormal signals over the left frontal lobe.
   (b) MRS showed that the NAA concentration over the left hippocampus (NAA/Cr: 1.31) was slightly lower than the corresponding part on the right (NAA/Cr: 1.36). The CHO concentration over the left hippocampus (CHO/Cr: 1.26) was slightly higher than the corresponding part on the right (CHO/Cr: 1.12).
   (c) SPECT showed that the volume of the left temporal lobe was smaller and the perfusion was significantly reduced compared to the contralateral side, and the cortical perfusion over the left frontal lobe (inferior frontal gyrus) was reduced.
7. *EEG* For details, see Figs. 2.55, 2.56, 2.57, 2.58, and 2.59.

[Case Review]

1. Case Characteristics
   (a) *Seizure characteristics* ① Cluster seizures. ② Irregular swaying and extension and flexion movements of both lower limbs. ③ Oropharyngeal automatisms after seizures. ④ Without aura.
   (b) *EEG characteristics* ① Interictal EEG showed sharp waves/spikes and slow waves over the left frontal region, the central region, and the temporal region. ② Ictal EEG showed periodic-like sharp waves over the left frontal and temporal region at the beginning.
   (c) *Imaging characteristics* ① MRI showed abnormal signals over the left frontal lobe. ② SPECT showed that the volume of the left temporal lobe was smaller and the perfusion was significantly reduced compared to the contralateral side, and the cortical perfusion over the left frontal lobe (inferior frontal gyrus) was reduced.
2. *Diagnosis and treatment strategy and follow-up results* The patient's MRI showed clear abnormal signals over the left frontal lobe, and the interictal and ictal EEGs both showed discharges over the left frontal and temporal regions; SPECT showed reduced cortical perfusion over the left inferior frontal gyrus. According to these information, it was considered that the epileptic focus was located over the left frontal lobe. A strip electrode was placed over the temporal lobe because of oropharyngeal automatism during the late ictal phase. Interictal IEEG showed extensive abnormal discharges, especially over the frontal lobe; the ictal IEEG showed that the seizure origin was extensively located over the left orbitofrontal region and dorsolateral frontal cortex. The left middle and inferior frontal gyrus and orbitofrontal region were resected. The surgical result was satisfactory because the seizure origin shown by the IEEG and the sites of the left frontal lobe with abnormal signals revealed by MRI were completely resected by the operation. After the surgery, the patient was seizure-free during a 3-year follow-up.

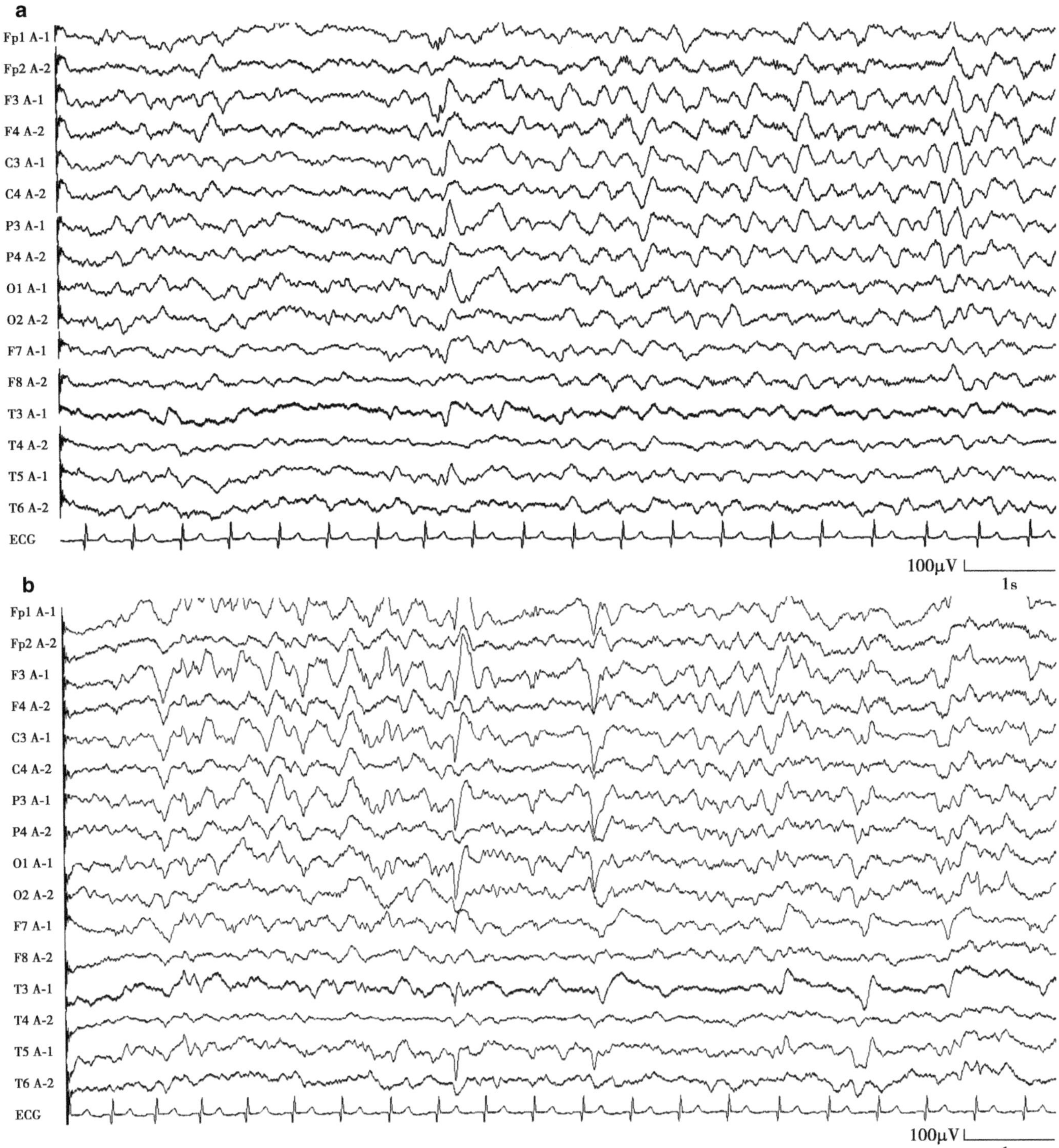

Fig. 2.55 Interictal scalp EEG. (**a**) The EEG was the background EEG of stage I of sleep and many 3.0–4.0 Hz slow waves of medium and high amplitude. Spikes of low amplitude were occasionally observed over the left hemisphere, especially over the left frontal region (Fp1 and F3). (**b**) The EEG was the background EEG of stage I of sleep, and showed irregular slow waves of high amplitude over the left frontal region (Fp1, F3), the central region (C3), the parietal region (P3), and the occipital region (O1), and positive spikes over the left caused by the activation of ear lobe electrode. (**c**) The EEG was the background EEG during the period of wakefulness, and showed sharp waves of medium and high amplitude over the left frontal region (Fp1 F3) and the temporal region (F7 T3, T3 T5, T5 O1). (**d**) The EEG was presented as the background EEG of stage II of sleep, and showed spikes of medium and high amplitude over the left frontal region (Fp1 F3), the central region (F3 C3, C3 P3), the temporal region (F7 T3, T3 T5, T5 O1) and the midline (Fpz Fz, Fz Cz)

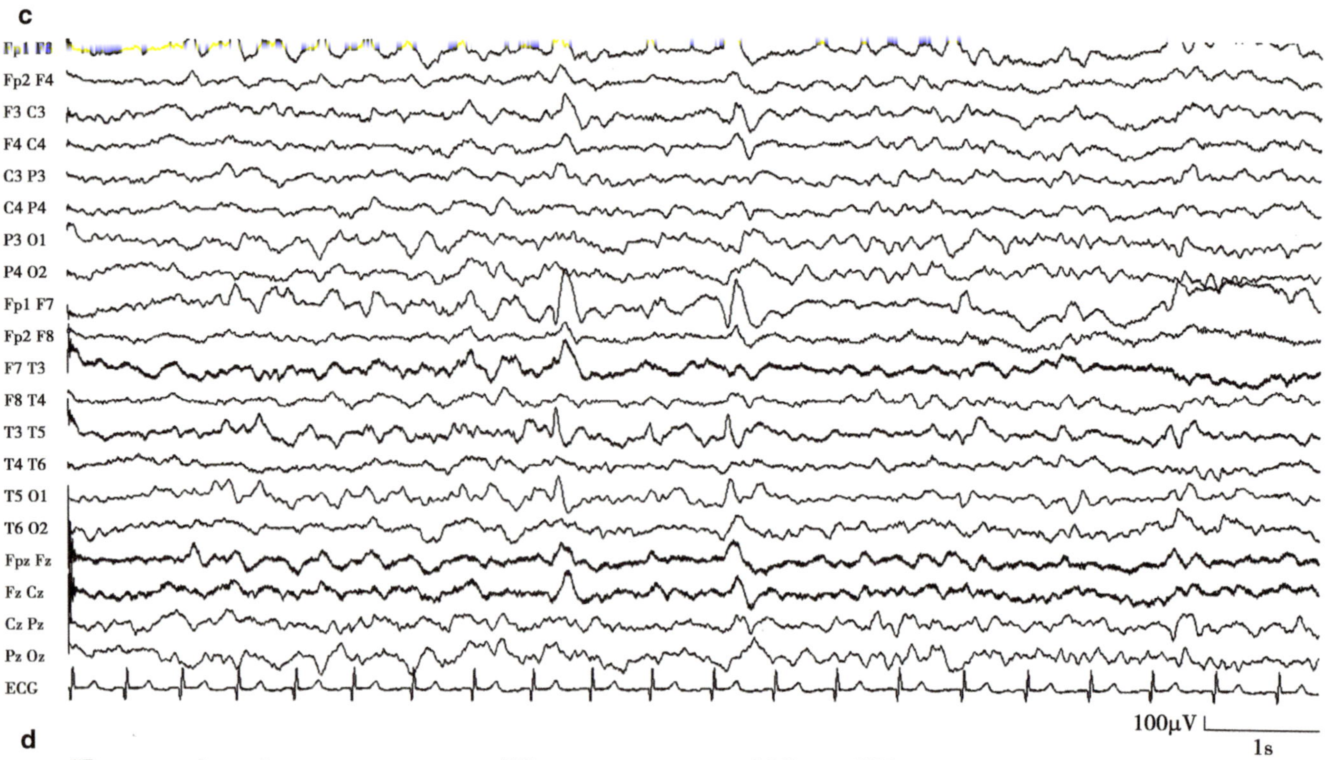

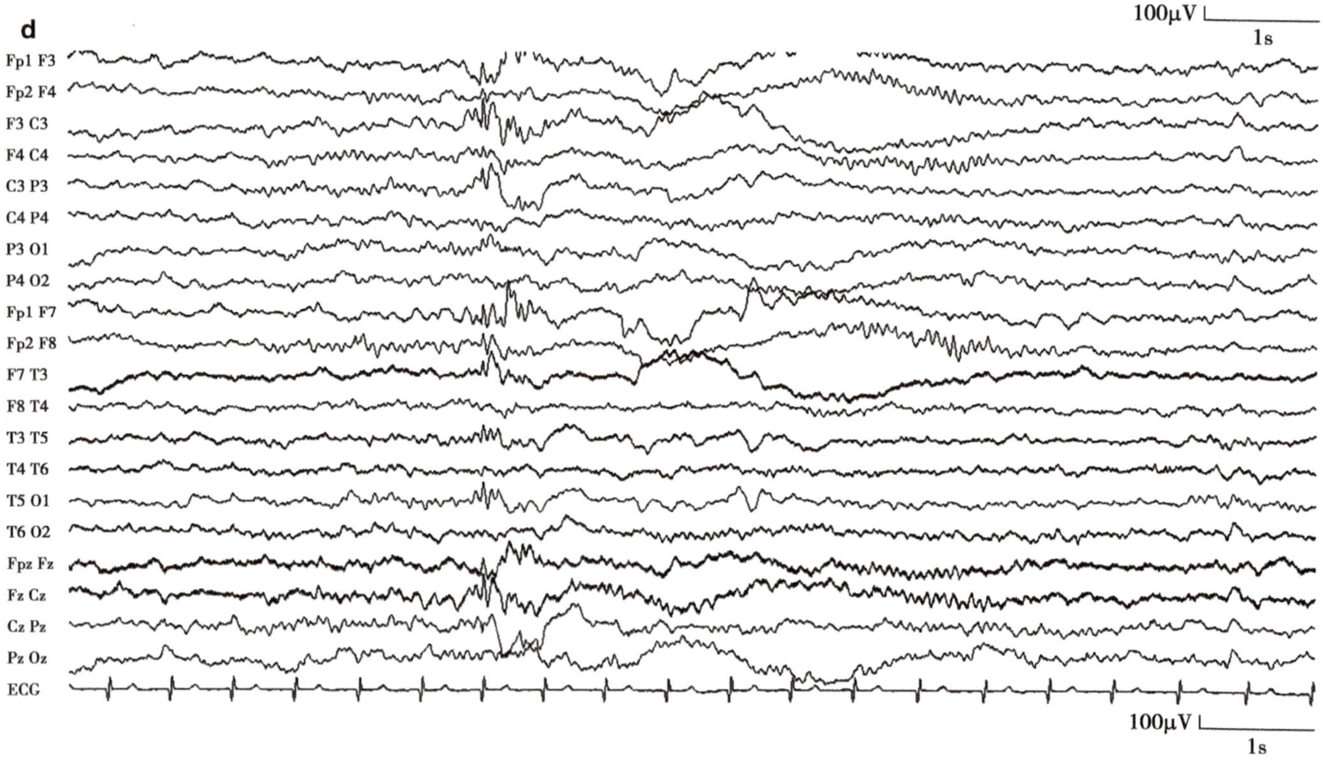

Fig. 2.55 (continued)

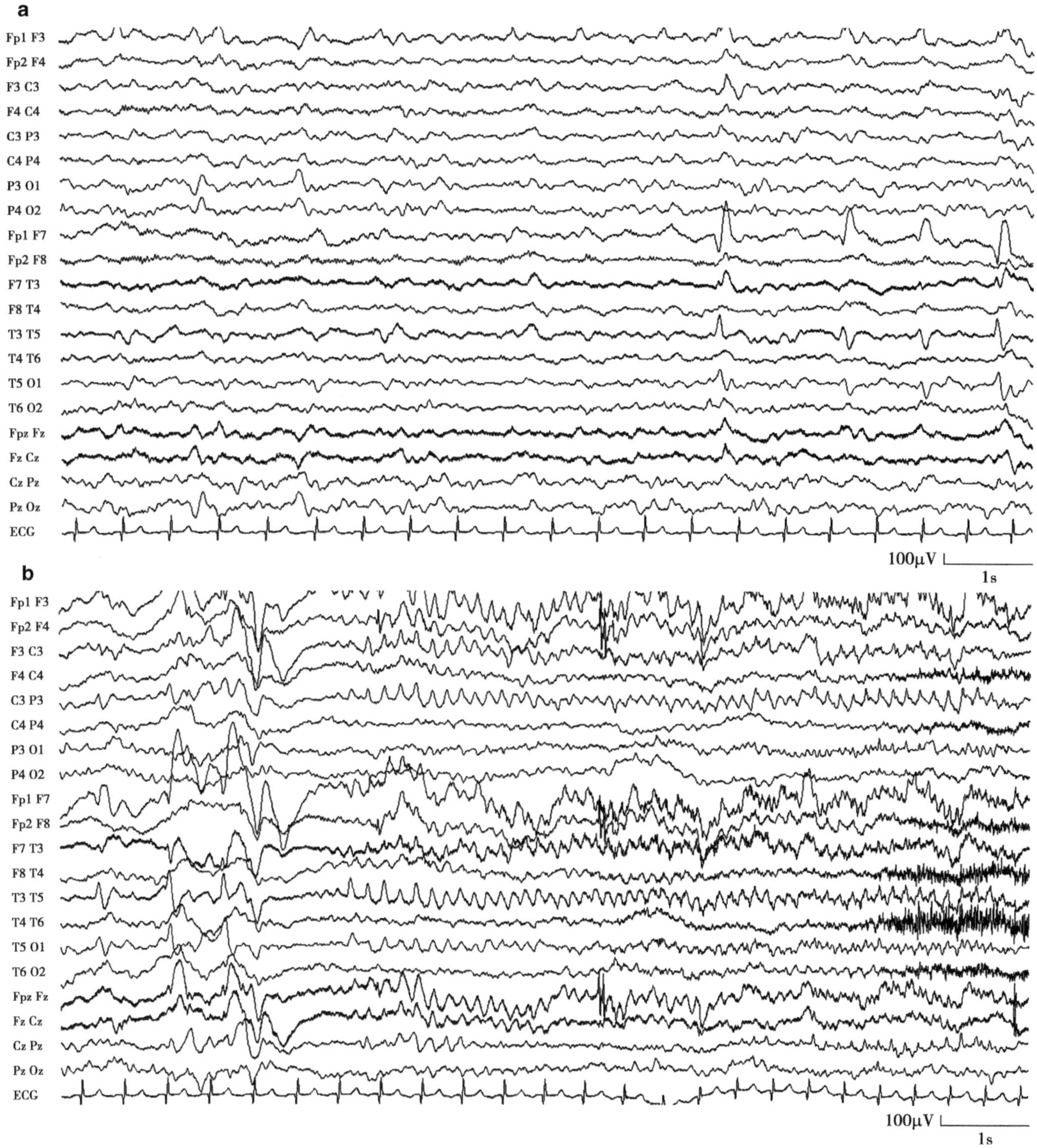

Fig. 2.56 Ictal scalp EEG. (**a**) The patient was asleep 15 s before the seizure. The background EEG of stage II of sleep showed periodic-like sharp waves of medium and high amplitude over the left frontal region (Fp1 F3, Fp1 F7) and the temporal region (F7 T3, T3 T5, T5 O1). (**b**) During the seizure, the patient opened his eyes and slightly raised her head. The EEG showed the rhythm of sharp waves of medium amplitude over the left frontal region (Fp1 F3, Fp1 F7), the central region (F3 C3, C3 P3), the temporal region (F7 T3, T3 T5, T5 O1), and the midline (Fpz Fz, Fz Cz) (**c**) The patient had irregular swaying and extension and flexion movements of both lower limbs without tonic convulsion of the limbs, and failed to answer questions. The EEG showed that each lead had flat waves of low amplitude, and electrode wobble artifact over the left frontal pole; 5.0–6.0 Hz irregular slow waves of medium and high amplitude were observed over the left frontal region (Fp1 F3, Fpz Fz) about 8 s later; in addition, EMG artifacts were observed especially over the bilateral temporal regions. (**d**) The seizure ended. The IEEG recovered to the background EEG

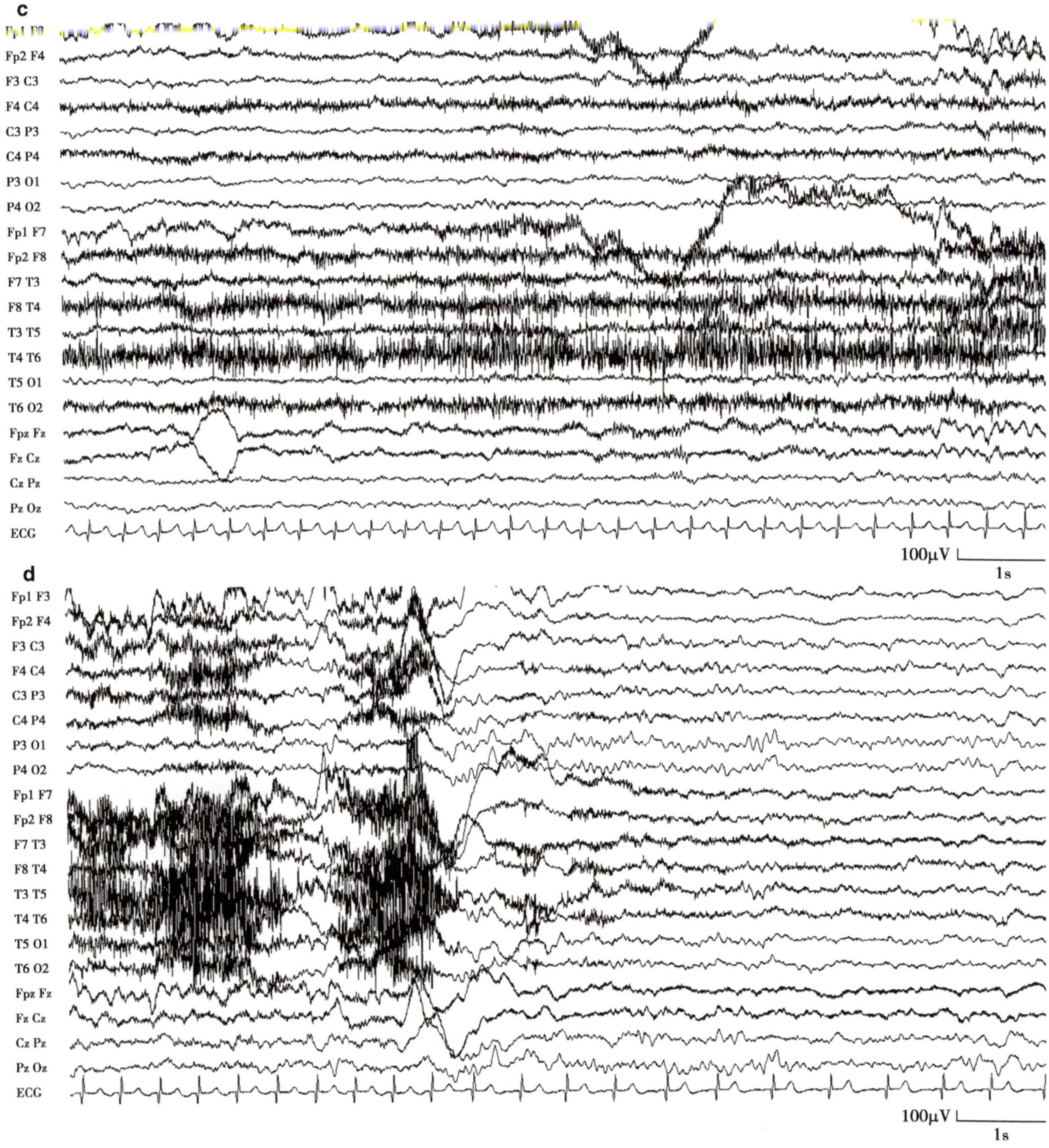

Fig. 2.56 (continued)

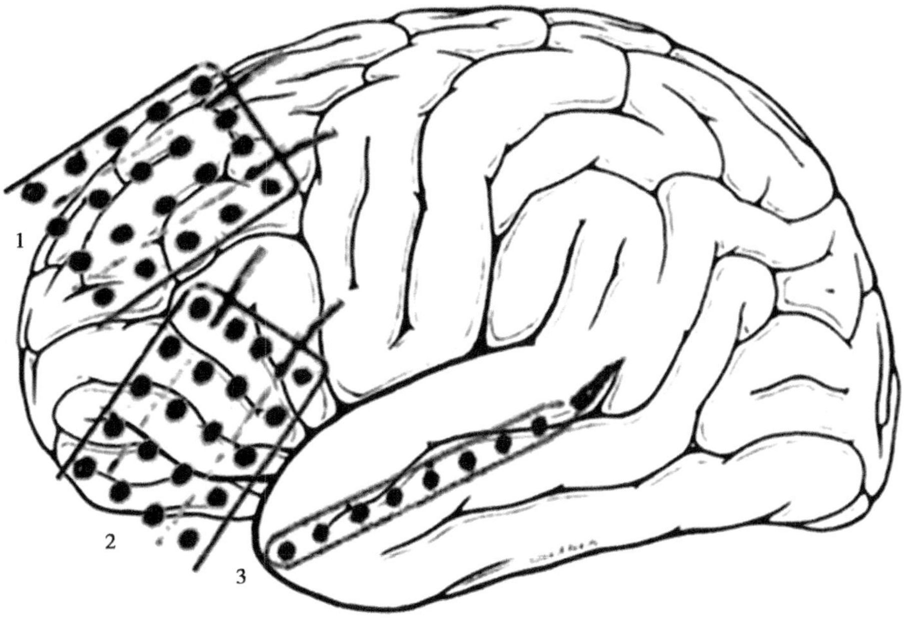

Fig. 2.57 Scheme of intracranial electrodes
Grid electrode 1: the left lateral frontal region (20 contacts); Grid electrode 2: the left orbitofrontal region (20 contacts); Strip electrode 3: the left temporal pole (8 contacts)

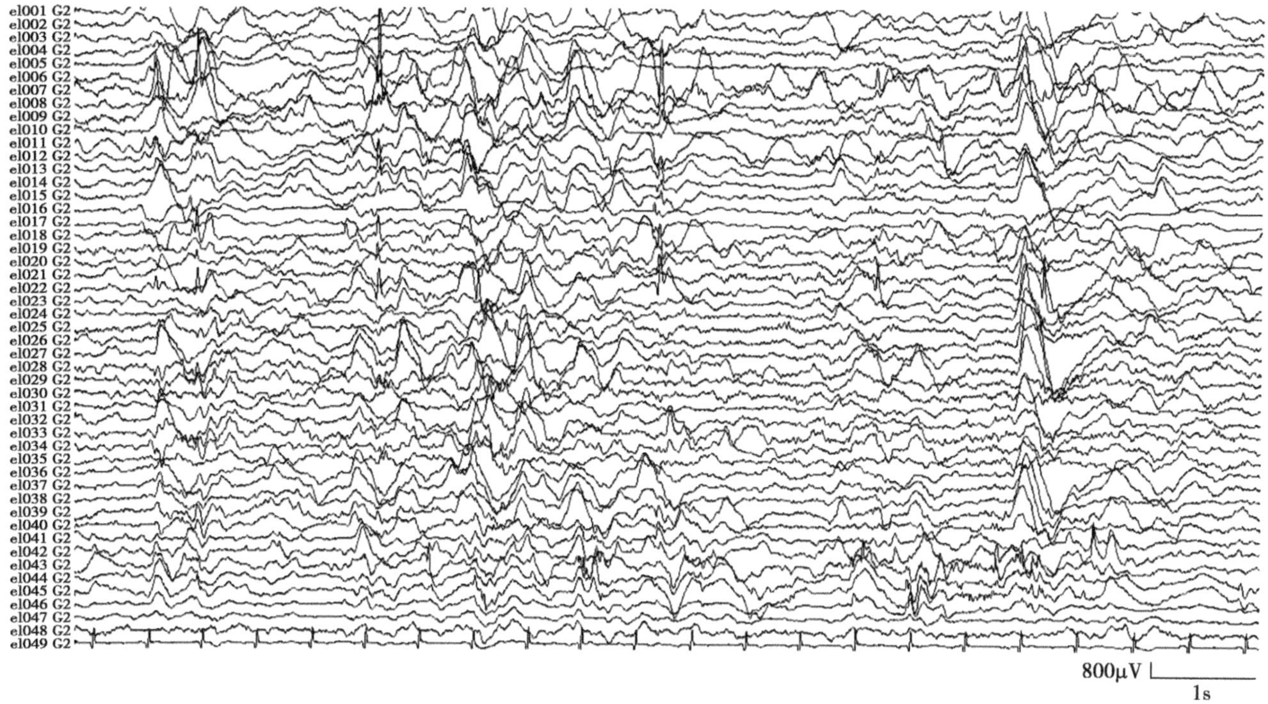

Fig. 2.58 Interictal intracranial EEG
Frequent spikes of high amplitude, spike-and-wave complexes, and slow waves were observed over the left lateral frontal region (contact numbers el006, el007, el008, el009, el011, el012, el013, el014, el015, el018, el019, el020), the orbitofrontal region (contact numbers el022, el027, el028, el029, el031, el032, el033, el034, el037, el038, el039, el040); and spikes of medium and high amplitude and the low amplitude fast activity were observed over the left temporal pole (contact numbers el042, el043, el044, el045, el046)

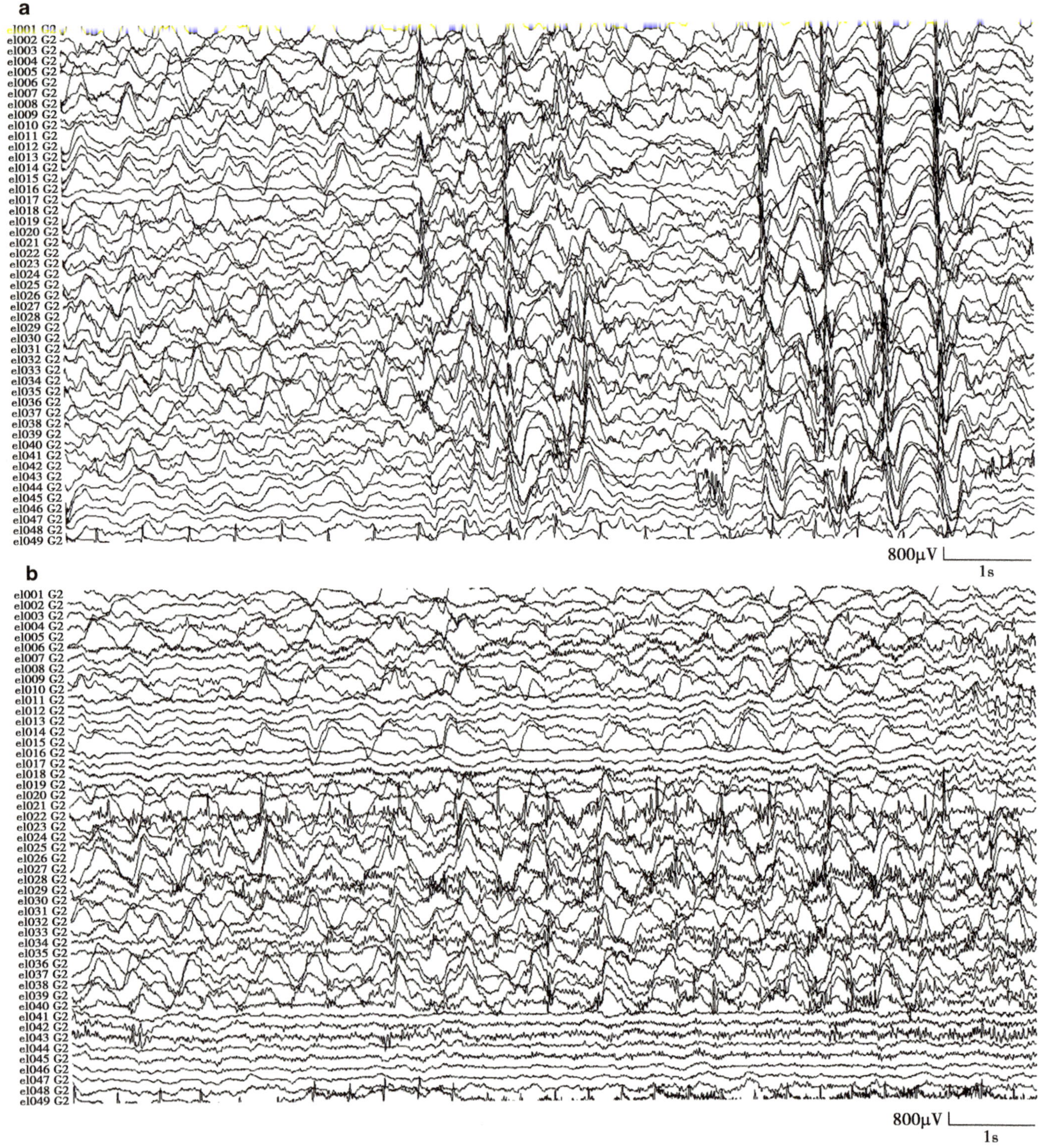

Fig. 2.59 Ictal EEG of intracranial electrodes. (**a**) Before the seizure, the patient was sleeping in the position of right lateral decubitus. The IEEG showed polyspike-and-wave complexes of high amplitude that were emitted rhythmically over the left lateral frontal region (contact numbers el006, el007, el008, el011, el012, el013, el014, el018, el019, el020), the orbitofrontal region (contact numbers el021, el022, el023, el024, el026, el027, el028, el029, el030, el033, el034, el035, el036, el037, el038), and the temporal pole (contact numbers el042, el043, el044, el045, el046). (**b**) During the seizure, the patient grasped the bed rail with the left hand, swayed slightly at the hip, and dorsiflexed both feet. The IEEG showed the low amplitude fast activity over the left lateral frontal region (contact numbers el006, el007, el018) and the temporal pole (contact numbers el042 and el043), and the rhythms of polyspike-and-wave complexes and low amplitude fast activity over the orbitofrontal region (contact numbers el021, el022, el026, el027, el028, el029, el032, el033, el034, el037, el038, el039, el040). (**c**) The patient still grasped the bed rail with his left hand, and his feet were dorsiflexed and shaken, which ended after about 6 s. The IEEG showed the rhythm of spikes of high amplitude over the left lateral frontal region (contact numbers el006, el007, el008, el011, el012, el013, el018) and the orbitofrontal region (contact numbers el021, el022, el026, el027, el038, el039, el040), and the low amplitude fast activity over the temporal pole (contact numbers el042 and el043). (**d**) The seizure ended. The IEEG showed the rhythm of slow waves of extremely high amplitude over the frontal region

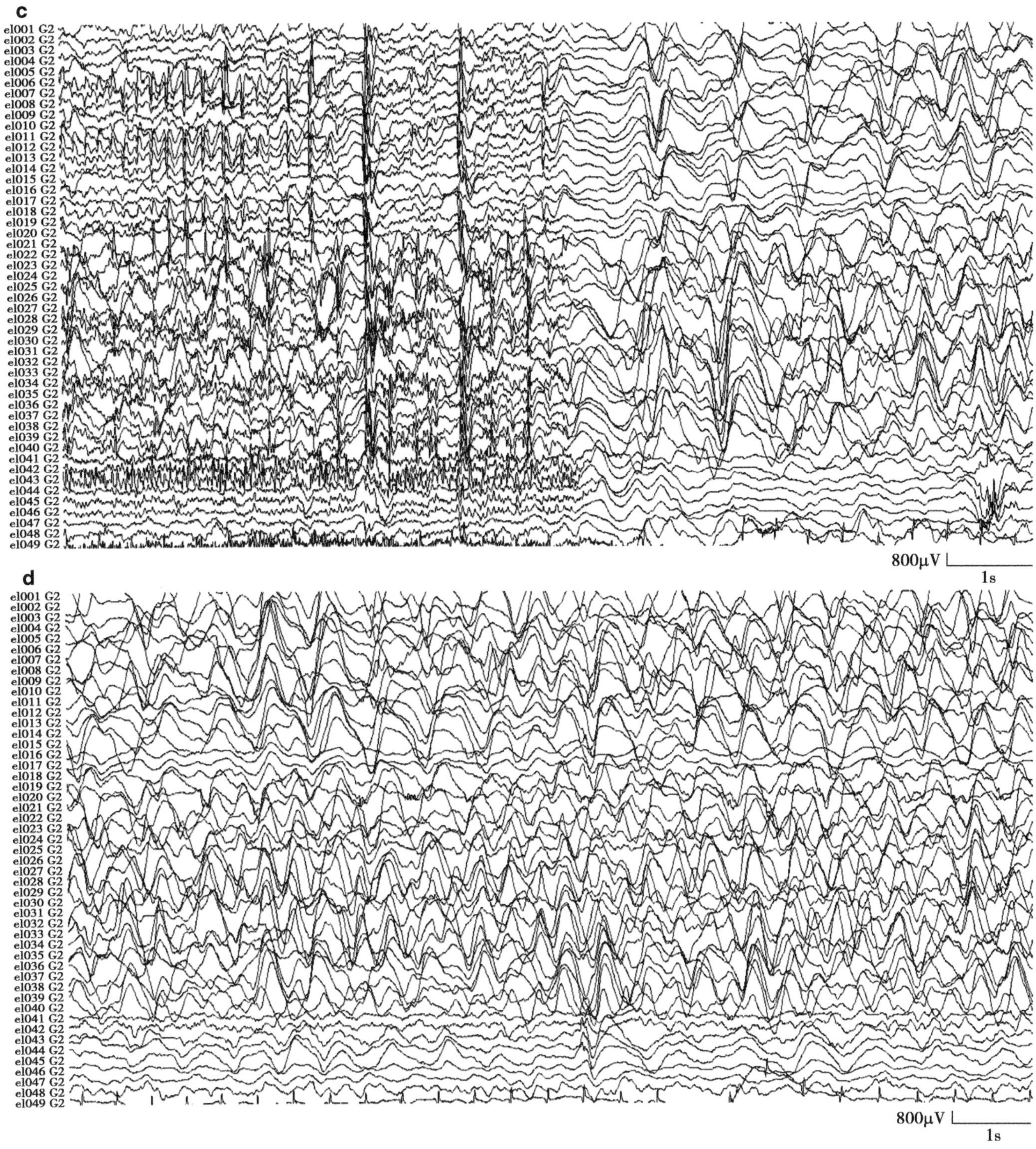

Fig. 2.59 (continued)

Case 2.13 Orbitofrontal Epilepsy

[Abstract of Medical Records]
Male, 8 years old.

1. *Chief complaint* Episodic unconsciousness for more than 2 years.
2. *History of present illness* The patient had episodic unconsciousness 2 years before admission, which were characterized by staring eyes, failure to answer questions, frightened expression, grasping of surrounding objects with both hands, straightening of the legs, and "grunting," which lasted for about half a minute and then resolved. All of the symptoms described above occurred during sleep, without aura before the seizure. The patient fell asleep after the seizure occurred. The frequency of seizures was more than 10 times a month, with no other types of seizures. He had taken multiple antiseizure medications orally while feeling the effect was poor. He is now taking carbamazepine at a dose of 200 mg t.i.d., topiramate at a dose of 75 mg b.i.d., and valproate at a dose of 250 mg t.i.d.
3. *Past history* The patient was delivered at full term and normally grew up, with no history of febrile convulsions and no family history.
4. *Physical examination* The patient has poor cognitive functions but no other positive signs in the rest of the neurological examinations.
5. *Imaging examination*
   (a) MRI showed no abnormalities.
   (b) MRS revealed that the NAA concentration (NAA/Cr: 1.33) over the left hippocampus was higher than that over the right side (NAA/Cr: 1.05); the Cho concentration (Cho/Cr: 1.07) over the left hippocampus was slightly higher than that over the right side (Cho/Cr: 1.05).
   (c) SPECT revealed diffuse hypoperfusion over the cortices of the left cerebral and cerebellar hemispheres.
6. *EEG* For details, see Figs. 2.60, 2.61, 2.62, 2.63, and 2.64.

[Case Review]

1. *Case Characteristics*
   (a) *Seizure characteristics* ① Seizures often occurred during sleep mainly characterized by hyperkinetic automatisms. ② The patient had panic expressions. ③ There was no aura before the seizure. ④ There was no information on the side of the seizure symptoms.
   (b) *EEG characteristics* ① Interictal EEG showed spikes, spike-and-wave complexes, and slow waves over the left frontal region, the central region, and the anterior temporal region. ② Ictal EEG showed spikes and rhythmic spike-and-wave complexes in relevant leads over the left frontal region and the temporal region.
   (c) *Imaging characteristics* MRI showed no obvious abnormalities.
2. *Diagnosis and treatment strategy and follow-up results* According to the patient's seizure symptoms and the interictal and ictal EEGs, the seizure focus was considered to be located in the frontal lobe. Since the EEG showed frequent spikes and rhythmic spikes over the left sphenoid, a piece of electrode was also implanted in the temporal lobe. The interictal IEEG showed significantly abnormal discharges over the left middle and inferior frontal gyrus; the ictal IEEG showed rhythmic spikes over the anterior part of the left inferior frontal gyrus, indicating clear seizure origin. The left middle and inferior frontal gyrus and orbitofrontal region were resected. After the surgery, the patient had only two seizures during a 1-year follow-up. The postoperative outcome was satisfactory because of the near complete resection of the epileptic focus. It should be noticed that the discharges collected by the electrode over the sphenoid do not only originate from the temporal lobe, but can also originate from the inferior frontal cortex or the lateral orbitofrontal region.

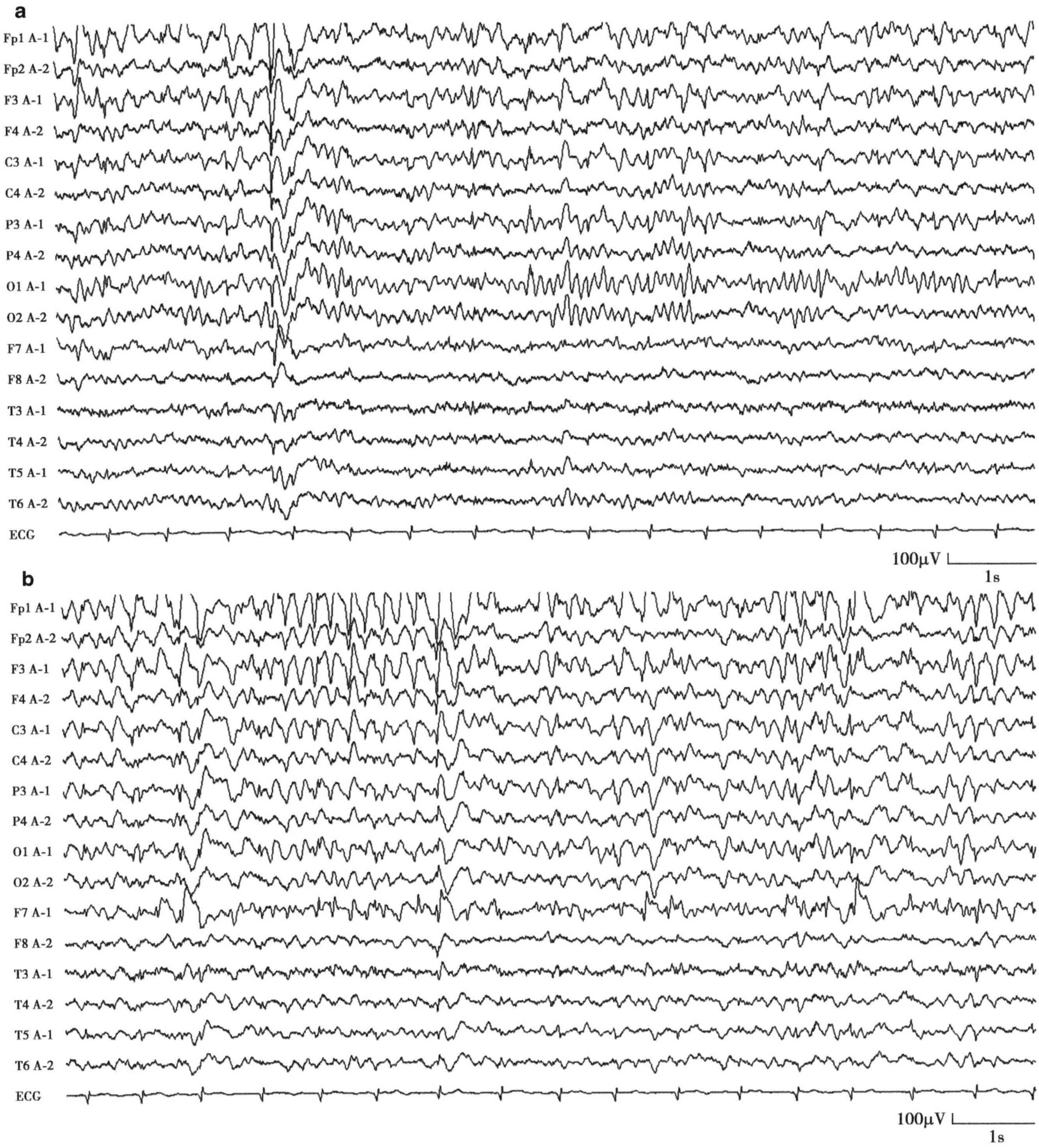

Fig. 2.60 Interictal scalp EEG. (**a**) The EEG showed a basic rhythm of 8.0 Hz, mixed with many 4.0–6.0 Hz slow waves of medium and high amplitude, especially over the left frontal region (Fp1, F3). Positive spikes due to the activation of ear lobe electrode were over the left leads. (**b**) Paroxysmal 4.0–5.0 Hz slow waves and spike-and-wave complexes were observed, especially over the left frontal region (Fp1, F3). (**c**) Persistent spikes of high amplitude were observed over the left sphenoid (Sph-L) and the left anterior temporal region (F7), which were phase-inverted; slow waves of high amplitude and sharp waves were observed over the left frontal region (Fp1 F3) and the central region (F3 C3)

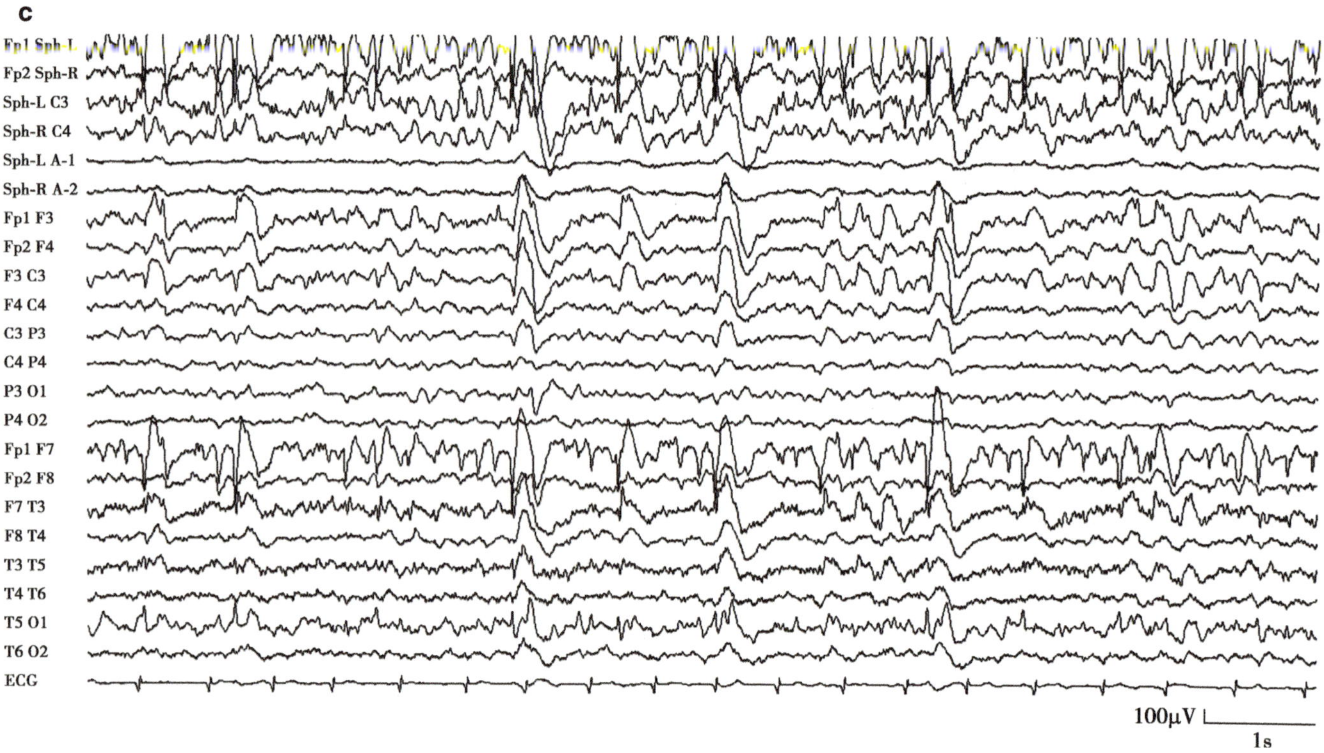

Fig. 2.60 (continued)

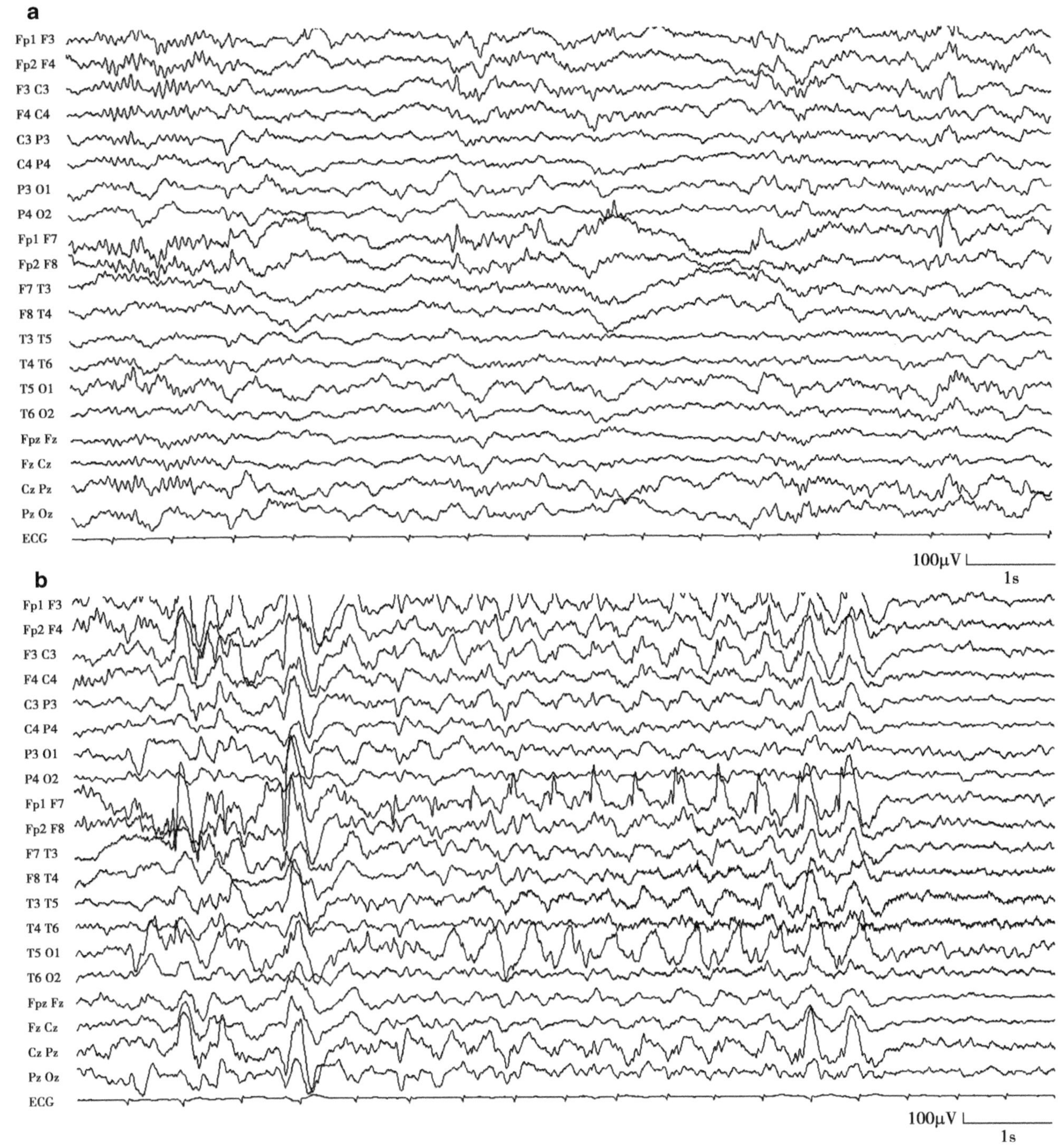

Fig. 2.61 Ictal scalp EEG. (**a**) Before the seizure, the patient was sleeping in a supine position. The EEG was the background EEG of stage II of sleep, and showed many spikes over the leads over the left frontal region (Fp1 F7). (**b**) At the time of seizure, the patient's body was turned to the left in lateral decubitus. The EEG showed rhythmic slow waves of medium and high amplitude and spike-and-slow-wave complexes over the left frontal region (Fp1 F3, Fp1 F7, F3 C3), the temporal region (T5 O1), and the midline (Cz Pz) in addition to the background EEG when the patient was asleep, especially over Fp1 F7. (**c**, **d**) About 8 s later, the patient continued to turn his body left in a prone position, with body twisting and stomping movements of both lower limbs. The EEG showed rhythmic 1.5–2.0 Hz spike-and-wave complexes of medium and high amplitude over the left frontal region (Fp1 F3, F3 C3), frontal and temporal region (Fp1 F7, T3 T5, T5 O1), and the midline (Cz Pz). (**e**, **f**) The patient sat up, grasped the bed rail with both hands, swayed back and forth, and failed to answer questions. The EEG showed that the wave amplitude of each lead was lower than before, and the emission of sharp waves of low and medium amplitude over the left frontal region (Fp1 F3, Fp1 F7, F3 C3), the central region (C3 P3), and the anterior temporal region (F7 T3); the left frontal region (Fp1 F3, Fp1 F7) were mixed with many EMG artifacts. (**g**) The patient sat up, grasped the bed rail with both hands, swayed back and forth, and failed to answer questions. The EEG showed that the wave amplitude of each lead was lower than before, and the sharp waves of low and medium amplitude over the left frontal region (Fp1 F3, Fp1 F7, F3 C3), the central region (C3 P3), and the anterior temporal region (F7 T3); the leads over the left frontal region (Fp1 F3, Fp1 F7) were mixed with many EMG artifacts. (**h**) At the end of the seizure, the patient lay down again and recovered his consciousness. The EEG gradually recovered to the background EEG when the patient was awake

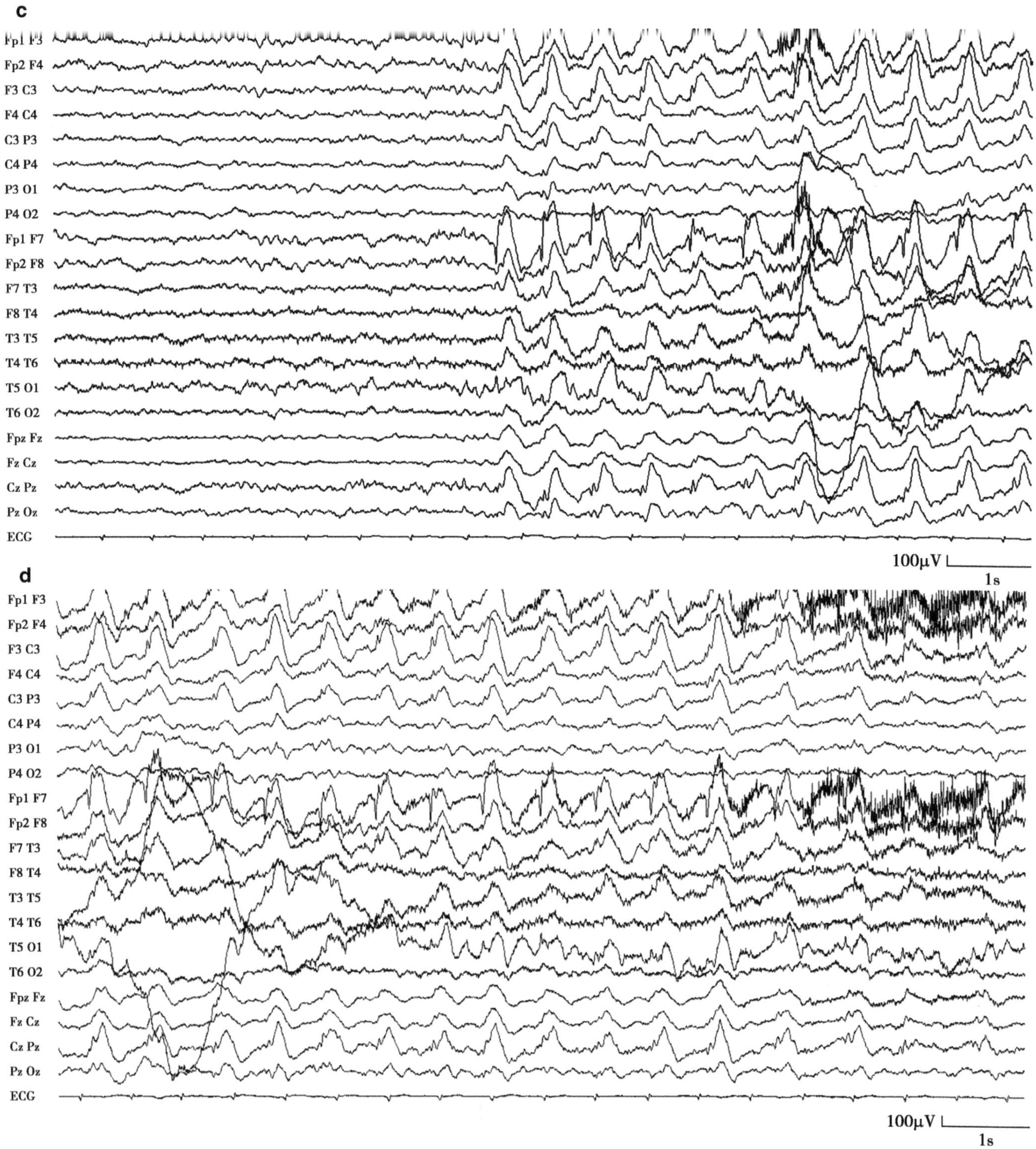

Fig. 2.61 (continued)

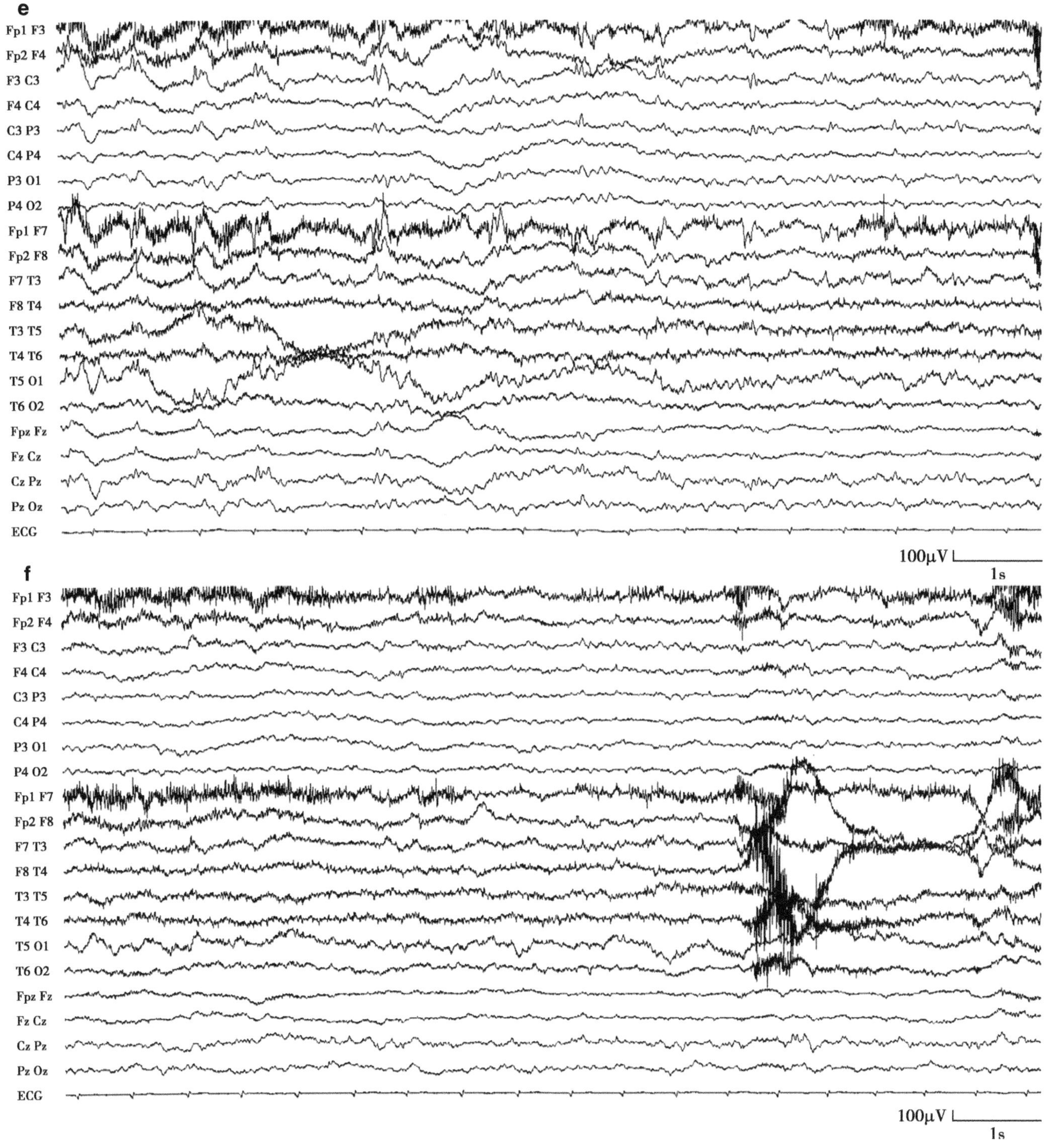

Fig. 2.61 (continued)

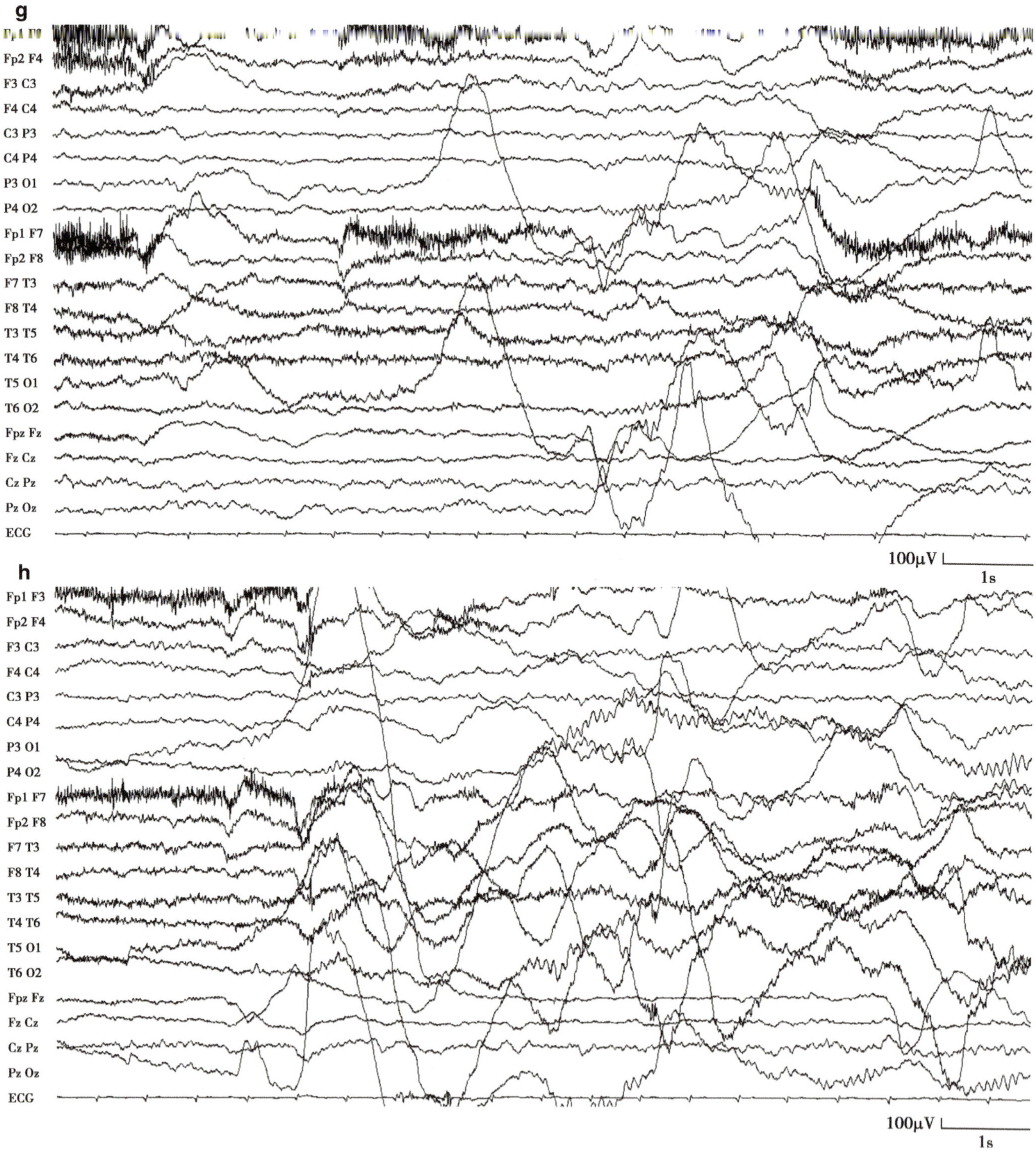

Fig. 2.61 (continued)

Fig. 2.62 Scheme of intracranial electrodes
Grid electrode 1: the left superior frontal gyrus (16 contacts); Grid electrode 2: the left middle and inferior frontal gyrus (32 contacts); Strip electrode 3: the temporal pole (16 contacts)

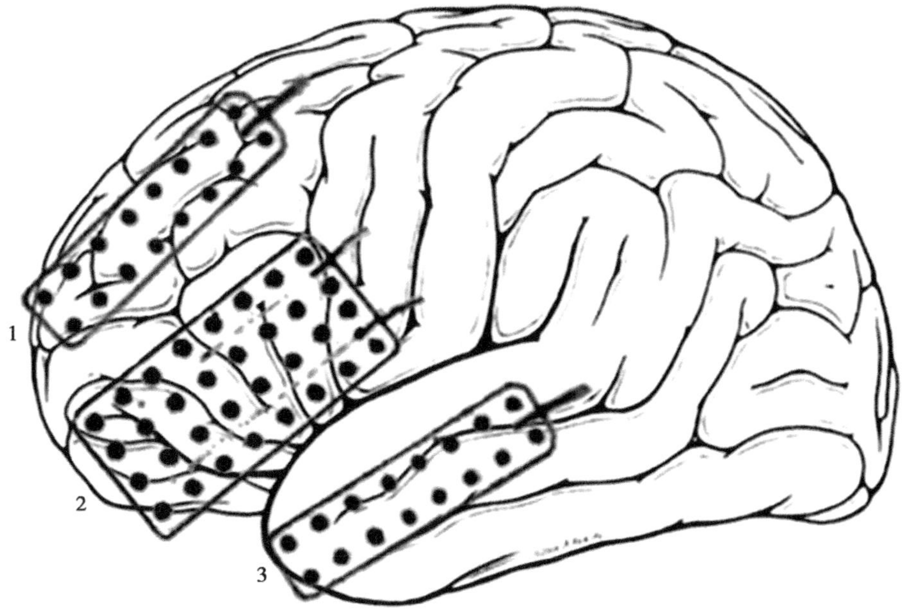

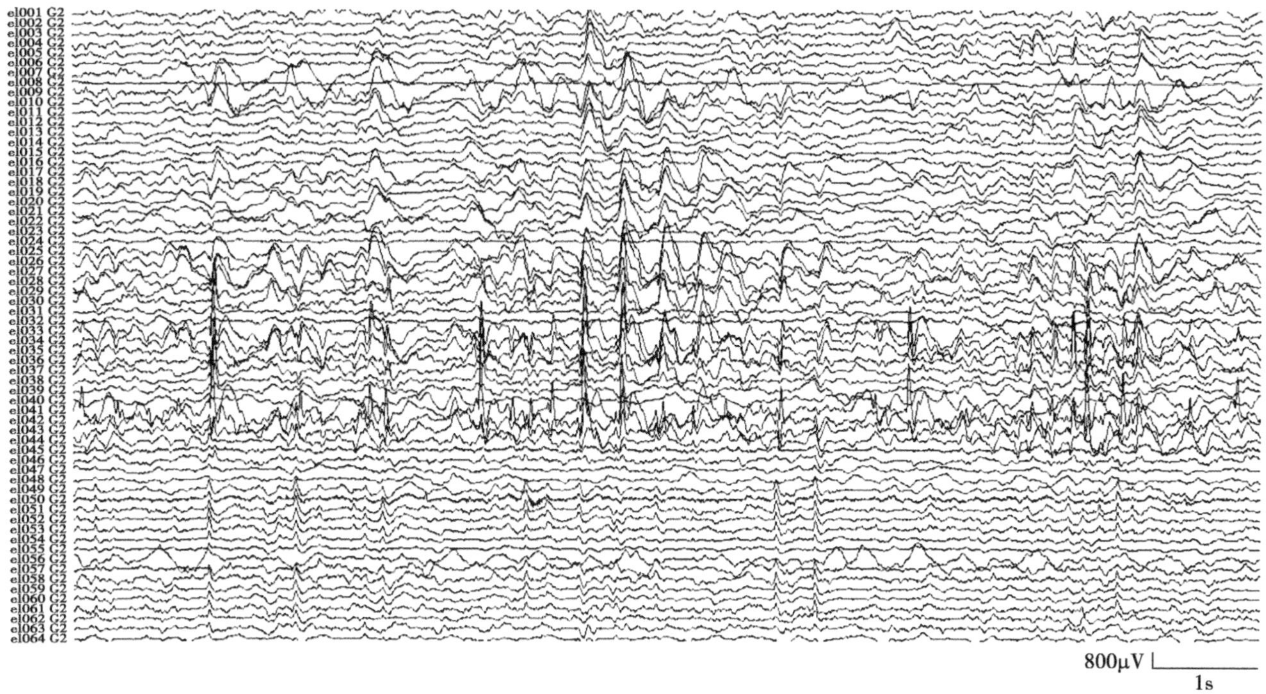

Fig. 2.63 Interictal intracranial EEG
The spike-and-wave complexes of high amplitude was often observed over the anterior part of the left middle and inferior frontal gyrus (contact numbers el025, el026, el027, el028, el029, el030, el033, el034, el035, el036, el041, el042, el043, el044)

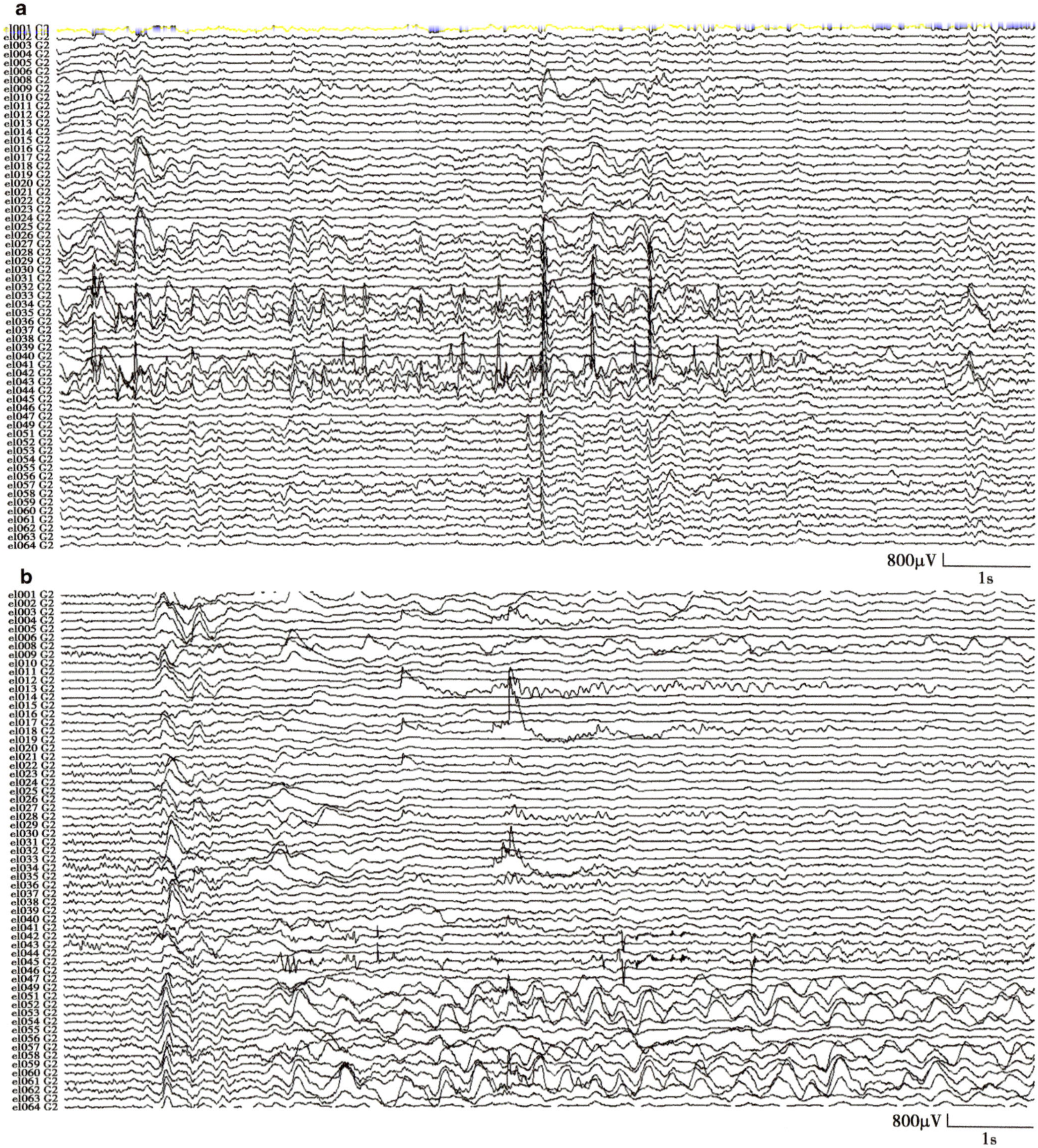

Fig. 2.64 Ictal EEG of intracranial electrodes. (**a**) The patient was asleep before the seizure. The IEEG showed rhythmic spikes over the left middle and inferior frontal gyrus (contact numbers el033, el034, el035, el041, el042, el043). (**b**) During the seizure, the patient suddenly sat up from the bed, turned his body slightly to the left, grasped clothes with both hands, and stomped on both lower limbs. The IEEG showed reduced electrical activity over the left frontal region and the rhythm of slow waves of high amplitude over the left temporal region (contact numbers el049, el051, el052, el053, el058, el059, el060, el061, el062). (**c**) With the help of his family members, the patient re-lay down but still fumbled and grasped clothes with both hands, repeatedly flexing and extending both lower limbs, turning both eyes to the left, and failed to answer questions. The IEEG showed the rhythms of fast activity of low amplitude, spikes and spike-and-wave complex with increasing amplitude over the left inferior frontal gyrus (contact numbers el034, el035, el036, el037, el041, el042, el043, el044). (**d**) The patient sat up slightly, crossed both lower limbs, swayed from side to side, and then lay down after about 7 s. The rhythm of slow waves of high amplitude was observed (especially over the prefrontal cortex) on the IEEG. (**e**) When the seizure was over, the patient could answer questions. The IEEG showed reducing wave amplitude of slow activities

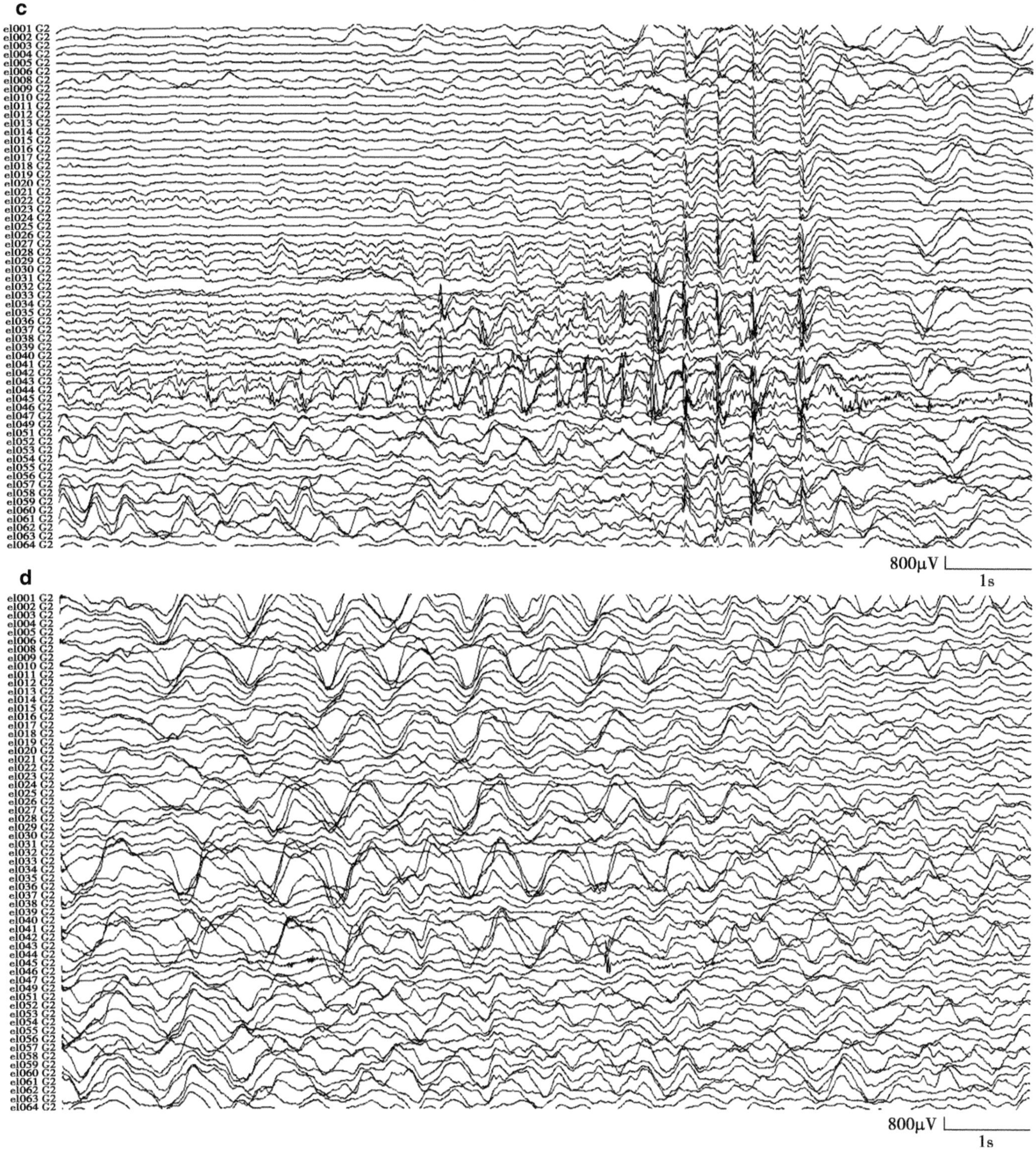

Fig. 2.64 (continued)

e

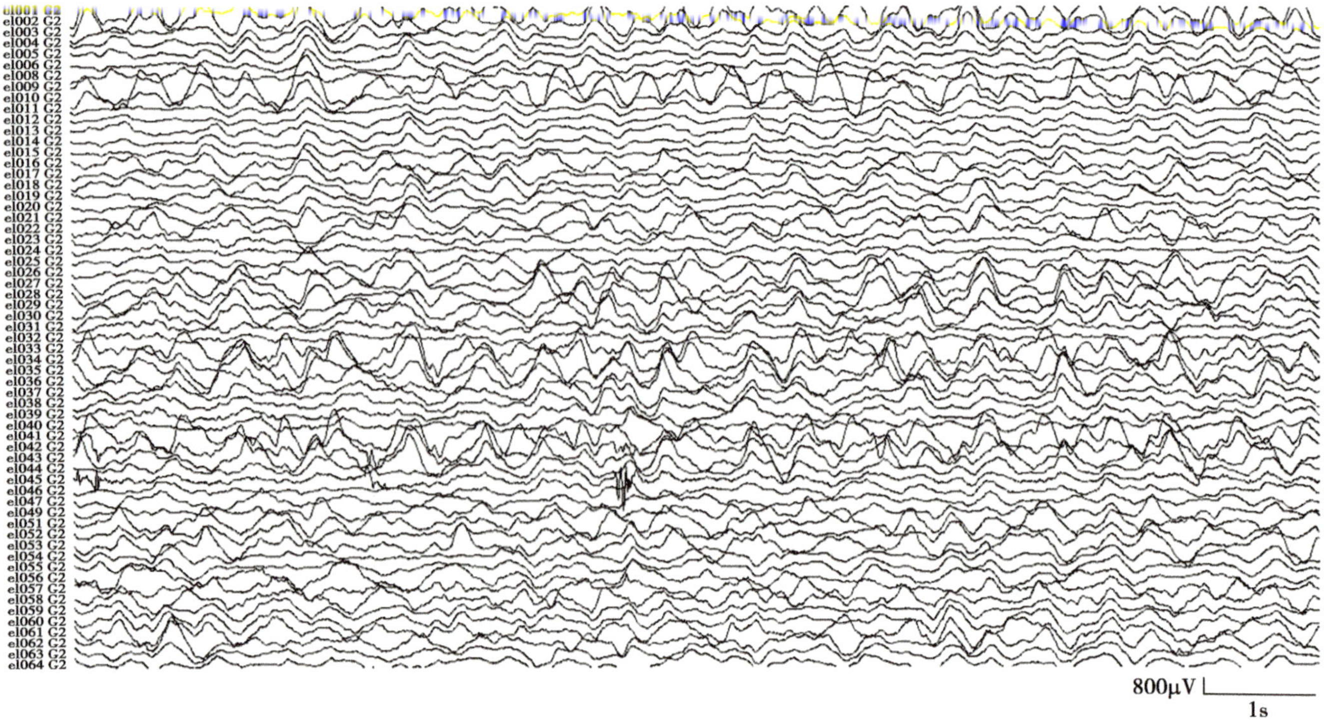

Fig. 2.64 (continued)

Case 2.14 Orbitofrontal Epilepsy

[Abstract of Medical Records]
Male, 37 years old.

1. *Chief complaint* The patient had recurrent episodes of unresponsiveness, limb movement, and speaking bestial words for 6 years.
2. *History of present illness* The patient suffered from a sudden onset of episodic nocturnal unresponsiveness without apparent cause 6 years ago, with wide-open eyes looking straight ahead, restless movements of the limbs, especially the upper limbs, and indiscriminate swearing, which lasted for about 5 s and then disappeared on its own. The symptoms of upturning of the eyeballs, clenched teeth, foaming at the mouth, and urinary and fecal incontinence were not observed. At that time, he did not go to the hospital nor take any medication for symptomatic treatment. Six months later, the abovementioned symptoms recurred during nighttime sleep. Seizures may occur both during daytime and nighttime sleep, each of which lasted for a few seconds to a few tens of seconds (usually no more than 1 min), and could occur 2–3 times a day. The interval between seizures was usually more than 10 days to 2 months, and the seizures were more likely to occur after exertion. After each seizure, there was a period of 2–3 min of unconsciousness before he was fully awake. He visited the hospital for many times and was diagnosed with epilepsy. After treatment with various antiseizure medications, the symptoms were effectively controlled. He is now taking sodium valproate and levetiracetam, but still has recurrent seizures.
3. *Past history* He has a history of hypertension.
4. *Personal and family history* No history of associated diseases.
5. *Imaging examination*
   (a) MRI showed abnormal signals over the right frontal lobe, and slightly larger left temporal angle of ventricles than the contralateral one.
   (b) MRS showed that the NAA concentration (NAA/Cr: 1.13) over the left hippocampus was lower than that over the right side (NAA/Cr: 1.48); the CHO concentration (Cho/Cr: 0.97) over the left hippocampus was slightly lower than that over the right side (NAA/Cr: 1.35).
   (c) SPECT showed that the perfusion over the right anterior temporal region was lower than the contralateral side; none of the local perfusion over the bilateral frontal cortices, the perfusion over the right basal ganglia, the perfusion over the left thalamus, and the perfusion over the right cerebellar hemisphere was satisfactory.
6. *EEG* For details, see Figs. 2.65, 2.66, 2.67, 2.68, and 2.69.

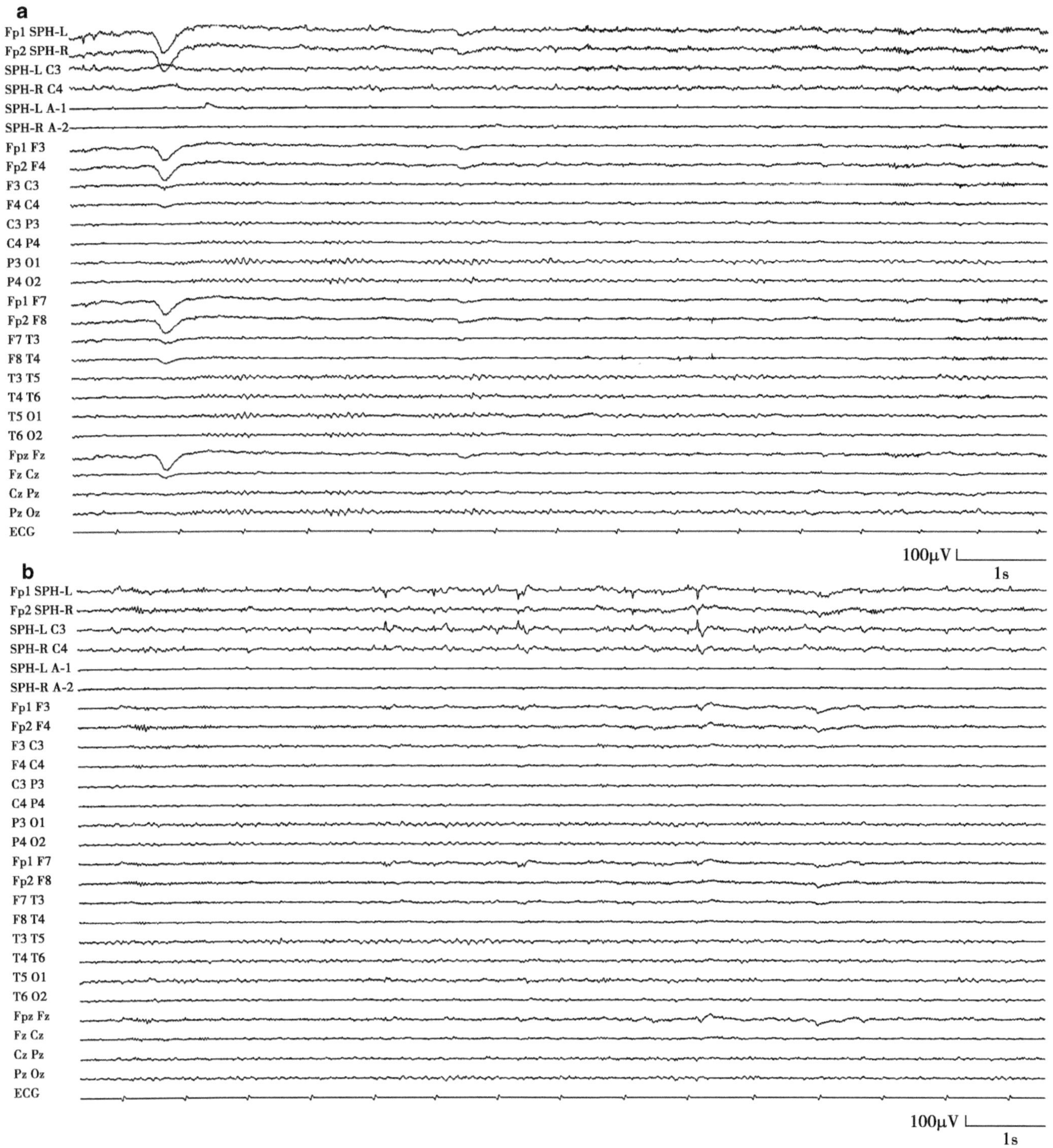

Fig. 2.65 Interictal scalp EEG. (**a**) The EEG had a basic rhythm of 11.0 Hz, and showed well formed α rhythms over the occipital cortex. (**b**) The patient was awake. The EEG had a basic rhythm of 11.0 Hz, and frequent sharp waves over the left sphenoid electrode. (**c**) The patient was asleep. The EEG showed bilaterally symmetrical peak waves and spindle waves, and phase-inverted sharp waves over the left sphenoid electrode

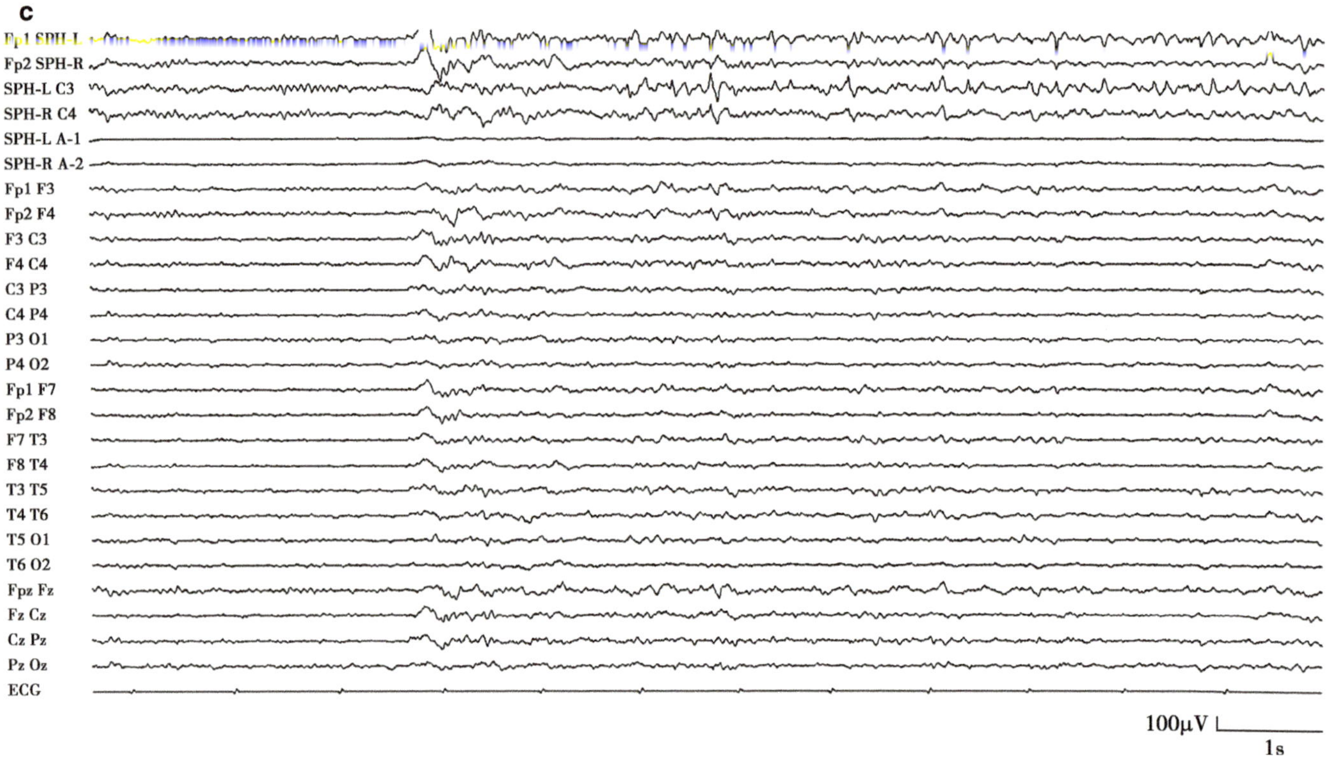

Fig. 2.65 (continued)

[Case Review]

1. Case Characteristics
   (a) *Seizure characteristics* ① The seizures occurred mostly at night. ② The seizures were brief. ③ The seizures are clustered (2–3 times a day). ④ Hyperactive automatism (kicking of both lower limbs, body twisting, repeated lifting of the hips off the bed) occurred during seizures. ⑤ The seizures were with vocalization (head clonus while speaking bestial words). ⑥ Consciousness was soon recovered after seizures. All of the above seizure characteristics were consistent with the characteristics of frontal lobe seizure, but the seizure symptoms did not suggest information on the side.
   (b) *EEG characteristics* ① Interictal EEG showed sharp waves over the left sphenoid electrode. ② Interictal EEG showed the low-voltage fast activity over all leads.
   (c) *Imaging characteristics* ① MRI showed abnormal signals over the right frontal lobe.
2. *Diagnosis and treatment strategy and follow-up results* The patient's seizure symptoms were not completely consistent with the sites of abnormal signals on the MRI, nor the manifestations of MEG and MRI were consistent. Therefore, it was considered to implant intracranial electrodes bilaterally to clarify the side. The sites covered by symptom related electrodes mainly included frontal pole, orbitofrontal region, and medial frontal areas. As both EEG and MEG revealed foci over the temporal lobe, electrodes should be implanted over the temporal lobe to exclude hypermotor seizure of temporal lobe origin. The interictal IEEG after implantation of intracranial electrodes showed that abnormal discharges were confined to the right orbitofrontal region. As the ictal IEEG revealed the origin over the right orbitofrontal region, the right orbitofrontal region was resected. After the surgery, the patient was seizure-free during a 2-year follow-up. The IEEG confirmed that the seizure origin was clear, which was completely resected. The patient hence had a good postoperative outcome.

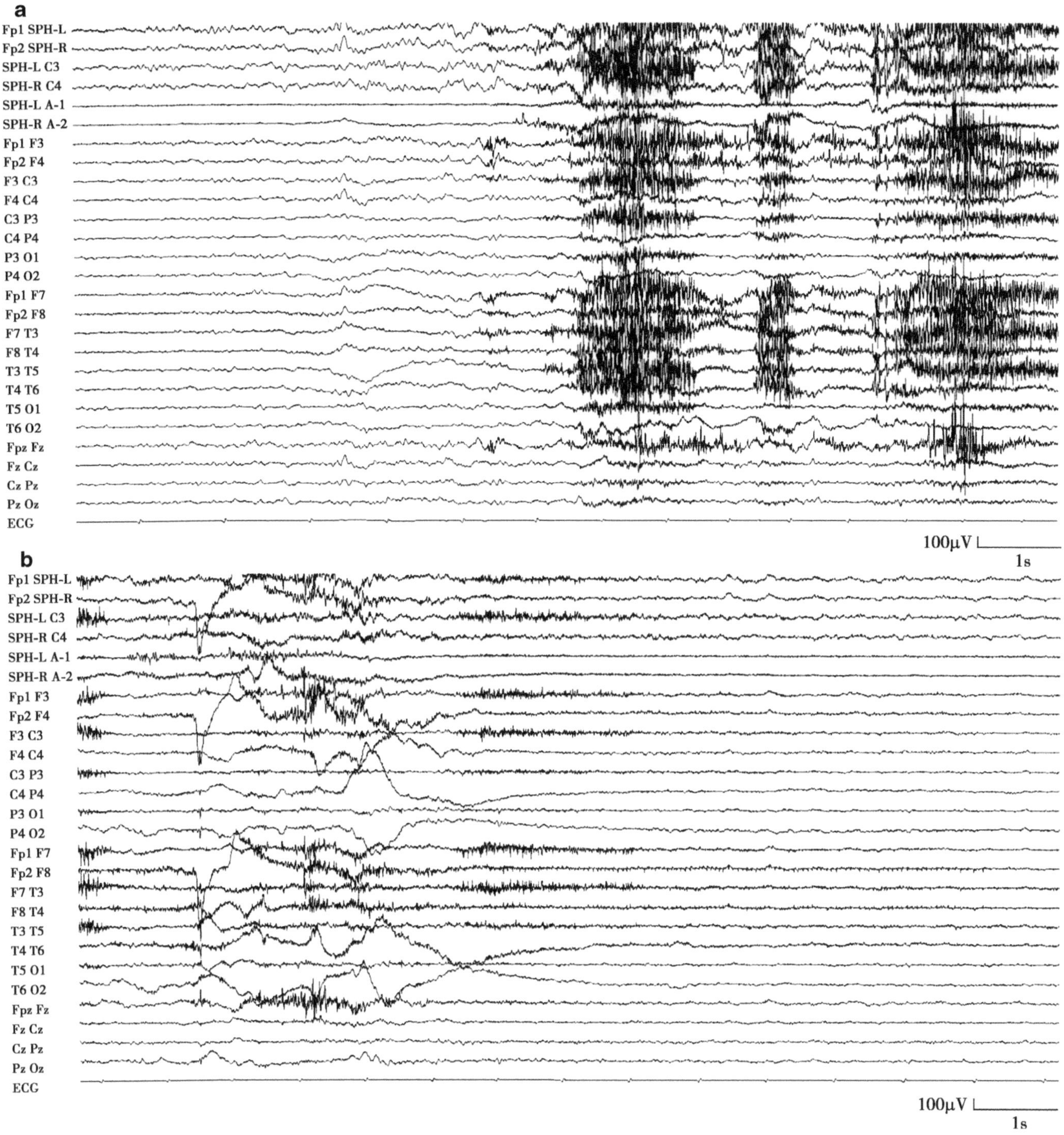

Fig. 2.66 Ictal scalp EEG. (**a**) Before the seizure, the patient was sleeping in the position of right lateral decubitus, and touched his face and scratched his head with both hands when waking. Mixed EMG artifacts were seen on the EEG. (**b**) The patient continued to touch his face and scratch his head. The low amplitude fast activities were observed on the EEG. (**c**) The patient was lying in the right lateral position and opened his eyes while being still and immobile, with a blank look. The rhythm of fast activities of low amplitude was observed on the EEG. (**d**) The patient's symptoms and the EEG presentation were the same as **c**. (**e**) The patient's right hand twitched rapidly, both lower limbs kicked, both upper limbs were elevated. The patient had head clonus with speaking bestial words. EEG showed numerous EMG artifacts and wobble artifacts mixed. (**f**) The patient twisted the body while repeatedly lifting the hip off the bed. His both lower limbs slowly kicked and twisted, especially on the left, with head clonus and oropharyngeal automatisms. EEG showed numerous EMG artifacts and wobble artifacts. (**g**) The patient was quiet and immobile in the supine position. EEG showed EMG artifacts and wobble artifacts mixed. (**h**) At the end of the seizure, the patient sat up and communicated with his family. The EEG recovered to the background activity

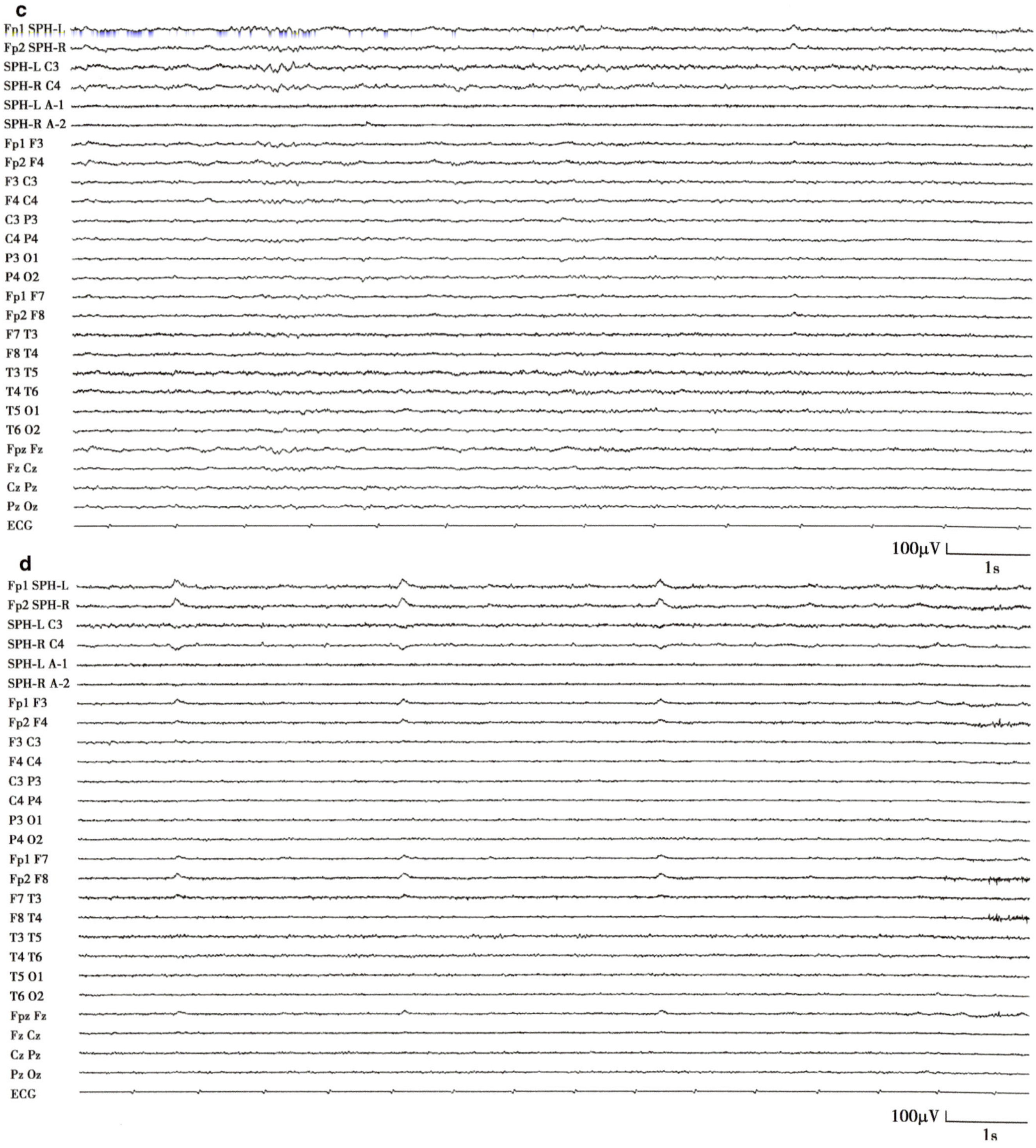

Fig. 2.66 (continued)

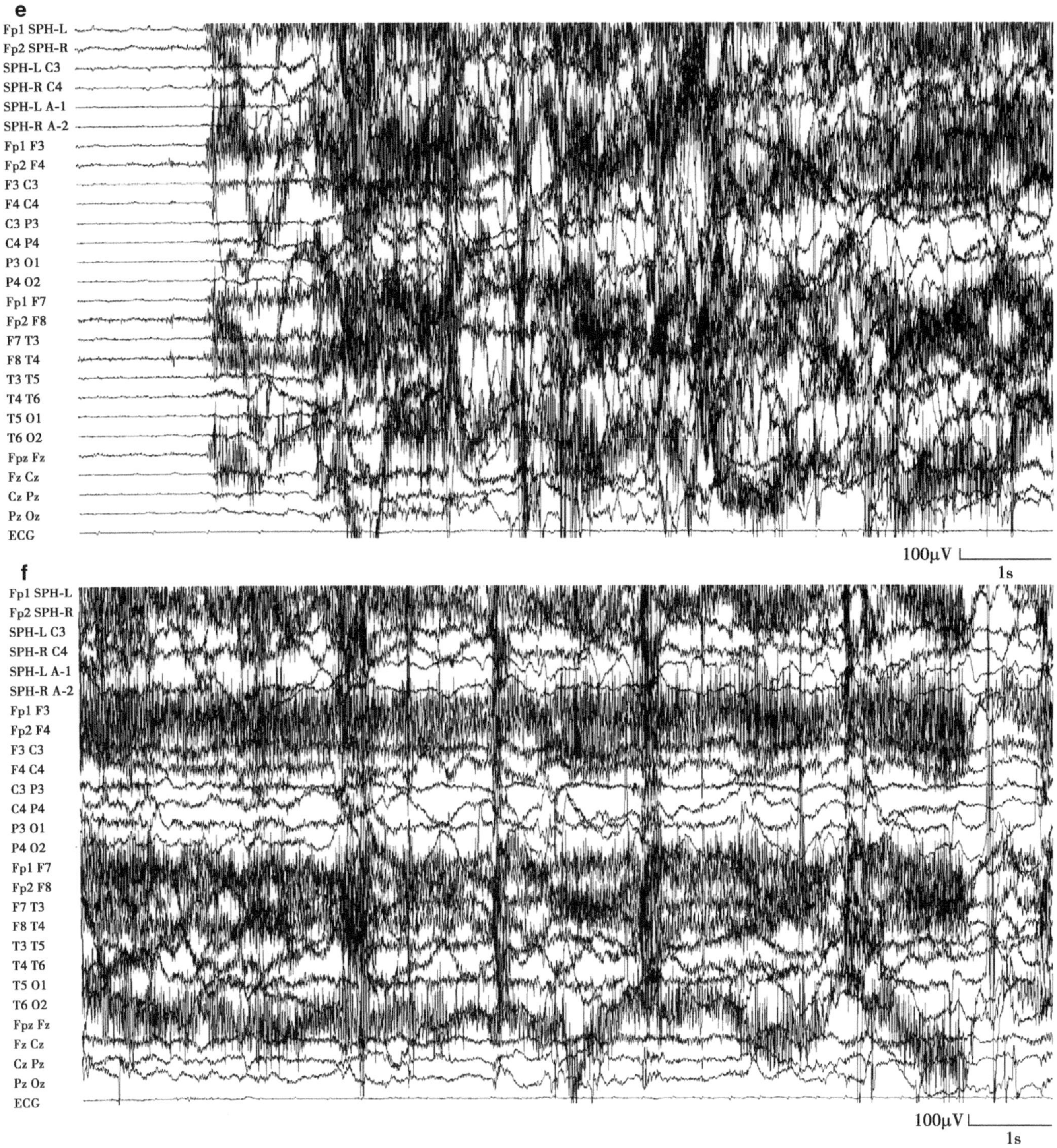

Fig. 2.66 (continued)

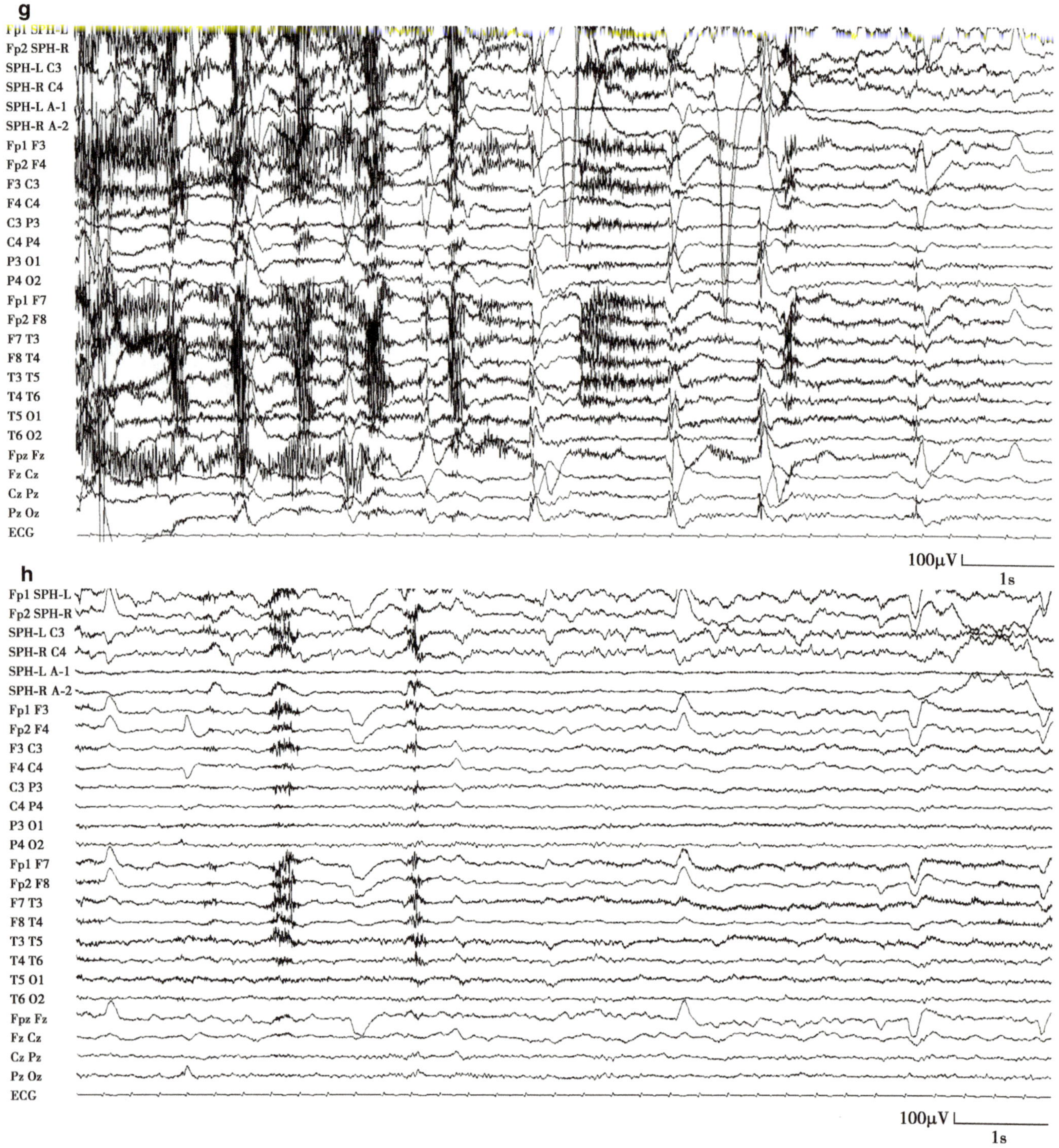

Fig. 2.66 (continued)

Fig. 2.67 Scheme of intracranial electrodes
Strip electrode 1: the left medial frontal cortex (8 contacts); Strip electrode 2: the right medial frontal cortex (8 contacts); Grid electrode 3: the left frontal pole (16 contacts); Grid electrode 4: the right frontal pole (16 contacts); Grid electrode 5: the left orbitofrontal region (16 contacts); Grid electrode 6: the right orbitofrontal region (16 contacts); Grid electrode 7: the left posterior frontal cortex (16 contacts); Grid electrode 8: the right posterior frontal cortex (16 contacts); Strip electrode 9: the left temporal region (8 contacts); Strip electrode 10: the right temporal region (8 contacts)

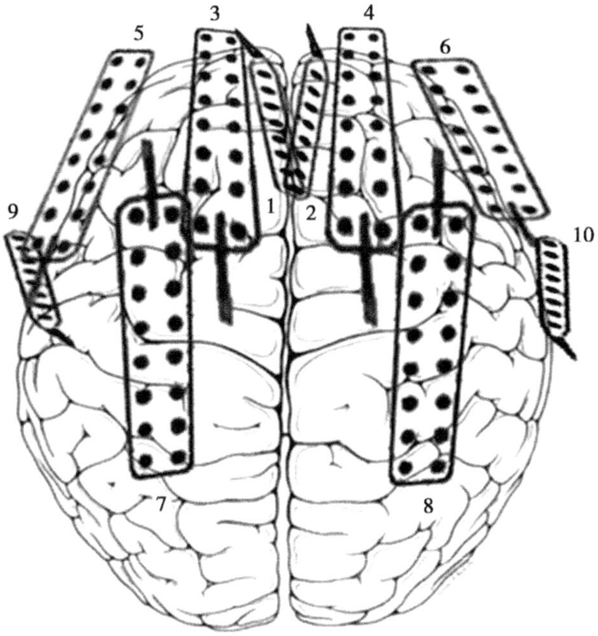

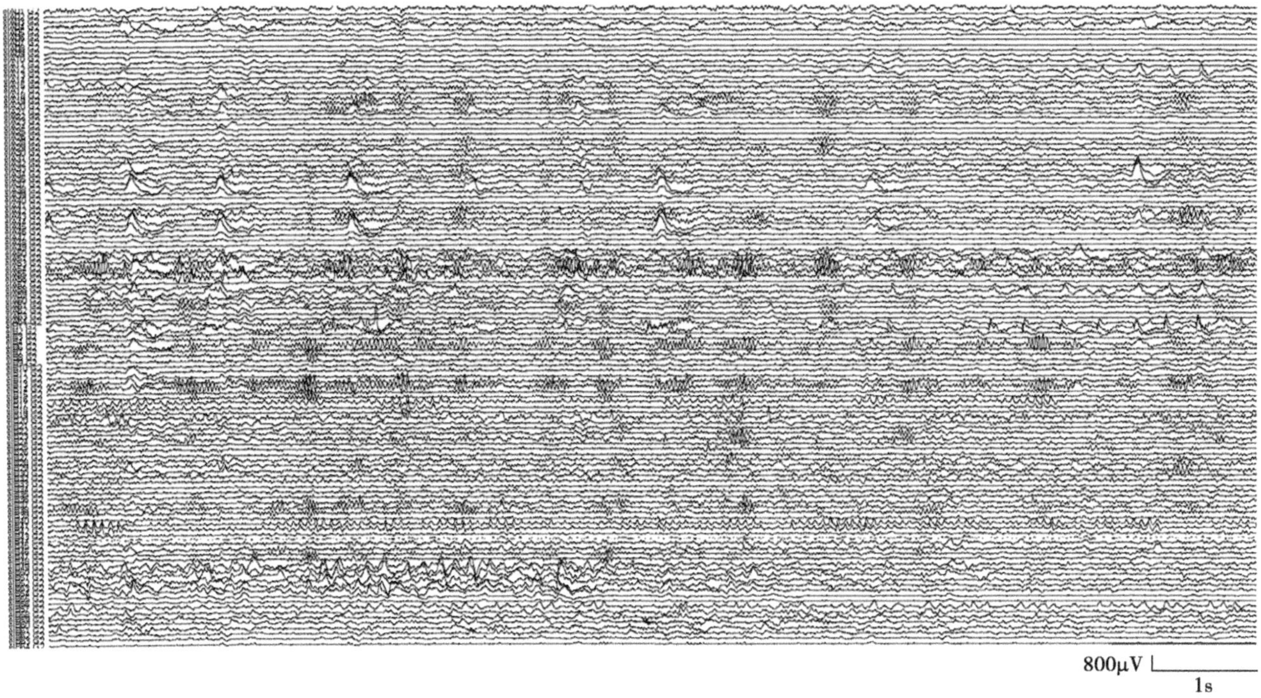

Fig. 2.68 Interictal intracranial EEG
Periodic sharp waves of high amplitude and the bursts of low amplitude fast activity were over the right orbitofrontal region (contact numbers elB1 and elB2)

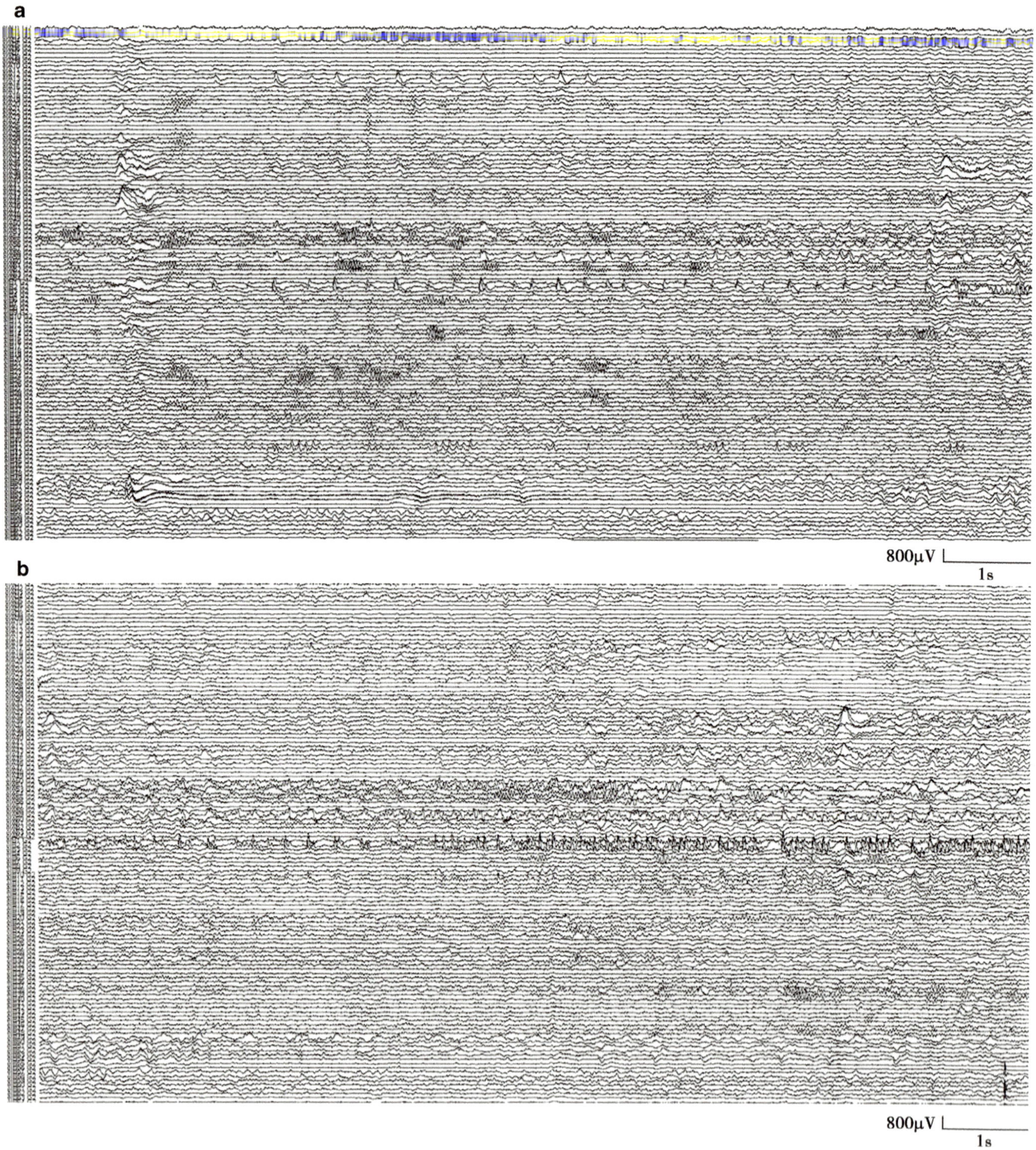

Fig. 2.69 Ictal EEG of intracranial electrodes. (**a**) The patient was quiet in the supine position before the seizure. The IEEG showed periodic sharp waves of high amplitude over the right orbitofrontal region (contact numbers elB01 and elB02). (**b**) The patient was quiet in the supine position. The IEEG showed periodic-like sharp waves of high amplitude in the right orbitofrontal region (contact numbers elB01 and elB02), which gradually developed into a rhythm of spikes of high amplitude and spread to the left orbitofrontal region (contact numbers elA50 and elA51). (**c**) The patient opened eyes after shaking both lower limbs a few times. The IEEG showed the rhythm of spikes of high amplitude over the right orbitofrontal region (contact numbers elB01, elB02, elB03), which spread to the ipsilateral medial frontal cortex (elA13) and frontal region (contact numbers elA34, elA35, elA45, elA46). (**d**) The patient blinked continuously and developed oropharyngeal automatism, followed by sudden elevation of the left upper limb, which was held down by his family member. Meanwhile, he turned the head to the left, with both eyes gazing upper left. The IEEG showed the low amplitude fast activity over the right frontal region (contact numbers elA33, elA34, elA35, elA42, elA43, elA44, elB1, elB2, elB3, elB33, elB34, elB35, elB36, elB37, elB41, elB42, elB43, elB44). (**e**) The patient blinked continuously and developed oropharyngeal automatism, followed by sudden elevation of the left upper limb, which was held down by his family member. Meanwhile, he turned the head to the left, with both eyes gazing upper left. The IEEG showed the low amplitude fast activity over the right frontal region (contact numbers elA33, elA34, elA35, elA42, elA43, elA44, elB1, elB2, elB3, elB33, elB34, elB35, elB36, elB37, elB41, elB42, elB43, elB44)

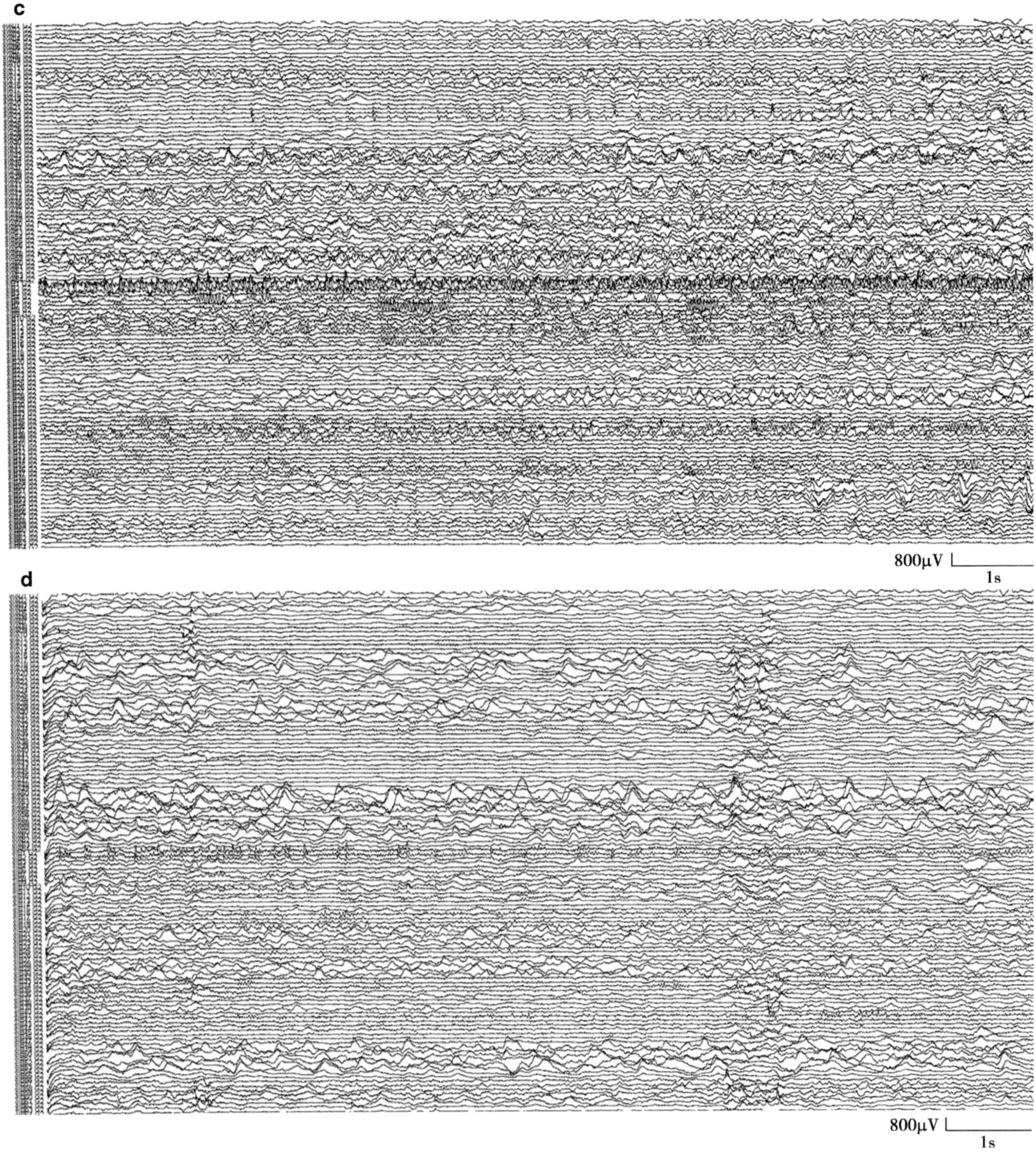

Fig. 2.69 (continued)

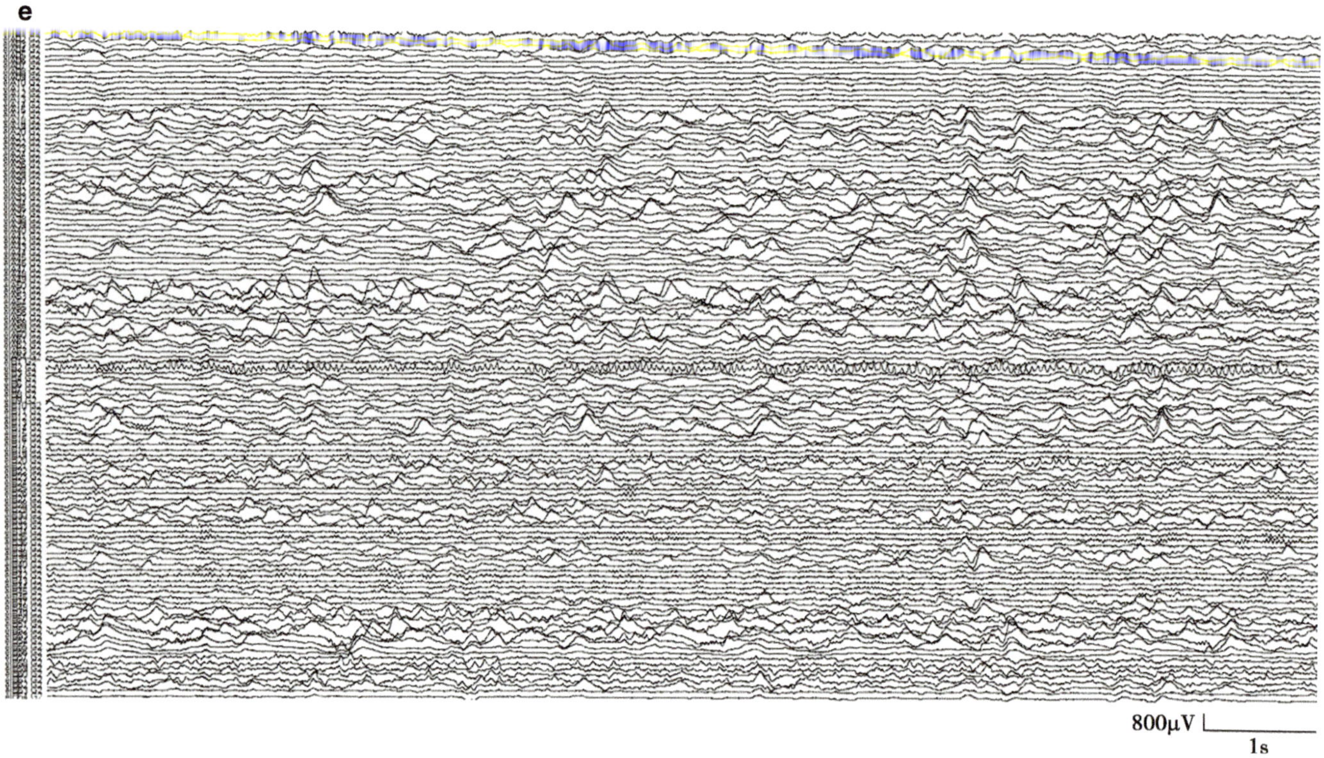

Fig. 2.69 (continued)

Cases of Frontal Pole Epilepsy

Case 2.15 Frontal Pole Epilepsy

[Abstract of Medical Records]
Male, 17 years old.

1. *Chief complaint* Paroxysmal convulsion for 13 years.
2. *History of present illness* The patient suddenly had rigid limbs and rotated in place, with loss of consciousness, but did not tumble 13 years ago, which lasted 30–40 s and then resolved.

   Since then he had frequent episodic twitching of the limbs, rarely with loss of consciousness. The seizures lasted from a few seconds to 1 min. At the time of admission, the seizures were mainly characterized by aimless walking, limb stiffness, and spinning; or by sudden sitting up during sleep. During the seizure, the patient was conscious but could not speak. The seizures occurred 3–10 times a day. The patient once took sodium valproate and was seizure-free for 4 years, while the seizure reoccurred after the discontinuation of drugs and could not be controlled any more. The seizures usually occurred during sleep, 3 to 10 times per day.
3. *Personal history* The patient had a history of neonatal hemolysis after birth.
4. *Family history* No history of associated diseases.
5. *Physical examination* No neurological abnormalities were found.
6. *Imaging examination* MRI showed localized cortical thickening over the right temporal lobe.
7. *EEG* For details, see Figs. 2.70, 2.71, 2.72, 2.73, and 2.74.

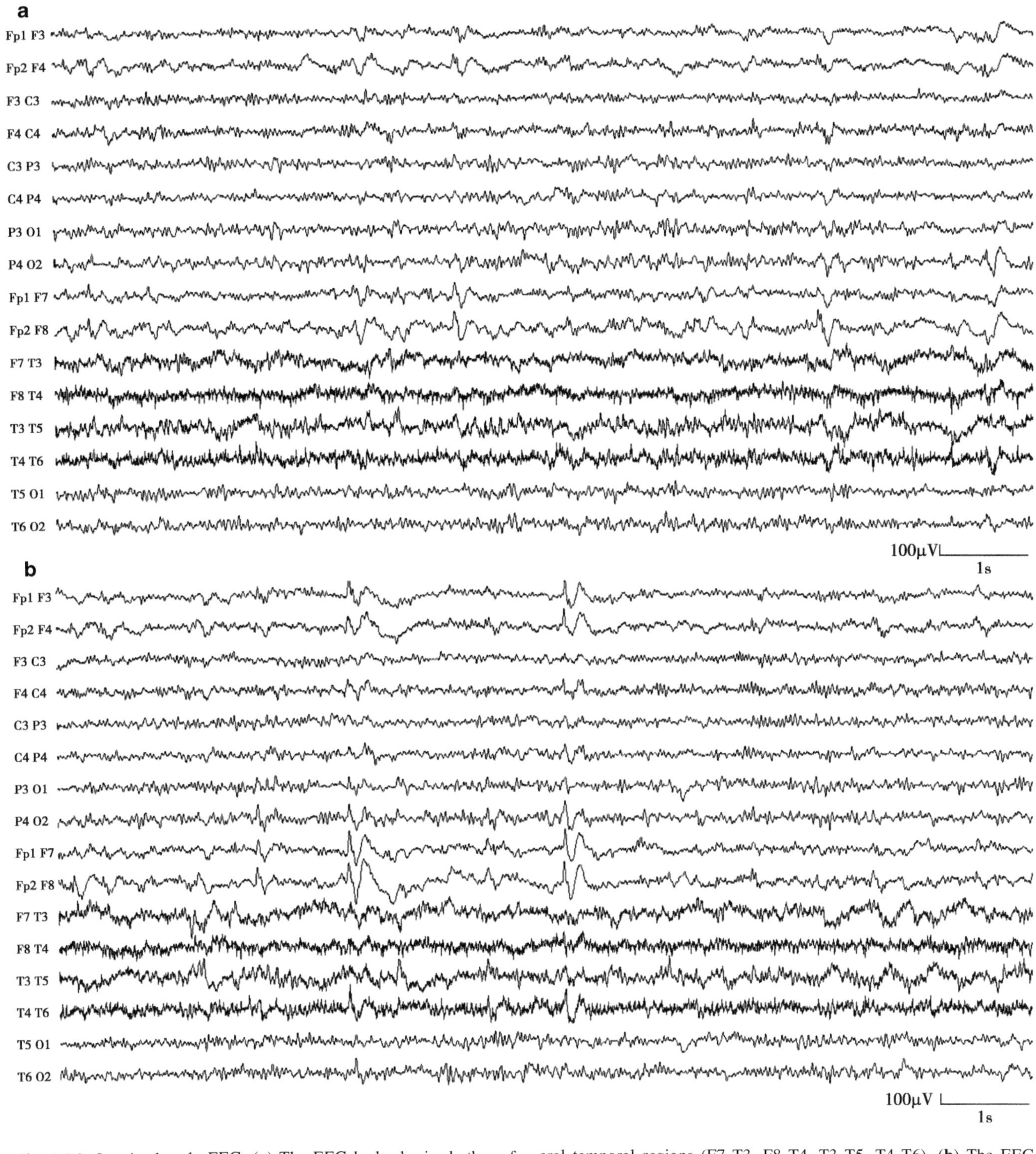

Fig. 2.70 Interictal scalp EEG. (**a**) The EEG had a basic rhythm of 9 Hz and showed many 18–25 Hz faster activities of low amplitude mixed in each lead. Irregular slow waves and sharp waves of medium amplitude were observed over the bilateral frontal regions (Fp1 F3, Fp2 F4, Fp1 F7, Fp2 F8), and EMG artifacts were observed over the bilateral temporal regions (F7 T3, F8 T4, T3 T5, T4 T6). (**b**) The EEG showed spike-and-wave complexes over the bilateral frontal poles (Fp1, Fp2), which sometimes spread to the right temporal (T4 T6) and parietal (P4 O2) regions

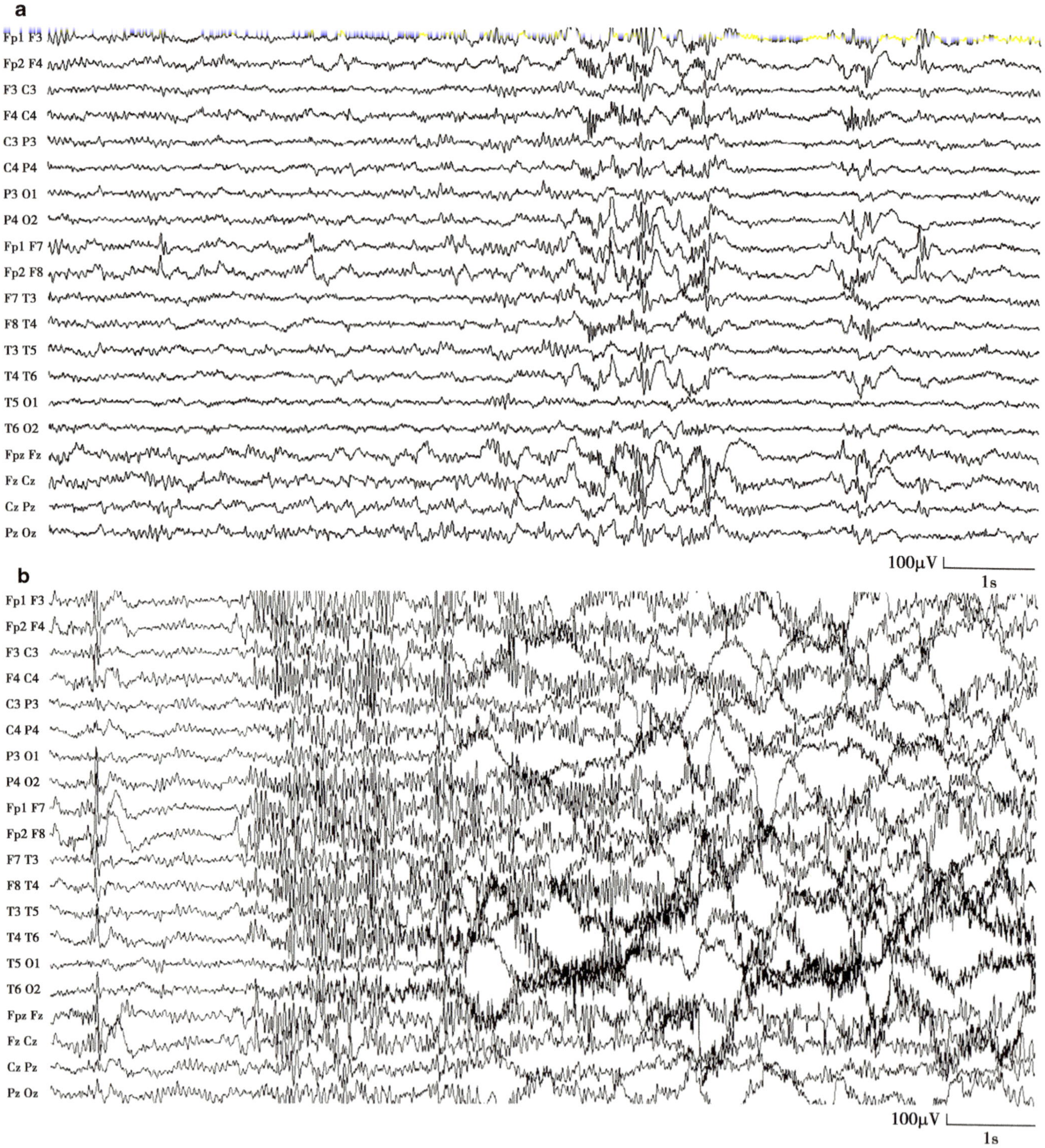

Fig. 2.71 Ictal scalp EEG. (**a**) Before the seizure, the patient was sleeping in a supine position with his hands on his chest and eyes closed. The EEG was presented as the background EEG of stage II of sleep, and showed spikes of high amplitude and spike-and-wave complexes over the bilateral frontal regions (Fp1 F3, Fp2 F4, Fp1 F7, Fp2 F8) and the frontal midline (Fpz Fz, Fz Cz), which spread to the right. (**b**) During the seizure, the patient opened his eyes and held his left hand with his right hand. The EEG showed spike-and-wave complexes of high amplitude over the bilateral frontal regions (Fp1 F3, Fp1 F7, Fp2 F4, Fp2 F8), followed by the rhythm of spikes of high amplitude bilaterally. A few EMG artifacts and electrode wobble artifacts were observed over the bilateral temporoparietal cortices. (**c**) The patient fumbled on the chest with both hands for about 15 s. The EEG showed the rhythm of spikes over the anterior head bilaterally (Fp1 F3, Fp2 F4, F3 C3, F4 C4, Fp1 F7, Fp2 F8, F7 T3, F8 T4), with artifacts same as before. (**d**) At the end of the seizure, the patient lay down in a supine position quietly again with his eyes closed. The EEG presentation recovered to that of the background EEG

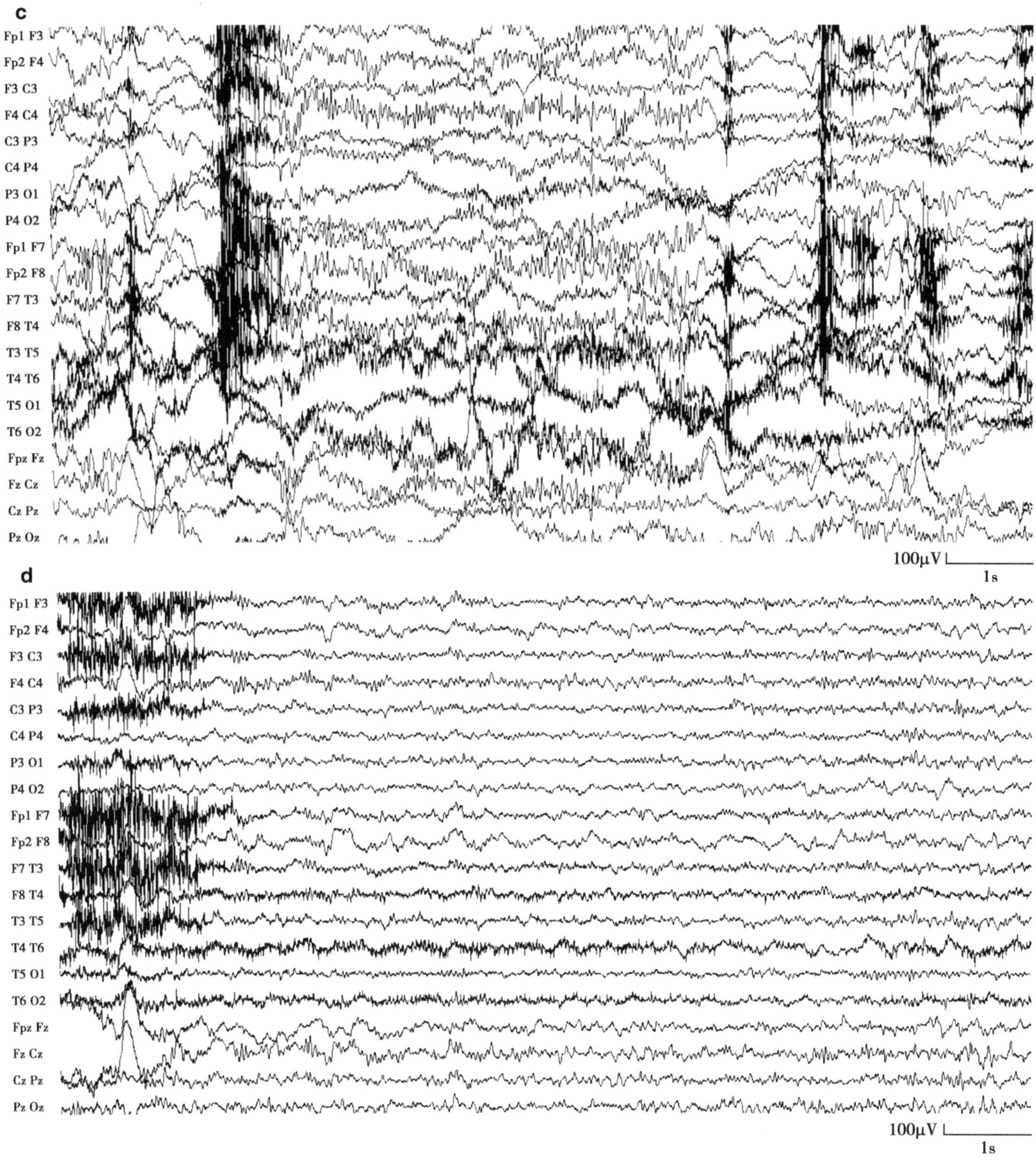

Fig. 2.71 (continued)

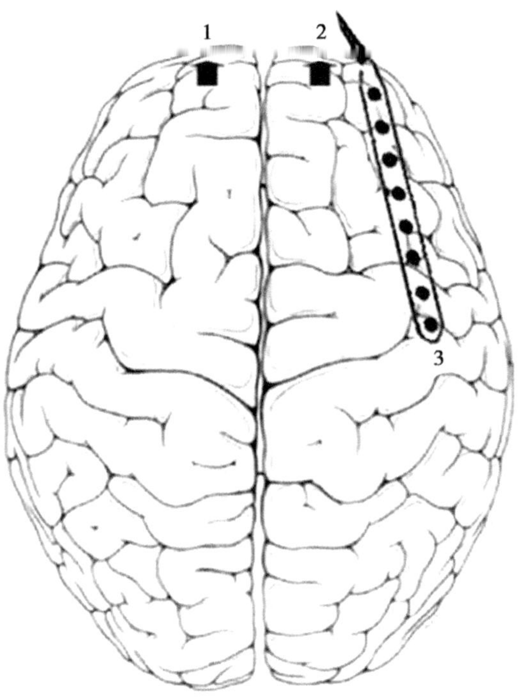

Fig. 2.72 Scheme of intracranial electrodes
Deep electrode 1: the left frontal pole region (8 contacts); Deep electrode 2: the right frontal pole region (8 contacts); Strip electrode 3: the right frontal region (8 contacts)

[Case Review]

1. Case Characteristics
   (a) *Seizure characteristics* ① Often during sleep. ② Cluster seizures (ranging from 3 to 10 seizures per day). ③ Transient seizure of automatism with or without loss of consciousness.
   (b) *EEG characteristics* ① Interictal EEG showed spike-and-wave complexes over the bilateral frontal regions, and the right temporal region. ② Ictal EEG showed spikes of high amplitude and spike-and-wave complexes over the bilateral frontal regions and the frontal midline, especially on the right.
   (c) *Imaging characteristics* MRI showed localized cortical thickening over the right temporal lobe.
2. *Diagnosis and treatment strategy and follow-up results* According to the patient's seizure characteristics and

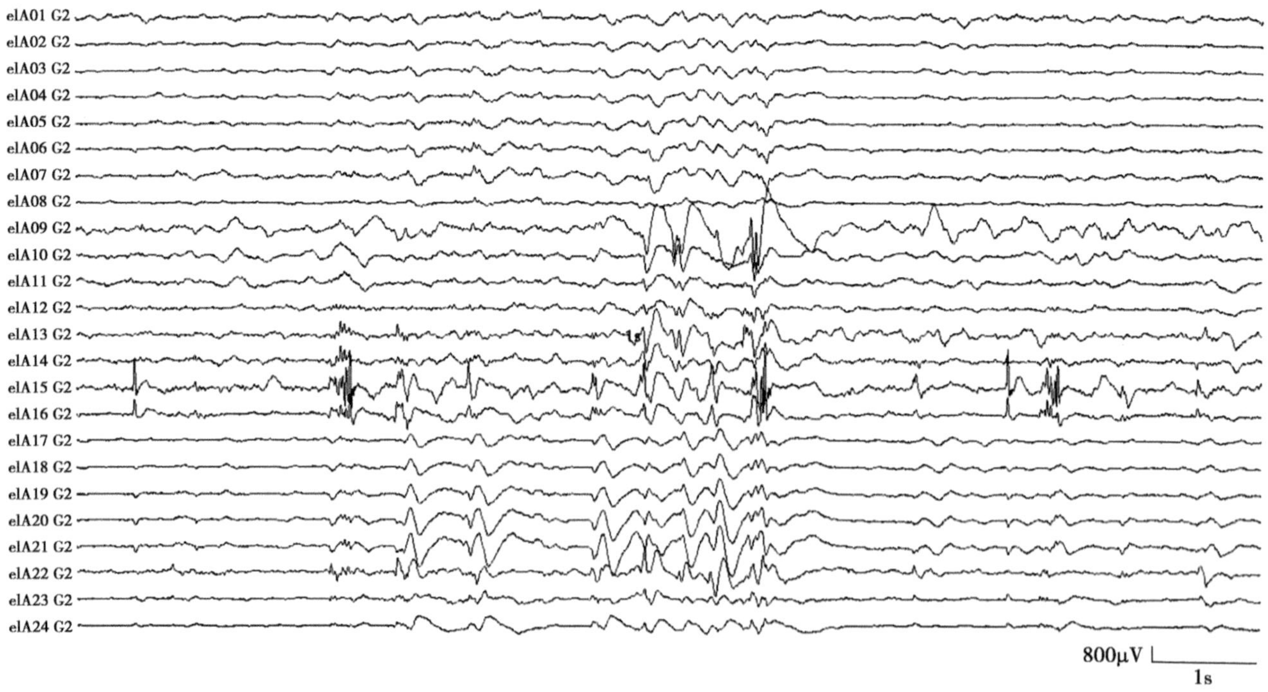

Fig. 2.73 Interictal intracranial EEG
Paroxysmal spike-and-wave complexes of high amplitude and rhythmic polyspikes were observed over the deep electrodes (contact numbers elA09, elA13, elA14, elA15, elA16) and strip electrodes (contact numbers elA19, elA20, elA21, elA22) over the right frontal region, especially over the deep electrodes (contact numbers elA09, elA15, elA16)

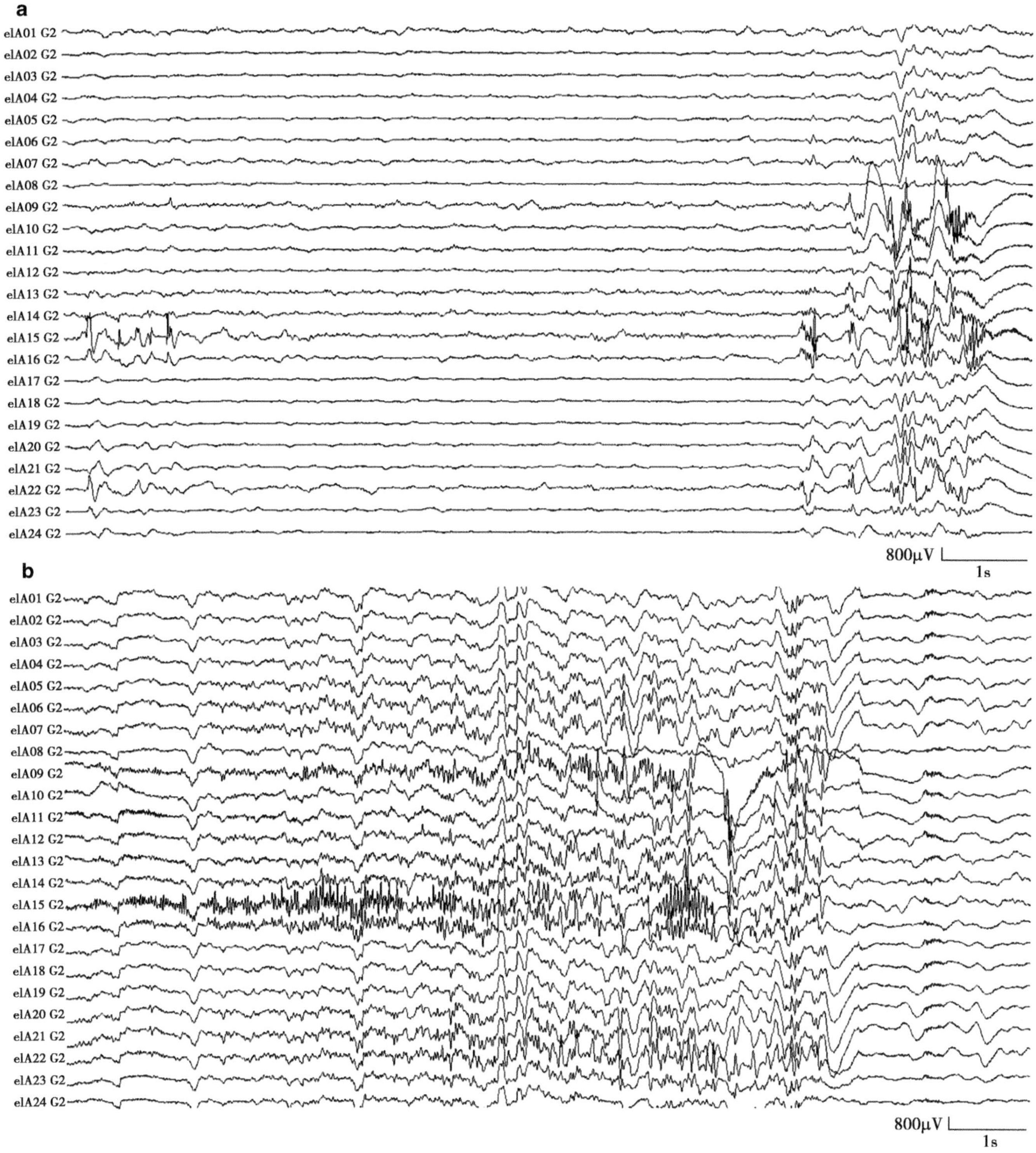

Fig. 2.74 Ictal EEG of intracranial electrodes. (**a**) The patient was supine with eyes closed before the seizure. The IEEG showed polyspike-and-wave complexes of high amplitude and spikes, with enhanced rhythm, over the deep electrodes (contact numbers elA09, elA10, elA13, elA14, elA15, elA16) and cortical electrodes (contact numbers elA21, elA22) over the right frontal region 2 s before the seizure, especially over the right deep electrodes (contact number elA15). (**b**) During the seizure, the patient opened his eyes, clasped his hands together, and fumbled on the chest. The IEEG showed the low amplitude fast activity over the deep electrodes over the right frontal pole region (contact numbers elA09, elA15, elA16), the amplitude of which gradually increased and developed into the rhythm of spikes. (**c**) The seizure ended. The IEEG recovered to the background EEG

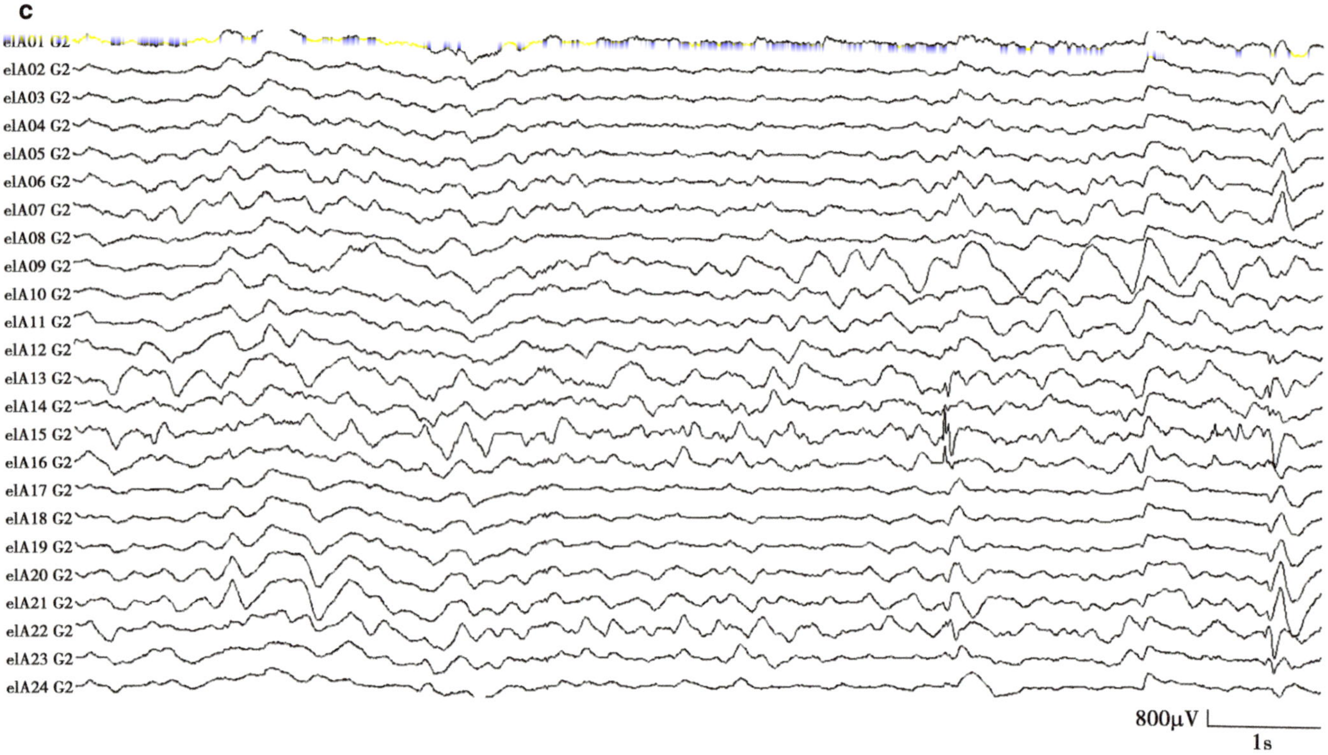

Fig. 2.74 (continued)

EEG characteristics, it was considered that the seizure foci might be located over the right frontal lobe, but MRI showed local cortical thickening over the right temporal lobe. Therefore, the strategy of implanting intracranial electrodes over the right frontal and temporal regions should be adopted. However, since it was not possible to implant a large number of intracranial electrodes at that time, a small number of electrodes were implanted over the frontal region because the foci were judged to be mainly over the frontal region based on the seizure symptoms. The postoperative interictal and ictal IEEGs showed polyspike-and-wave complexes over the deep and strip electrodes over the right frontal region, indicating a clear seizure origin. The epileptic focus over the right frontal pole region was then resected. During a 3-year follow-up, the patient was seizure-free when taking medication and experienced recurrent seizures due to discontinuation of medication at his own discretion, which disappeared when the patient resumed medication. As the seizure origin of the patient was limited and the epileptic focus was clear, the postoperative outcome was satisfactory.

Cases of Temporal Lobe Epilepsy

3

Li Liping, Liu Jing, Zhai Yi, Du Wei, Piao Yuanyuan, and Yu Tao

Overview of Temporal Lobe Epilepsy

Anatomy of Temporal Lobe

Temporal lobe epilepsy (TLE) is the most clinically common type of intractable epilepsy that has been extensively studied in clinical and basic research. Seizures originating from different structures of the temporal lobe have different symptoms. Depending on anatomic and clinical characteristics, TLE can be classified into medial temporal lobe epilepsy and neocortical temporal lobe epilepsy. The temporal lobe is closely connected in function to other brain regions and structures via cortical connections, limbic system, and extensive fiber connections. The upper part of the temporal lobe is delimited from the frontal lobe by the lateral fissure, and the posterior part of temporal lobe is separated from the lateral occipital cortex by an imaginary line from the superior margin of the parieto-occipital sulci to the anterior occipital notch (about 4 cm anterior to the occipital pole). The lateral temporal lobe is divided into the superior temporal gyrus, the middle temporal gyrus, and the inferior temporal gyrus by the superior temporal sulcus and the inferior temporal sulcus, which are distributed by longitude. In the posteromedial part of the superior temporal gyrus, the short transverse gyrus that passes into the lateral fissure and forms the inferior wall of the lateral fissure is the transverse temporal gyri, which is the auditory center (areas 41 and 42). The posterior part of the superior temporal gyrus is the auditory language center, which is area 22. The base of the temporal lobe is mainly composed of the gyrus lateral occipito-temporalis (fusiform gyrus) and the medial parahippocampalis gyrus. The structure of the medial temporal lobe includes the hippocampal, the parahippocampal gyrus, and the amygdala complex. The hippocampal is a collective term that includes the hippocampus, the dentate gyrus, and a number of cortices closely related to the parahippocampal gyrus. The parahippocampal gyrus, together with the cingulate cortex and olfactory cortex, forms the limbic lobe, which influences the activity of visceral organs, emotional responses, behavioral activity, and state of mind. The amygdala complex is a subcortical mass of gray matter located in the medial temporal lobe, deep in the uncus of gyrus parahippocampalis. The amygdala complex is a part of the rhinencephalon and also an important structure of the limbic system, involved in olfactory recognition and visceral and endocrine responses due to emotion and motivation, as well as somatosensory and somatomotor activities.

Clinical Manifestations

1. Aura: An aura is actually a sensory seizure that can occur alone but mostly appears before a focal seizure with loss of consciousness or secondarily generalized tonic-clonic seizures, which lasts a few seconds to 1–2 minutes and is followed by loss of consciousness. The type of aura is related to the seizure onset site and contributes to the localization of the seizure origin but rarely has a lateralization value. The aura can be mainly divided into experiential phenomena (including déjà vu, jamais vu, memory loss, and anticipation of seizures), specific visceral sensations (the feeling of stomach gas rising), hallucinations

L. Liping (✉) · L. Jing · Z. Yi
Department of Neurology, Beijing, China
e-mail: Lilp@xwhosp.org

D. Wei · P. Yuanyuan · Y. Tao
Department of Neurosurgery, Beijing, China

Y. Wang (ed.), *Electroencephalogram for Presurgical Epilepsy Evaluation*, https://doi.org/10.1007/978-981-95-8003-3_3

(visual, auditory, olfactory, and gustatory hallucinations and illusion), emotional discomfort (mainly fear), and other physical discomfort (e.g., palpitation, dizziness). Among them, stomach gas rising, fear, jamais vu and déjà vu are the most common auras before a seizure occurs to TLE patients.

2. Automatism: The most common automatisms include oropharyngeal automatisms (including chewing, swallowing, smacking lips, etc.) and hand automatisms (fumbling, tapping, rubbing, and grasping with one or both hands). The relatively uncommon automatisms include vocalizations (grunting, crying, and shouting without words), self-talking (spontaneously speaking more than two words during a seizure), blinking, spitting or drinking, and somatic automatisms (excessive movements). In addition, more rare forms of automatisms include laughing and leaving behaviors such as walking aimlessly during a seizure. Rarely, automatisms involve whistling. Post-seizure automatisms include postictal coughing and nose rubbing.
3. Motor symptoms: Early non-tonic head deviation, deviation tonic (with eyes and head deviated to one side by an angle greater than 90°), staring to one side, partial clonus (twitching of one corner of the mouth), general tonic (no postural or deviation manifestations but may be characterized by elevation of the hands with increased muscular tone), postural tonic (asymmetric extension or flexion of the head, shoulders, or upper or lower limbs), figure-4 sign, dystonia-like posture, tremor (mild shaking of the hands or head), and asymmetric limb clonus at the end of the seizure.
4. Language: During the seizure, speech ceases, followed by postictal aphasia.
5. Autonomic symptoms: Shortness of breath, increased heart rate, pale or flushed face, sweating, urinary incontinence, and piloerection during the seizure.
6. Changes in consciousness: Consciousness involves cognition, comprehension, emotion, and memory. The patient with focal seizure and loss of consciousness inability recalls the process of seizures, which are typically characterized by movement arrest and staring for 30 s to 1–2 min.
7. Others: Some patients experience premonitory symptoms before the seizure, including headache, personality changes, irritability, anxiety, or nervousness that last for minutes, hours or days, but these symptoms are not seizures and their presence can indicate that the patient may be about to have a seizure.

In addition, emotional disorders and psychiatric disorders occur at a high rate in patients with temporal lobe epilepsy. It is important to distinguish whether co-morbidities or seizures cause emotional or psychiatric disorders. Psychiatric symptoms or cognitive impairment lasting several hours or even days that occur in a minority of patients are likely to be non-convulsive status epilepticus.

EEG Characteristics

EEG is currently the most effective examination method for diagnosing and identifying seizure types and plays a critical role during the preoperative evaluation of medically intractable focal epilepsy. Applying electrodes to sphenoid in addition to the standard EEG monitoring in TLE patients can improve the diagnostic accuracy and increase the positive rate of EEG in TLE patients by 25–28%. The frequency of abnormal discharges during nonrapid eye movement (NREM) sleep is usually significantly higher than that during wakefulness. EEG during sleep is hence more conducive to analyzing the frequency and location of interictal epileptic discharge (IED).

The interictal EEG of TLE patients shows IEDs in unilateral or bilateral temporal region, with 50% of the patients showing spikes on the bilateral temporal regions. Spikes may also appear on the frontal and parietal lobes. Isolated spikes confined to the unilateral temporal region with scalp electrodes might be related to a temporal lobe cortical lesion, and the frequency of IED is closely related to the extent of the lesion, with a high frequency of IED suggesting a larger lesion. The spikes on the unilateral temporal region shown on the interictal EEG correlate well with the side of seizure origin, with about 85% of TLE patients having unilateral temporal IEDs consistent with the side of seizure origin. However, sometimes the site of IEDs does not exactly correspond to the side of origin of the epileptiform abnormal ictal discharge (ID); therefore, ictal EEG recording is still required for the preoperative evaluation.

The ictal EEG in TLE patients can be divided into: 1. rhythmic activity; activities of α wave (8–13 Hz), θ wave (4–7 Hz), and δ wave (0.1–3.5 Hz); 2. activity of paroxysmal rhythmic fast waves. Frequency >13 Hz; and 3. continuous epileptiform discharges. The continuous three or more spikes and spike-and-wave complexes; 4. irregular electrical activity. Nonrhythmic electrical activity of irregular and mixed-frequency waveforms; 5. suppression of electrical activity, with wave amplitude ≤10 μV. The EEG electrical activity at the onset of the seizure is difficult to be identified due to electromyographic (EMG) artifacts during the seizure. The presence of rhythmic changes and continuous epileptiform discharges or markedly reduced wave amplitude on the EEG a few seconds before the seizure may suggest the site of seizure onset. About 76.0–85.0% of the ictal EEGs allows for lateralization. For example, the dominant rhythmic activity on one side during the seizure and the slow wave activity on one side after the seizure are of high value to lateralization. In nearly 80.0% of patients with medial temporal lobe epilepsy (MTLE), rhythmic α, θ, or δ wave activities can be seen over the temporal region within 30 s of seizure onset. It is rare to see such electrical activity in other leads on the ipsilateral hemisphere simultaneously. Among these, rhythmic θ and δ wave activities are most common in TLE patients with hippocampal sclerosis, while paroxysmal rhythmic fast activity is most common in TLE patients without hippocampal sclerosis.

Cases of Medial Temporal Lobe Epilepsy

Case 3.1 Medial Temporal Lobe Epilepsy

[Abstract of Medical Records]
Female, 23 years old.

1. *Chief complaint*: Episodic loss of consciousness for 5 years.
2. *History of present illness*: There are two seizure types. Type I: episodic palpitation and chest discomfort with clear consciousness ending in about 20 s, with 2–3 seizures per month. Type II: generalized convulsions secondary to the first seizure type, 1 seizure per month on average. She once took phenobarbital and phenytoin sodium, the effect of which were both poor. She is now taking carbamazepine 200 mg/dose tid and sodium valproate 400 mg/dose tid.
3. *Personal and family history*: No history of associated diseases.
4. *Imaging examination*: MRI showed right hippocampal sclerosis.
5. *EEG*: For details, see Figs. 3.1 and 3.2.

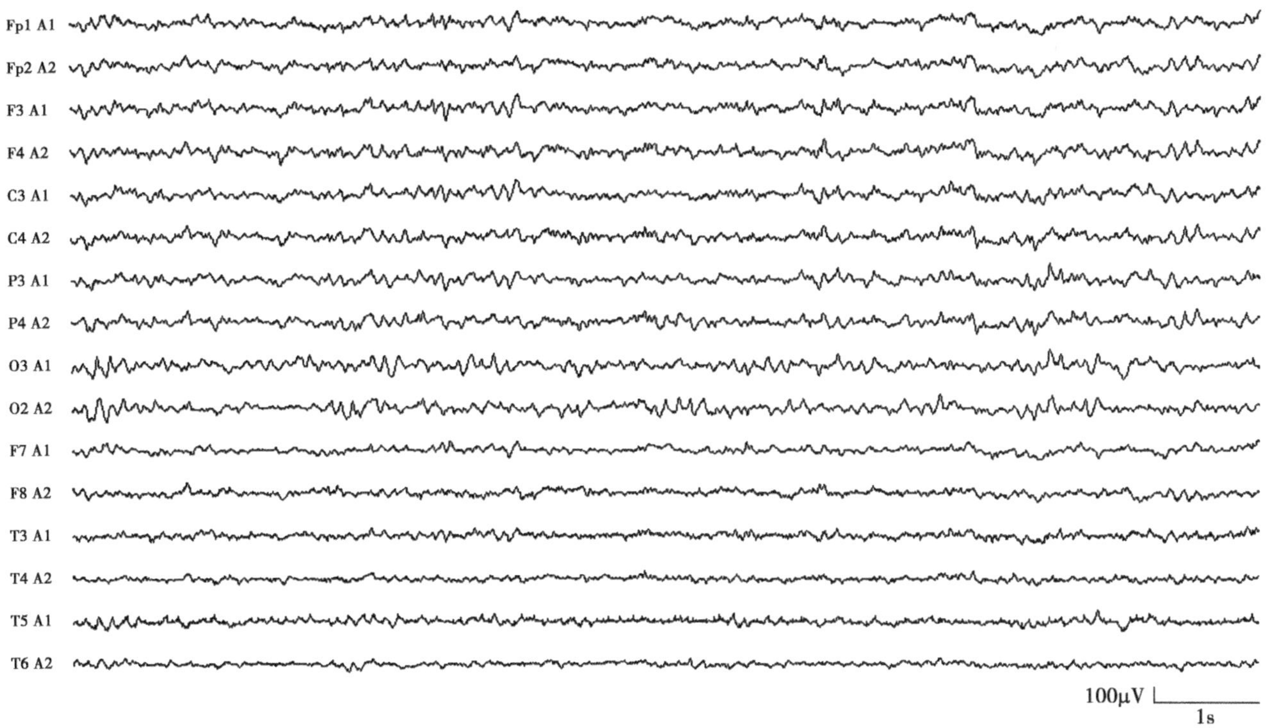

Fig. 3.1 Interictal scalp EEG. (**a**) 9.0–11.0 Hz α waves mainly over the occipital region had poor amplitude modulation. (**b**) The EEG of stage II of sleep showed scattered phase-inverted spikes over the right sphenoid electrode (Sph-R). (**c**) The EEG of stage II of sleep showed sharp waves over the right temporal region (F8, T4)

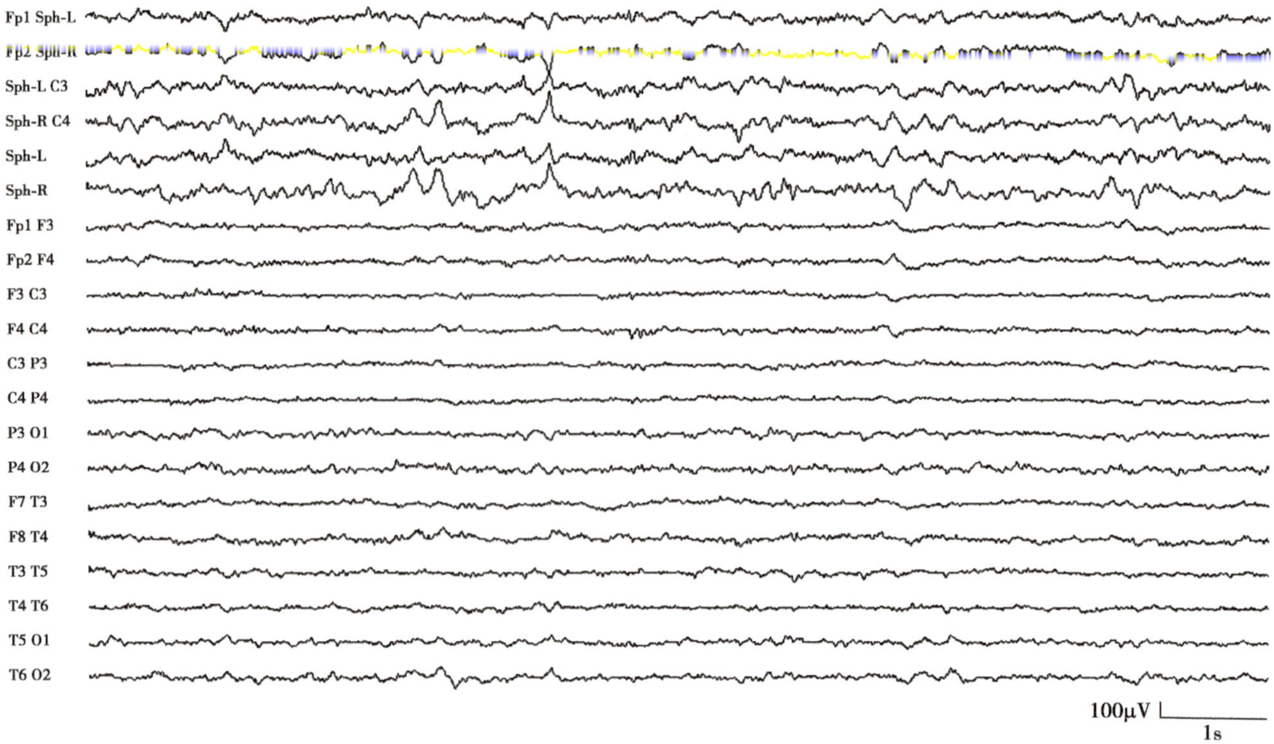

Fig. 3.2 Ictal scalp EEG. (**a**) Before the seizure, the patient had an aura (feeling chest tightness), lifted the blanket by herself, got up to look at the watch, and then lay down. The EEG showed electrode wobble artifacts and EMG artifacts. (**b**) The patient had involuntary movements of both hands, and the concurrent EEG showed EMG artifacts. α wave rhythms were seen, followed by fast activity of low amplitude in all leads. (**c**) The patient had slight movements of both hands and both lower limbs, and the concurrent EEG showed the rhythm of 3.0–5.0 Hz slow waves of medium and low amplitude over the right temporal region, followed by a rhythm of sharp waves that spread to the right frontal region. (**d**) When the patient lay down without any movements, the EEG showed 4.0–5.0 Hz slow waves of medium amplitude over the right frontal and temporal regions, which evolved into fast activity with α wave rhythm 3 s later. (**e**) The patient's symptoms were the same as in **d**. The EEG showed a gradual increase in amplitude and a gradual decrease in rhythmic frequency of the sharp waves over the right frontal and temporal regions. (**f**) The patient's symptoms were the same as in **d**. The EEG showed a gradual increase in amplitude and a gradual decrease in frequency of the sharp waves rhythm over the right frontal and temporal regions. (**g**) The patient's symptoms were the same as in **d**. The EEG showed rhythmic sharp waves and slow waves over the right frontal and temporal regions

[Case Review]

1. Case Characteristics
   (a) *EEG characteristics*: The interictal EEG showed sharp waves over the right sphenoid electrode and over the right temporal region. The ictal EEG showed the rhythms of slow waves and sharp waves over the right temporal region, which spread to the right frontal region and then evolved into fast activity and sharp rhythm.
   (b) *Imaging characteristics*: The patient's MRI showed right hippocampal sclerosis.
2. *Diagnosis and treatment strategy and follow-up results*: The MRI, interictal EEG, and ictal EEG were consistent, which supported the origin from the right temporal lobe. The patient was seizure-free for 3 years since the resection of temporal lobe and the drug has been discontinued.

Case 3.2 Medial Temporal Lobe Epilepsy

[Abstract of Medical Records]

Male, 48 years old.

1. *Chief complaint*: Dialeptic seizures for 3 years and episodic twitching for one and a half years.
2. *History of present illness*: The patient was suddenly dialeptic and dull looking 3 years ago without any apparent inducement, accompanied by involuntary chewing and sometimes fumbling movements of hands, which lasted for about 1 min and then resolved. One and a half years ago, the patient suffered from episodic limb twitching. He had been treated with sodium valproate, with poor effects. Seizures occurred 1–2 times per day.
3. *Personal and family history*: No history of associated diseases.
4. *Imaging examination*: MRI showed no obvious abnormalities.
5. *EEG*: For details, see Figs. 3.3 and 3.4.

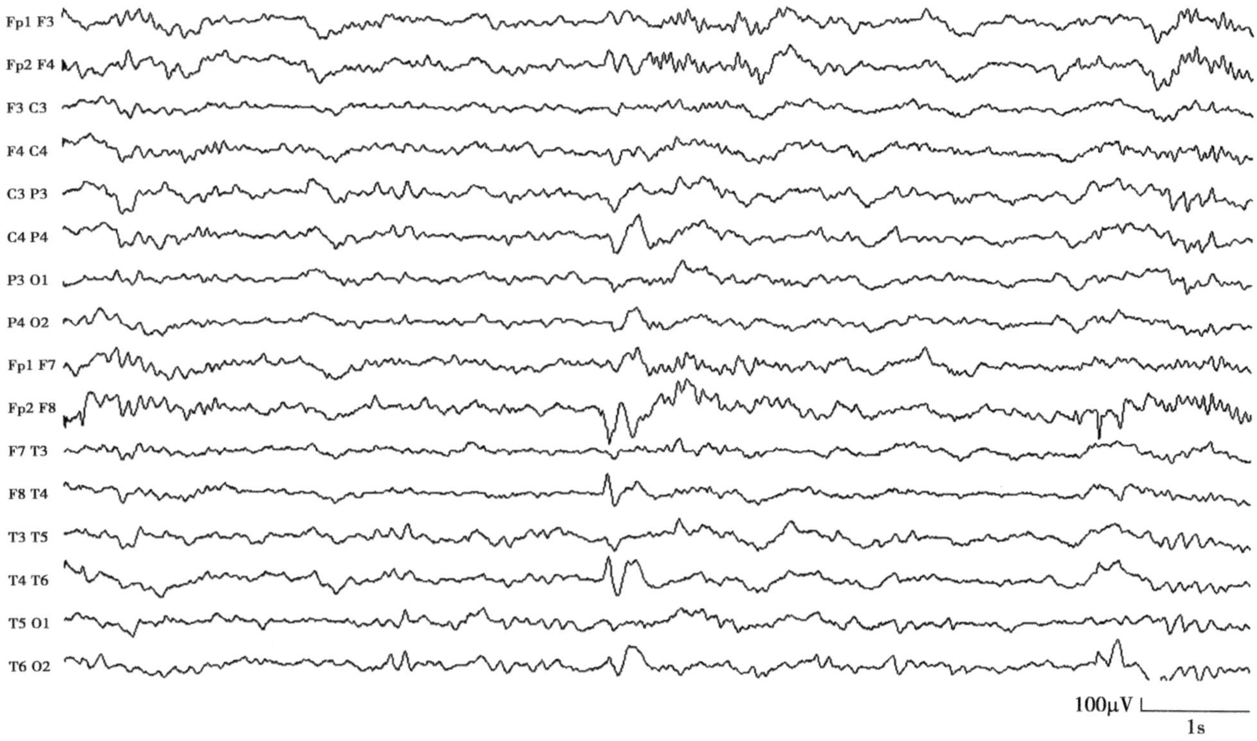

Fig. 3.3 Interictal scalp EEG. (**a**) The patient was conscious with eyes closed. The EEG showed a basic rhythm of 10.0 Hz with good amplitude modulation, mainly over the occipital region. (**b**) The EEG of stage II of sleep showed phase-inverted sharp waves over the right sphenoid electrode and sharp waves of low amplitude over the right anterior temporal region. (**c**) The EEG of stage II of sleep showed sharp waves and spikes over the right sphenoid electrode

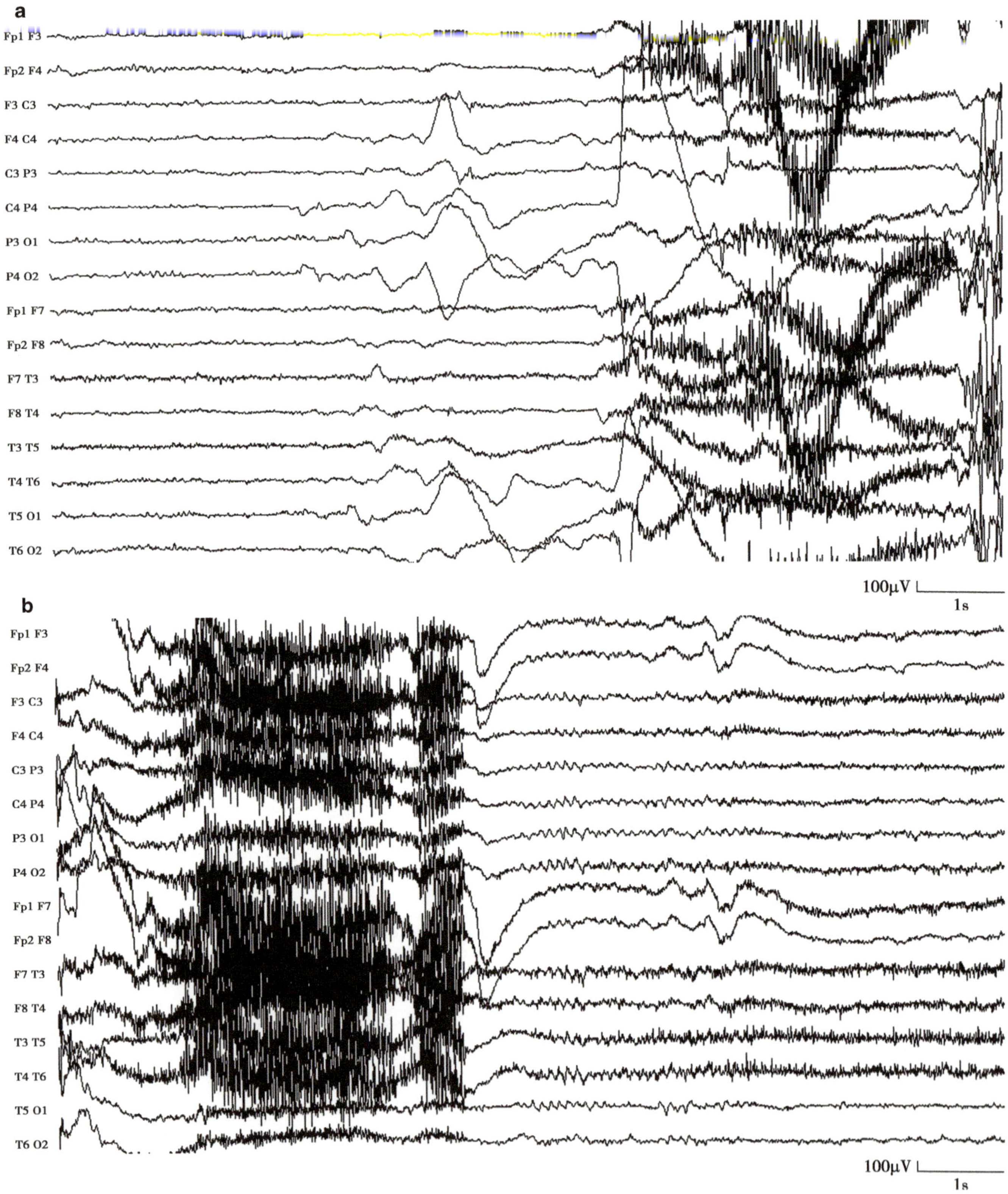

Fig. 3.4 Ictal scalp EEG. (**a**) Before seizure, the patient was lying on the left side with eyes closed in the awake state, and both upper limbs were flexed on the chest; during the seizure, he opened eyes, had a slightly sluggish expression, and started chewing 2 s later. The EEG showed fast activity of low amplitude, followed by mixed EMG artifacts. (**b**) The patient kept chewing with glassy eyes, raised head, and turned slightly to the left, with involuntary slow flexion and extension of the right lower limb. The EEG showed the rhythm of slow waves over the right frontal region, mixed with EMG artifacts. (**c**) The patient's symptoms were basically the same as in **b**. Sometimes there were involuntary movements of both upper limbs. The EEG showed the rhythm of sharp waves over the right temporal region and the rhythm of slow waves over the right frontal region with EMG artifacts. (**d**) The patient's symptoms were the same as in **c**. EMG artifacts were seen on the EEG

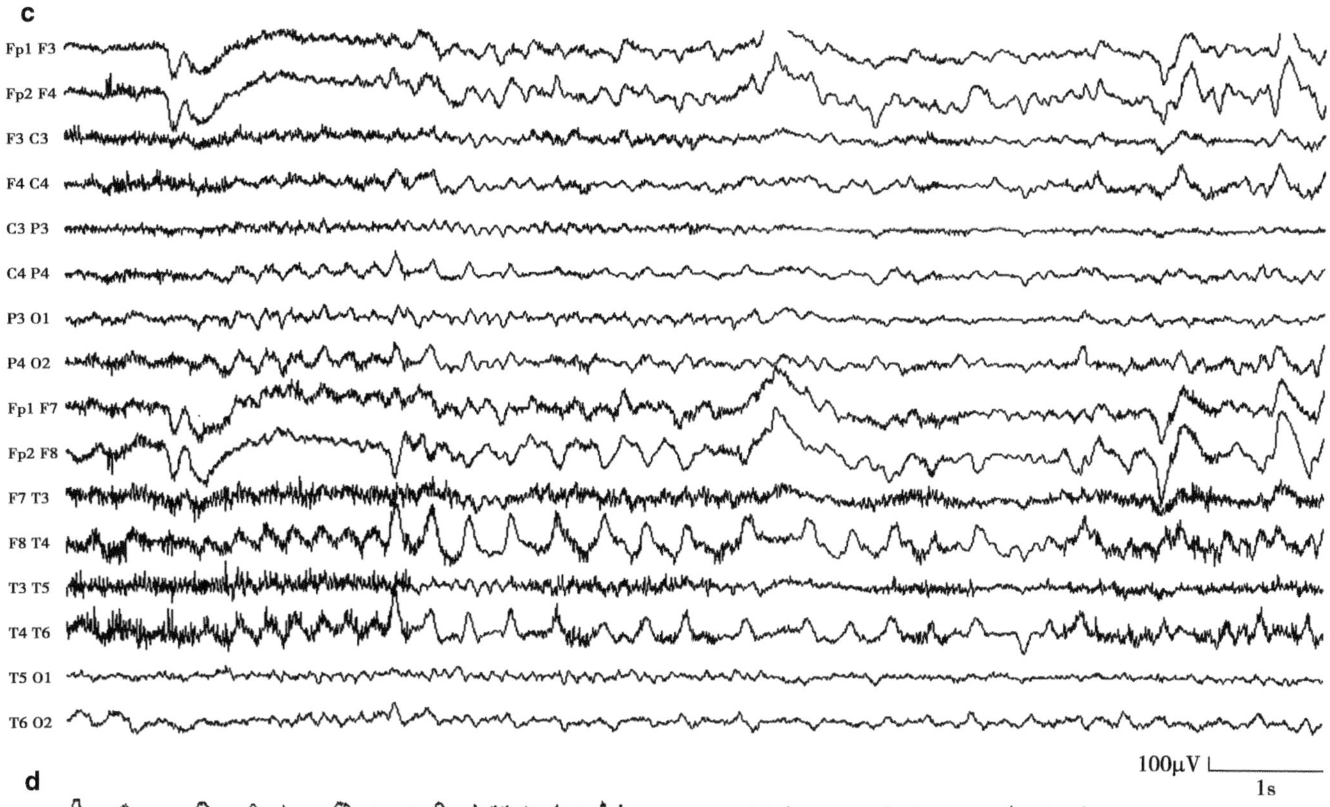

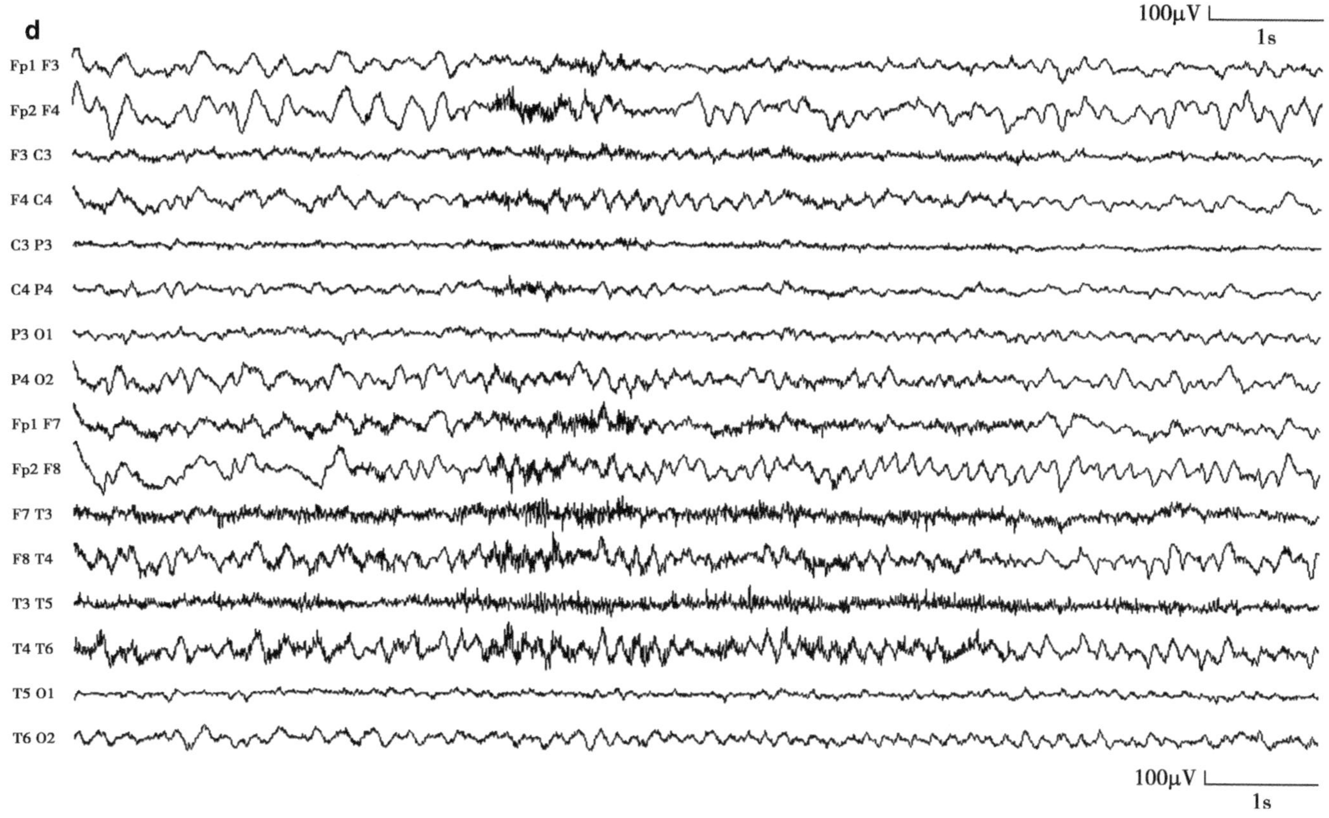

Fig. 3.4 (continued)

e

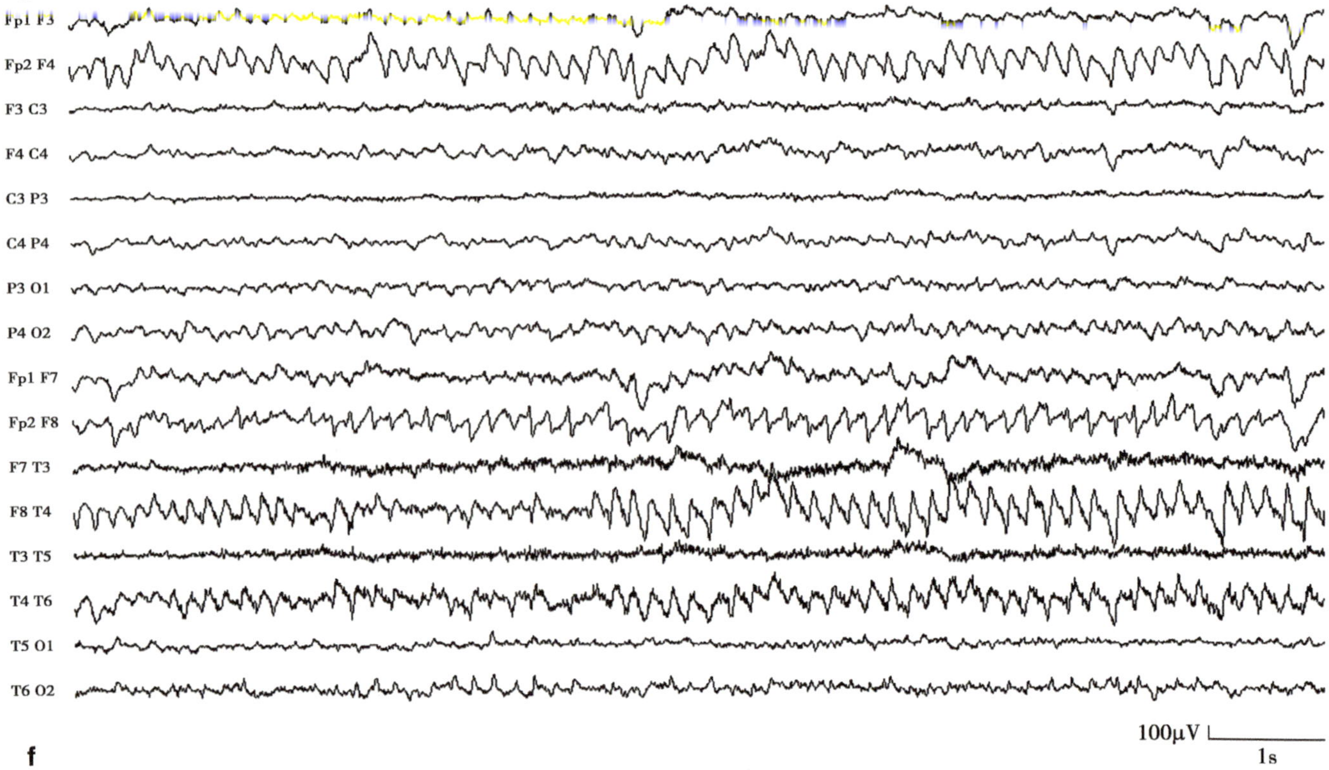

f

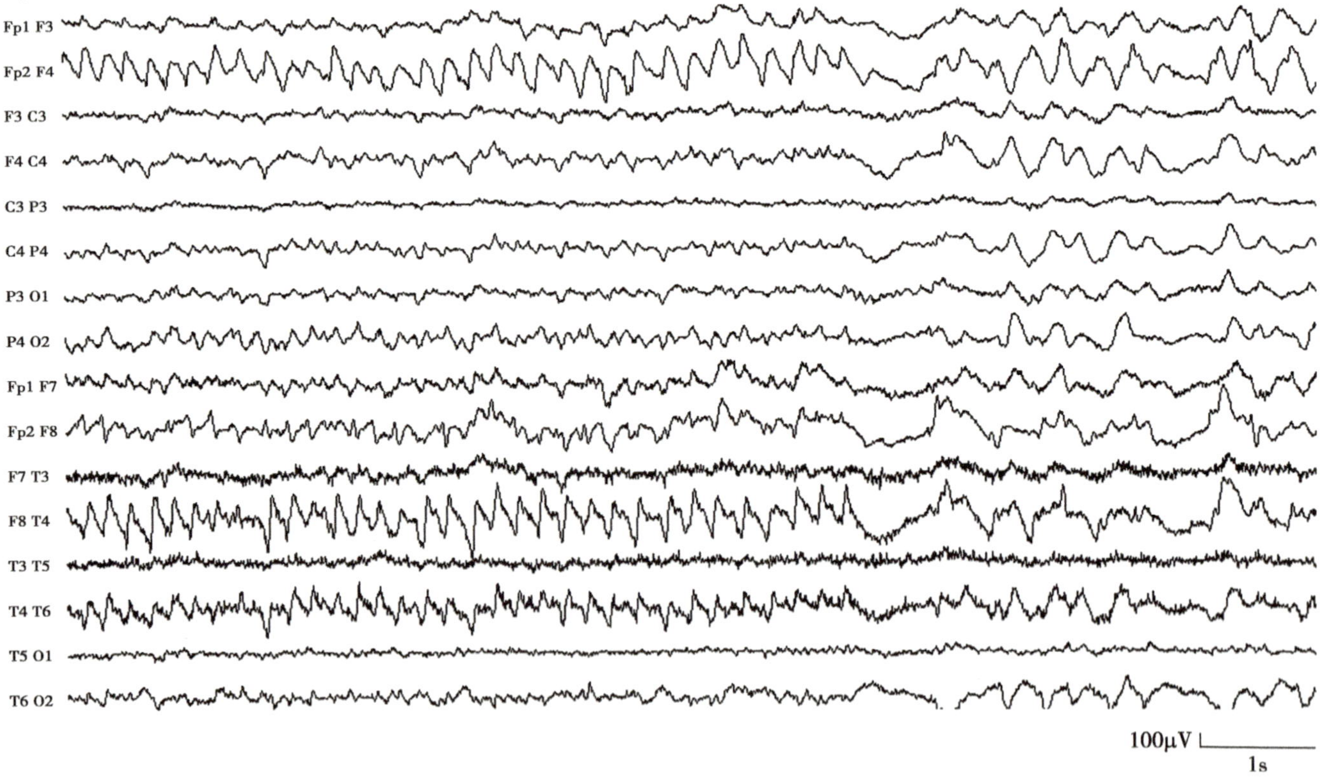

Fig. 3.4 (continued)

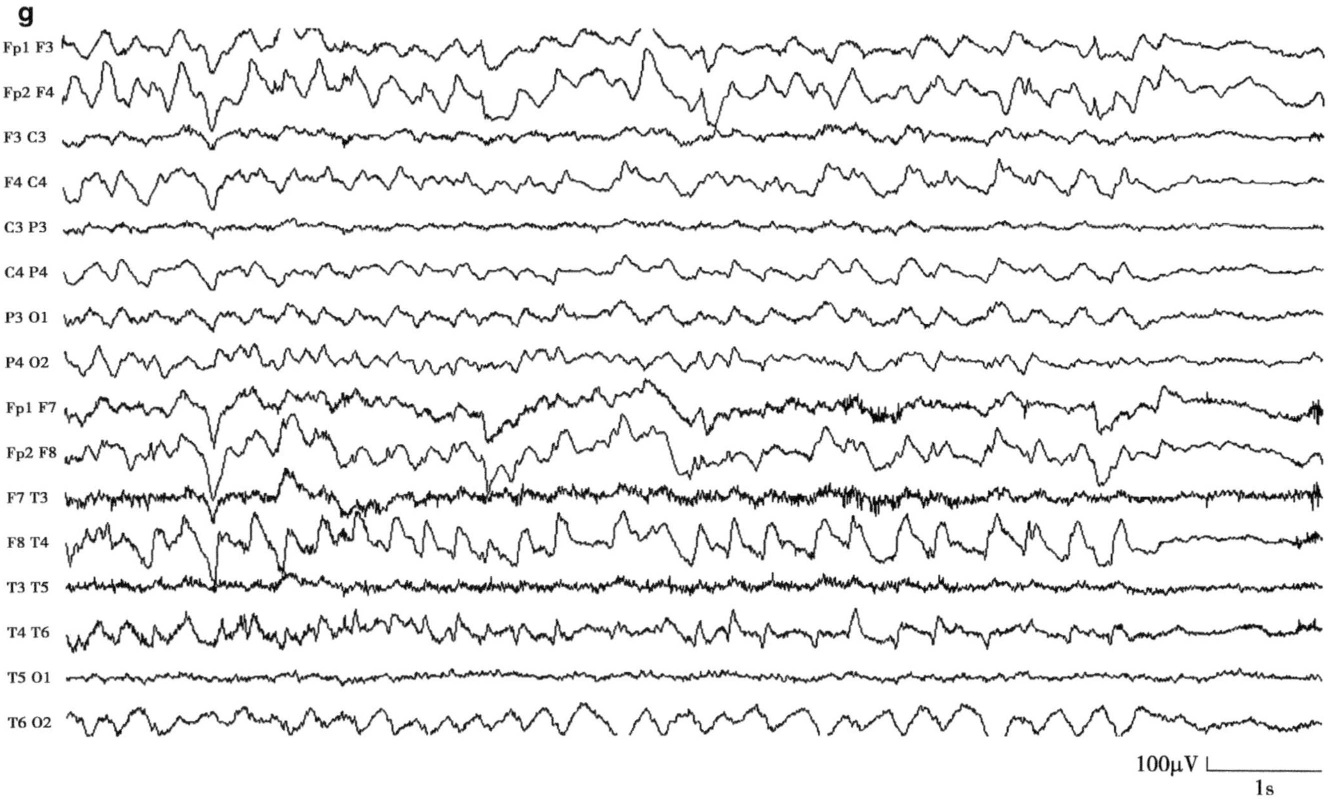

Fig. 3.4 (continued)

[Case Review]

1. Seizure characteristics
   (a) *Seizure characteristics*: The patient had staring eyes, constantly chewing, accompanied by automatic movements of both hands.
   (b) *EEG characteristics*: The interictal EEG showed phase-inverted sharp waves over the right sphenoid electrode. The interictal EEG showed flat waves of low amplitude. Artifacts showed up when the patient opened his eyes, followed by noticeable EMG artifacts caused by chewing movements (automatism). However, under the artifact masking, the sharpening slow wave activity was still visible, mainly over the right temporal region, which spread to the right frontal region and gradually formed a rhythm.
2. *Diagnosis and treatment strategy and follow-up results*: In combination with the clinical characteristics of the patient's dialeptic seizure and the interictal and ictal EEG, it was considered the patient had a right temporal lobe epilepsy of medial origin. The right anterior temporal lobe and medial structures were resected. After the surgery, the patient was seizure-free during a 1-year follow-up.

Case 3.3 Medial Temporal Lobe Epilepsy

[Abstract of Medical Records]
Female, 22 years old.

1. *Chief complaints*: Episodic loss of consciousness for 14 months.
2. *History of present illness*: The patient began to experience episodic disorders of consciousness without any inducement 14 months ago, manifested as lip smacking, fist clenching with the right hand, fumbling with the left hand, and haziness. Each seizure lasted for several seconds and then resolved spontaneously. Before the seizure, the patient felt panic and nausea. Initially, she had a seizure during sleep once in half a month. In the past 6 months, she experienced similar seizures during the daytime. Currently, the patient was taking carbamazepine and topiramate orally but still experienced 3.4 seizures per month, mostly at night. During the course of disease, the patient's diet, sleep, and urination and defecation were normal, without dizziness, headache, or limb twitching.
3. *Past history*: The patient had tuberculous meningitis at 10 months old.
4. *Physical examination*: The patient was conscious and articulate and had normal higher cortical functions, cerebral nerve examination results (negative), Grade 5 muscular strength of four limbs, slightly high flexor tension of right foot, and normal tone of other muscles. Her tendon reflexes were normal, and bilateral pathological signs were negative.
5. Imaging examination:
   (a) MRI showed the possibility of the left hippocampal sclerosis.
   (b) MRS showed that the concentration of NAA and Cho over the left hippocampus was lower than that on the contralateral side.
   (c) The cerebral blood flow perfusion imaging showed reduced perfusion over the left temporal pole cortex and poor perfusion over the left cerebral cortex and left thalamus.

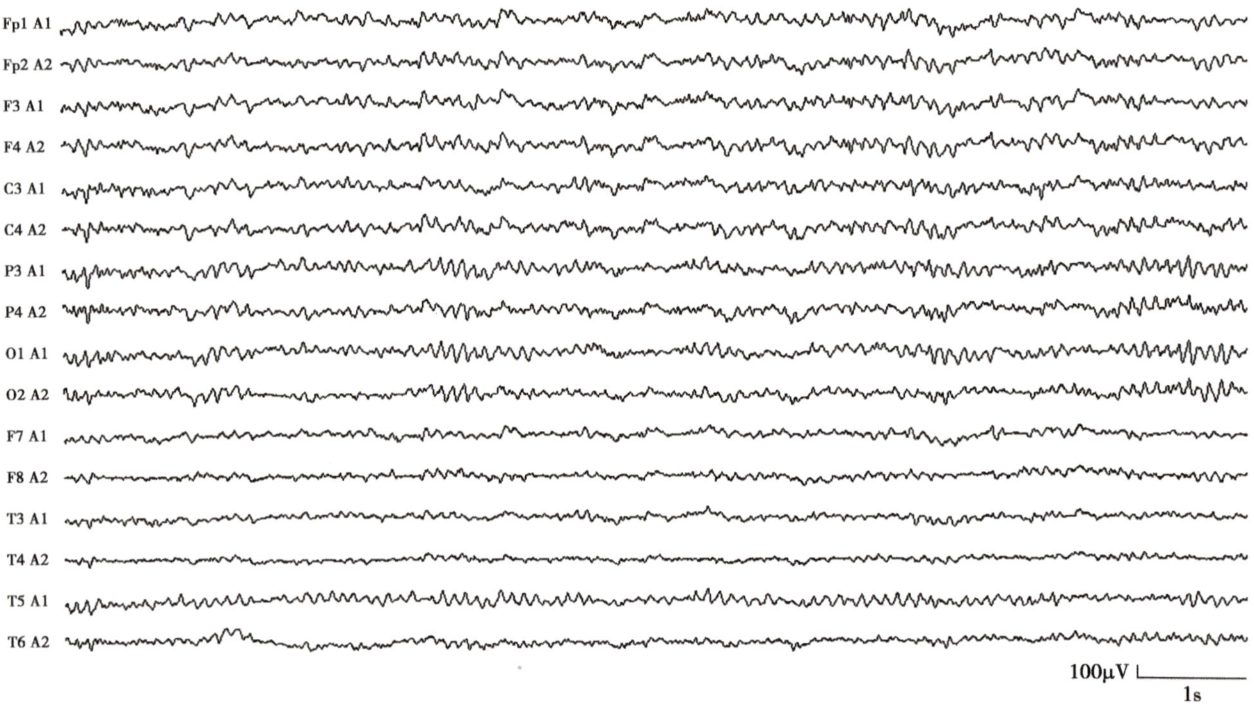

Fig. 3.5 Interictal scalp EEG. (**a**) The patient was conscious with eyes closed. The EEG showed sharp waves over the left sphenoid electrode and slow sharp waves over the left temporal region, which spread to the left frontal area. (**b**) Upon the activation of the left ear lobe electrode, positive sharp waves showed up over the left frontal and central area, and negative sharp waves showed up over the left anterior, middle, and posterior temporal region. (**c**) Sharp waves showed up over the left frontal area, and sharp-and-wave complexes showed up over the left temporal area. (**d**) When the patient was awake with eyes closed, sharp waves were seen over the left sphenoid electrode, and spike-and-wave complexes were seen over the left temporal area, which spread to the left frontal area

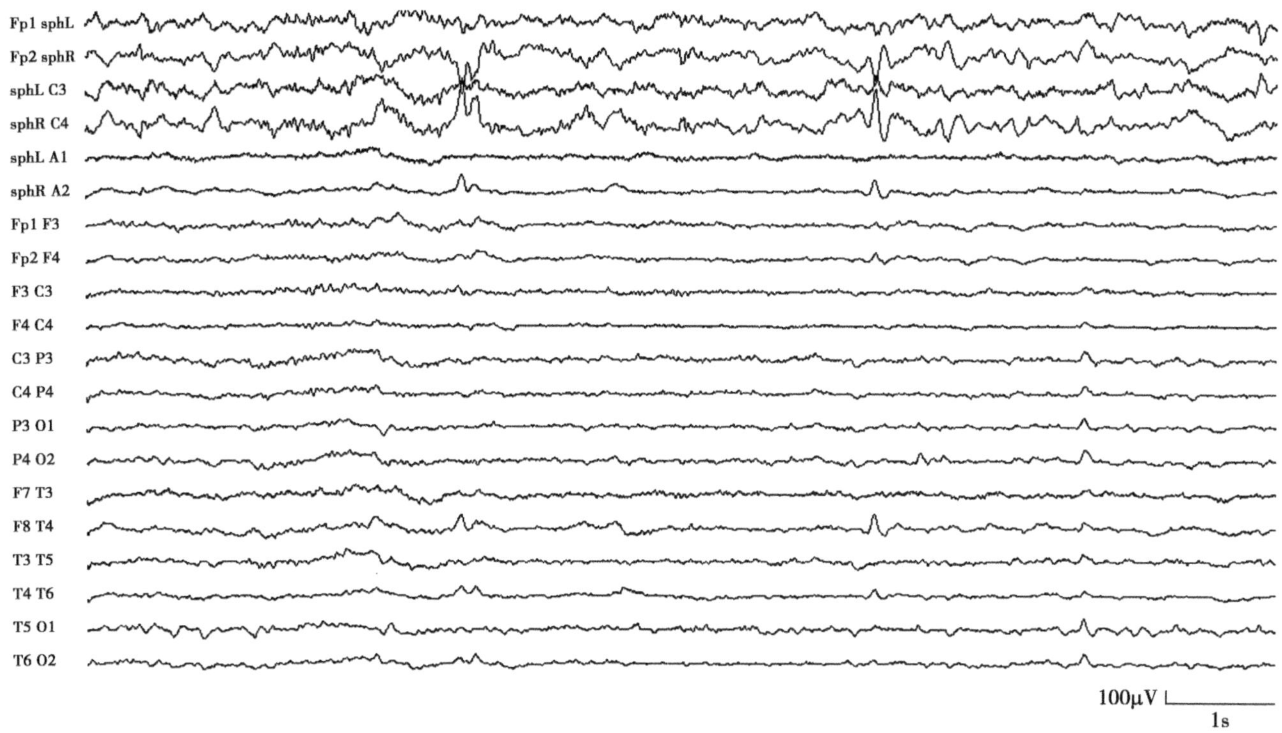

Fig. 3.6 Ictal scalp EEG. (**a**) The patient was reading a book in a supine position before the seizure and suddenly put down the book in his hand at the onset of the seizure, having a sluggish expression and blinking. The EEG showed a mixture of spike rhythm and slow waves over left sphenoid electrode, while the rhythm of slow waves appeared over the left posterior temporal area and bilateral parietal and occipital region simultaneously. (**b**) The patient smacked his lips 5 s later, raised the right upper limb once, and lifted head once involuntarily, followed by involuntary movements of both lower limbs. The EEG showed the rhythm of sharp waves over the left sphenoid electrode and the left temporal region, which spread to the left central and parietal region. (**c**) The patient had a slightly painful expression and slightly turned her head to the right. The right upper limb was flexed and stiffened, accompanied by lip smacking for 5 s. The EEG showed numerous mixed EMG artifacts. (**d**) The patient had a few mild clonus of the right upper limb and still smacked his lips and involuntarily raised and lowered the left lower limb. EEG showed numerous EMG artifacts. (**e**) The patient had a blank expression. The right upper limb was slightly stiffened and flexed in front of the chest, accompanied by raising head, moving legs, twisting body, and left hand automatism from time to time. The EEG showed the rhythm of sharp waves over the left hemisphere. (**f**) The patient's symptoms were basically the same as in **e**, characterized by continuously lifting legs and body when she was in a supine position and keeping swallowing. The EEG manifestation was basically the same as in **e**. (**g**) The patient constantly raised her head and smacked her lips. The EEG manifestation was basically the same as in **e**. (**h**) The patient shrugged her shoulders, lightly kicked with both lower limbs, and fumbled with both hands in front of the chest till the seizure ended. The EEG showed a mixture of 3.0–5.0 Hz slow waves of high amplitude and wobble artifacts over the left hemisphere

6. *EEG*: For details, see Figs. 3.5 and 3.6.

[Case Review]

1. Case Characteristics
   (a) *Seizure characteristics*: The patient experienced oropharyngeal automatism with involuntary movements of the limbs, which was generally characterized by increased muscular tone, occasionally with mild clonus, and mainly the left upper limb. As the seizure progressed, the patient showed automatism in both hands and repeated pedaling-like movements of both lower limbs, suggesting symptoms of the involvement of bilateral temporal and frontal lobes.
   (b) *EEG characteristics*: Interictal EEG showed spike-and-wave complexes over the left frontal region and the left temporal region. The ictal EEG first showed wave amplitude depression, followed by the rhythm of slow waves and sharp waves mainly over the left posterior temporal region, which spread extensively.
2. *Diagnosis and treatment strategy and follow-up results*: The patient received the resection of the left anterior temporal lobe and medial structures and was seizure-free during a 4-year follow-up postoperation.

Case 3.4 Medial Temporal Lobe Epilepsy

(Same patient as Case 3.1 with another seizure)

[Abstract of Medical Records]
Female, 23 years old.

1. *Chief complaint*: Episodic loss of consciousness for 5 years.
2. *History of present illness*: There are two seizure types. Type I: episodic palpitation and chest discomfort with clear consciousness ending in about 20 seconds, with 2–3 seizures per month. Type II: generalized convulsions secondary to type I seizure, 1 seizure per month on average. She once took phenobarbital and phenytoin sodium, the effect of which were both poor. She is now taking carbamazepine 200 mg/dose t.i.d and sodium valproate 400 mg/dose t.i.d.
3. *Personal and family history*: No history of associated diseases.
4. *Imaging examination*: The brain MRI showed right hippocampal sclerosis.
5. *EEG*: For details, see Figs. 3.7 and 3.8.

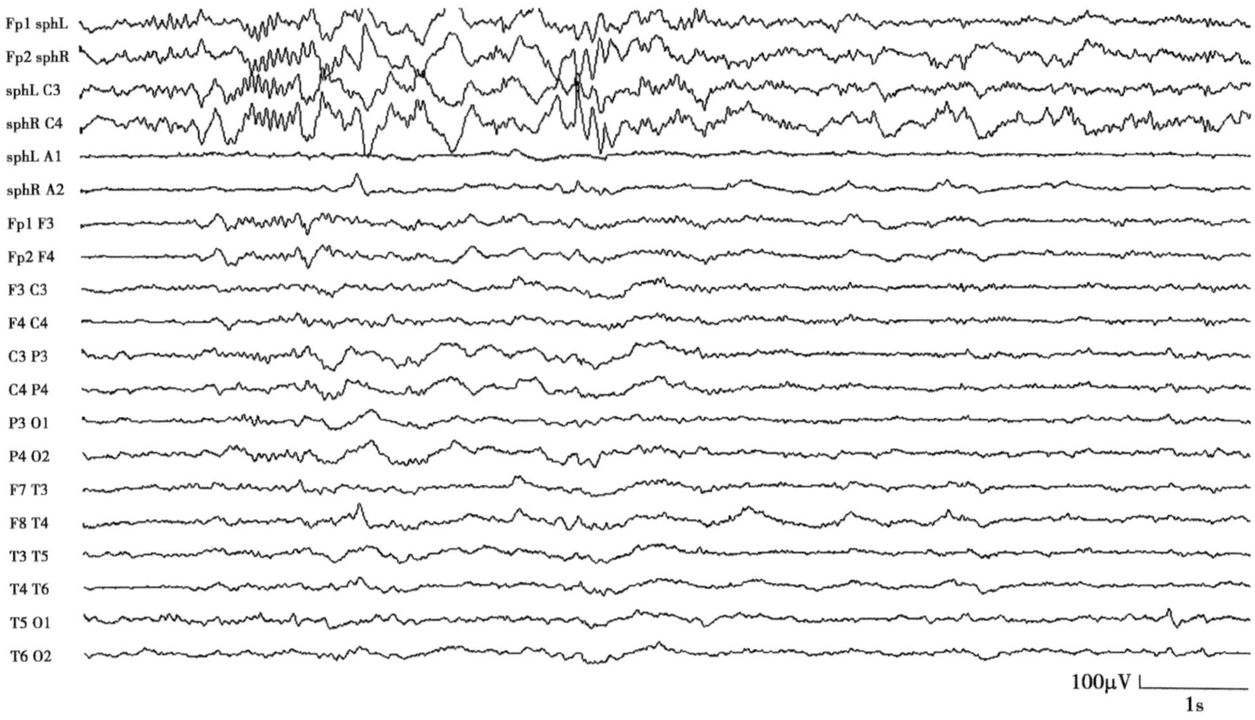

Fig. 3.7 Interictal scalp EEG. (**a**) The patient was awake with eyes closed. The basic rhythm of EEG was 9.0 Hz. (**b**) The EEG of stage II of sleep showed sharp waves over the right sphenoidal electrode. (**c**) The EEG of stage II of sleep showed sharp waves and sharp-and-wave complexes over the right temporal region

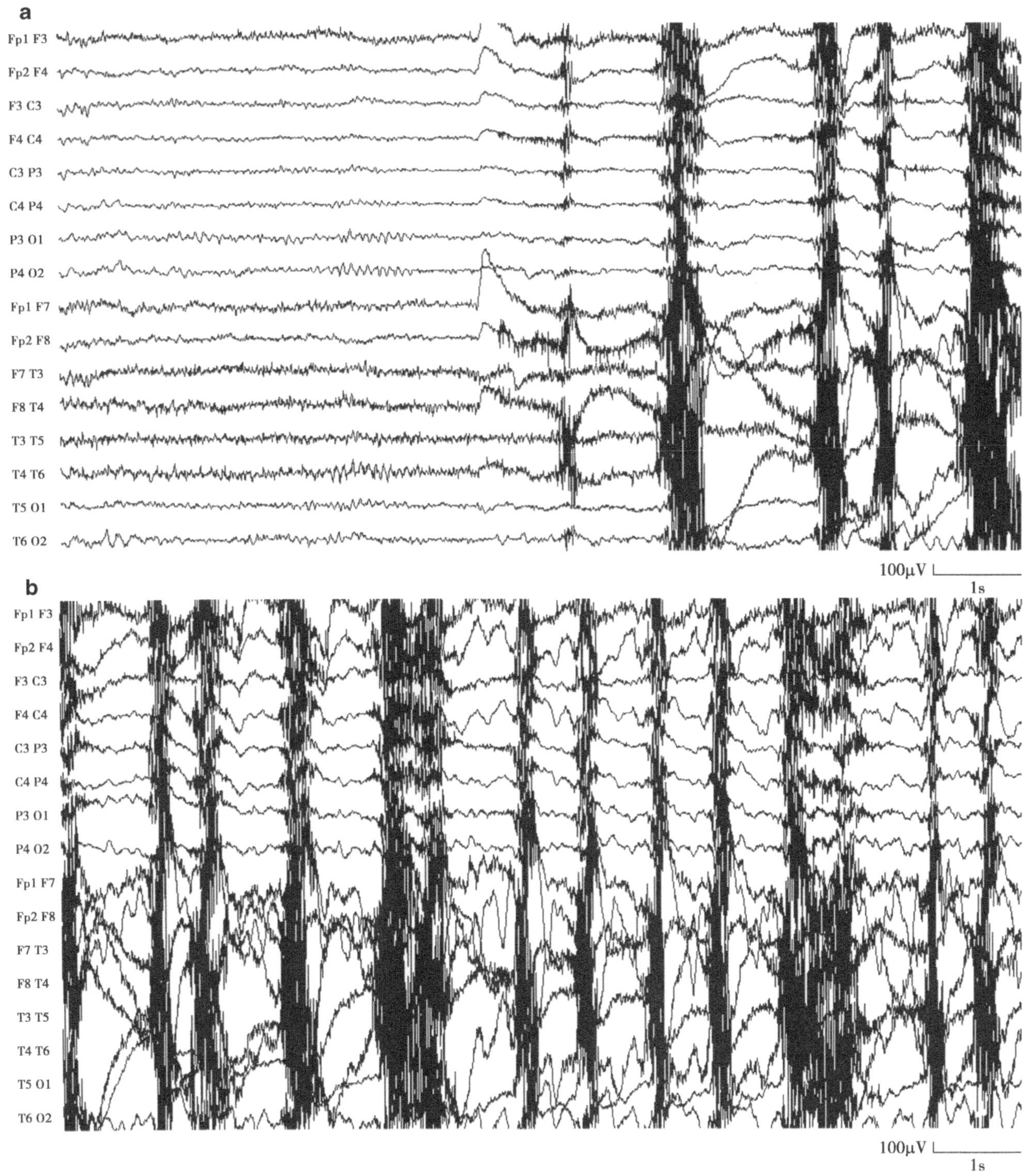

Fig. 3.8 Ictal scalp EEG. (**a**) Before the seizure, the patient was lying awake and felt chest tightness and discomfort and indicated to her family member that a seizure was about to come. The EEG showed slow waves over the right posterior temporal region and artifacts over the left temporal and parietal leads during wakefulness. (**b**) The patient had no obvious movements. The EEG showed irregular slow waves over the right frontal region (F2 F4, Fp2 F8) and sharp waves of low amplitude over the right temporal region (T4 T6, T6 O2). (**c**) The patient suddenly screamed, with the mouth corners twitching to the left, followed by mouth opening and backward tilting of the head. The EEG showed the rhythm of sharp waves over the right frontal and temporal region and a few spike-and-wave complexes over the right frontal region (Fp2 F4), followed by EMG artifacts and wobble artifacts. (**d**) The patient tilted her head backwards and wide opened the mouth, with tonic flexion first and then limbs tonic extension. EEG showed numerous EMG artifacts and wobble artifacts. (**e**) The patient had tonic limbs, with clonus 5 s later. The EEG presentation was the same as **d**. (**f**) The patient's symptoms changed from tonic clonus to clonus. The EEG showed rhythmic artifacts and wobble artifacts. (**g**) The clonic rhythm gradually decreased. The EEG showed spike-and-wave complexes and polyspike and wave complexes with EMG artifacts and wobble artifacts, while the EMG artifacts were less than before. (**h**) At the end of clonus, the patient fell into a stupor state. The EEG was mixed with EMG artifacts

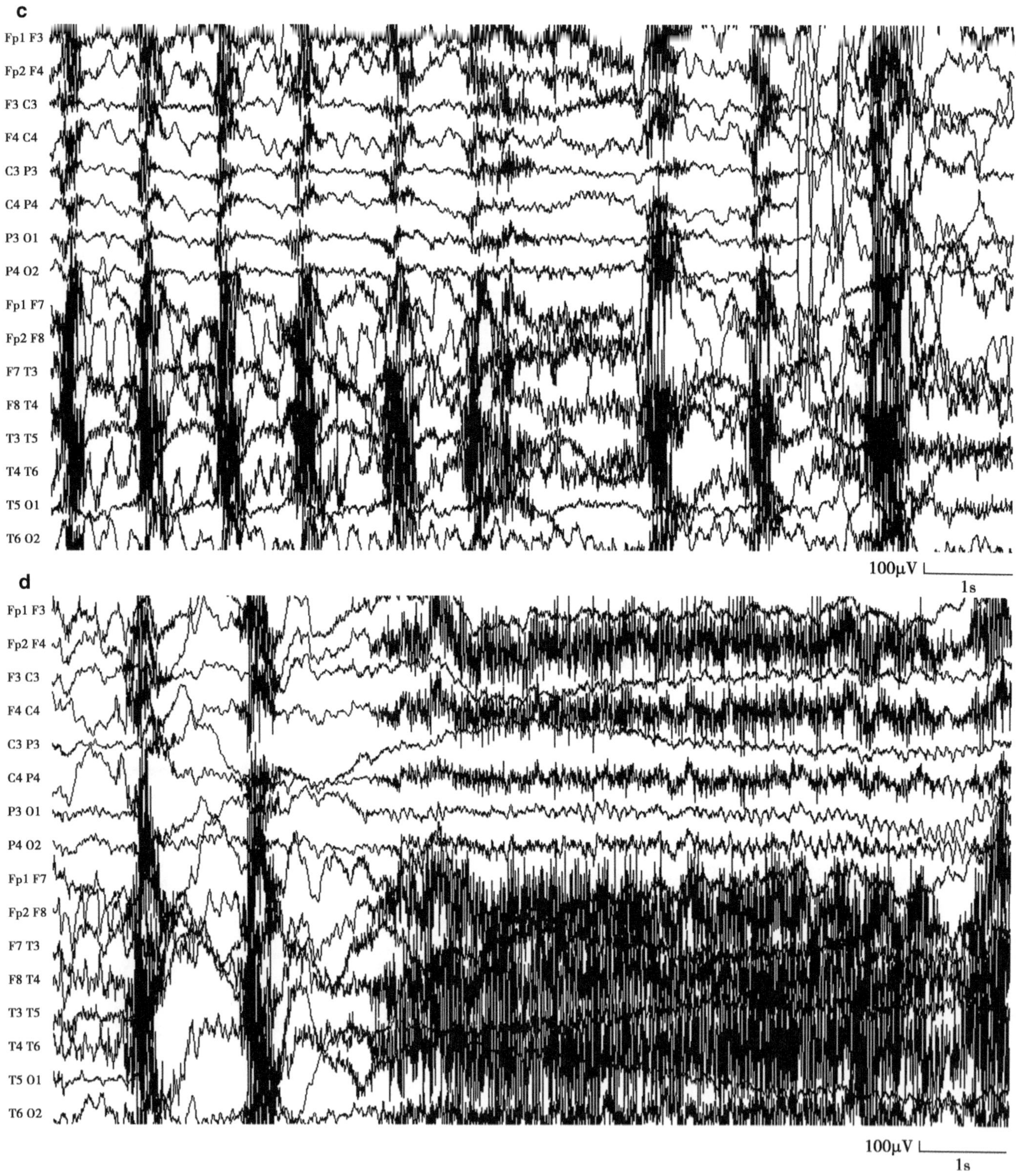

Fig. 3.8 (continued)

[Case Review]

1. Case Characteristics
   (a) *Seizure characteristics*: This patient showed the seizure symptoms of typical medial temporal lobe epilepsy.
   (b) *EEG characteristics*: The interictal EEG showed limited spikes over the right temporal electrode and the right sphenoidal electrode; the ictal EEG showed rhythmic slow wave activity especially over the right temporal region, which involved the right frontal region and gradually increased to form the rhythm of sharp waves. The duration of the whole process was short, and the EEG changes were mainly over the temporal and prefrontal regions, which did not noticeably spread to the periphery.
2. *Diagnosis and treatment strategy and follow-up results*: It was combined with the characteristics of the patient's seizures, EEG characteristics, and imaging findings to confirm that the patient had signs of hippocampal sclerosis, and a selective right hippocampal amygdala resection was performed. The patient was followed up for 3 years without seizures, and the drug has been discontinued.

Case 3.5 Medial Temporal Lobe Epilepsy

[Abstract of Medical Records]
Female, 36 years old.

1. *Chief complaint*: Episodic loss of awareness with twitching for 16 years.
2. *History of present illness*: The patient suddenly screamed at night during sleep without any obvious inducement 16 years ago, followed by loss of awareness and twitching of the limbs, which lasted for more than 10 min and then resolved. After resolution, she had two more seizures in the same way on the same day. Afterwards, she was treated at a clinic with unknown medication and had no further seizures for about 1 year. Fifteen years ago, the patient was irritated and then screamed again, accompanied by twitching, loss of awareness, and generalized tonic clonus, which lasted more than 10 min and then resolved. Since then, the patient experienced irregular seizures, sometimes up to 2–6 times a day. Thirteen years ago, she took phenytoin sodium for more than 1 year, which caused hairy all over the body, and hence discontinued the medication. The effect of taking sodium valproate and topiramate was unsatisfactory. The patient is now taking carbamazepine at a dose of 500 mg/d, with an average of 1 seizure every 2–3 days, which is characterized by loss of awareness, generalized tonic clonus, and occasional urinary incontinence.
3. *Past history*: The patient was born at term without any history of hypoxia or trauma. She suffered from whooping cough, pyrexia, and convulsions twice at 2 years old, which resulted in strabismus and amblyopia in her right eye. Strabismus was surgically corrected later.
4. *Personal and family history*: No history of associated diseases.
5. *Physical examination*: The patient had poor computing power. The intelligence examination revealed slightly lower intelligence.
6. Imaging examination:
   (a) MRI revealed right hippocampal sclerosis.
   (b) SPECT revealed localized hypoperfusion over the right frontoparietal junction and the bilateral medial temporal cortices and slight hypoperfusion over the right frontal and temporal cortices over a large area.
7. *EEG*: For details, see Figs. 3.9 and 3.10.

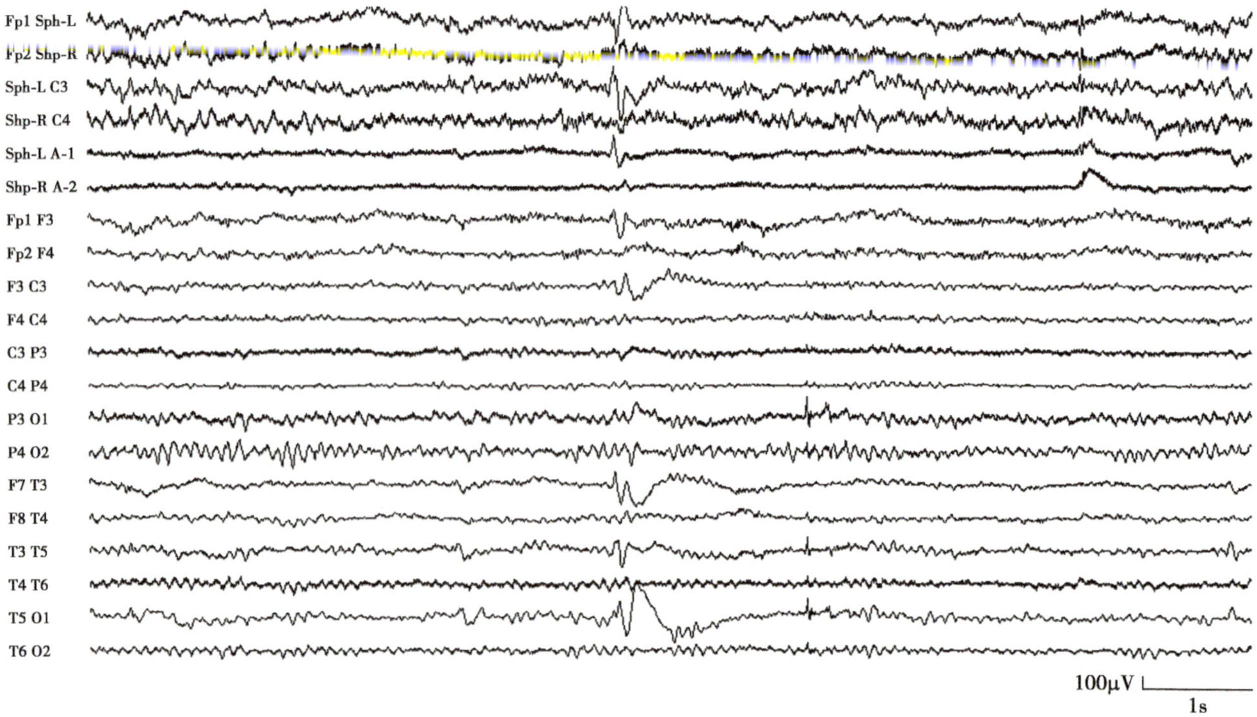

Fig. 3.9 Interictal scalp EEG. (**a**) The background EEG during wakefulness showed the rhythm of 9.0–10.0 Hz α waves over the occipital region. (**b**) The EEG showed sharp waves of high amplitude over the right posterior frontal, central, parietal, occipital, and temporal regions. (**c**) The EEG showed phase reversing spikes over the right sphenoidal electrode and the right temporal region. (**d**) The EEG showed spike-and-wave complexes over the bilateral sphenoid electrodes and spikes over the bilateral frontal regions and right temporal region. (**e**) The EEG showed spike-and-wave complexes of high amplitude, mainly on the right

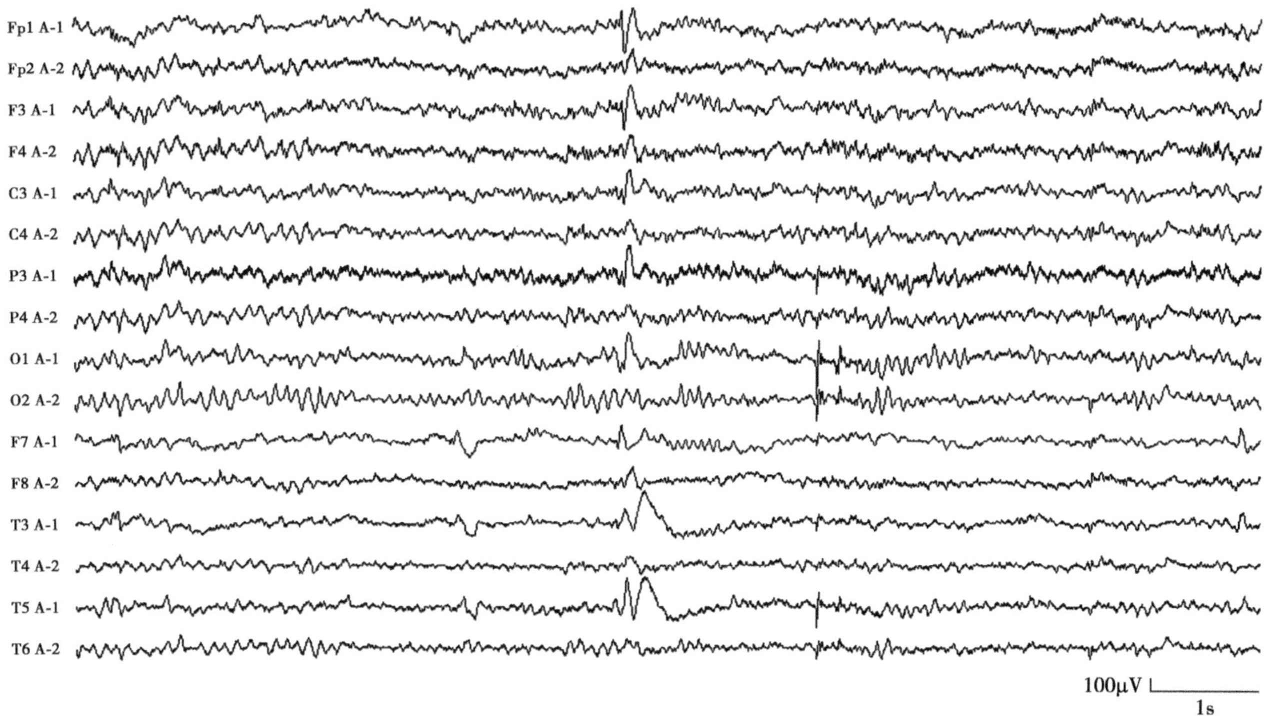

Fig. 3.10 Ictal scalp EEG. (**a**) The patient was awake without limb movements. The EEG was the background EEG when the patient was awake. (**b**) The patient had no limb movements. The EEG showed fast activities of low amplitude for 4 s and the rhythm of 2.0–5.0 Hz slow waves of medium and low amplitude mainly over the right hemishpere. (**c**) 5 s later, the patient opened his eyes and swallowed. The EEG showed irregular slow-wave rhythm over the right temporal region, sharp wave rhythm over the right sphenoid electrode, followed by the rhythm of spike-and-wave complexes over the bilateral frontal and parietal leads. Slow waves mixed with spikes were seen over other electrodes, mainly on the right. (**d**) The patient was lying flat on her back with the upper limbs moving around. 10 s later, her head was tilted to the left and the mouth corners were tilted to the left. The EEG showed the rhythms of slow waves and sharp-and-wave complexes, with increased amplitude and decreased frequency, followed by the rhythm of 8.0–9.0 Hz sharp waves over the right sphenoid electrode and over the right temporal region, mixed with EMG artifacts and wobble artifacts. (**e**) The patient still turned head to the left while making sound. The corners of her mouth twitched to the left, and the left upper limb was elevated and flexed, with the five fingers being extended. The EEG showed EMG artifacts and wobble artifacts. (**f**) The patient's mouth corners twitched to the left; the lower limbs were straight and the hands were clenched. The left upper limb was flexed in front of the chest, and the right upper limb was elevated in clonus. The EEG showed numerous EMG artifacts and wobble artifacts. (**g**) The patient opened the mouth while making sound, with the jaw twitching, hands clenched, the upper limbs flexed in front of the chest, the lower limbs being straight, followed by generalized tonic clonus. The EEG showed numerous EMG artifacts and wobble artifacts. (**h**, **i**) The patient's symptoms and the EEG presentation were basically same as in **g**. (**j**) The patient's symptoms were the same as in **g**. The patient recovered with muscle relaxed and fell into sleep while snoring. The EEG showed numerous EMG artifacts and wobble artifacts

[Case Review]

1. Pathological characteristics
   (a) *Seizure characteristics*: During this seizure, swallowing only briefly occurred in the early stage, followed by the deflection of head and eyes to the left and left facial twitching that progressed to bilateral tonic-clonic seizure.
   (b) *EEG characteristics*: The patient's interictal EEG showed spikes and spike-and-wave complexes mainly over the right temporal region and also spike-and-wave complexes over the whole leads. Amplitude reduction was seen on the ictal EEG, followed by extensive slow wave rhythm on the right, during which the spike-and-wave rhythm was seen mainly over the right temporal region.
   (c) *Imaging characteristics*: MRI revealed right hippocampal sclerosis.
2. *Diagnosis and treatment strategy and follow-up results*: Although MRI revealed right hippocampal sclerosis, the EEG and seizure characteristics were significantly different from those of common temporal lobe epilepsy. Considering that the seizure originated from the temporal lobe, rapidly spread to the broader cortex on the right, and progressed into a bilateral tonic-clonic seizure, the right anterior temporal lobe and medial structure were surgically resected. The seizures disappeared during a 3-year follow-up after surgery.

Case 3.6 Medial Temporal Lobe Epilepsy

[Abstract of Medical Records]
Male, 44 years old.

1. *Chief complaint*: Episodic loss of awareness for more than 20 years.
2. *History of present illness*: The patient complained of episodic loss of awareness without any obvious inducement 20 years ago, manifested by flexion of both upper limbs, extension of lower limbs with convulsions, eyes on the turn, froth at the mouth, cyanosis of lips, and urinary incontinence, which lasted for 3–5 min and then resolved. The patient fell asleep and could not recall after waking up. The seizures occurred 4–5 times a year, all at night during sleep. He orally took phenytoin sodium. The seizures above did not occur again, but there were minor seizures characterized by straightening of the eyes, unresponsiveness, making licks, swallowing, and retching. The patient experienced dizziness and discomfort in the upper abdomen before the seizure, which occurred 7–8 times a month. Sometimes the patient stared blankly, looked around, and smacked lips, all of which lasted 1–2 min and then resolved. Seizures occurred both during the day and night. Treatment with carbamazepine had no significant resolving effects. The patient discontinued phenytoin sodium 7 years ago due to its toxicity and replaced it with topiramate, which failed to control the seizures. Three years ago, he started the treatment of carbamazepine combined with topiramate by gradually increasing the dosage, which was ineffective; then he was treated with oxcarbazepine, which was also ineffective; since then, he has been treated with gabapentin till now, while the seizure still occurred frequently up to 2–3 times a day at an interval of 1–2 days. Since the onset of the disease, the patient experienced significant memory loss, no weight change, good appetite, poor sleep, and normal bladder and bowel functions.
3. *Past history*: The patient was born at full-term by normal delivery. He did not have a history of trauma. He suffered from encephalitis at 3–4 months old, the details of which are unknown.
4. *Family history*: No family genetic history.
5. *Physical examination*: No neurological abnormalities were found.
6. Psychological test report: The results of the Wechsler Adult Intelligence Scale-Revised by China (WAIS-RC) showed verbal intelligence quotient (VIQ) = 77, performance intelligence quotient (PIQ) = 79, full intelligence quotient (FIQ) = 76; the impression of the WAIS-RC IQ test showed marginal intelligence.
7. Imaging examination.
   (a) MRI was consistent with the bilateral hippocampal sclerotic changes.
   (b) MRS revealed that the NAA concentration (NAA/Cr: 1.18) over the left hippocampus was slightly higher than that over the right side (NAA/Cr: 1.10); the Cho concentration (NAA/Cr: 1.27) over the left hippocampus was slightly higher than that over the right side (NAA/Cr: 1.00).
   (c) The cerebral blood flow perfusion imaging (interictal) SPECT showed localized hypoperfusion over the left frontal and temporal junction cortex and poor perfusion over the bilateral temporal regions, mainly on the right.
8. *EEG*: For details, see Figs. 3.11, 3.12, 3.13, and 3.14.

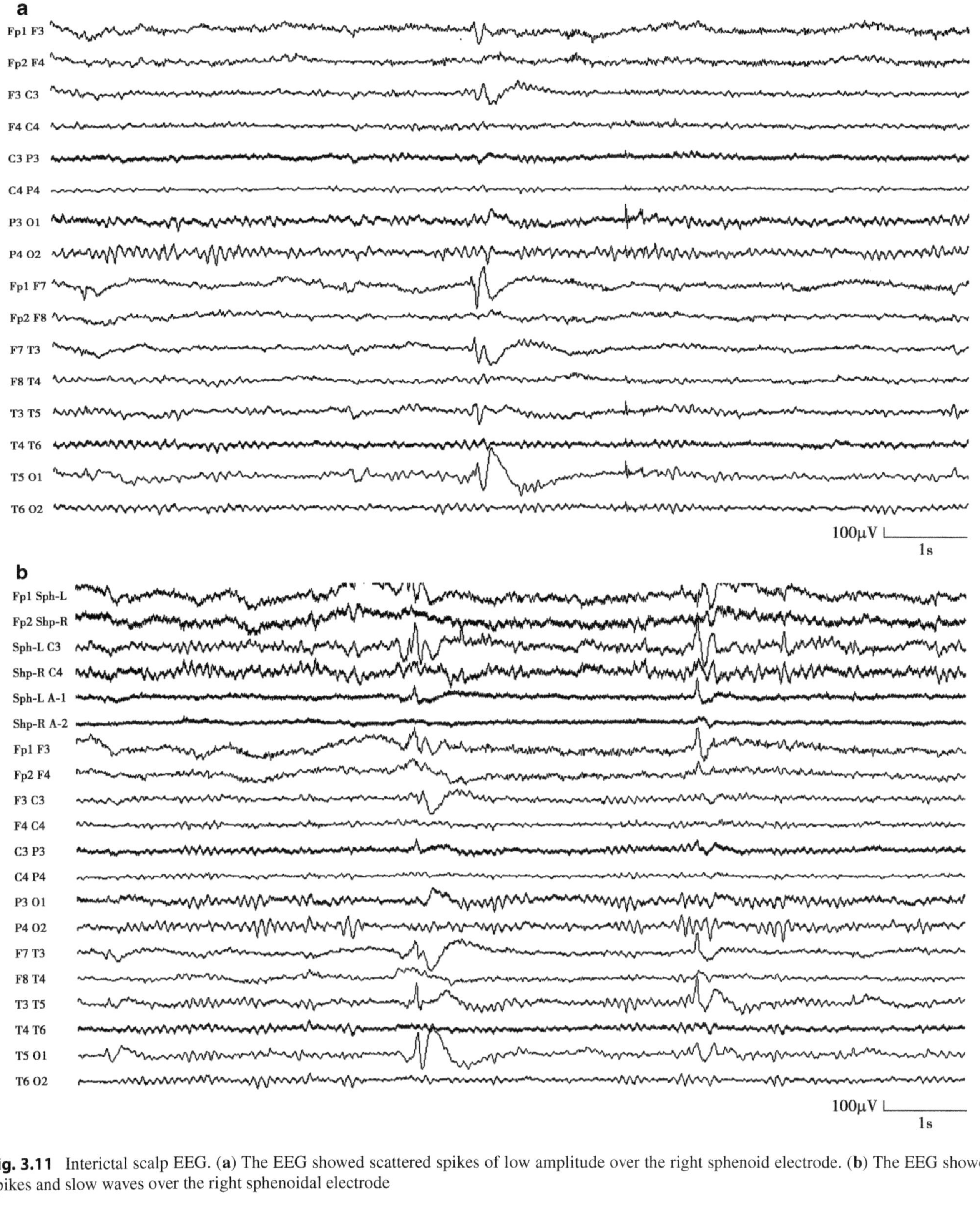

Fig. 3.11 Interictal scalp EEG. (**a**) The EEG showed scattered spikes of low amplitude over the right sphenoid electrode. (**b**) The EEG showed spikes and slow waves over the right sphenoidal electrode

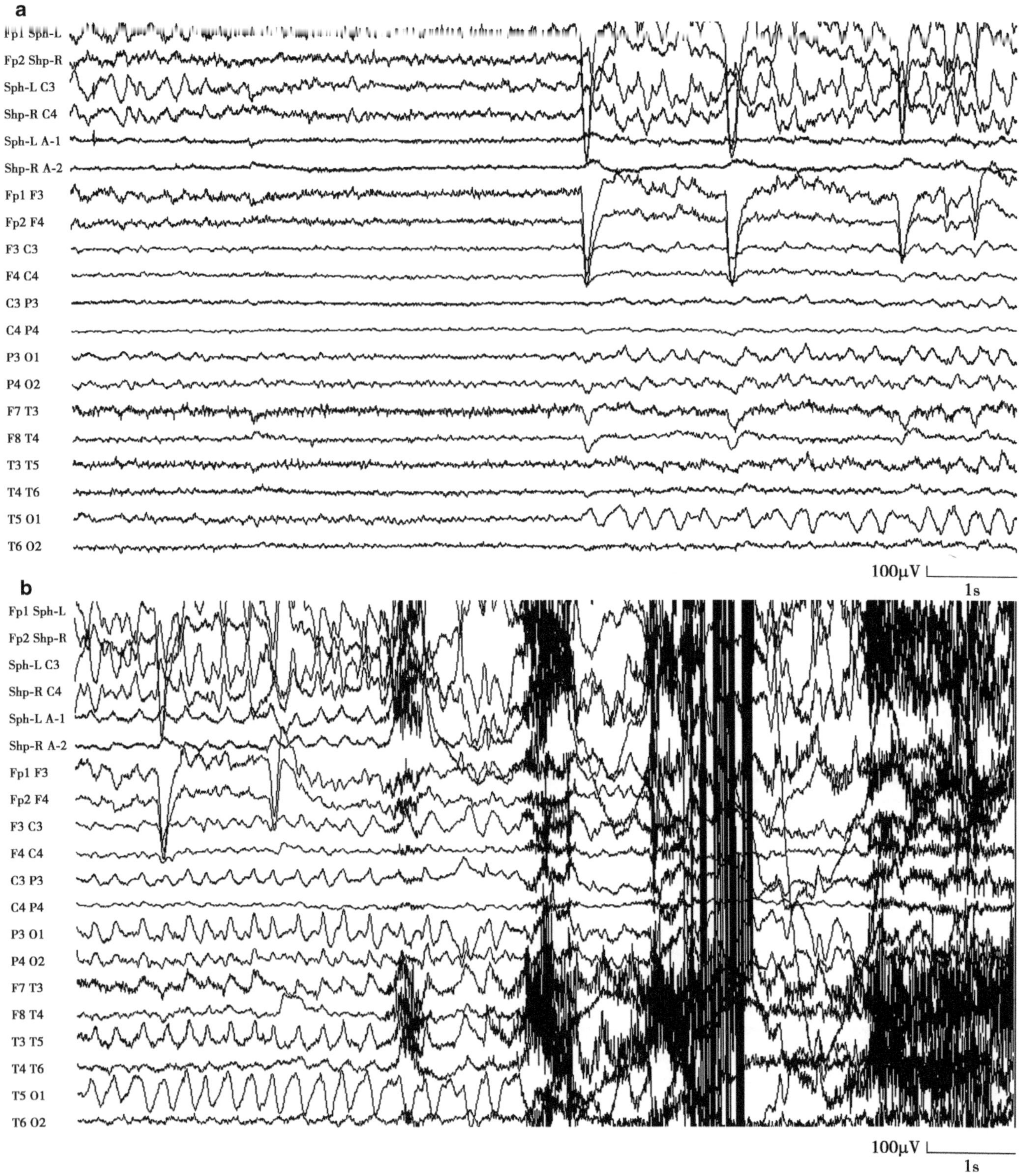

Fig. 3.12 Ictal scalp EEG. (**a**) The patient was asleep before the seizure and woke up from sleep without obvious auras. The EEG was shifted from stage II of sleep to fast activity of low amplitude. The rhythm of slow waves was seen over the bilateral sphenoidal electrode. (**b**) The patient smacked lips and fumbled with the right hand during the seizure. The EEG showed sharp waves of medium amplitude in bilateral sphenoid electrodes, followed by the rhythm of sharp waves over the right sphenoid electrode and sharp waves over the right temporal region. (**c**) The patient was still smacking lips and the expression was dull. The EEG showed the rhythm of sharp waves over the right sphenoidal electrode and a mixture of rhythmic sharp waves and slow waves over the right temporal region. (**d**) The patient's manifestation was the same as in **c**. The EEG showed the rhythm of sharp waves over the right sphenoid electrode. Mixed EMG artifacts can be seen. (**e**) The patient's manifestation was the same as in **c**. The EEG showed mixed EMG artifacts in all leads and the rhythm of slow waves over the right posterior temporal region and the midline

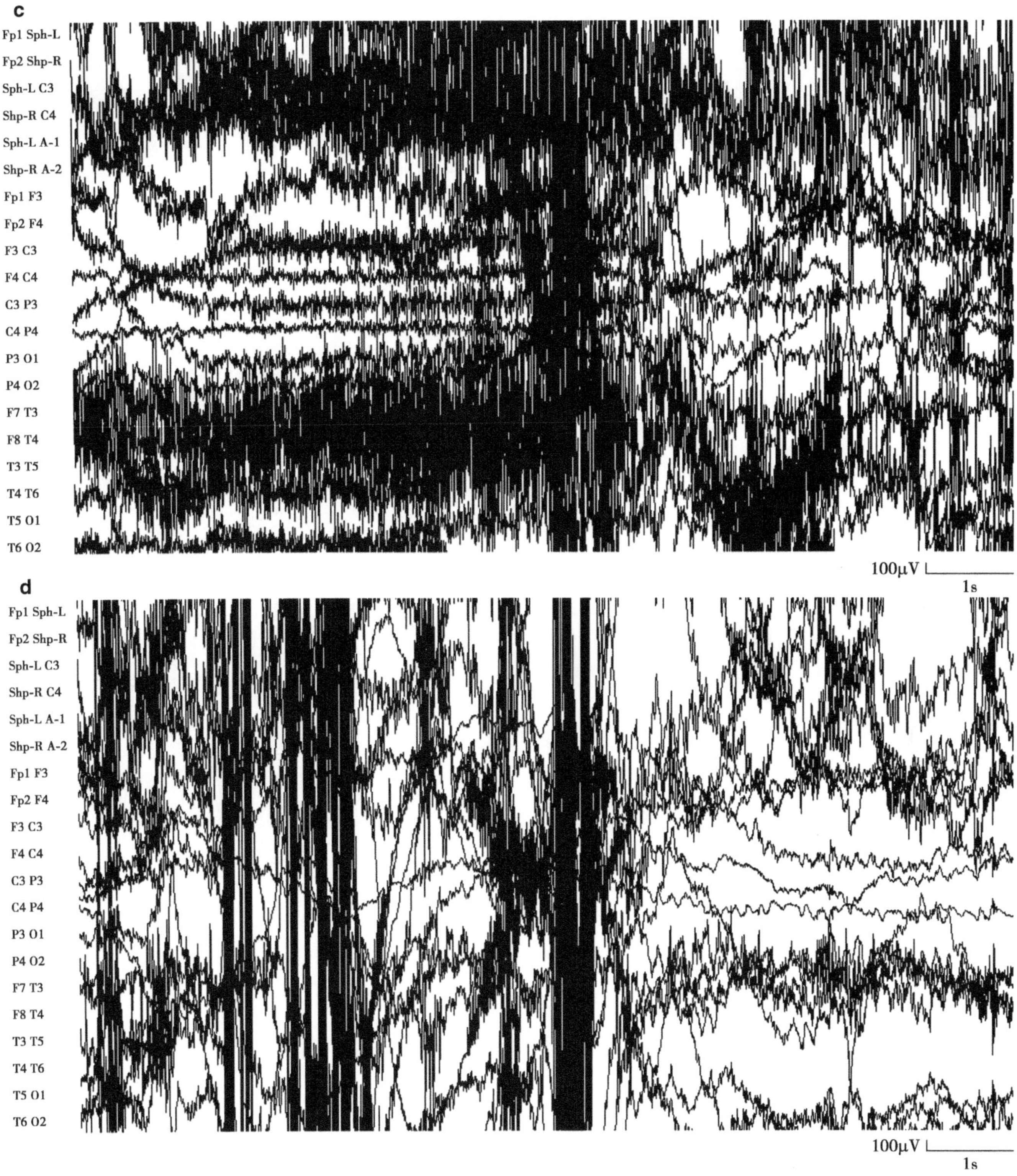

Fig. 3.12 (continued)

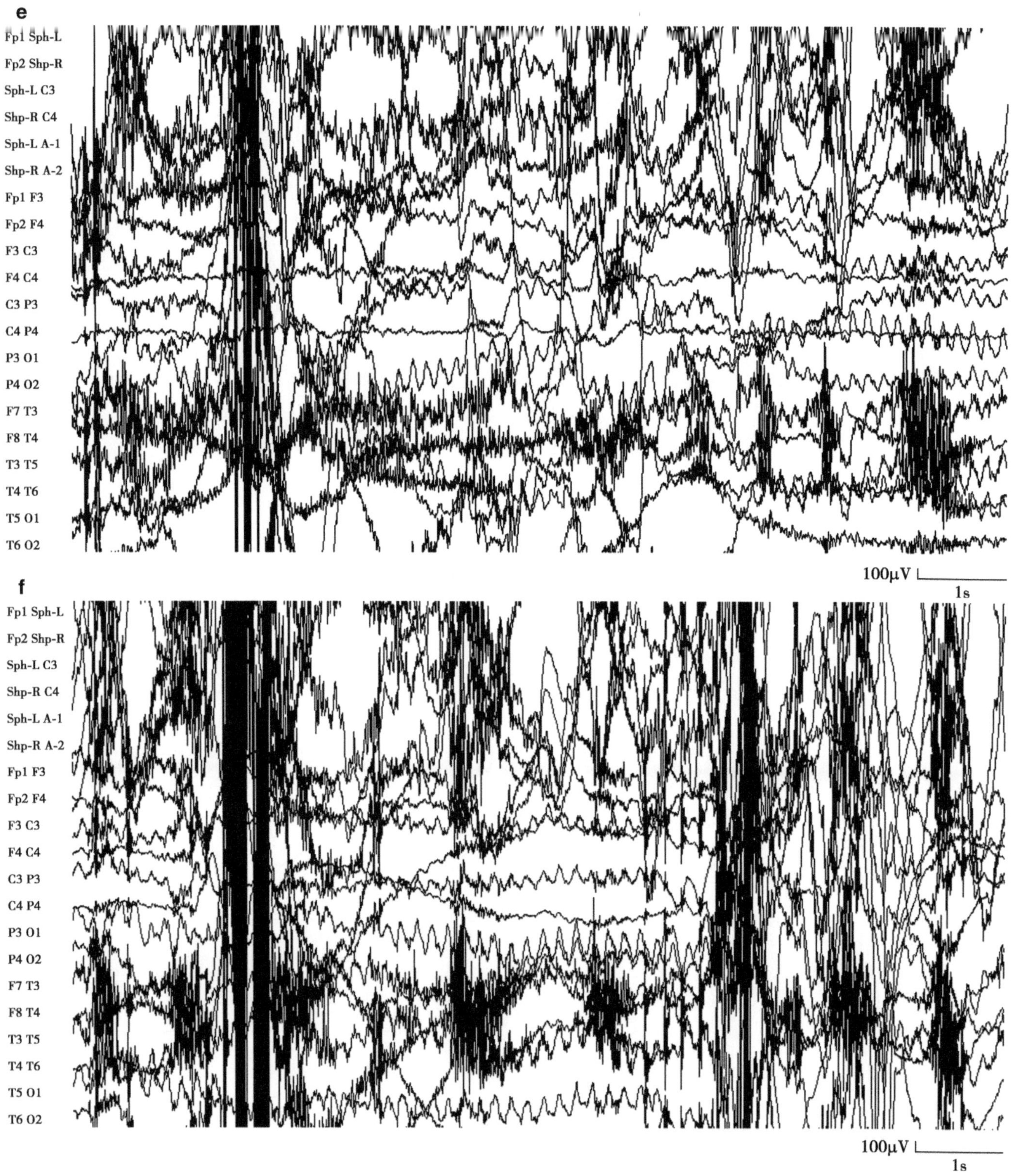

Fig. 3.12 (continued)

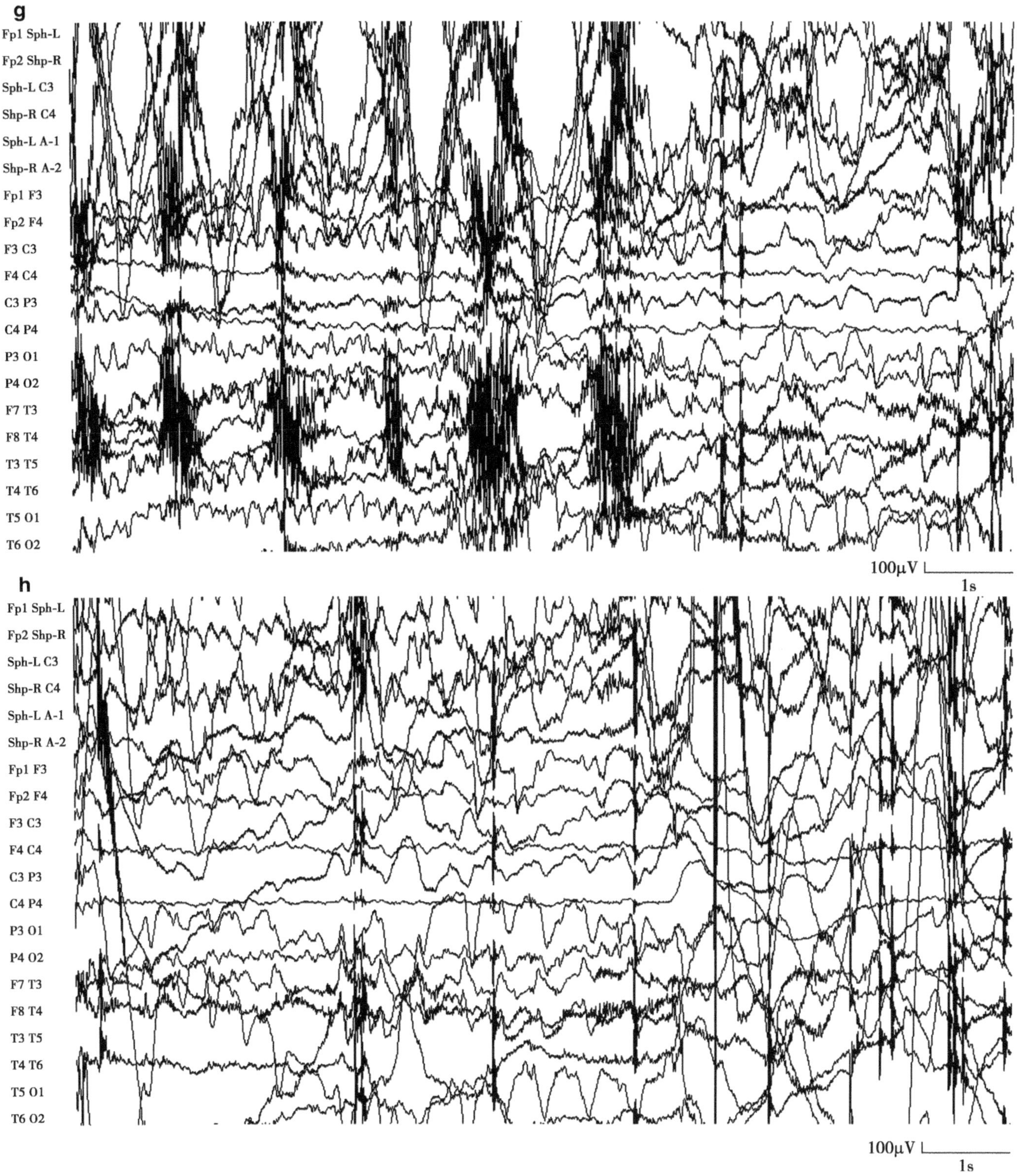

Fig. 3.12 (continued)

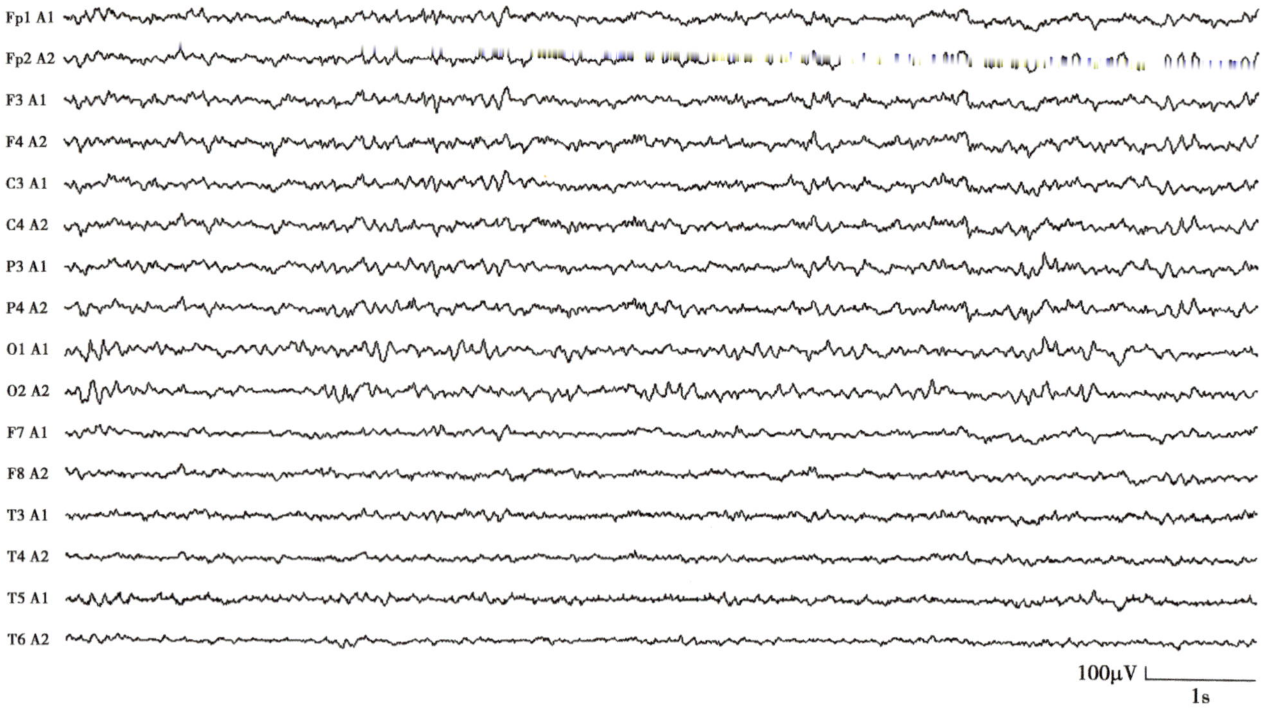

Fig. 3.13 Scheme of intracranial electrodes
Depth electrode 1: the left hippocampus (6 contacts); depth electrode 2: the right hippocampus (6 contacts); strip electrode 3: the left temporal pole (8 contacts); strip electrode 4: the right temporal pole (8 contacts)

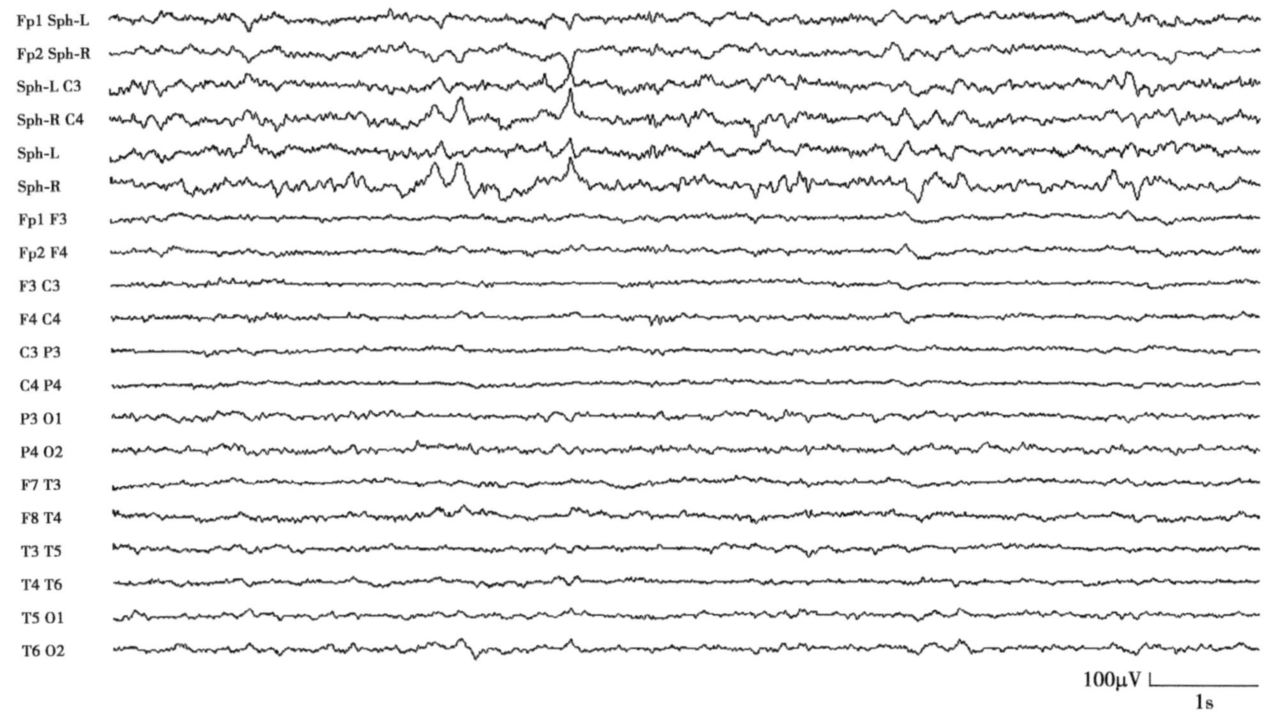

Fig. 3.14 Ictal EEG of intracranial electrodes. (**a**) The patient was awake without any movements. The IEEG showed a shift from spikes to the fast activity of low amplitude over the right hippocampus (contact number elA08). (**b**) The patient did not have any movement. The IEEG showed that the fast activity of increasing amplitude in right hippocampus (contact number elA08). The rhythm of sharp waves was seen over the left hippocampus (contact numbers elA04 and elA05), and the fast activities of low amplitude over the left temporal region (contact number elA20) changed to the rhythm of sharp waves. (**c**, **d**) The patient did not have any movement. The IEEG presentation was basically the same as in **b**. (**e**) The patient had some face-touching behaviors. The IEEG showed an increasing rhythm of spikes over the right hippocampus (contact number elA08), and the characteristics for the rest of the leads were basically the same as in **d**. (**f**) The patient moved his body on the bed, with both upper limbs flexed in front of the chest. The IEEG showed the low amplitude fast activities over the right hippocampus and right temporal pole and the rhythm of slow waves over the left hippocampus and left temporal pole. (**g**) The patient had a sluggish expression. The IEEG showed the rhythm of fast activities over the right hippocampus (contact numbers elA08, elA09, elA10), the rhythm of spike-and-wave complexes over the left hippocampus (contact number elA05), the rhythm of slowed sharp-like waves over the left temporal region (contact numbers elA19, elA20, elA21), and the low amplitude fast activities over the right temporal region (contact numbers elA25 and elA26). (**h**) The patient's symptoms were the same as described in **g**. The EEG showed the rhythm of spike-and-wave complexes over the right hippocampus and right temporal region. (**i**) The patient's symptoms were the same as described in **g**. The EEG showed the rhythm of spike-and-wave complexes over the right hippocampus and right temporal region. (**j**) The patient's symptoms were the same as described in **g**. The EEG showed the rhythm of polyspike and wave complexes over the bilateral hippocampus (contact numbers elA01, elA08, elA09, elA10) and the rhythm of spike-and-wave complexes over the right temporal region. (**k**) The patient's symptoms were the same as described in **g**. The patient did not respond to the calls of his family members at the end of the clinical seizure. The IEEG showed polyspikes on the left hippocampus and rhythmic spikes on the left temporal region

[Case Review]

The patient's MRI showed bilateral hippocampal sclerosis, while the scalp EEG and the ictal symptoms were insufficient to lateralize from which the seizure originated. In such cases, it was necessary to implant intracranial electrodes to monitor the EEG thereof. To distinguish the side from which the temporal lobe seizure originated, it was preferable to bilaterally and symmetrically implant depth electrodes and strip electrodes into the hippocampus. It was conducive to identifying the side of seizure origin and determining whether it was a medial temporal or neocortical origin and whether it was an ipsilateral hippocampal—ipsilateral cortical spreading pattern or a trans-ipsilateral hippocampal—contralateral hippocampal/cortical spreading pattern. In addition, patients with bilateral temporal lobe epilepsy needed to receive relevant neuropsychological assessment before surgery to comprehensively evaluate the impact of surgery on the patient's cognitive function. The patient underwent right anterior temporal lobe and medial structural resection. The patient was seizure free during a 5-year follow-up after surgery.

Case 3.7 Medial Temporal Lobe Epilepsy

[Abstract of Medical Records]
Female, 37 years old.

1. *Chief complaint*: Episodic loss of awareness and behavioral arrest of movements for 16 years.
2. *History of present illness*: Sixteen years ago, the patient developed dizziness without obvious inducement, followed by loss of awareness and termination of movements 1–2 s later, which resolved spontaneously after 2–3 s, without limb twitching and incontinence. The patient subsequently had seizures once to twice a month or once every 2–3 months, with the same manifestation and no diagnosis and treatment. Seizures occurred frequently 14 years ago, one seizure every 2–3 days, accompanied by rubbing hands or face. It usually occurred before and after menstruation. She was treated at a local hospital and given oral antiseizure medications such as carbamazepine, but the effect was poor. Sometimes it was secondary to twitching of the limbs, turning of the eyes upward, and clenched teeth, and similar generalized tonic-clonic seizures occurred 2–3 times a year. Two years ago, she started to take traditional Chinese medicines (exact composition unknown) and carbamazepine (100 mg per dose, t.i.d.). One month ago, she had four grand mal seizures within 1 month and came to our hospital. She then orally took oxcarbazepine at a dose of 450 mg bid and clonazepam at a dose of 0.5 mg once per night. No grand mal seizure occurred in 1 month. The current seizure type is mainly characterized by dialeptic seizure with rubbing hands together or rubbing the face, each lasting 2–3 s before resolving, at a frequency of 1 seizure every 2–3 days or 3–4 times a day. She has been orally taking oxcarbazepine (450 mg/dose bid), clonazepam (0.5 mg/dose, once per night), and traditional Chinese medicines.
3. *Past history*: The patient has no history of obstructed labor and birth trauma. She had carbon monoxide poisoned of unknown extent at 6 years old.
4. *Physical examination*: No neurological abnormalities were found.
5. Imaging examination:
   (a) MRI revealed paranasal sinusitis and multiple cysts over the left ethmoidal cellules and maxillary sinus.
   (b) Cranial MRS revealed that the NAA concentration (NAA/Cr: 1.56) over the left hippocampus was slightly higher than that over the right side (NAA/Cr: 1.11); the Cho concentration (Cho/Cr: 1.12) over the left hippocampus was slightly higher than that over the right side; the right hippocampus was slightly smaller compared with the contralateral hippocampus.
   (c) SPECT revealed poor diffuse perfusion over the bilateral cerebral cortices, with localized hypoperfusion over the right parietal lobe.
6. *EEG*: For details, see Figs. 3.15, 3.16, 3.17, 3.18, and 3.19.

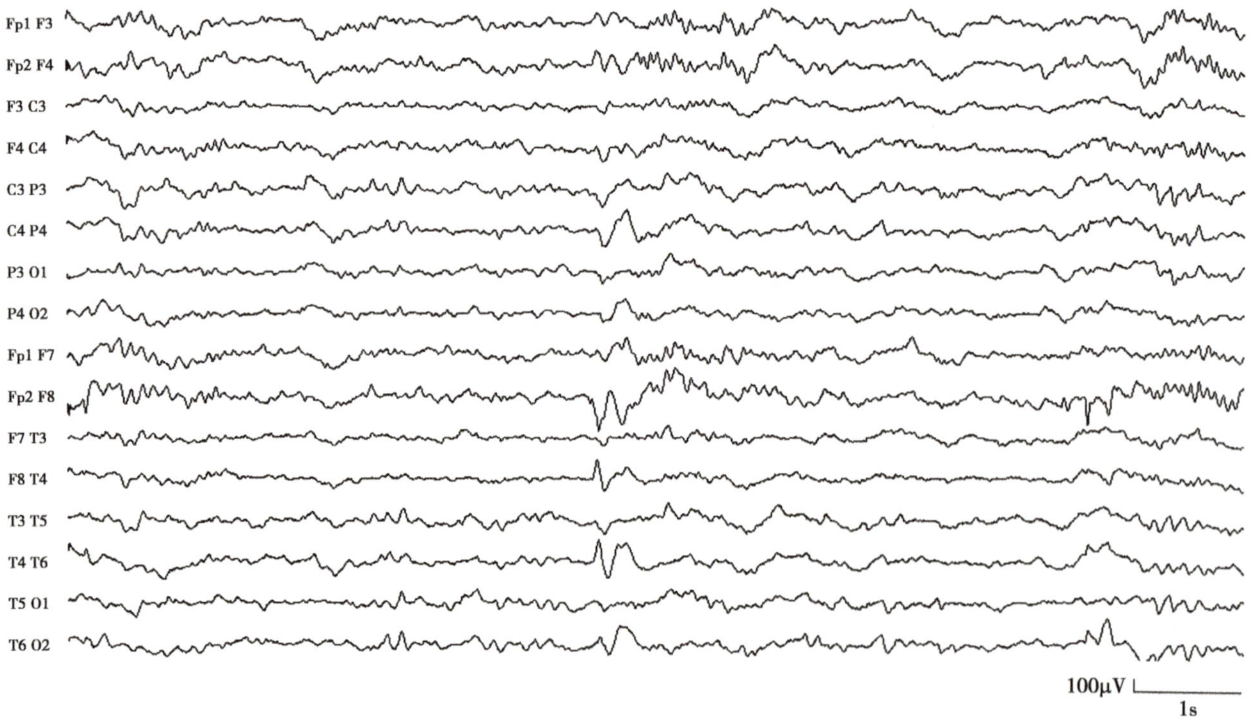

Fig. 3.15 Interictal scalp EEG
The EEG showed sharp waves over the right sphenoidal electrode and sharp waves and slow waves over the right temporal region

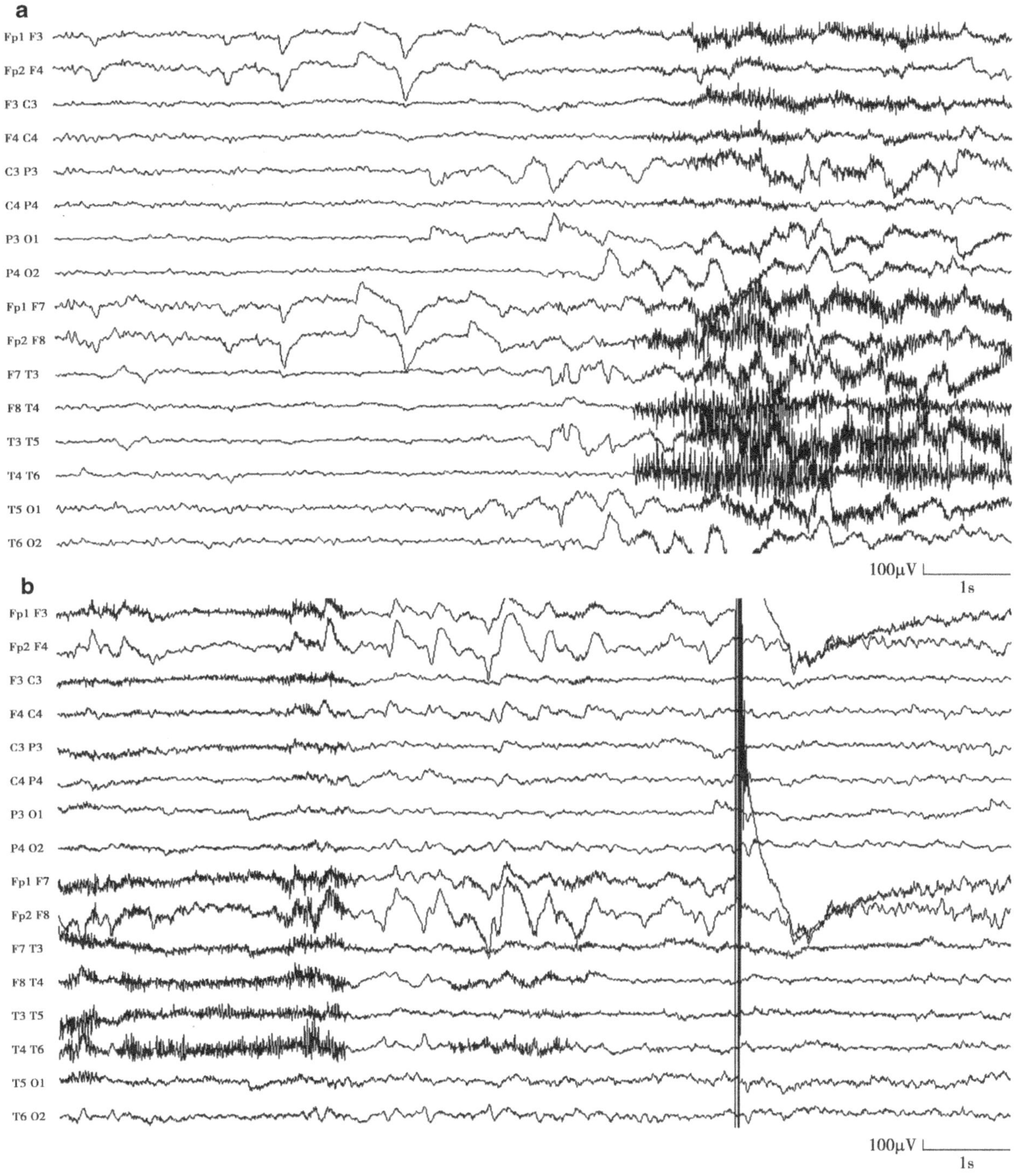

Fig. 3.16 Ictal scalp EEG. (**a**) The patient was awake before the seizure and opened her eyes with a slow blink during the seizure. The EEG showed the disappearance of α activities and a mixture of slow waves and fast activity of low amplitude with blink artifacts. (**b**) The patient had a sluggish expression without any limb movement. The EEG still showed low amplitude fast activities. (**c**) The patient slowly turned head to the left and right involuntarily, accompanied by involuntary flexion and extension of the lower limbs and fumbling for clothes with both hands. The EEG showed a mixture of slow waves and EMG artifacts over the bilateral temporal regions and the rhythm of fast activities over the right posterior temporal region. (**d**) The patient moved the lower limbs involuntarily and fumbled with both hands in front of the chest. The EEG showed the rhythm of fast activity over the right posterior temporal region, which extended to the contralateral side, and the rhythm of sharp waves and slow waves in bilateral sphenoidal electrode. (**e**) The patient turned the toes outwards and fumbled with both hands. The EEG showed slow waves of high amplitude and slow sharp waves with increasing amplitude in bilateral sphenoidal electrode, and a mixture of the rhythm of fast activity and slow waves was seen over the bilateral posterior temporal regions. (**f**) The patient turned head to the right with right upper limb elevated. Mixed EMG artifacts were seen on the EEG. (**g**) The patient's right upper limb was flexed and elevated, and both lower limbs were tonic and abducted, gradually followed by flexed upper limbs and abducted lower limbs with clonus. The IEEG presentation was the same as **f**. (**h**, **i**) The patient had tonic-clonic limbs. The IEEG presentation was the same as **f**. (**j**) The patient had tonic-clonic limbs. The clonus slowed down and stopped after about 30 s. The IEEG presentation was the same as **f**

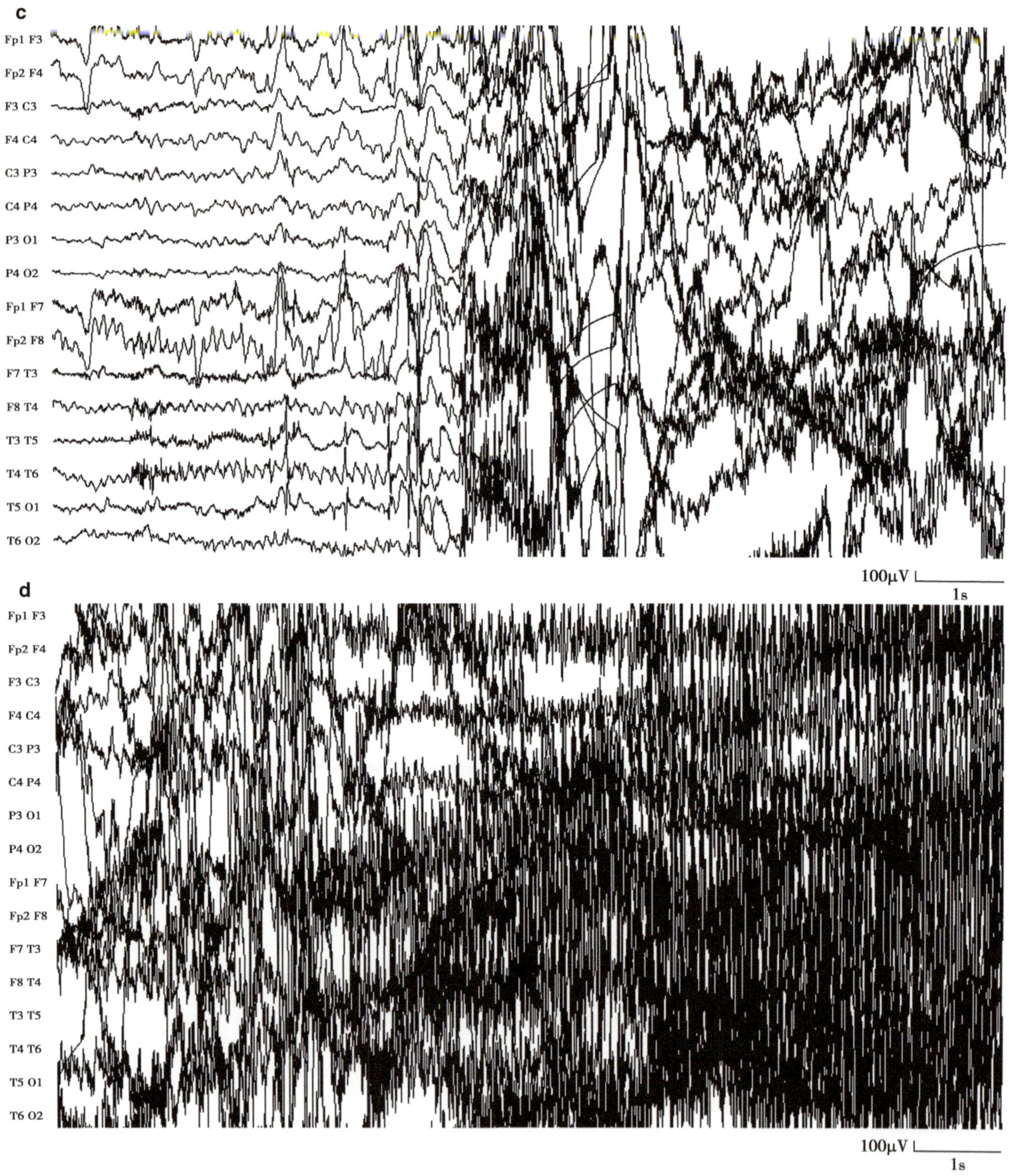

Fig. 3.16 (continued)

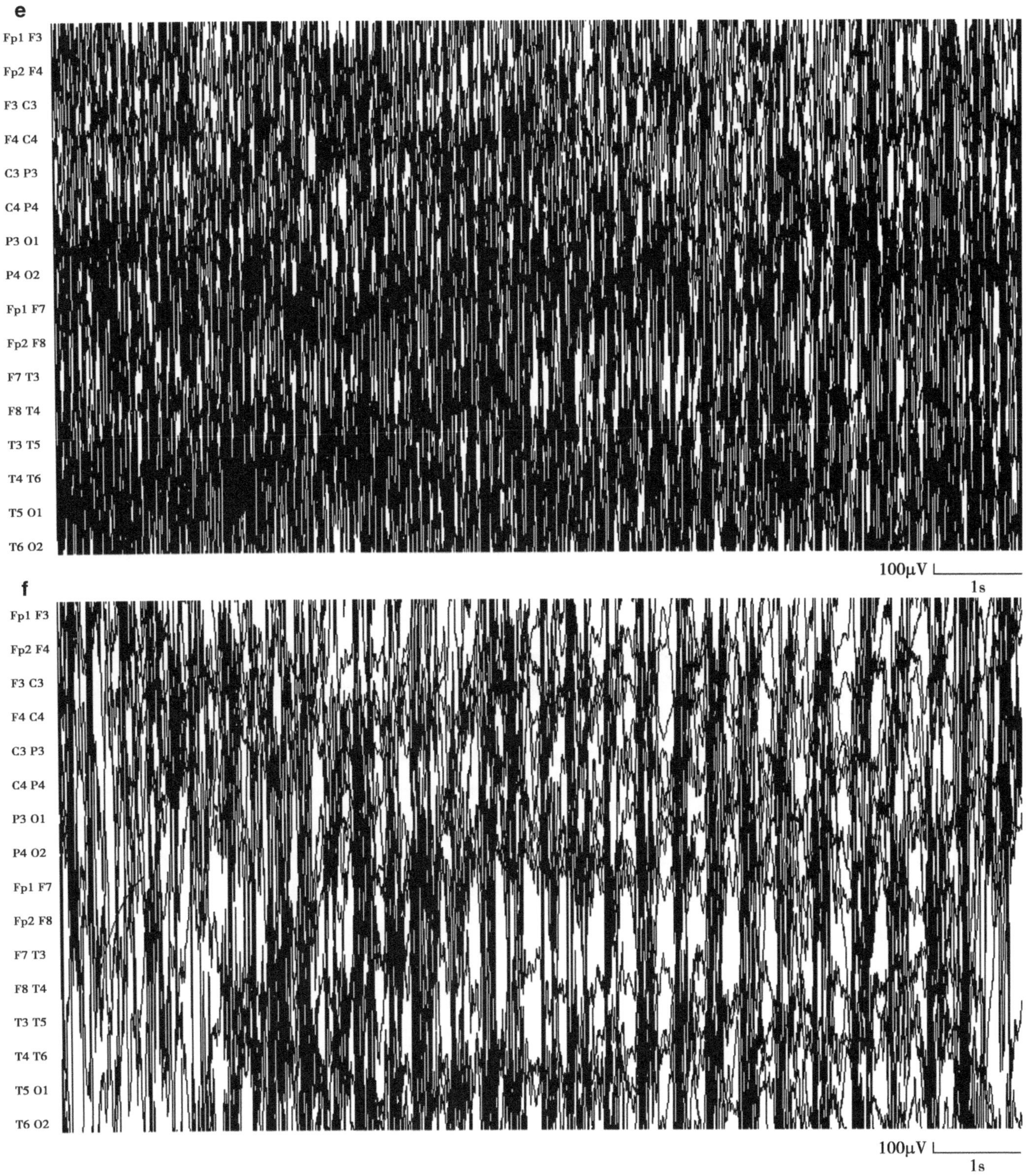

Fig. 3.16 (continued)

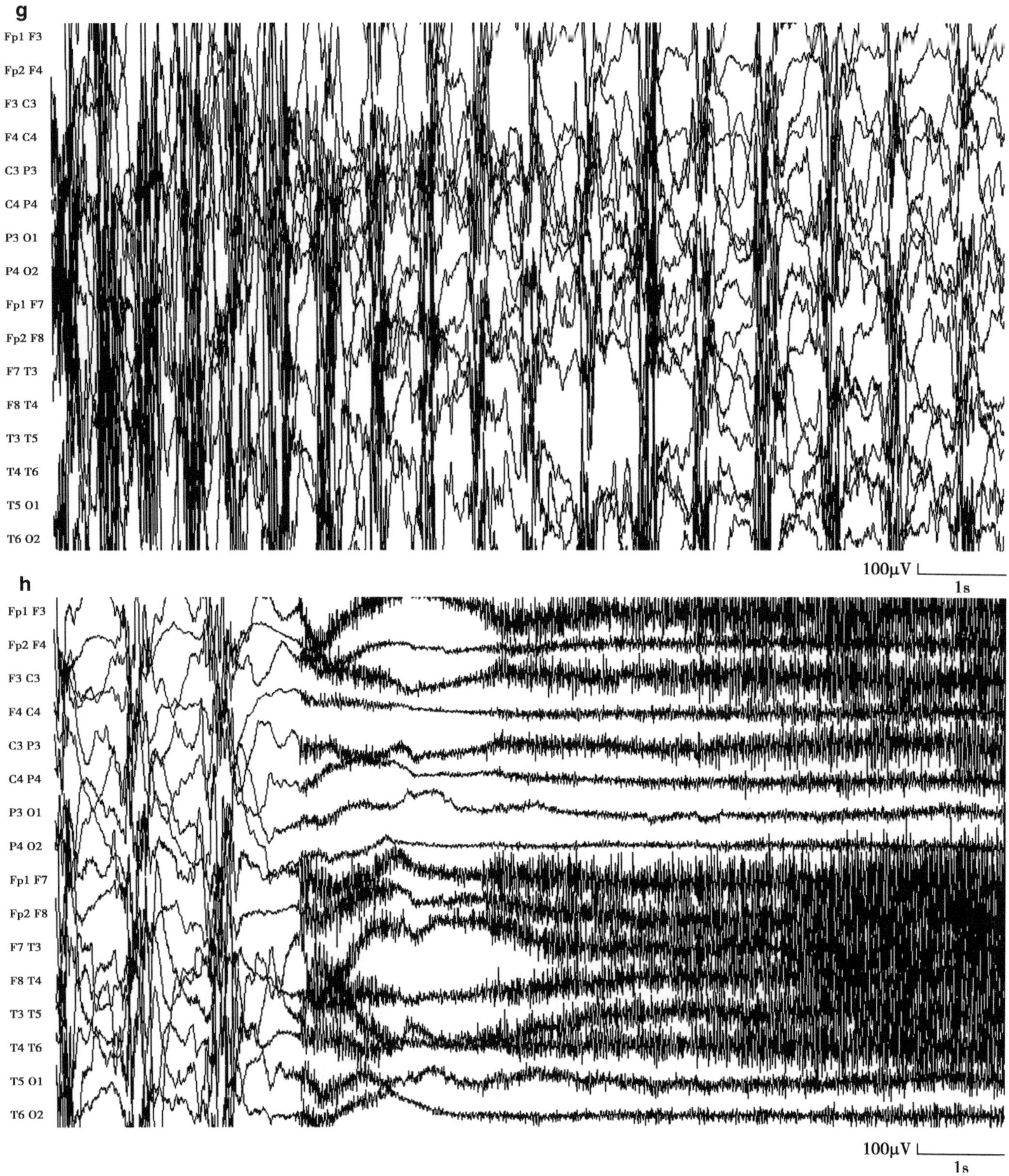

Fig. 3.16 (continued)

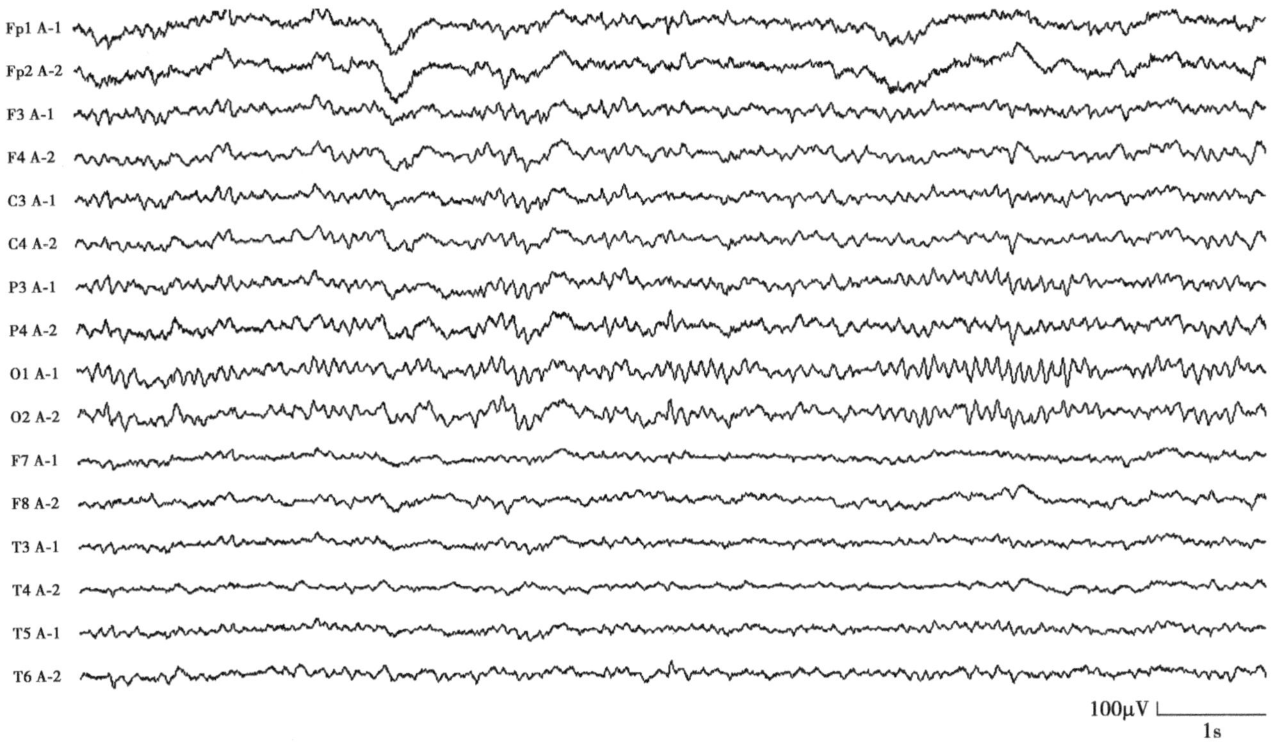

Fig. 3.17 Scheme of intracranial electrodes
Depth electrode 1: the left hippocampus (6 contacts); depth electrode 2: the right hippocampus (6 contacts); strip electrode 3: the left temporal pole (8 contacts); strip electrode 4: the right temporal pole (8 contacts); strip electrode 5: the left posterior temporal region (6 contacts); strip electrode 6: the right posterior temporal region (6 contacts)

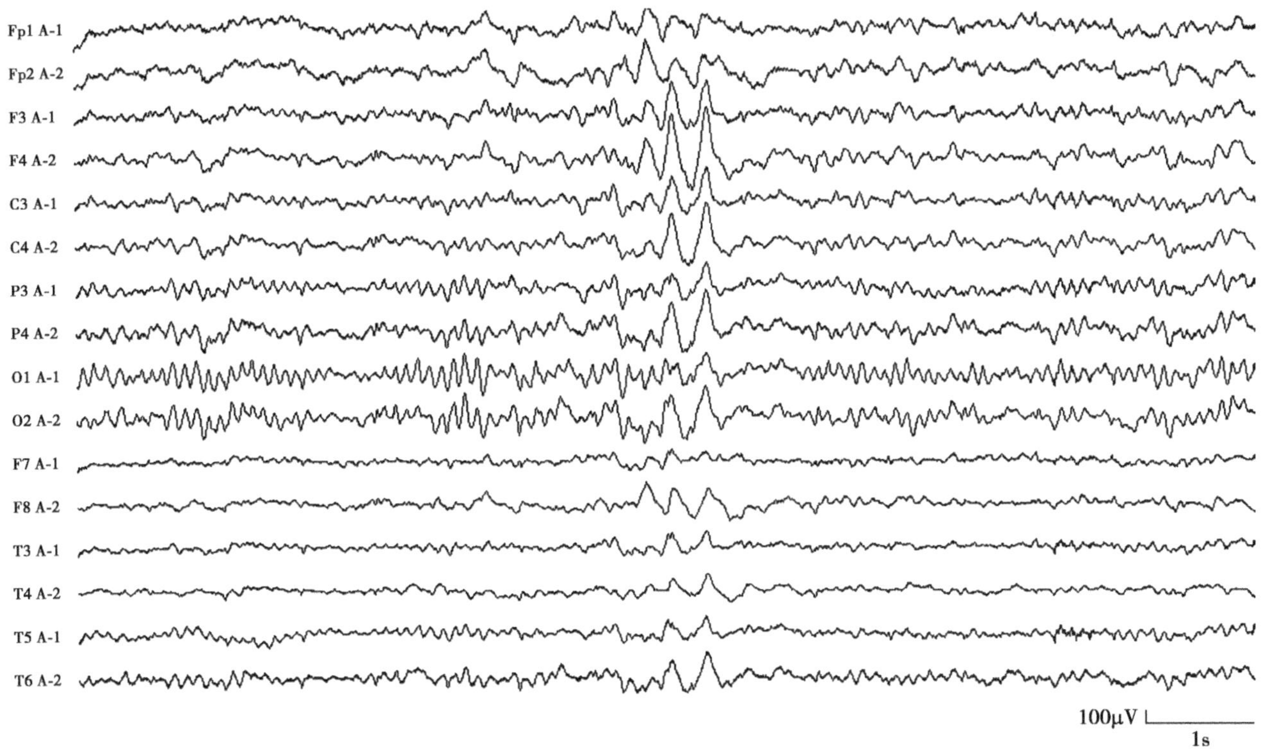

Fig. 3.18 Interictal intracranial EEG. (**a**) The EEG showed a burst of spike-and-wave complexes and spikes over the right hippocampus (contact numbers elA10, elA11, elA12), the right temporal pole (contact numbers elA25, elA26, elA27, elA28), and the right temporal region (contact numbers elA37, elA38, elA39, elA40). (**b**) The EEG showed rhythmic spike-and-wave complexes over the right hippocampus (contact numbers elA07, elA08, elA09) and rhythmic spike-and-wave complexes and sharp waves over the right temporal pole (contact numbers elA25, elA26, elA27, elA28). (**c**) Sharp waves and spike-and-wave complexes were seen over the right hippocampus (contact numbers elA07, elA08, elA09) and the right temporal pole (contact numbers elA25, elA26, elA27, elA28); spike-and-wave complexes were seen over the left hippocampus (contact numbers elA01, elA02, elA03, elA04)

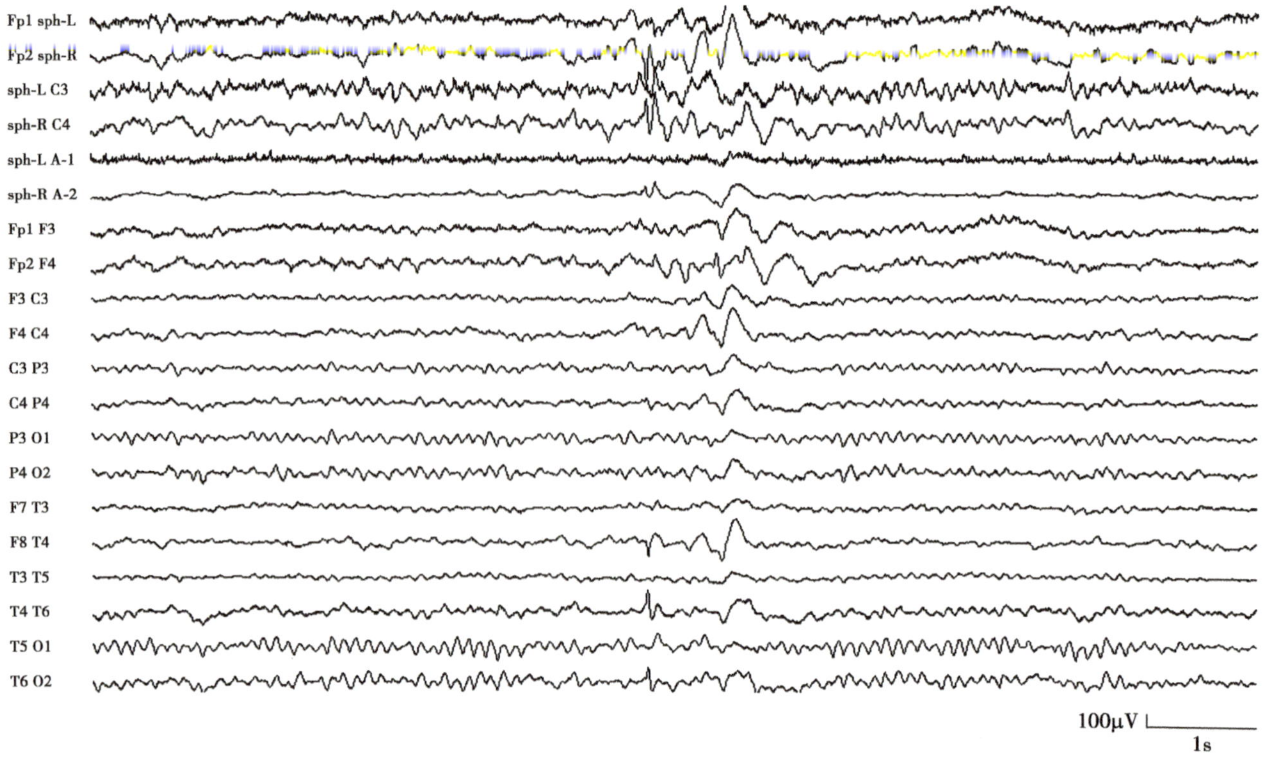

Fig. 3.19 Ictal EEG of intracranial electrodes. (**a**) The patient was asleep before the seizure. The IEEG showed spike-and-wave complexes and polyspike and wave complexes on the right hippocampus (contact numbers elA07, elA08, elA10, elA11, elA12), the right temporal pole (contact numbers elA23, elA24, elA25, elA26, elA27), and the right posterior temporal region (contact numbers elA37, elA38, elA39). (**b**) The patient was still asleep. The IEEG showed the rhythm of fast activities over the right hippocampus lead (contact numbers elA11 and elA12) and spike-and-wave complexes of high amplitude over the right temporal pole (contact numbers elA24, elA25, elA26, elA27, elA28), which gradually developed into the rhythm of spikes and showed the low amplitude fast activities over the right posterior temporal region (contact numbers elA35, elA36, elA37, elA38, elA39, elA40). (**c**) The patient opened eyes with a blank expression. The IEEG showed the rhythm of spike-and-wave complexes over the right posterior temporal region and the right temporal pole and the rhythm of sharp waves over the right hippocampus. (**d**) The patient moved her body to the right, and the seizure ended. The IEEG showed the rhythm of spike-and-wave complexes over the right hippocampus and mainly over the right posterior temporal region. The rhythm of slow waves was seen over the contralateral side

[Case Review]

The EEG of the patient at seizure onset showed a sudden disappearance of brain electrical activity from the background EEG, followed by the appearance of slow waves. It was difficult to distinguish between the right and left sides at the stage and was not until more than 30 seconds later that low-amplitude fast activity appeared over the right posterior temporal region. The application of intracranial electrodes made it easier to lateralization. The burst of fast activity and the rhythm of spike-and-wave complexes appeared first over the right hippocampus, posterior temporal region and temporal pole, and then spread to the contralateral temporal lobe. The right anterior temporal lobe and medial structures were resected. During a 7-year follow-up after the operation, two seizures occurred in the first year after the operation before seizure freedom.

Case 3.8 Medial Temporal Lobe Epilepsy

[Abstract of Medical Records]
Male, 35 years old.

1. *Chief complaint*: episodic recurrent loss of consciousness for 10 years.
2. *History of present illness*: Ten years ago, the patient had a sudden loss of awareness without obvious inducement and fell to the ground with tonic limbs, followed by limb twitching, cyanosis of lips, and urinary incontinence, which lasted 2–3 min and then resolved. Later on, the seizures occurred in this pattern 1–2 times a week, sometimes with swallowing and fumbling. Before the seizure, there was sometimes a feeling of fever on the head, without headache or temperature increase. Later, the seizures occurred in another type: dialeptic seizure, lasting about 1 min.
3. *Personal and family history*: No history of associated diseases.
4. *Imaging examination*: MRI showed atrophy of right hippocampus and enlarged right temporal angle of ventricle.
5. *EEG*: For details, see Figs. 3.20, 3.21, 3.22, 3.23, and 3.24.

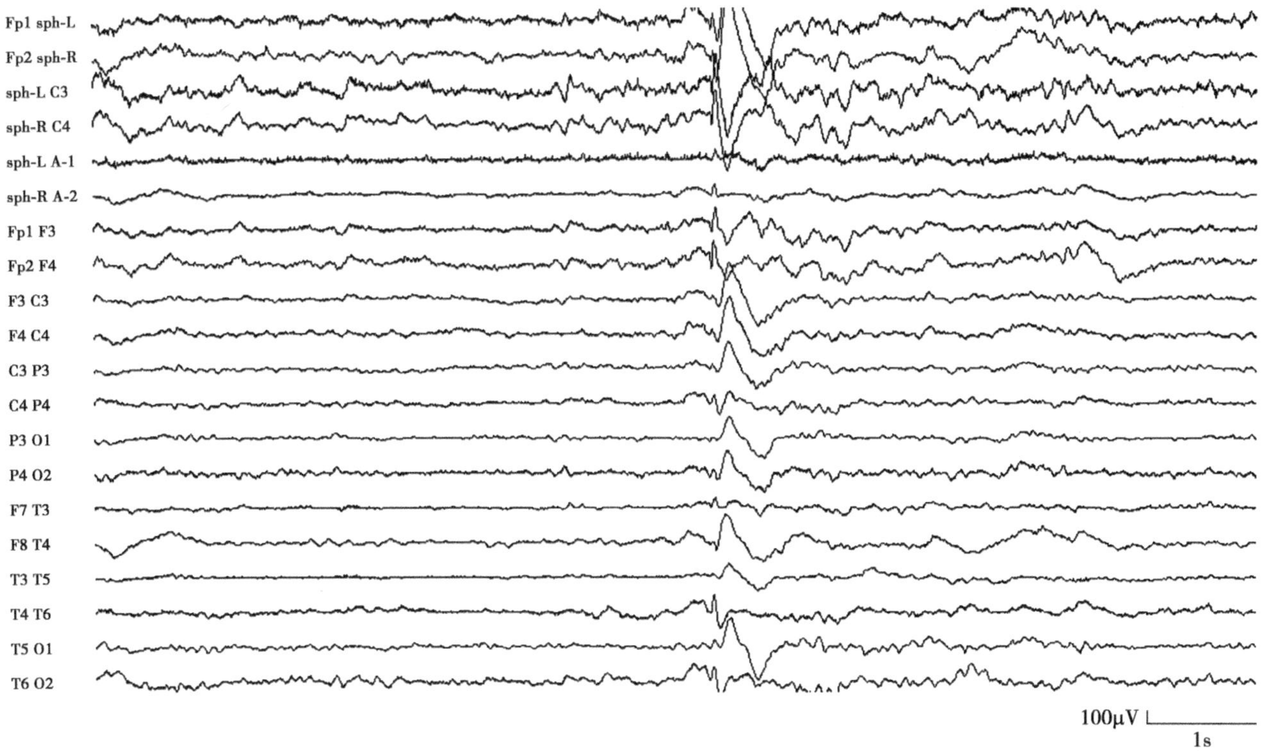

Fig. 3.20 Interictal scalp EEG. (**a**) The EEG during wakefulness showed sharp waves of low amplitude over the bilateral sphenoidal electrode. (**b**) Sharp waves were seen over the right sphenoidal electrode and over the right anterior temporal region

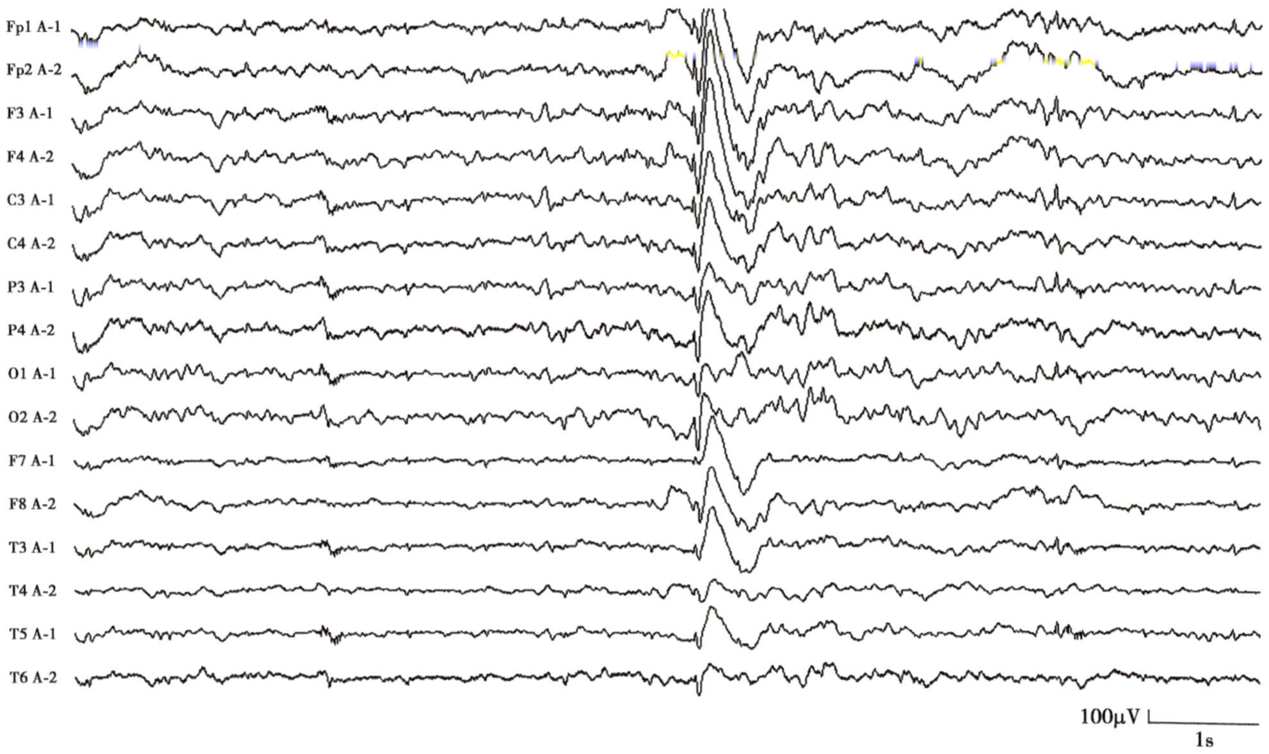

Fig. 3.21 Ictal scalp EEG. (**a**) The patient was awake and lying on his back without obvious auras. The EEG showed irregular slow waves of high amplitude in bilateral sphenoidal electrodes and over the bilateral middle temporal regions. (**b**) The patient swallowed in a somewhat painful expression. The EEG showed irregular slow waves in bilateral sphenoidal electrodes and over the bilateral temporal regions, gradually mixing with fast activity. (**c**) The patient kept blinking. The EEG showed sharp waves and slow waves of high amplitude over bilateral sphenoidal electrode and slow waves of low and medium amplitude over the remaining electrodes. (**d**) The patient kept blinking. The patient's EEG manifestations were the same as shown in **c**. (**e**) The patient kept blinking, and the jaw twitched with head turning to the right while being clonic. The EEG showed the rhythm of slow waves over the central area of bilateral posterior frontal regions, mixed with EMG artifacts over the bilateral frontal and temporal regions. (**f**) The patient looked to the left and twitched his mouth corner to the right. The EEG showed mixed EMG artifacts over the bilateral frontal and temporal regions. The rhythm of slow waves was seen over the remaining electrodes. (**g**) The patient twitched his mouth corner to the right and flexed and elevated the right upper limb. The EEG was basically the same as in **f**. (**h**) The patient twitched his mouth corner to the right, with nystagmus. The EEG was basically the same as in **f**. (**i**) The patient had a head-to-right with trunk clonus. The EEG was basically the same as in **f**. (**j**) The patient had a head-to-right with trunk clonus. The EEG showed mixed EMG artifacts over the bilateral frontal and temporal regions. The rhythm of slow waves was seen over the other electrodes. At the end of the seizure, voltage reduction was seen in all leads

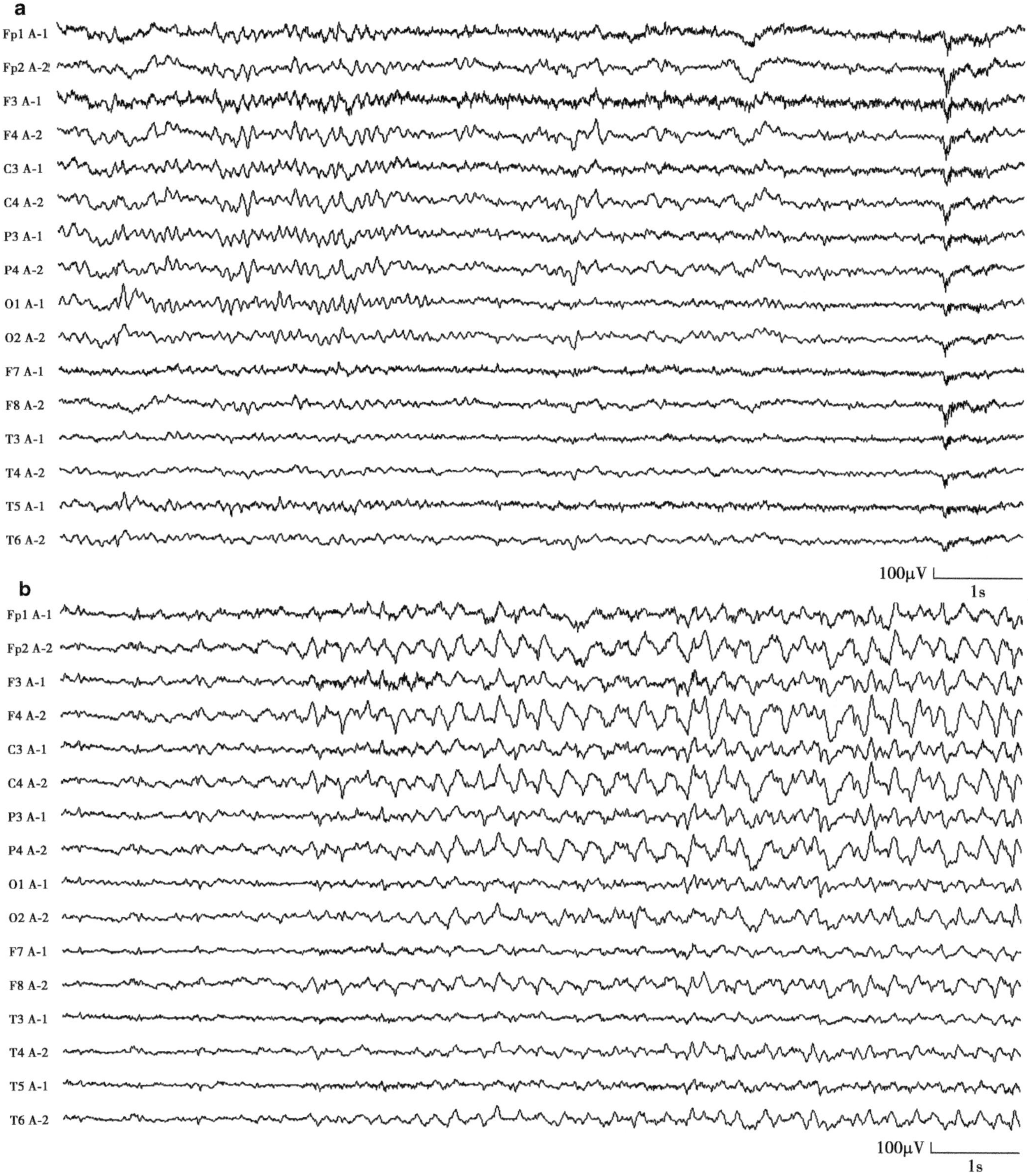

Fig. 3.22 Scheme of intracranial electrodes
Strip electrode 1: the left longitudinal frontal fissure (eight contacts); strip electrode 2: the left frontal pole (eight contacts); strip electrode 3: eight contacts over the right longitudinal frontal fissure (eight contacts); strip electrode 4: the right frontal pole (eight contacts); strip electrode 5: the left temporal pole (eight contacts); strip electrode 6: the left temporal base (eight contacts); strip electrode 7: the right temporal pole (eight contacts); strip electrode 8: the + right temporal base (eight contacts)

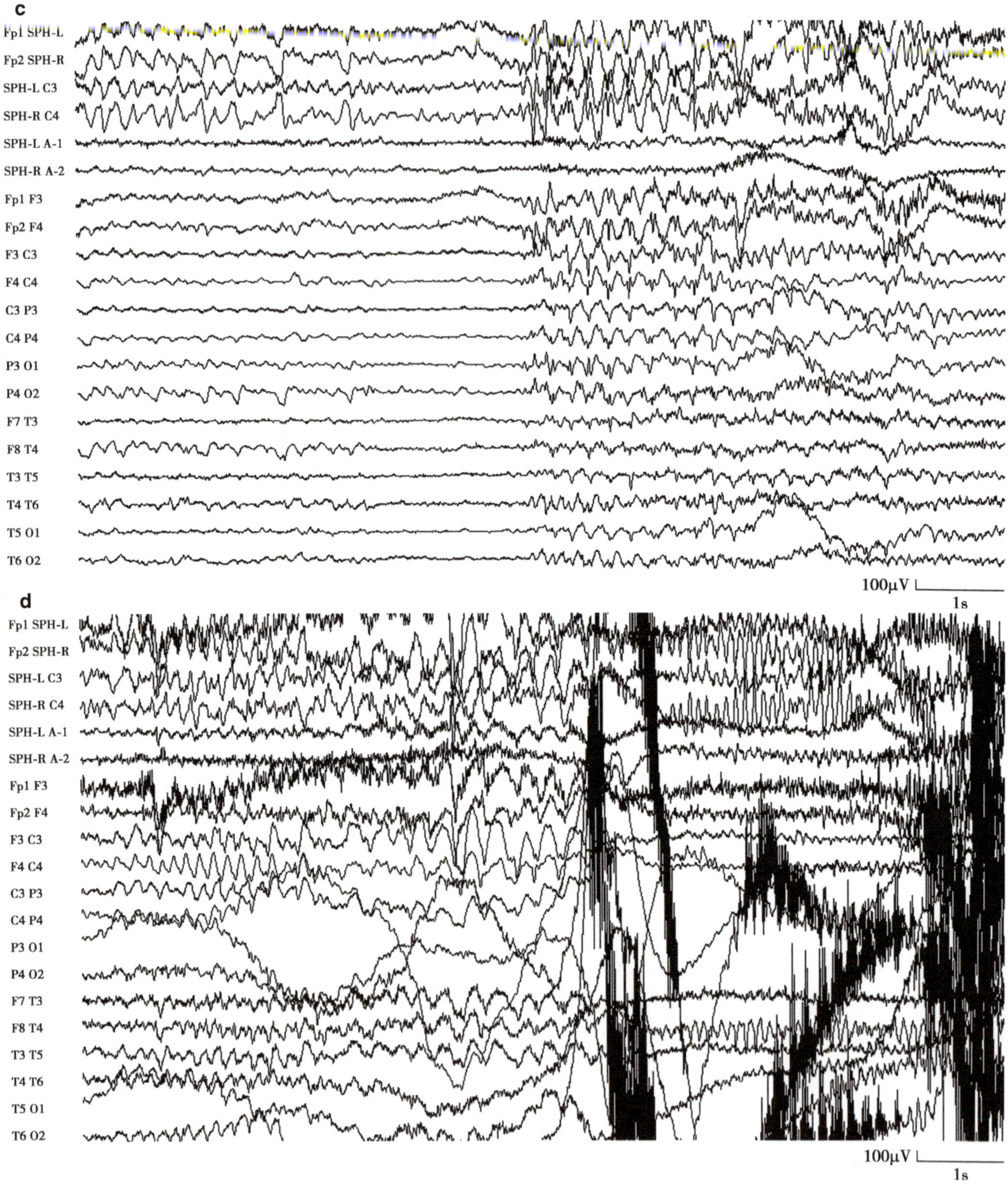

Fig. 3.22 (continued)

e

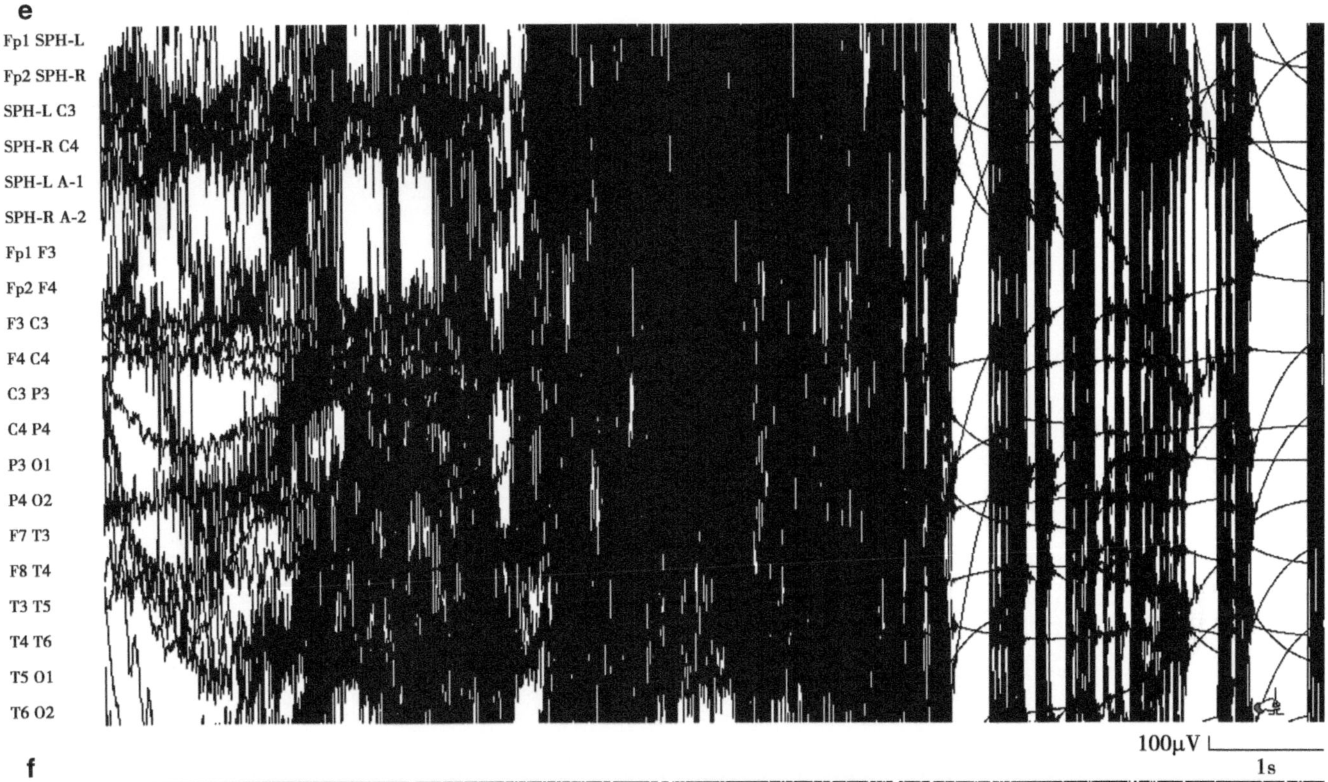

f

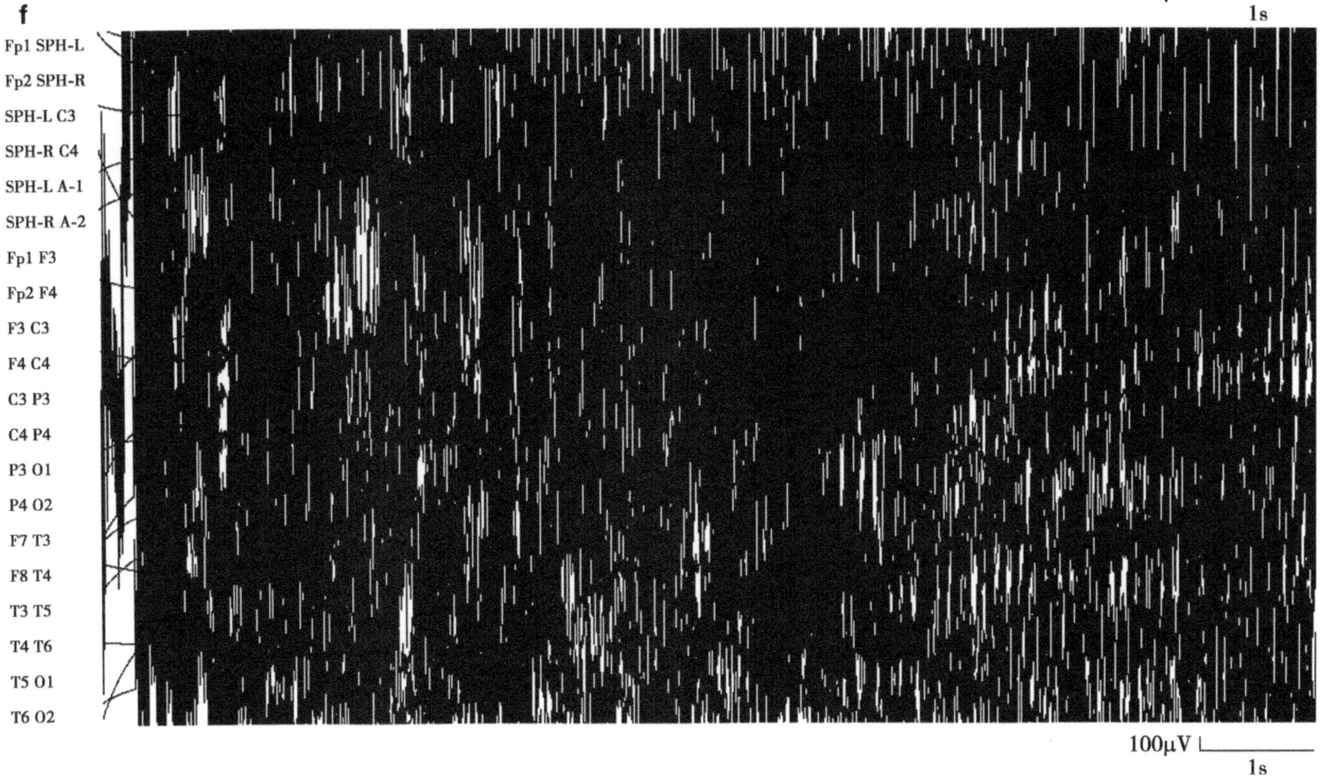

Fig. 3.22 (continued)

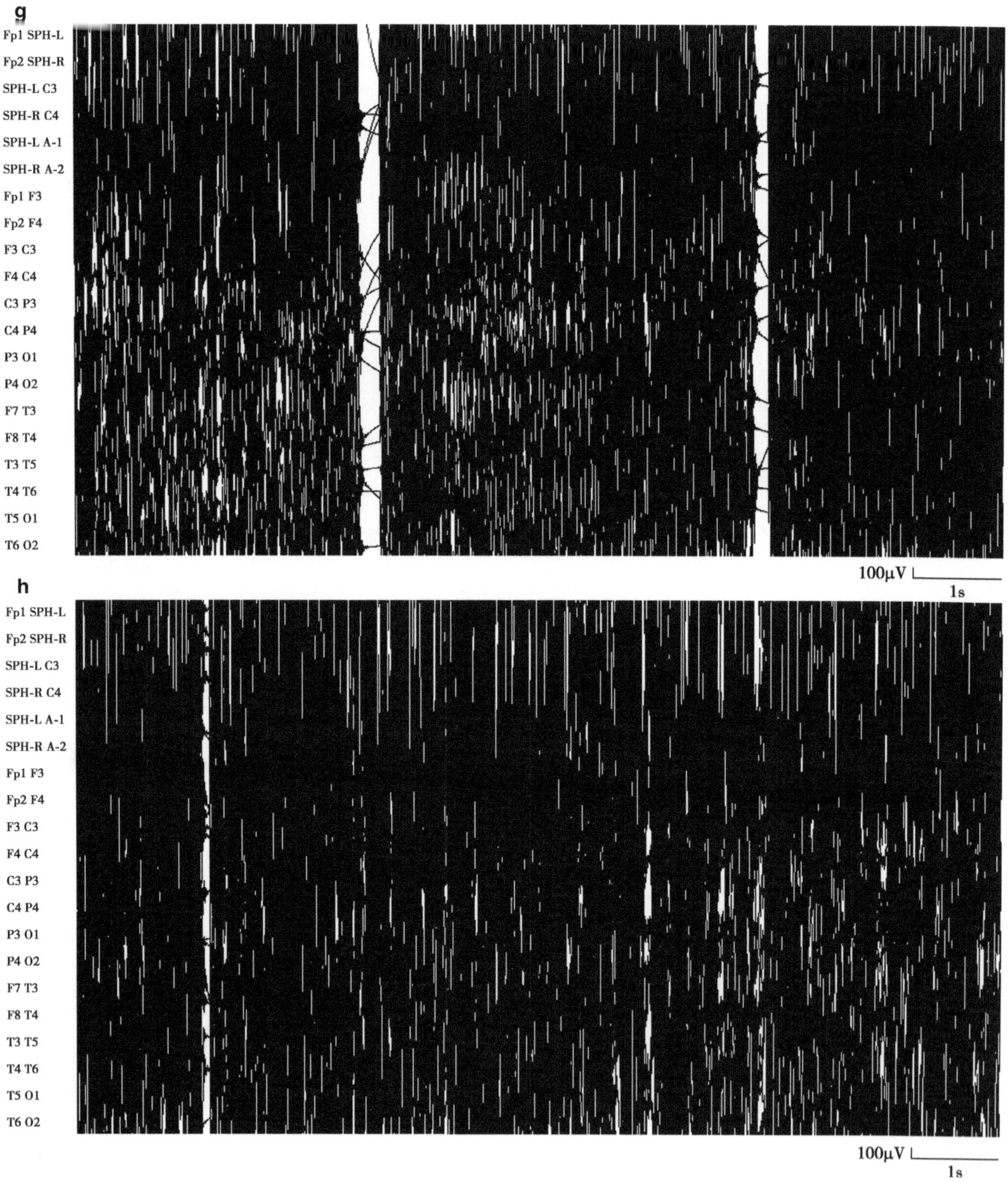

Fig. 3.22 (continued)

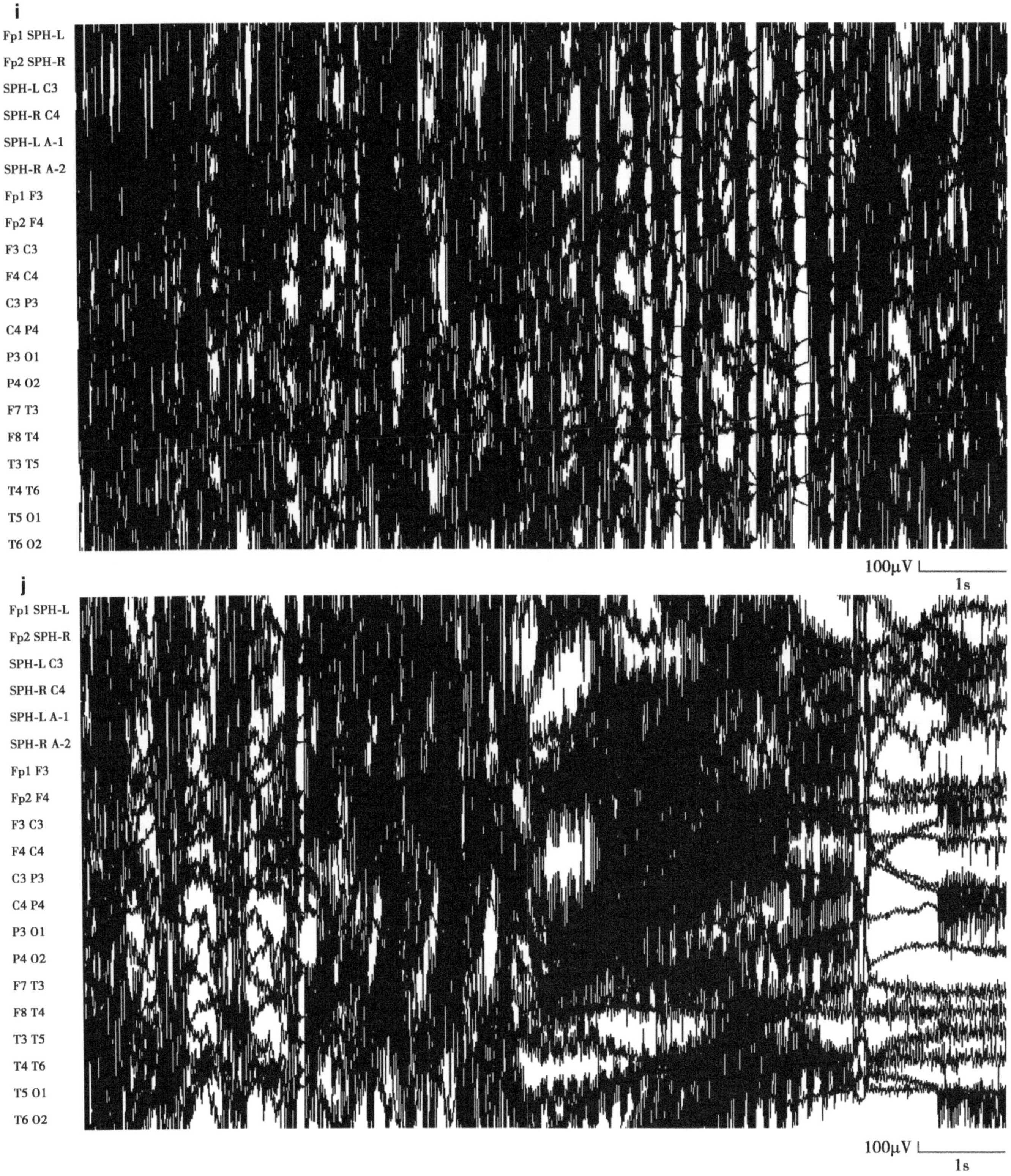

Fig. 3.22 (continued)

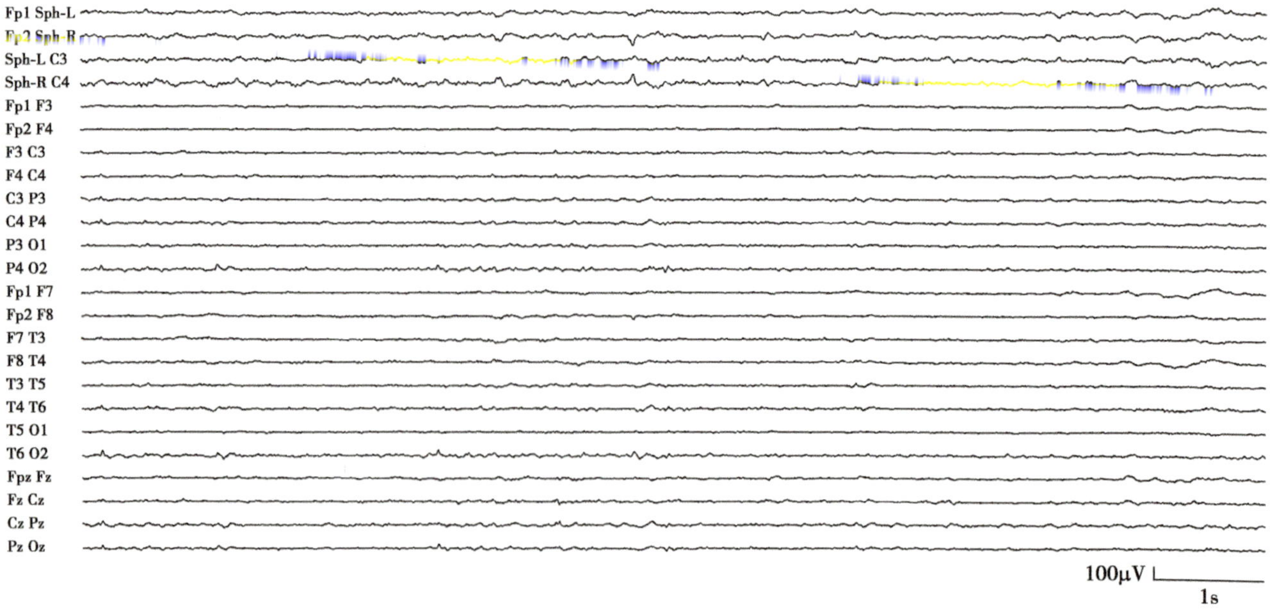

Fig. 3.23 Interictal intracranial EEG
The EEG showed repetitive sharp waves over the right temporal pole (contact numbers elB15 and elB16) and sharp waves and slow waves over the right frontal pole (contact numbers elA28, elA29, and elA30)

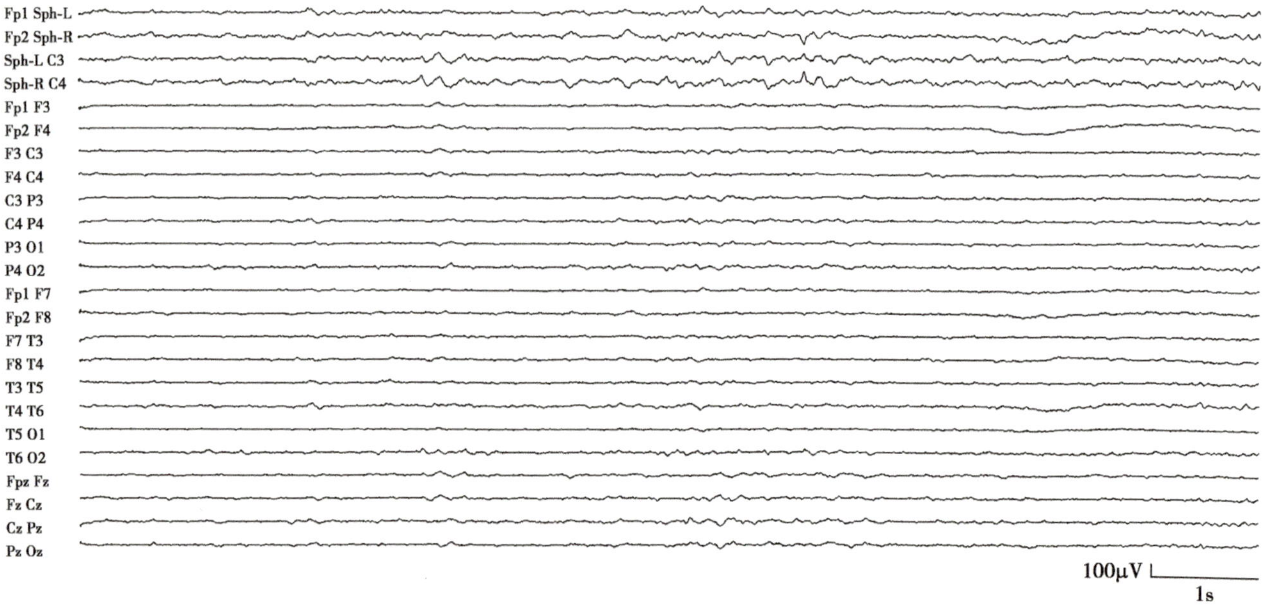

Fig. 3.24 Ictal EEG of intracranial electrodes. (**a**) The patient opened eyes in a painful expression. The IEEG showed the rhythm of spike-and-wave complexes over the right temporal base (contact numbers elB26, elB27, elB28). (**b**) The patient involuntarily flexed and extended the right lower limb with painful expression. The IEEG showed the rhythm of spike-and-wave complexes over the right temporal base lead (contact numbers elB25, elB26, elB27, elB28), which gradually spread to the right temporal pole (contact numbers elB16, elB17, elB18). (**c**) The patient looked to the left with smacking lips. The IEEG showed that the rhythm of spike-and-wave complexes spread from the right temporal pole and temporal base to the left temporal base and the right frontal pole. (**d**) The patient curled up and smacked lips in a painful and dull expression. The IEEG showed that the rhythm of spike-and-wave complexes spread from the right temporal region to the left temporal region and the right frontal region and gradually spread to the left frontal longitudinal fissure and frontal region. (**e, f**) The patient curled up and smacked lips with a painful and dull expression. The IEEG showed that the rhythm of spike-and-wave complexes spread from the right temporal region to the left temporal and the right frontal and gradually spread to the left frontal longitudinal fissure and frontal region. (**g**) The patient's upper limbs were straightened and elevated with clonus, and the lower limbs were tonic. The IEEG showed that the rhythm of spike-and-wave complexes over the right temporal pole and the temporal base gradually disappeared, and the rest of the leads were basically the same as in **f**. (**h**) The patient mainly had clonus in both upper limbs. The IEEG showed the rhythm of spike-and-wave complexes over the left temporal pole, temporal base and right frontal pole, the rhythm of spikes over the left longitudinal frontal fissure, and the rhythm of irregular slow waves in right temporal base

[Case Review]

The interictal EEG showed that the sharp waves were clearly seen in bilateral sphenoidal electrodes when the patient was awake. The ictal EEG of scalp electrodes first showed irregular slow waves in bilateral sphenoidal electrodes and in bilateral temporal regions, which were gradually mixed with fast activities. Later, the rhythm of slow waves of bilateral leads was still seen in EMG artifacts. The lateralization features of EEG were unclear and appeared to be more pronounced over the left temporal region, and the appearance of right-sided symptoms of corner of the mouth later in the seizure also seemed to indicate a left epileptic focus. For temporal lobe epilepsy where lateralization cannot be determined, it was proposed to use intracranial electrodes to determine the origin of the seizure. In this case, intracranial electrodes showed that the seizure originated over the medial area of the right temporal base (near the gyrus parahippocampalis), which gradually spread to the right temporal region and left temporal base. The application of intracranial electrodes modified the lateralization diagnosis on scalp EEG and avoided misjudgment. Because the patient had less frequent automatism and atypical auras, electrodes were also implanted to the bilateral frontal lobes in order to exclude frontal lobe epilepsy. The right anterior temporal lobe and medial structures were resected. The patient remained seizure-free during a 4-year follow-up after surgery.

Case 3.9 Medial Temporal Lobe Epilepsy

[Abstract of Medical Records]
Male, 46 years old.

1. *Chief complaint*: Episodic tonic limbs with convulsions and dialeptic seizures for 25 years.
2. *History of present illness*: The patient had episodic flexion of the upper limbs and extension or flexion of the lower limbs 25 years ago (at 21 years old), accompanied by tonic convulsion, eyes rolling upward, unresponsiveness, and head turn to one side (side not known). Each seizure lasted 3–4 minutes, and the seizure frequency ranged from over 10 times per month to 1 time every 1–2 months, 80% of which occurred at night during sleep. There was also another type of seizure: the patient suddenly experienced dialeptic seizure, stared blankly, and failed to respond to calls during an activity, accompanied by smacking lips, swallowing, and fumbling. Occasional palpitation occurred before the seizure, which resolved after a few minutes and occurred 1–2 times a month. The treatment with a variety of antiseizure medications was ineffective. He is taking phenytoin sodium 0.2g/day and carbamazepine 0.3g/day. The drug has been discontinued on his own in the last 6 days.
3. *Past history*: The patient was born at term and had normal development. He had a history of head trauma 33 years ago and denied a history of febrile convulsions, encephalitis, or meningitis. He denied a family history of epilepsy.
4. *Physical examination*: No neurological abnormalities were found.
5. *Psychological test report*: IQ was moderate to low, with VIQ = 92, PIQ = 83, FIQ = 88.
6. *Imaging examination*:
   (a) MRI revealed abnormal right hippocampus.
   (b) SPECT revealed localized hypoperfusion over the cortices of the right parietal lobe, frontal lobe, temporal lobe, and temporal pole.
7. *EEG*: For details, see Figs. 3.25, 3.26, 3.27, 3.28, and 3.29.

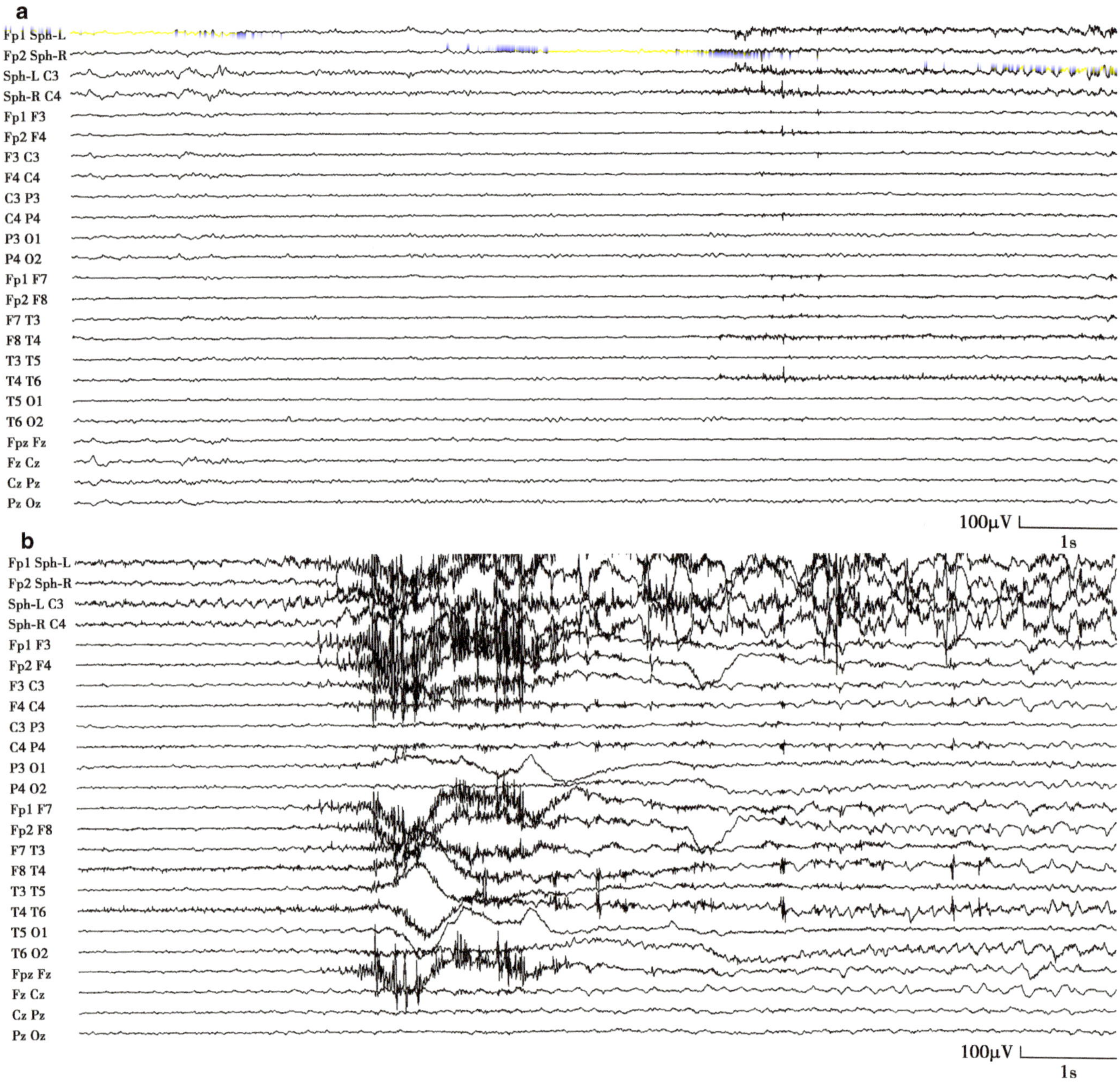

Fig. 3.25 Interictal scalp EEG. (**a**) Sharp waves were seen over the left sphenoidal electrode and over the left temporal region. (**b**) Multiple slowed sharp waves were seen over the right sphenoidal electrode, and the slow waves of low amplitude were seen over the right temporal region

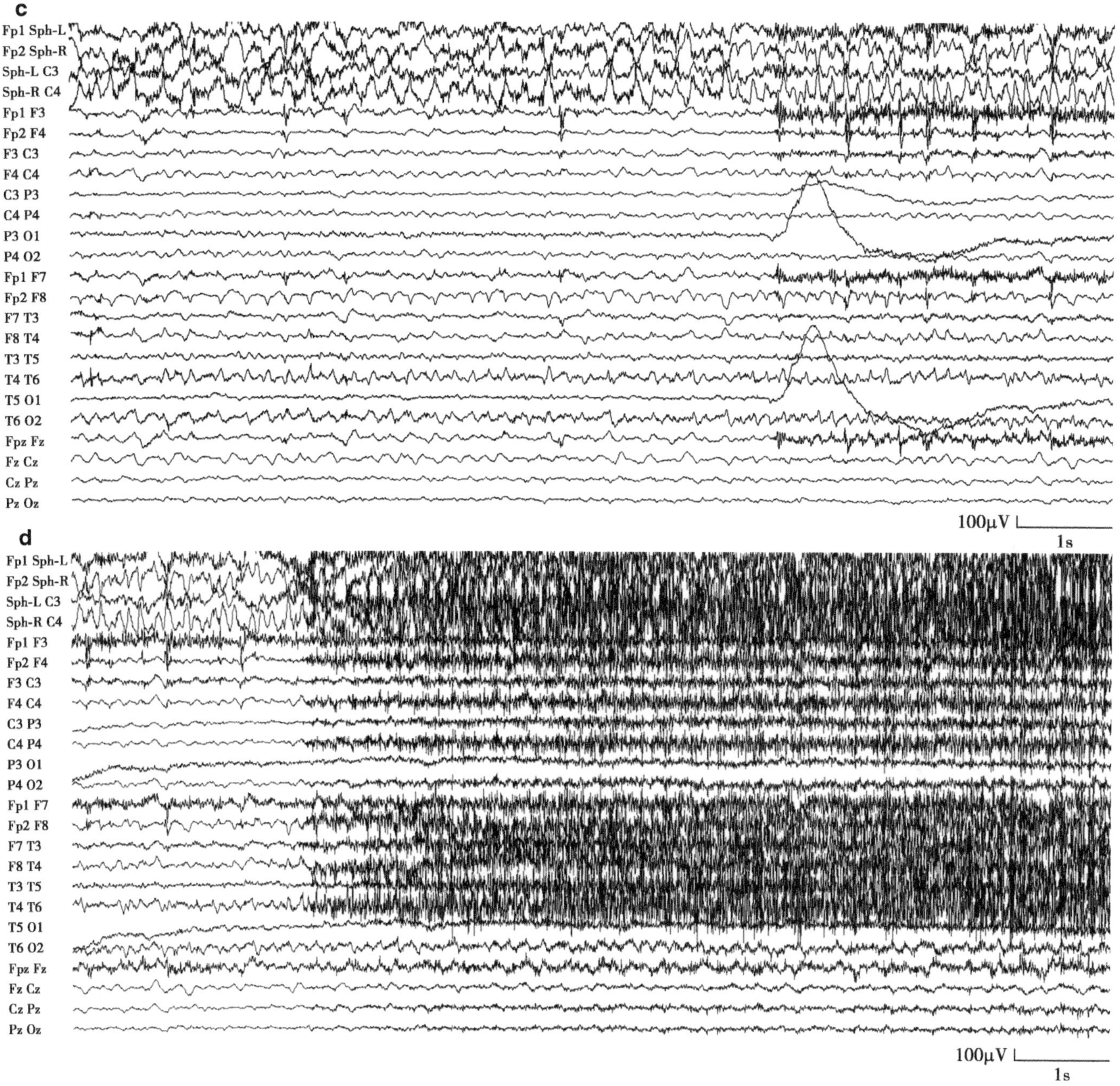

Fig. 3.25 (continued)

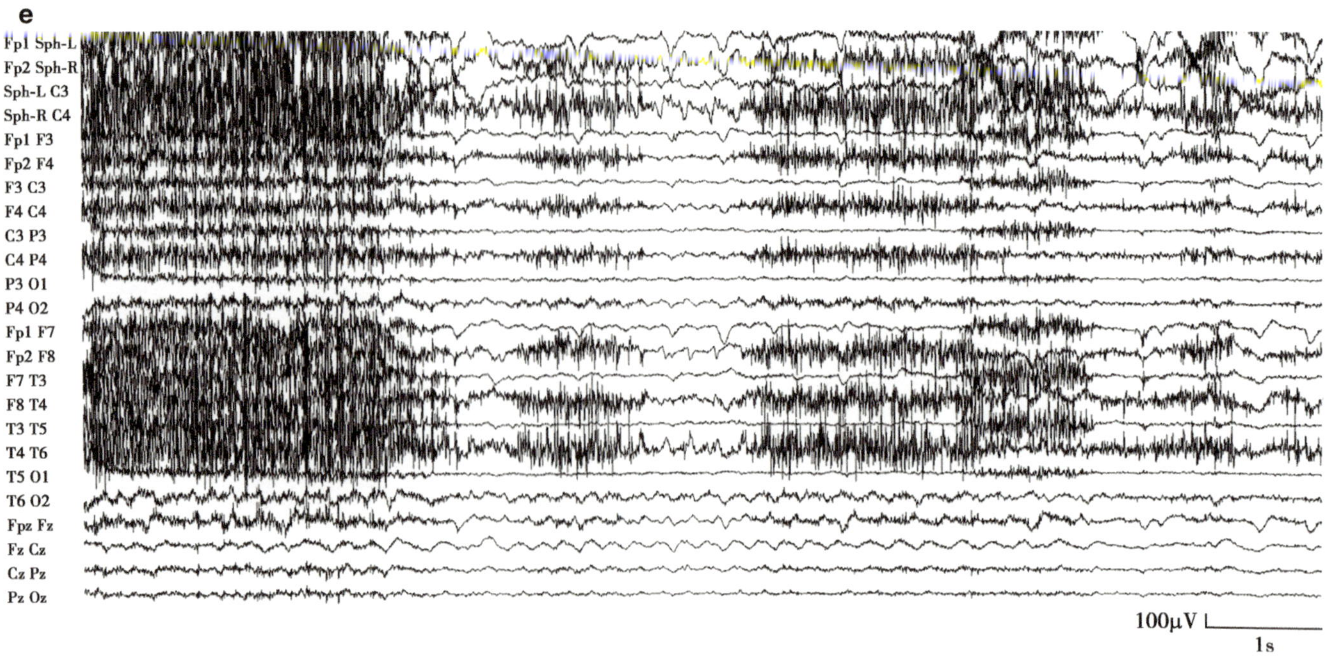

Fig. 3.25 (continued)

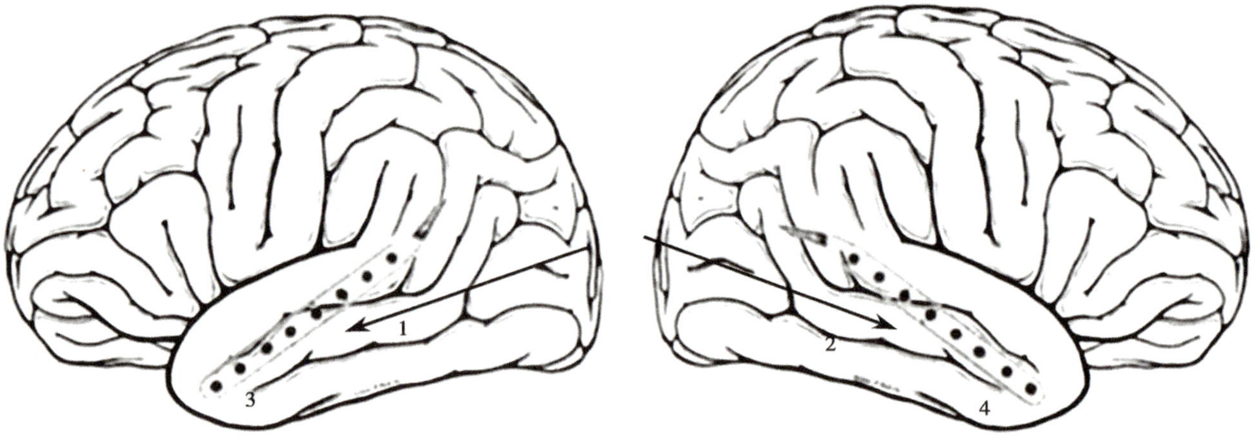

Fig. 3.26 Ictal scalp EEG. (**a**) Before the seizure, the patient was lying asleep on the right side. The EEG showed the stage II sleep. (**b**) The patient woke up during the seizure, with involuntary flexion and extension movements of the left upper and lower limbs. The EEG showed sharp waves over the left sphenoidal electrode, mixed with EMG artifacts over the bilateral frontal and temporal regions. (**c**) The patient had no obvious movements. The EEG showed the rhythm of sharp waves in bilateral sphenoidal electrodes, mixed with EMG artifacts in frontal and temporal regions and then the rhythm of sharp waves in bilateral temporal regions, mainly over the left temporal region. (**d**) The patient's body was slightly tilted backward with both lower limbs being abducted and stiffened. The EEG showed a gradually increasing rhythm of sharp waves in bilateral sphenoidal electrodes and over the left temporal region. (**e**) The patient had slight limbs clonus and slightly tilted backward. The EEG was basically the same as in **d** but with more EMG artifacts. (**f**) The patient still had limbs clonus, with the left upper limb being flexed, stiffened and elevated 6 s later. The EEG showed the rhythm of slow waves over the bilateral frontal and temporal regions mixed with EMG artifacts. (**g**) The patient's upper limbs were elevated and the lower limbs were stiff, with head tilted back. The EEG showed mixed EMG artifacts over the bilateral frontal and temporal regions. (**h**) The patient's body shook slightly and the left hand moved involuntarily. The EEG showed wobble and EMG artifacts, mainly over the bilateral frontal and temporal regions. (**i**) The patient had involuntary movements of the upper limbs while chewing. The EEG was basically the same as in **h**

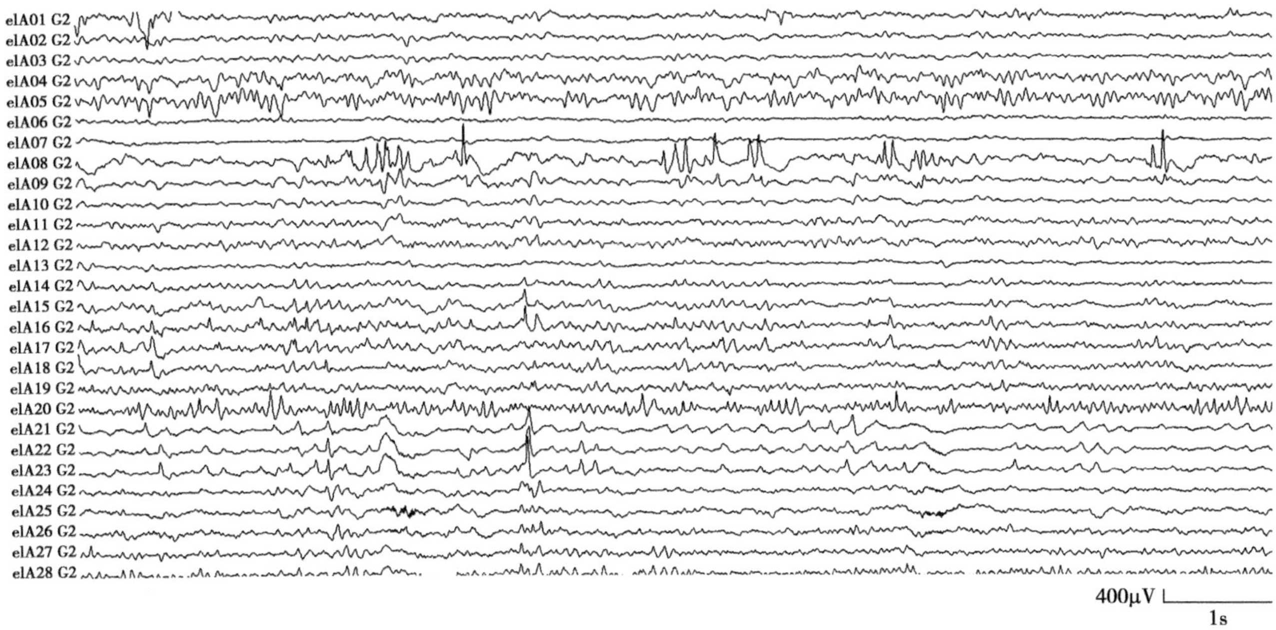

Fig. 3.27 Scheme of intracranial electrodes
Depth electrode 1: the left hippocampus (eight contacts); depth electrode 2: the right hippocampus (eight contacts)

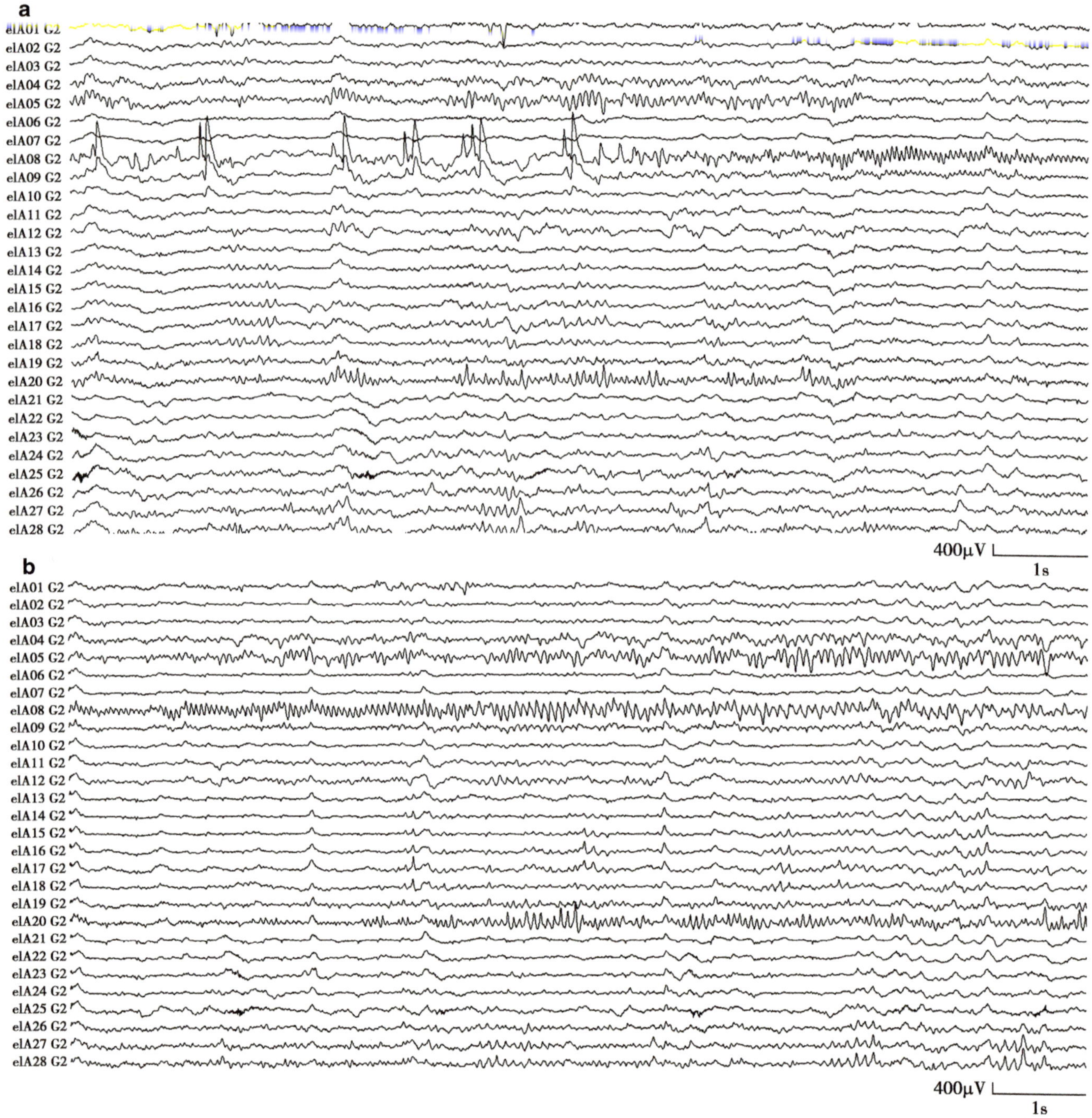

Fig. 3.28 Interictal intracranial EEG. (**a**) Spike-and-wave complexes were seen over the left hippocampus (contact numbers el002, el003, el004, el005), and spikes were seen over the right hippocampus (contact numbers el009 and el010). (**b**) Spikes of high amplitude and spike-and-wave complexes were seen over the left hippocampus (contact numbers el002, el003, el004, el005), and spikes of high amplitude and spike-and-wave complexes were seen over the right hippocampus (contact numbers el009, el010, el011, el012), which were asynchronous bilaterally

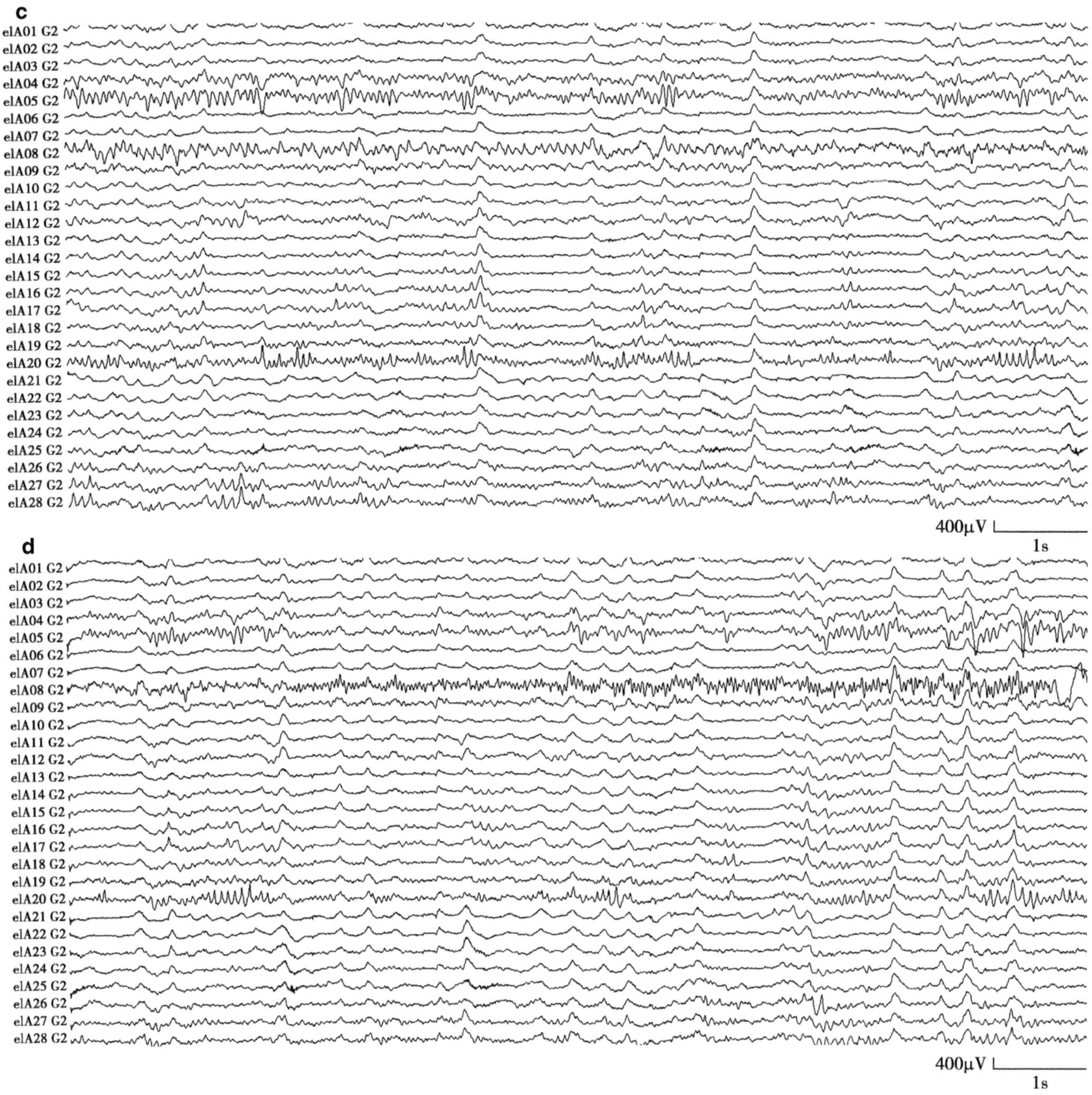

Fig. 3.28 (continued)

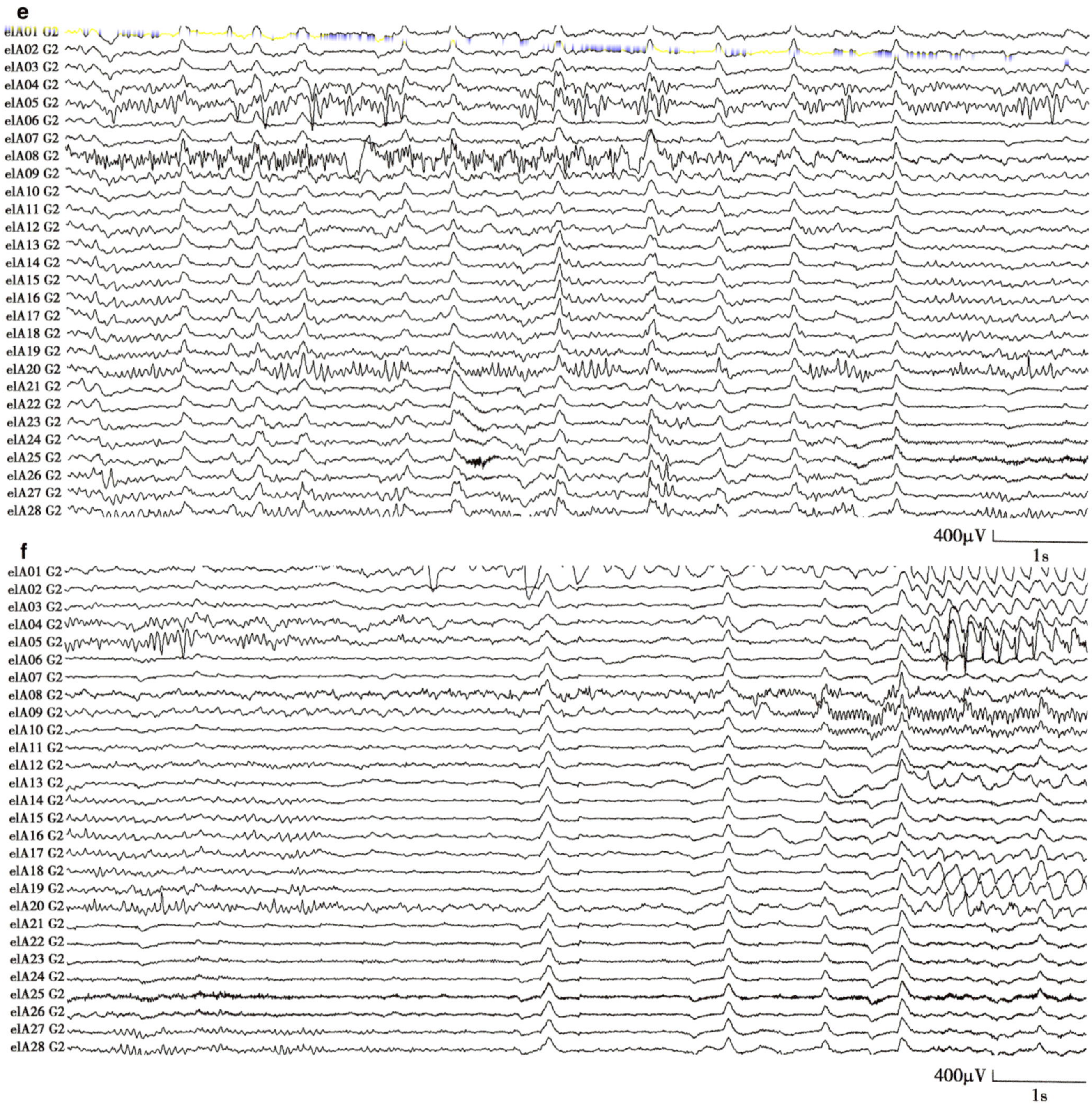

Fig. 3.28 (continued)

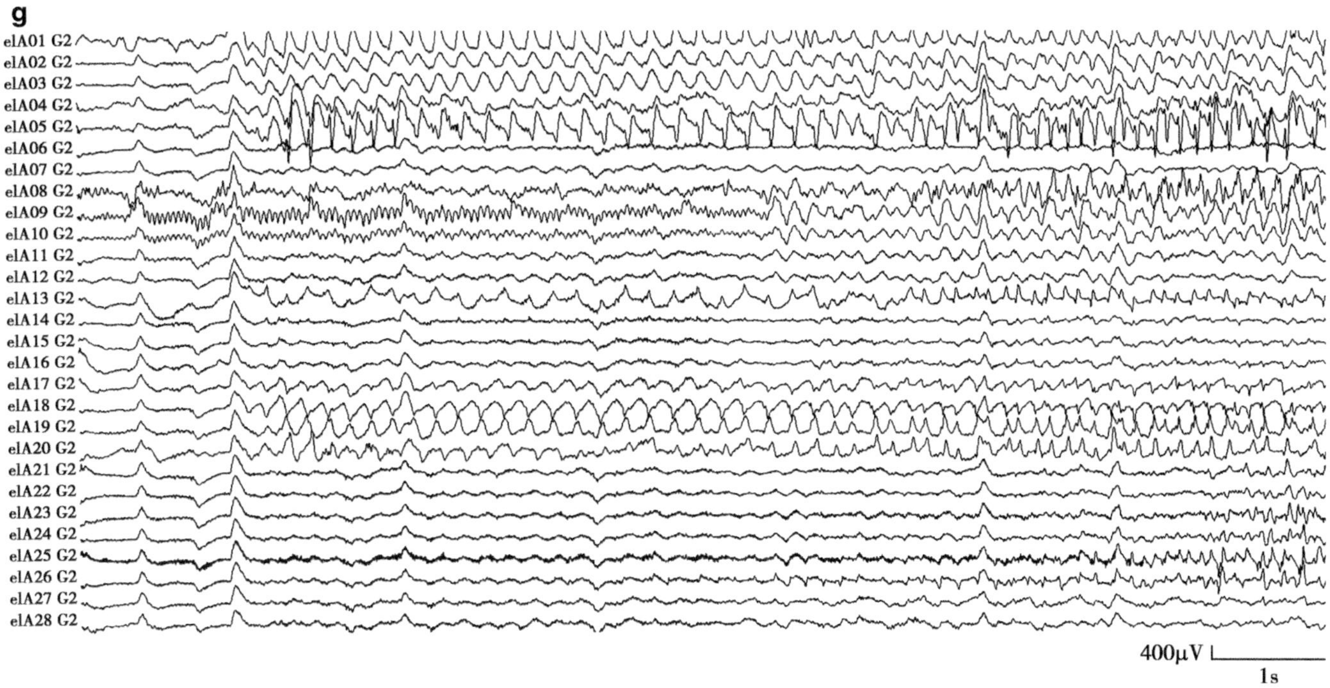

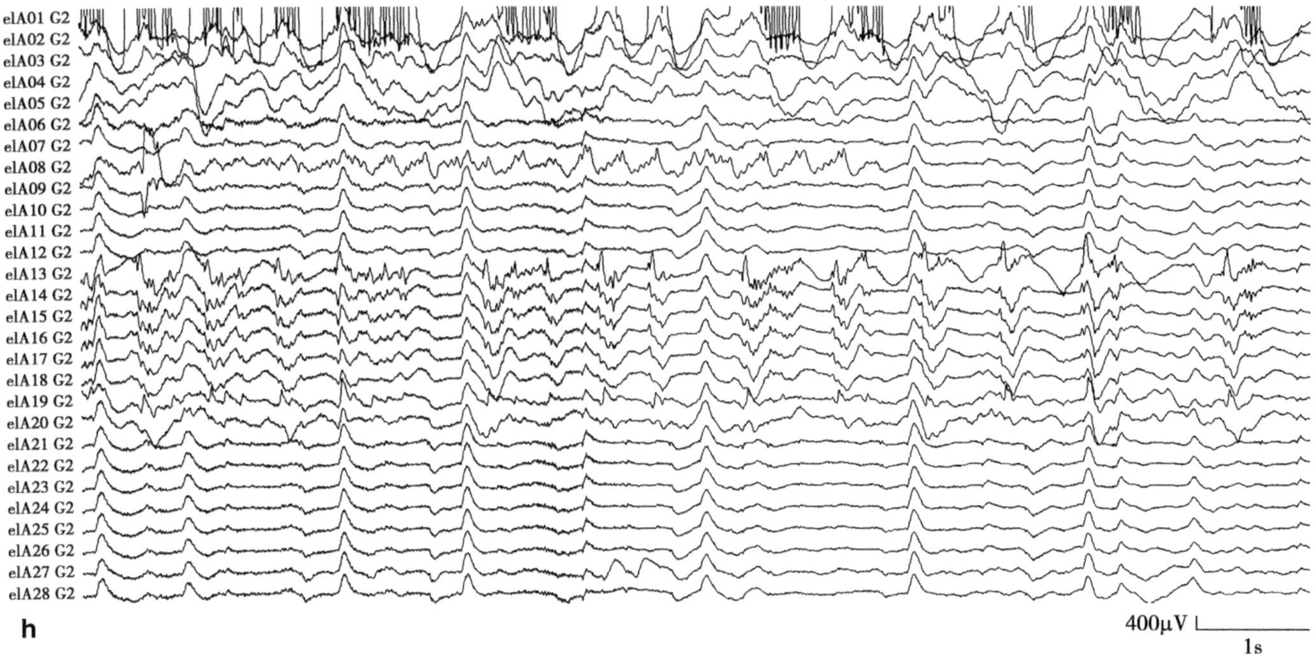

Fig. 3.28 (continued)

[Case Review]

The patient's interictal EEG of the bilateral sphenoidal eletrodes showed independent spikes and slow waves. At the beginning of the seizure, the EEG showed continuous sharp waves of high amplitude over the left sphenoidal electrode at an early stage, followed by a rhythm of sharp waves of high amplitude in bilateral sphenoidal eletrodes. Since the lateralization diagnosis on the scalp EEG was not clear, intracranial electrodes needed to be implanted. The electrodes over the bilateral hippocampus clearly showed that the burst of spike-and-wave complexes recorded by the electrodes over the right hippocampus was 2.5 s earlier than over the left hippocampus. Therefore, it was possible to definitively locate the seizures originating over the right hippocampus. The right anterior temporal lobe and medial structures were resected. The patient remained seizure-free during a 2-year follow-up after surgery.

Cases of Lateral Temporal Lobe Epilepsy

Case 3.10 Lateral Temporal Lobe Epilepsy

[Abstract of Medical Records]
Female, 16 years old.

1. *Chief complaint*: Episodic loss of consciousness with limb twitching for 6 years.
2. *History of present illness*: The patient started to walk aimlessly and could not respond to calls without any apparent inducement 6 years ago, which lasted for about 1 min and then resolved, and she was unable to recall the course of the seizure. Since then, the seizure occurred once per month, all of which occurred during the daytime in a pattern basically the same as before. Five years ago, the seizures began to manifest as fumbling by hands, staring blankly, making sound, and failing to respond to calls, which lasted for about 1 min and then resolved. The seizures occurred once every 10 days or so. Three years ago, she developed seizures with limb twitching, which manifested as loss of consciousness and fumbling with both hands in front of the chest, followed by falling to the ground, with the upper limbs flexed and the lower limbs extending, accompanied by clonus, lip cyanosis, foaming at the mouth, clenching of the teeth, but without incontinence or tongue bite, which lasted about 1 min and then resolved. After this, the patient felt restless and fumbled with both hands and occasionally wandered and talked to herself, which lasted for 3–5 min. She then fell asleep for about half an hour and woke up as usual. The patient had seizures mostly during the day, almost every day, without

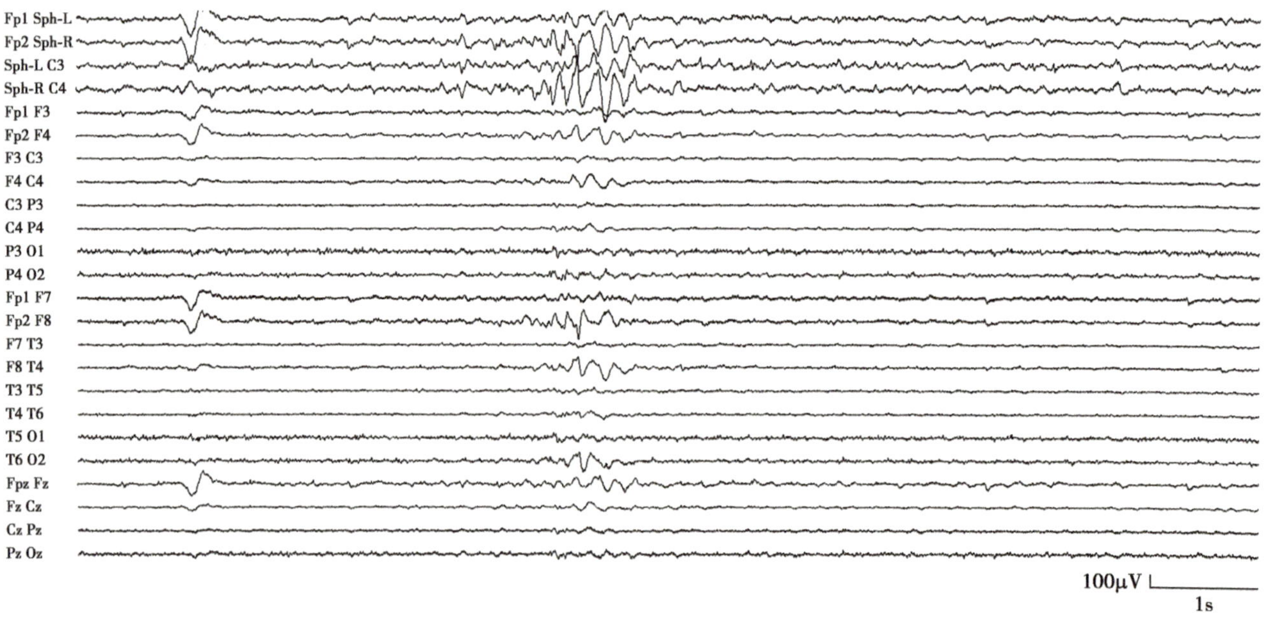

Fig. 3.29 Ictal EEG of intracranial electrodes. (**a**) The patient was asleep before the seizure. The IEEG showed sharp waves over the left hippocampus (contact numbers el003, el004, el005) and spikes over the right hippocampus (contact numbers el009 and el010). (**b**) The patient suddenly lifted his coat. The IEEG showed spike-and-wave complexes over the right hippocampus (contact numbers el009, el010, el011, el012, el013), followed by the rhythm of spikes (contact numbers el009, el010, el011, el012). (**c**) The patient was lying on the right side, with both upper limbs flexed in front of the chest and the body twisted to the right. The IEEG showed a gradually increasing rhythm of spikes over the right hippocampus (contact numbers el009, el010, el011, el012). Spike-and-wave complexes and the spike rhythm were seen over the left hippocampus (contact numbers el002, el003, el004, el005). (**d**) The patient's right upper limb was flexed and stiffened. The IEEG showed a gradually increasing rhythm of spikes of high amplitude in bilateral hippocampus. (**e**) The patient's head was gradually tilted back and deflected to the right with slight body clonus. The IEEG was basically the same as in **d**. (**f**) The patient had generalized clonus at decreasing speed. The IEEG showed the rhythm of spikes over the left hippocampus and rhythmic spikes over the right hippocampus. (**g**) The clonus stopped and the patient had involuntary movements of both lower limbs. The IEEG showed the sudden disappearance of rhythmic spikes over the right hippocampus and the formation of the rhythm of spike-and-wave complexes over the left hippocampus

aura. The patient was diagnosed with epilepsy at a local hospital when she first had a seizure 6 years ago and took phenytoin sodium orally, which failed to well control the seizure. She once took various medications (details unknown). A year ago, she started taking carbamazepine (200 mg/dose bid) and valpromide (400 mg/dose b.i.d.), during which the above-mentioned seizures with limb twitching occurred about once a month, and the seizures with hand fumbling occurred 1–2 times a day. Since the onset of the disease, the patient became more stubborn and irritable than before. The bladder and bowel functions were normal; there was no significant change in body weight.

3. *Past history*: No history of associated diseases.
4. *Personal and family history*: No history of associated diseases.
5. *Physical examination*: No neurological abnormalities were found.
6. *Auxiliary examination*: Blood concentration: sodium valproate 42.13 μg/mL (50–100 μg/mL); carbamazepine 5.88 μg/mL (4–12 μg/mL).
7. *Imaging examination*:
   (a) MRI revealed abnormal signals over the left temporal lobe.
   (b) DSA did not show any significant abnormality.
   (c) fMRI revealed activation over the primary motor cortex of the left cerebral hemisphere and no activation over the lesioned area of the left temporal lobe during the right-hand finger-finger test.
8. *EEG*: For details, see Figs. 3.30 and 3.31.

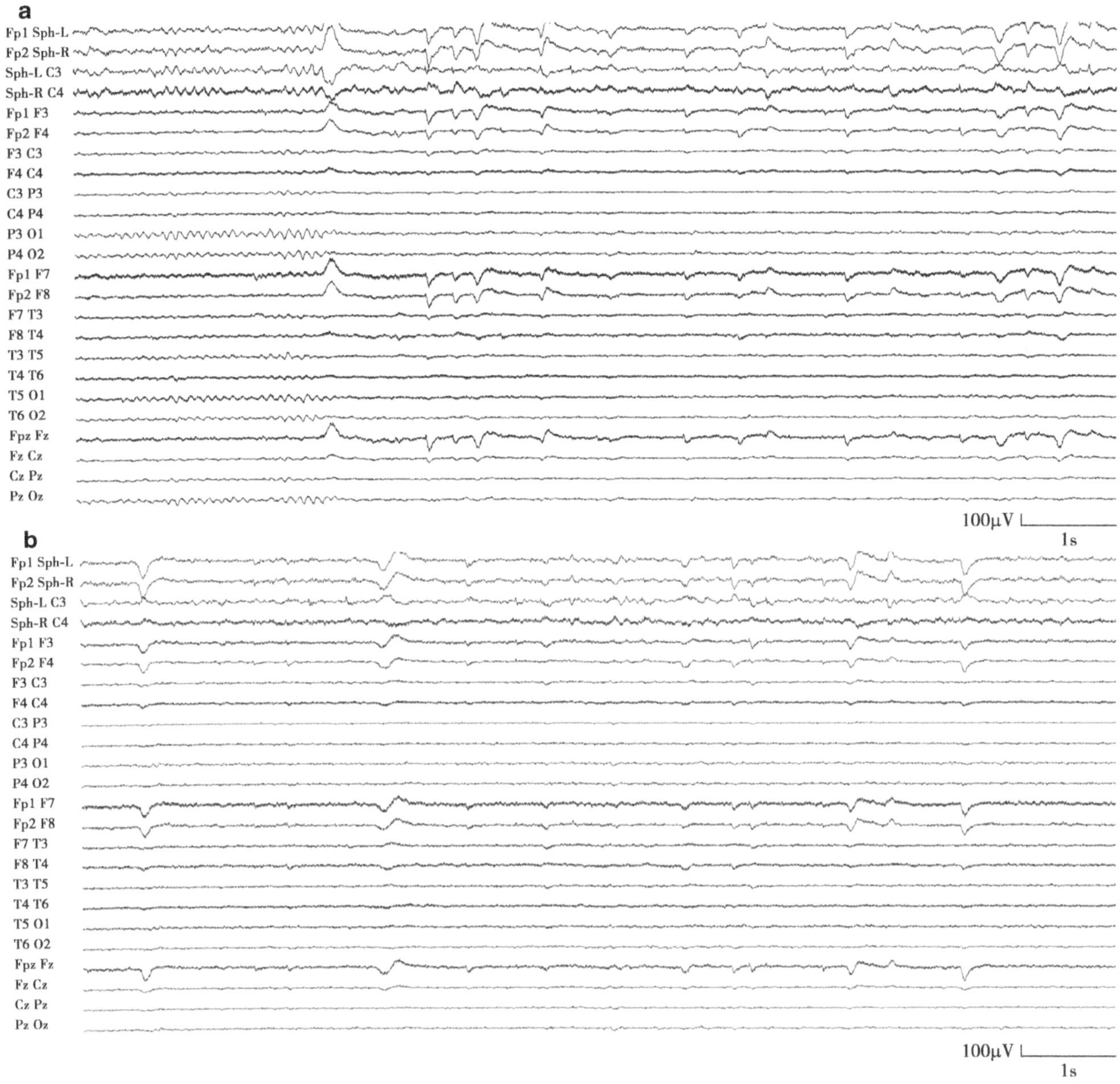

Fig. 3.30 Interictal scalp EEG. (**a**) The background EEG during wakefulness had a basic rhythm of 9–11 Hz. (**b**) Sharp waves and slow sharp waves were seen over the right sphenoidal electrode, and slow sharp waves and slow waves were seen over the right temporal region

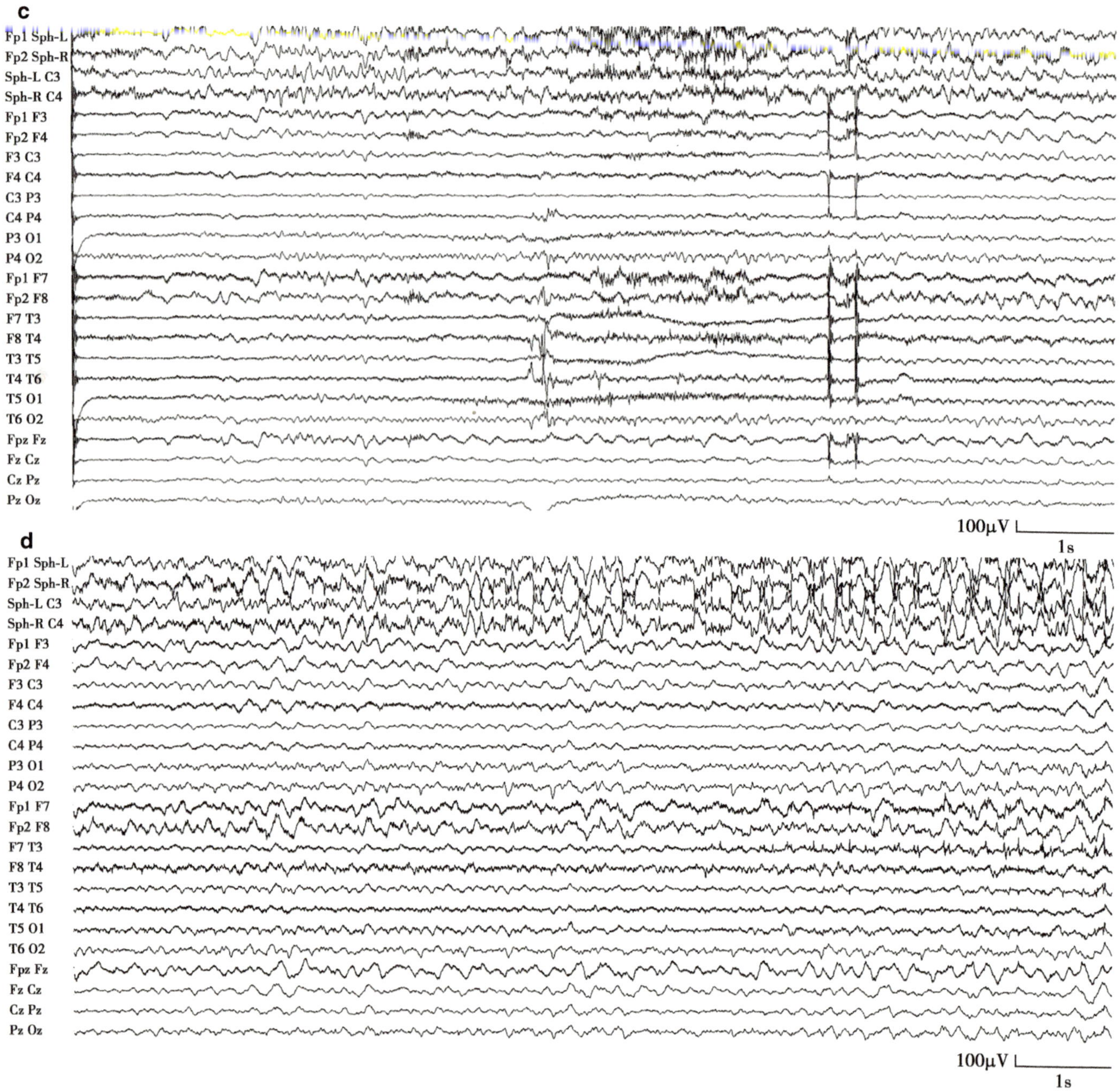

Fig. 3.30 (continued)

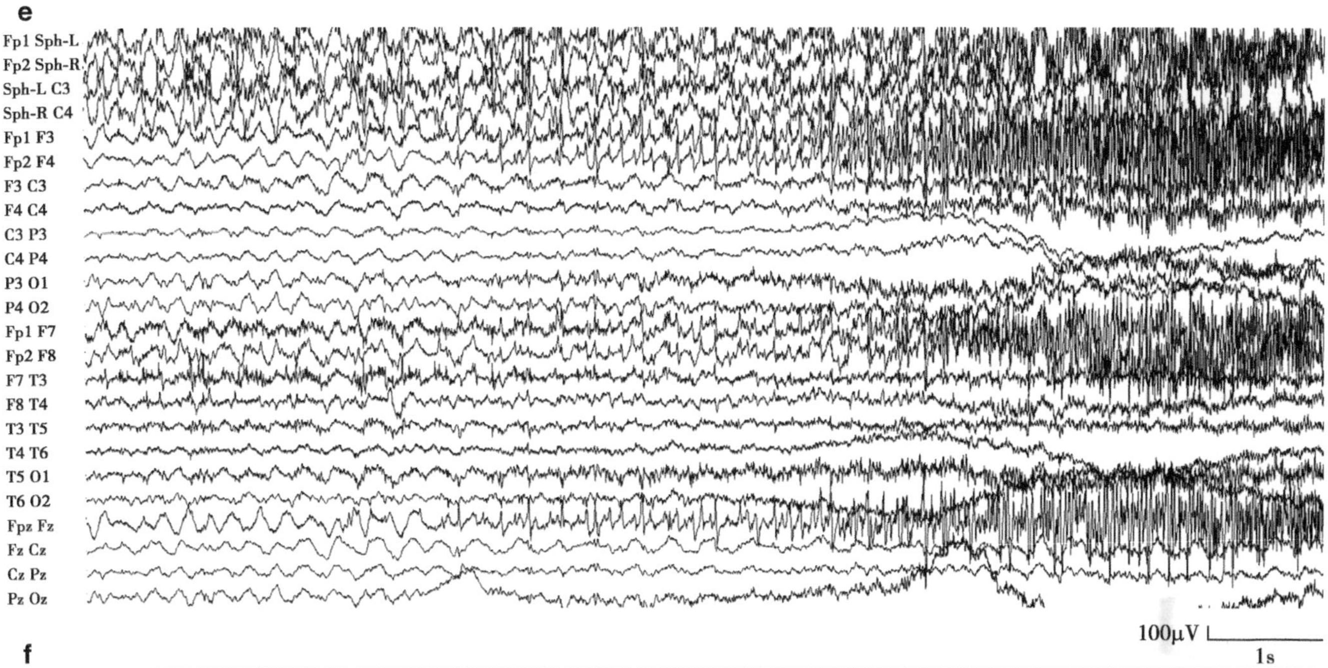

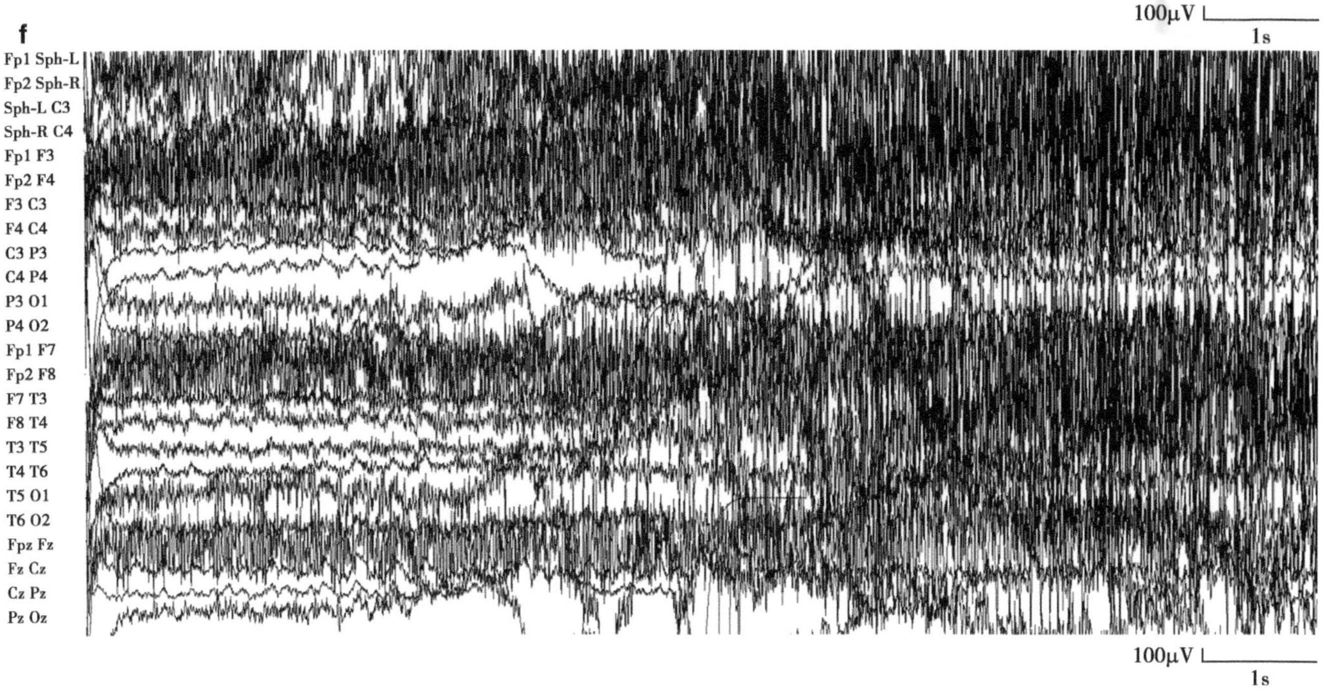

Fig. 3.30 (continued)

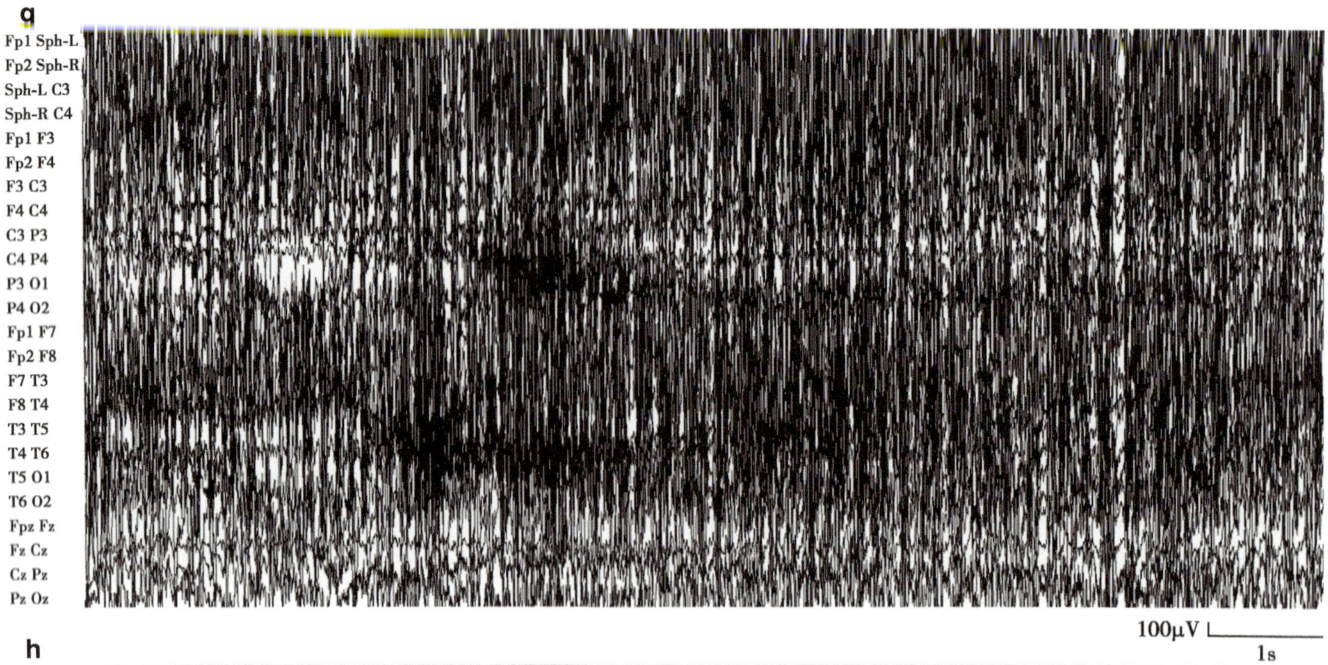

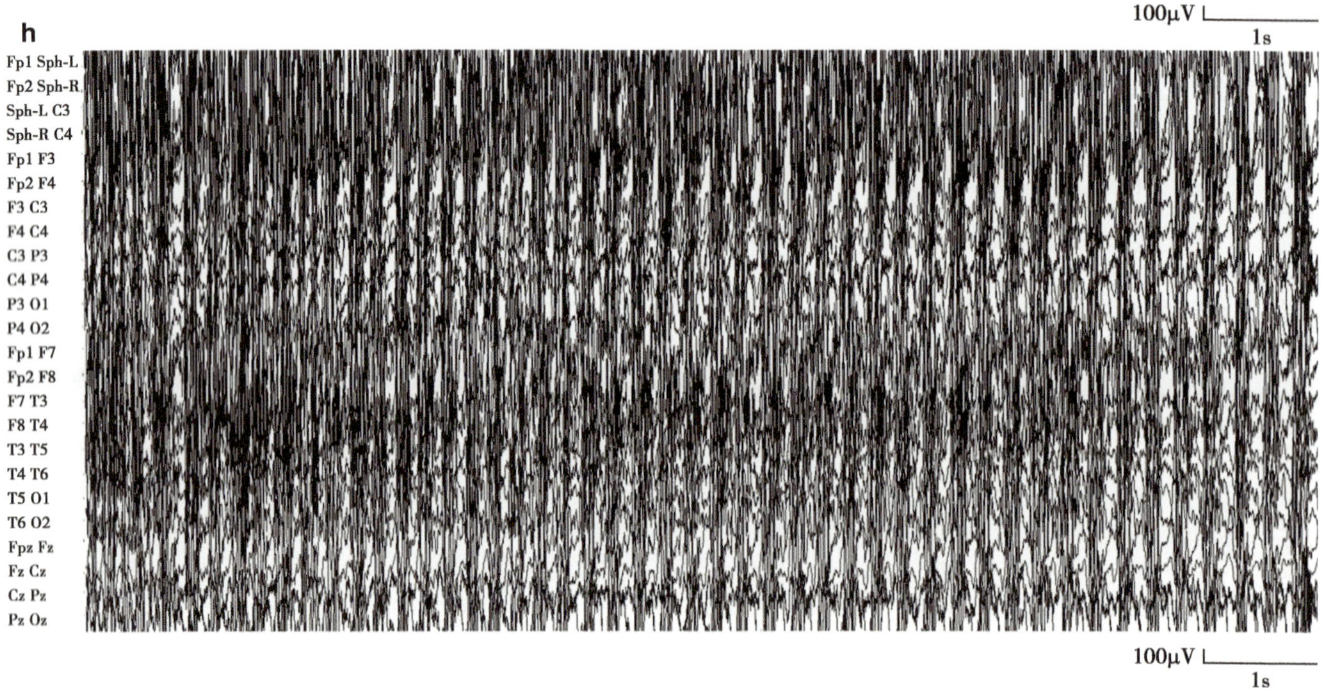

Fig. 3.30 (continued)

i

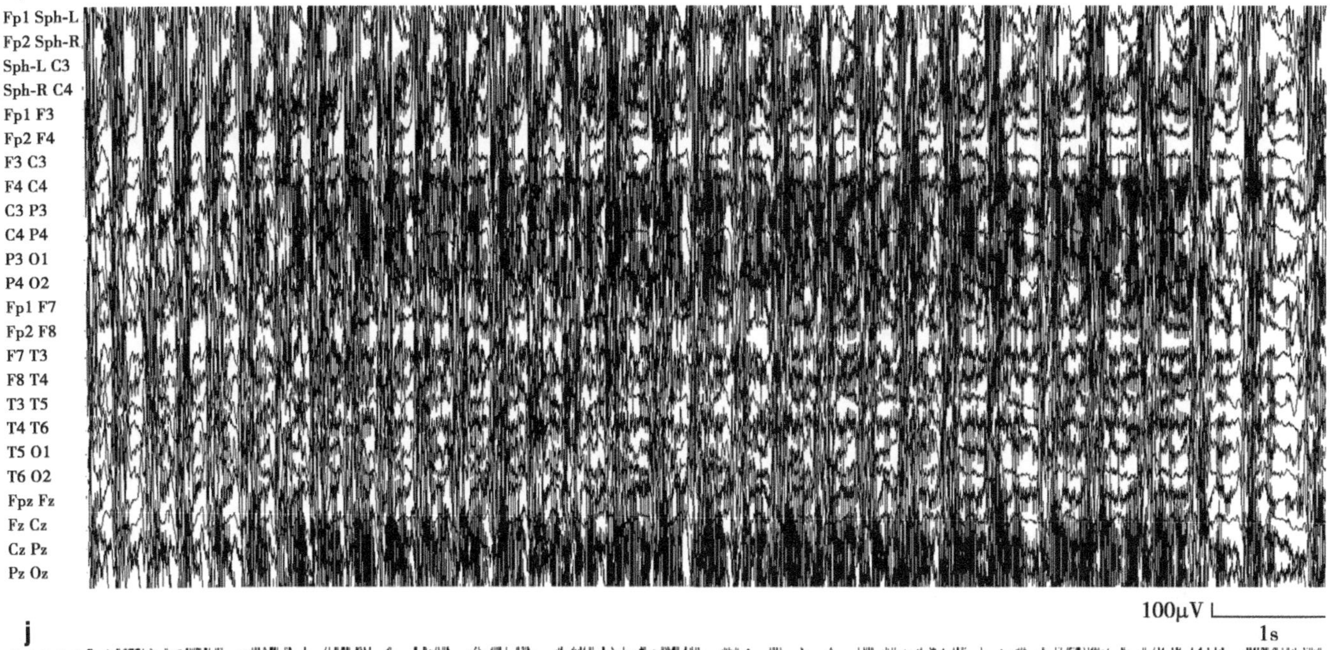

j

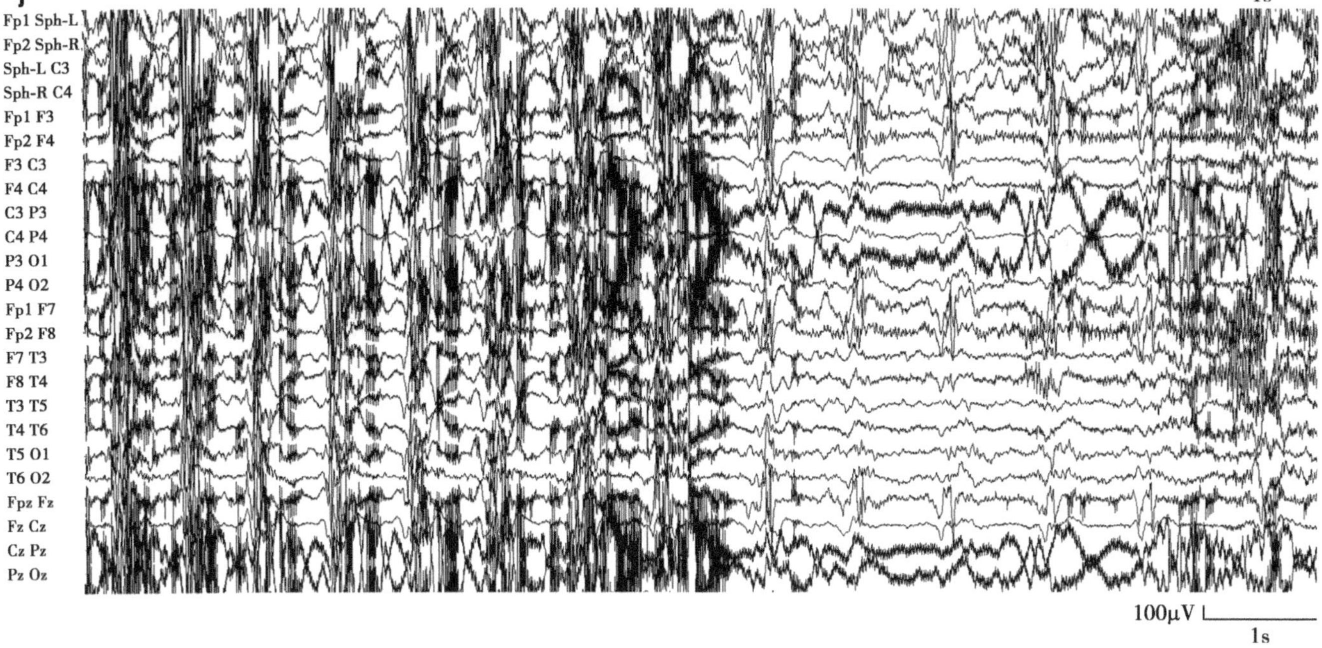

Fig. 3.30 (continued)

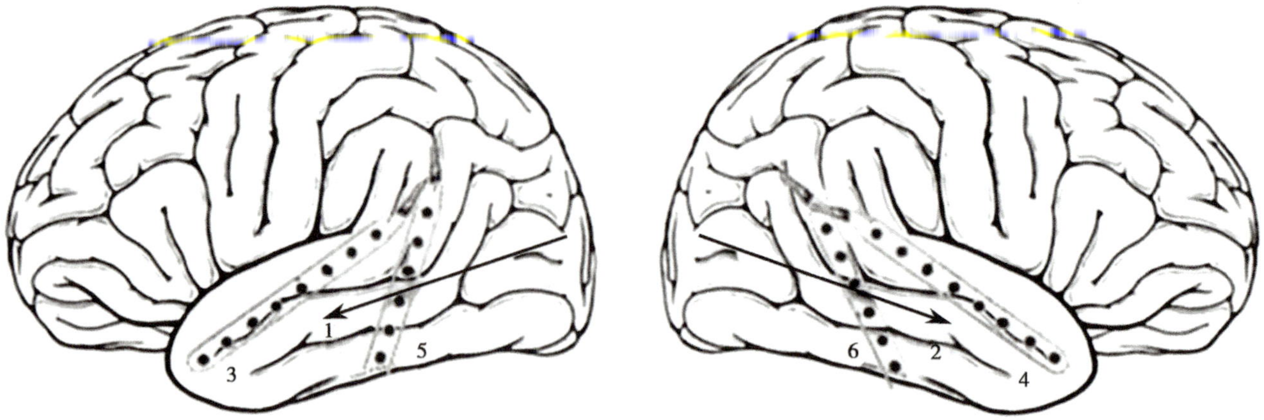

Fig. 3.31 Ictal scalp EEG. (**a**) The patient lay flat quietly 10 s before the seizure. Then, the patient lifted the left arm and tried to grasp something with hands. The EEG showed fast activity of low amplitude for 5 s and a slow rhythm over the left Fp1 F3 lead, followed by decreasing frequency and increasing wave amplitude in all leads. (**b**) The patient was restless, and her hands were pressed against the chest by her family members. The EEG showed the rhythm of slow waves over the bilateral frontal and parietal regions, and mixed EMG artifacts were seen. (**c**) The patient's eyes were glassy and the body was tonic. The EEG showed the rhythm of sharp waves in bilateral sphenoidal electrode, and a mixture of sharp waves/spikes and sharp waves/spike-and-wave complexes over the bilateral frontal, temporal, and parietal leads. (**d**) The patient stared to the right and had tonic clonus, followed by vocalization, rightward tilting of the mouth corners, lifting up of the lower limbs, clenching of the hands and flexion of the upper limbs in front of the chest, secondary to a generalized tonic-clonic seizure. The EEG showed sharp waves and slow waves over the bilateral frontal, temporal, and parietal regions and mixed EMG artifacts and artifacts 5 s later. (**e**) The patient extended the lower limbs, twitched the mouth corners, and made sound. The whole body was tonic and clonic. EEG showed EMG artifacts and wobble artifacts mixed. (**f**) The patient's symptoms and the EEG were basically same as in **e.** (**g**) The clonus intensity of the patient was reduced. The EEG was basically the same as in **e.** (**h**) The clonus intensity of the patient was reduced. The EEG showed spike-and-waves complexes, together with EMG artifacts and artifacts. (**i**) As the clonus intensity decreased, the patient's seizure ended 4 s later. The patient then fell asleep. The EEG was basically the same as in **h**

[Case Review]

The interictal EEG showed noticeable sharp waves, sharp-and-waves complexes, and slow waves over the right sphenoidal electrode and over the right temporal region. EEG changed bilaterally at the onset of seizures, which differed from the EEG change process of typical medial temporal epilepsy with a slightly more pronounced characteristics on the left during the seizure, and MRI revealed that the patient had a clear left temporal region lesion. A standard resection of the left temporal region was performed directly. The seizures disappeared during a 3-year follow-up after surgery.

Case 3.11 Lateral Temporal Lobe Epilepsy

[Abstract of Medical Records]
Female, 28 years old.

1. *Chief complaint*: Episodic loss of consciousness with twitching for 10 years.
2. *History of present illness*: The patient had episodic loss of consciousness and limb rigidity 10 years ago with involuntary chewing movements that lasted several minutes. Six months later, a similar seizure occurred again, preceded by a feeling of confusion in the surroundings and a feeling that people were talking somewhere far away. She took sodium valproate (dosage unknown), which was ineffective. There were intermittent seizures that each lasted from more than 10 seconds to 2 min at a frequency of 1–2 times per day or once every 20 days approximately. Later, she changed to take carbamazepine at a dose of 200 mg t.i.d., but the effect remained unsatisfactory.
3. *Past history*: The patient once fell from the second floor at 2 years old and was in a coma for 1 day.
4. *Personal and family history*: No relevant personal or family history.
5. *Physical examination*: No neurological abnormalities were found.
6. *Imaging examination*: MRI showed no abnormalities over the caudal part of the bilateral hippocampus.
7. *EEG*: For details, see Figs. 3.32 and 3.33.

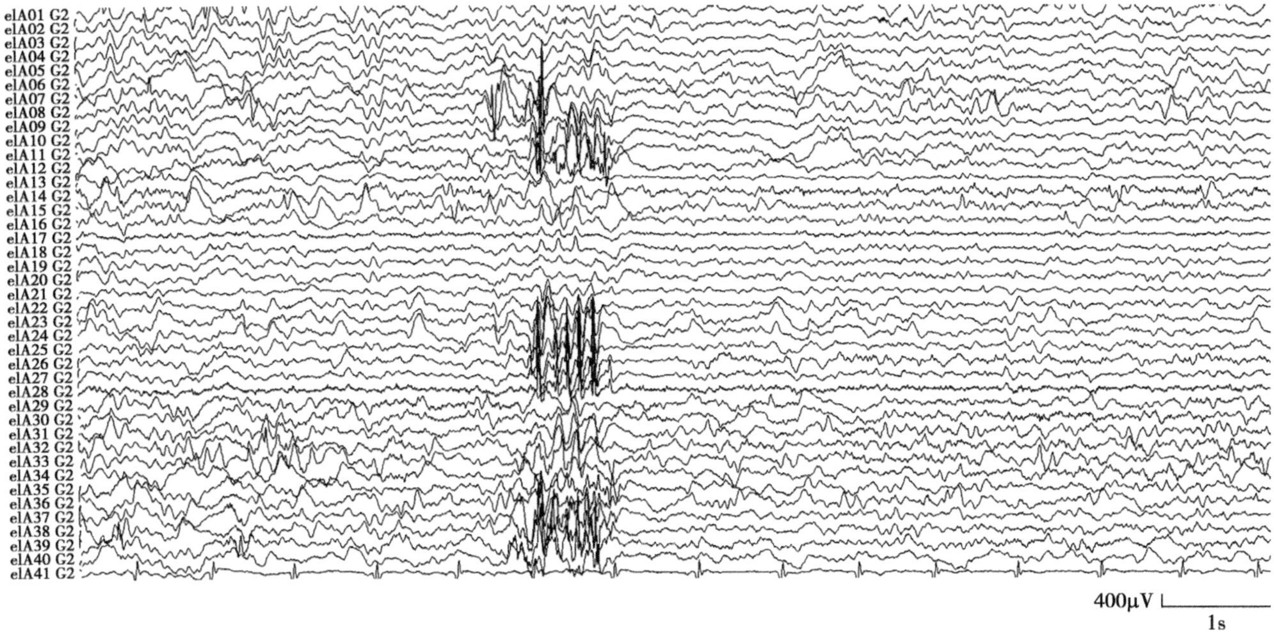

Fig. 3.32 Interictal scalp EEG. (**a**) The background EEG during wakefulness showed the rhythm of 10.0–12.0 Hz α activities over the occipital region, with poor amplitude modulation. (**b**) Sharp waves and slow waves were seen over the left sphenoidal electrode. (**c**) Slowed sharp waves were seen over the left sphenoidal electrode

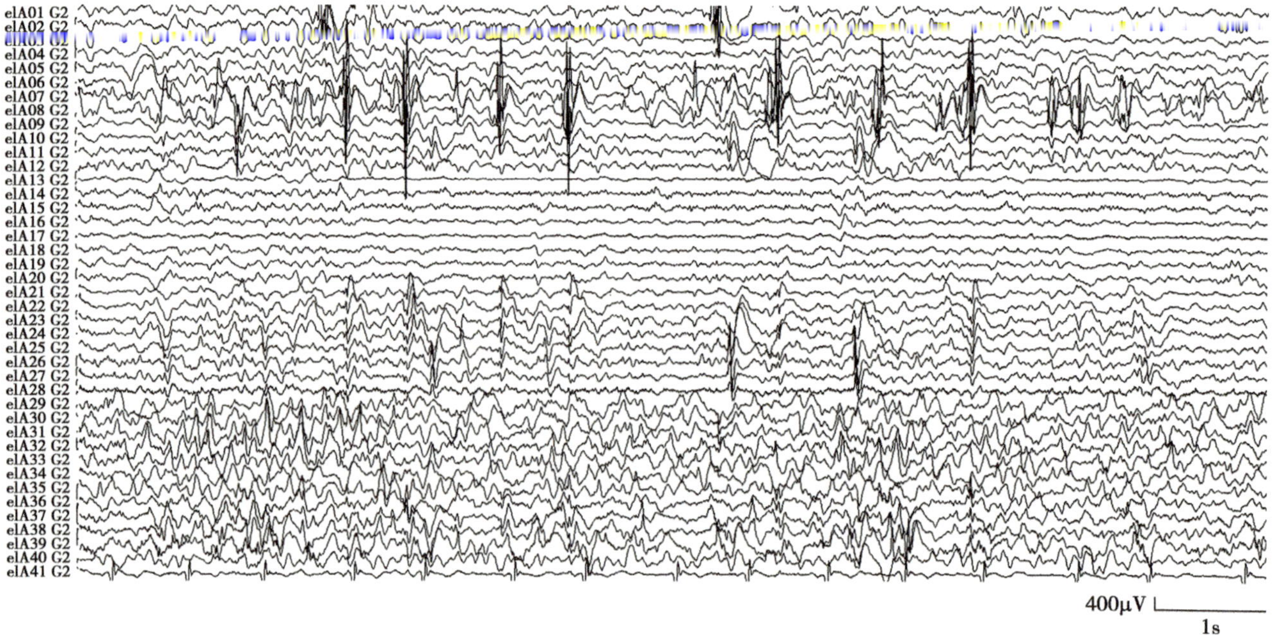

Fig. 3.33 Ictal scalp EEG. (**a**) The patient was awake and sitting on the bed; 4 s before the seizure, the patient had an aura and without any other obvious movements. The EEG was presented as the background EEG during wakefulness for 4 s, followed by the rhythm of 6.0–7.0 Hz slow wave of medium and high amplitude over the right sphenoidal electrode (Sph-R) with gradually increased amplitude, which developed into the rhythms of slow waves and sharp waves. The waves then spread to the right middle temporal region (T4), right posterior temporal region (T6), and contralateral side. (**b**) The patient rubbed her left hand continuously with his right hand and flexed the upper limbs in front of the chest with slight stiffness 6 s later. The EEG showed sharp waves of high amplitude and the rhythm of sharpened slow waves over the right sphenoidal electrode and over the right frontal region. The rhythm of slow waves of medium amplitude was seen over the remaining leads, mainly on the right. (**c**) 6 s later, the left lower limb was flexed, the right upper limb was bent in front of the chest, and the left upper limb was bent and elevated, with slight clonus. The EEG showed that the rhythm of sharp waves over the right sphenoidal electrode evolved into the rhythm of spikes. Slow waves and sharpened slow waves were seen over the remaining leads, mainly on the right. (**d**) The patient's symptoms were the same as described in **c**. The EEG showed the rhythm of spikes over the right sphenoidal electrode and the rhythm of sharp waves over the right frontal and temporal regions. The mixed slow waves, sharp waves, and sharpened slow waves can be seen over the remaining leads. (**e**) The patient was restless and fumbled with her left hand. She sat up 6 s later and tried to get out of bed. The EEG presentation was the same as **d**. (**f**) The patient sat on the side of the bed with the help of her family member, then got up and stood beside of the bed, and then sat on the bed again. The EEG showed the rhythm of sharp waves over the right sphenoidal electrode and the rhythms of sharp waves and slow waves over the bilateral frontal and temporal regions. (**g**) The patient fumbled with both hands. The EEG presentation was the basically same as **f**. (**h**) The patient was restless and involuntarily fumbled in front of the chest, grasping the chest and instruments, and arranging the sleeves. The EEG presentation was the basically same as in **f**. Each lead showed slightly decreased wave amplitudes compared with before and was mixed with EMG artifacts. (**i**) The patient turned head around as if looking for something. The EEG showed slight decrease in wave amplitudes in each lead compared with before and the rhythm of 7.0–8.0 Hz slow wave of low amplitude over the bilateral frontal and central leads. There were artifacts, together with sharp waves and slow waves, over the bilateral sphenoidal electrode. (**j**) The patient's symptoms and the EEG presentation were the same as in **i**. (**k**) The patient's symptoms and the EEG presentation were the same as in **i**; 7 s later, the EEG recovered the background EEG during wakefulness

[Case Review]

The patient had an auditory aura, which was clinically considered as the involvement of temporal lobe cortex. The lateralization features of the interictal EEG were not clear. The ictal EEG showed rhythmic activity mainly over the right sphenoidal electrode, which gradually developed into the rhythm of spikes. The rhythmic activity over the temporal region gradually spread to the frontoparietal region and then to the contralateral temporal and frontal regions. In terms of clinical manifestations, also became right-handed automatism, followed by increased muscular tone of upper limbs, mainly on the left side, with slight clonus. As the abnormal EEG rhythm spread to the contralateral side, the patient showed automatism over the contralateral hand, as well as automatism in both hands, with noticeable loss of consciousness. In this case, the patient's seizure symptoms and the ictal EEG presentation had clear definitive features for lateralization. In consideration of the patient's aura, seizure symptoms, and the obvious spreading process of EEG, the right anterior temporal lobe, hippocampus, and amygdala were resected. After the surgery, no seizure occurred to the patient during a 2-year follow-up.

Other Cases of Temporal Lobe Epilepsy

Case 3.12 Bilateral Temporal Lobe Epilepsy

[Abstract of Medical Records]
Male, 21 years old.

1. *Chief complaint*: Episodic facial and the limb twitching with unconsciousness for 4 years.
2. *History of present illness*: The patient suddenly suffered from limb twitching and loss of consciousness 4 years ago, which was diagnosed with encephalitis at that time, and he was hospitalized for treatment. After discharge from the hospital, he orally took carbamazepine at a dose of 300 mg t.i.d. but still had frequent seizures. One pattern of seizure was characterized by loss of consciousness with limb twitching. Sometimes seizure occurred every day. After taking 5 drugs including carbamazepine, sodium valproate, phenobarbital, lamotrigine, and clonazepam, he still had seizures. The seizure mainly manifested as absence of mind, laughing, left-sided facial twitching, and head and eyes turned to the left, which lasted 1–2 min. He felt blank before the seizure and showed unresponsiveness after the seizure. Another seizure pattern was characterized by tonic clonus of the limbs in addition to the symptoms above. The frequency of seizures was variable and related to stress, fatigue, and weather changes. Sometimes the seizures occurred once a few months, sometimes several times a day.
3. *Past history*: The patient was delivered at term with no postnatal asphyxia. There was no febrile convulsion. He grew normally but was involved in a car accident 10 years ago. There was no family history of epilepsy.
4. *Physical examination*: He was conscious and articulate and had memory loss, no abnormalities in cranial nerves, normal muscular tone, Grade 5 muscular strength, and negative bilateral pathological signs. Neuropsychological examination showed a verbal IQ of 66, PIQ of 77, and FIQ of 68, indicating mild dysgnosia.
5. Imaging examination:
   (a) MRI showed that the left hippocampus was small in volume.
   (b) MRS showed that the level (NAA/Cr: 1.13) over the left hippocampus was slightly lower than that over the right side (NAA/Cr: 1.40); the Cho concentration (Cho/Cr: 0.5) over the left hippocampus was slightly lower than that over the right side (Cho/Cr: 1.06).
   (c) SPECT showed a heterogeneous reduction of cortical perfusion over the cerebral hemispheres bilaterally.
6. *EEG*: For details, see Figs. 3.34, 3.35, and 3.36.

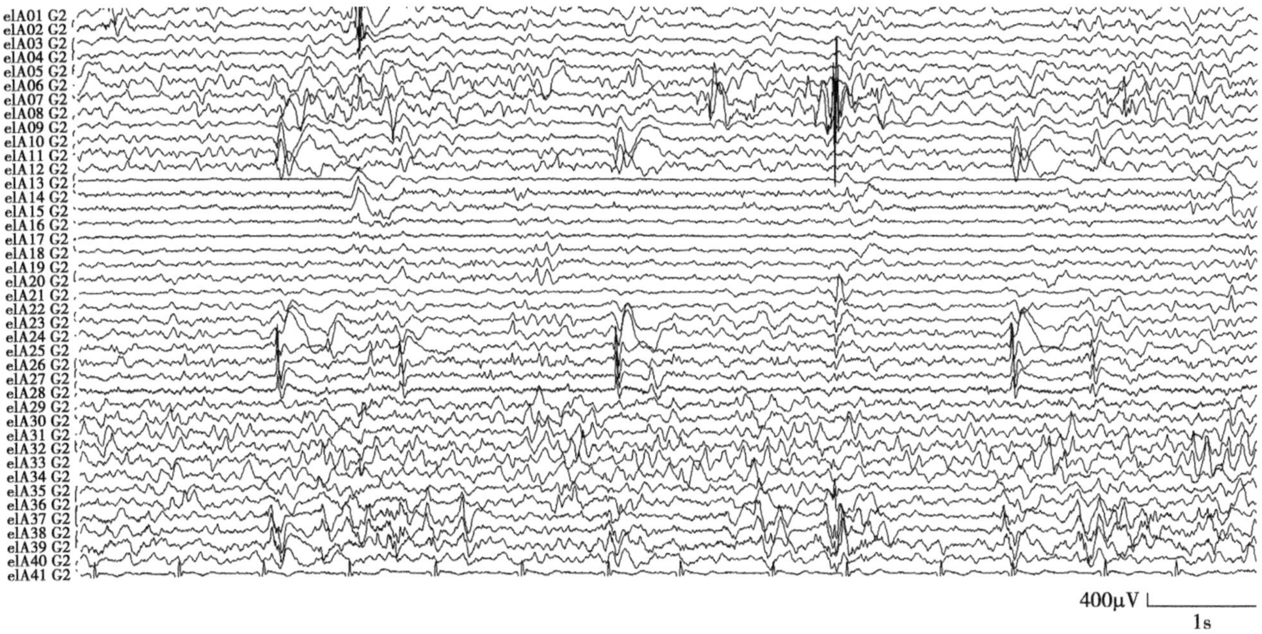

Fig. 3.34 Interictal scalp EEG. (**a**) The background EEG during wakefulness had a basic rhythm of 10.0–12.0 Hz. (**b**) The EEG of stage II sleep showed sharp waves and sharp-and-wave complexes over the right sphenoidal electrode and over the right temporal region. (**c**) Sharp waves were seen over the left sphenoidal electrode

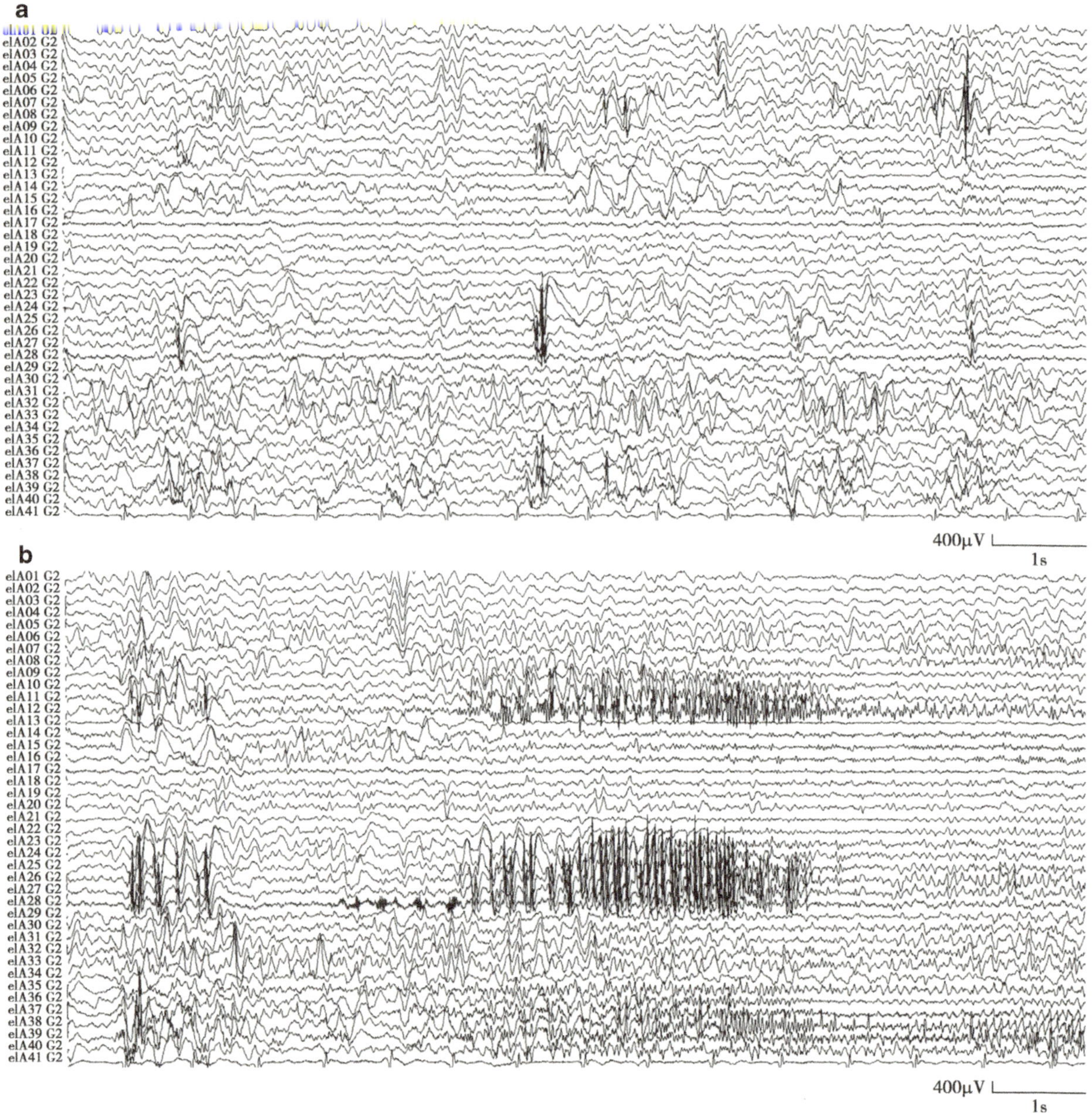

Fig. 3.35 Ictal scalp EEG 1. (**a**) Before the seizure, the patient was lying flat, with eyes open and the left upper limb flexed in front of the chest. The EEG showed the rhythm of slow waves of low amplitude over the left sphenoidal electrode 4 s before the seizure. Later, the wave amplitude gradually increased until the rhythm of sharp waves of high amplitude was reached. (**b**) 7 s later, the patient had a pleasant expression and smiled. The EEG showed the rhythm of sharp waves over the left sphenoidal electrode and over the left temporal region. (**c**) The patient was lying flat, with a pleasant expression and smiling, and then pursed his lips. The EEG showed the rhythm of sharp waves over the bilateral sphenoidal electrode and sharp waves and slow waves over the bilateral frontal and left temporal region. (**d**) The patient looked dull and had no limb movements. The EEG presentation was the basically same as **c**. (**e**) The patient's symptoms and the EEG presentation were basically same as **c**. (**f**) The patient's breathing rate increased, manifesting as a long deep breath. The EEG showed the rhythm of sharp waves over the bilateral sphenoidal electrode, and the rhythm of slow waves mixed with spikes over the bilateral frontal, temporal, and parietal leads. (**g**) The patient's symptoms and the EEG presentation were basically same as **f**. (**h**) The patient turned his head slowly to the right and looked right with both eyes. The EEG was basically the same as in **f**. (**i**) The patient's symptoms were basically same as described in **h**, with swallowing. The EEG presentation was basically same as **f**, accompanied by EMG artifacts and wobble artifacts. (**j**) The first 8 s, it was same as **i**. 8 s later, the patient suffered from twitching in the left upper limb with vocalizing. The EEG presentation was basically same as **f**, accompanied by many EMG artifacts and wobble artifacts (mainly the EMG artifacts). (**k**) The patient's right upper limb was raised and twitched, and the head was turned to the right with vocalization. The EEG was basically the same as **j**. (**l**) The patient's symptoms were the same as described in **k**. The EEG showed numerous EMG and wobble artifacts (mainly the EMG), and slow waves of low and medium amplitude only over the leads over the central, parietal, and occipital regions bilaterally. (**m**) The patient lowered the right upper limb and flexed it in front of the chest, while turning his head to the right. The EEG showed numerous EMG and wobble artifacts (mainly the EMG). (**n**) The first 3 s, the patient's symptoms were the same as described in **m**. 3 s later, the patient lay flat quietly with his head over the center position, and the seizure ended. The EEG showed numerous EMG and wobble artifacts (mainly the wobble)

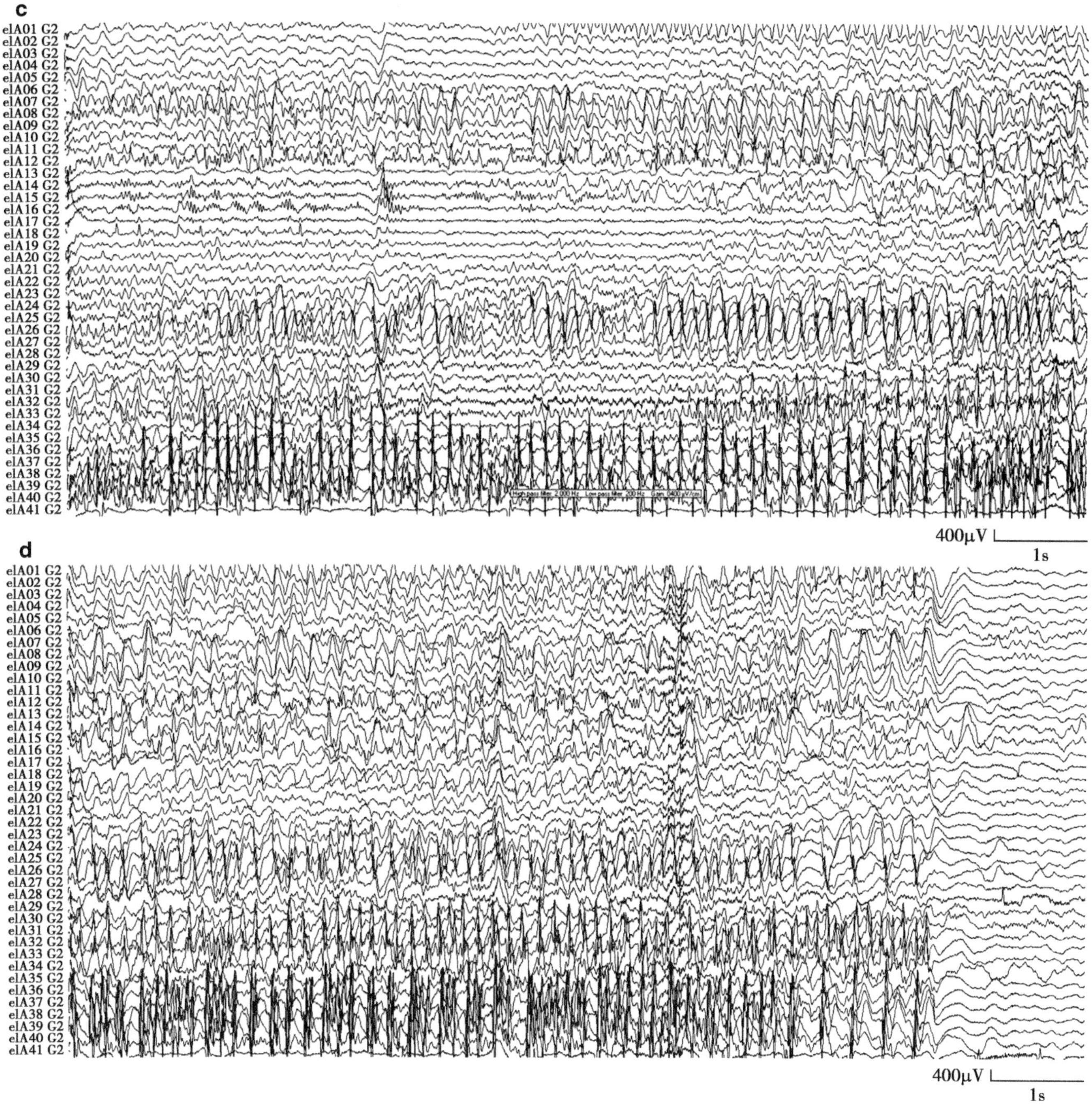

Fig. 3.35 (continued)

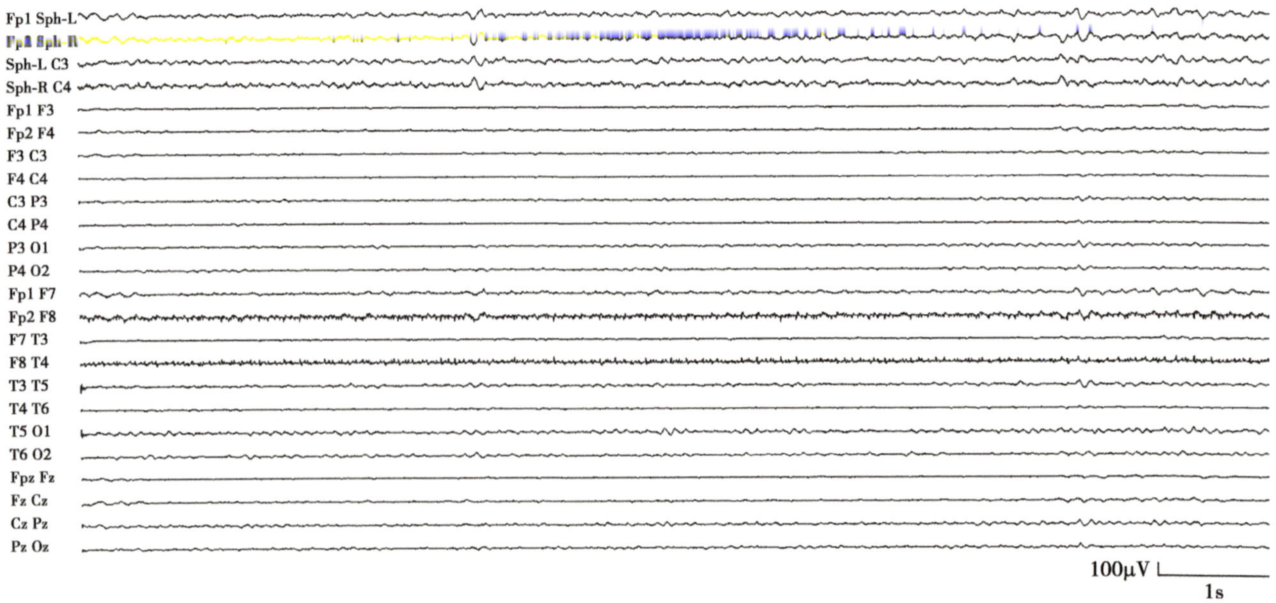

Fig. 3.36 Ictal scalp EEG 2 (this group of pictures is another seizure recorded from this patient). (**a**) Before the seizure, the patient was lying and talking to someone with his arms crossed in front of his chest. 6 s later, he stopped talking and was dazed, with no movement of the limbs. The EEG showed 5.0–6.0 Hz slow waves of low amplitude over the right sphenoidal electrode 6 s before the seizure. Later, the wave amplitude gradually increased until the rhythm of sharp waves of high amplitude was formed. (**b**) The first 7 s, the patient's symptoms were the same as described in **a**. 7 s later, he looked right. The EEG showed 5.0–6.0 Hz sharp waves of high amplitude over the right sphenoidal electrode, which spread to the bilateral frontal and temporal regions and the contralateral sphenoidal electrode. (**c**) The first 6 s, the patient's symptoms were the same as described in **b**. 6 s later, he smiled and had a pleasant expression. The EEG showed the rhythms of 5.0–6.0 Hz slow waves and sharpened slow waves over the bilateral sphenoidal electrodes and in bilateral frontal and temporal regions. Over the right sphenoidal electrode and right frontal and temporal regions, slow waves were mixed with sharp waves. (**d**) The first 3 s, the patient's symptoms were the same as described in **c**. 3 s later, he looked from the right to the front and stared, with no limb movements. The EEG showed slow waves and sharp waves in bilateral sphenoidal electrode and in bilateral frontal and temporal regions, mainly on the right. (**e**) The patient's symptoms were the same as described in **d**. His family put his upper limbs flat. The muscular tone of the left upper limb was slightly higher. The EEG was the same as **d**. (**f**) The patient gazed to the left s. 4 s later, he turned the head left like a gear. The EEG presentation was the same as **d**. (**g**) The patient's symptoms were the same as described in **f**. He continued to turn the head to left, with limb clonus. The EEG showed many EMG and wobble artifacts (mainly the EMG), and a few slow waves of medium and low amplitude only over the leads over the central, parietal, and occipital regions bilaterally. (**h**) The patient's head was turned to the left, and the left upper limb was elevated with clonus of an increasing amplitude. 3 s later, the patient turned the body to the left, extended the left upper limb, vocalized, and then developed into generalized tonic clonus, severe on the left. The EEG showed numerous EMG a and wobble artifacts (mainly the EMG). (**i**) The first 4 s, the patient's symptoms were the same as described in **h**. 4 s later, he elevated the right upper limb and then flexed and elevated both upper limbs, followed by generalized tonic clonus. The EEG showed numerous EMG and wobble artifacts (mainly the EMG)

[Case Review]

The bilateral sphenoidal eletrodes recorded frequently independent sharp waves during the interictal period. Two seizures were recorded, both exhibiting symptoms and EEG characteristics of temporal lobe origin, but originating from different sides of the temporal lobe, with the first from the left side and the second from the right side. This case suggests that it is important to record as many habitual clinical seizures as possible during preoperative evaluation. Normally, it is considered necessary to record at least 3 seizures, especially when seizures of bilateral origin need to be excluded. Besides, more clinical seizures should be recorded to avoid misjudgment. Conclusion: The seizure onset zone of this patient was of independent origin from bilateral temporal lobes, for which resection surgery was not applicable.

Case 3.13 Multilobar Fronto-Temporal Lobe Epilepsy

[Abstract of Medical Records]
Female, 21 years old.

1. *Chief complaint*: Episodic seizures for more than 3 years.
2. *History of present illness*: She was diagnosed with viral encephalitis and symptomatic epilepsy 3 years ago due to fever and recurrent seizures. Since then, she has been treated with various medications (e.g., phenytoin sodium, carbamazepine, and topiramate), which were ineffective. The present seizure manifested in two patterns: 1. Dialeptic seizure and speechless. The seizure, each lasting about 30 seconds, occurred 2–3 times a month; 2. Sudden shouting, with the head and eyes both turned right, followed by generalized tonic-clonic seizure, occurred about once every 3 months.
3. *Physical examination*: No neurological abnormalities were found.
4. *Imaging examination*: MRI showed no obvious abnormalities.
5. *EEG*: For details, see Figs. 3.37, 3.38, 3.39, 3.40, and 3.41.

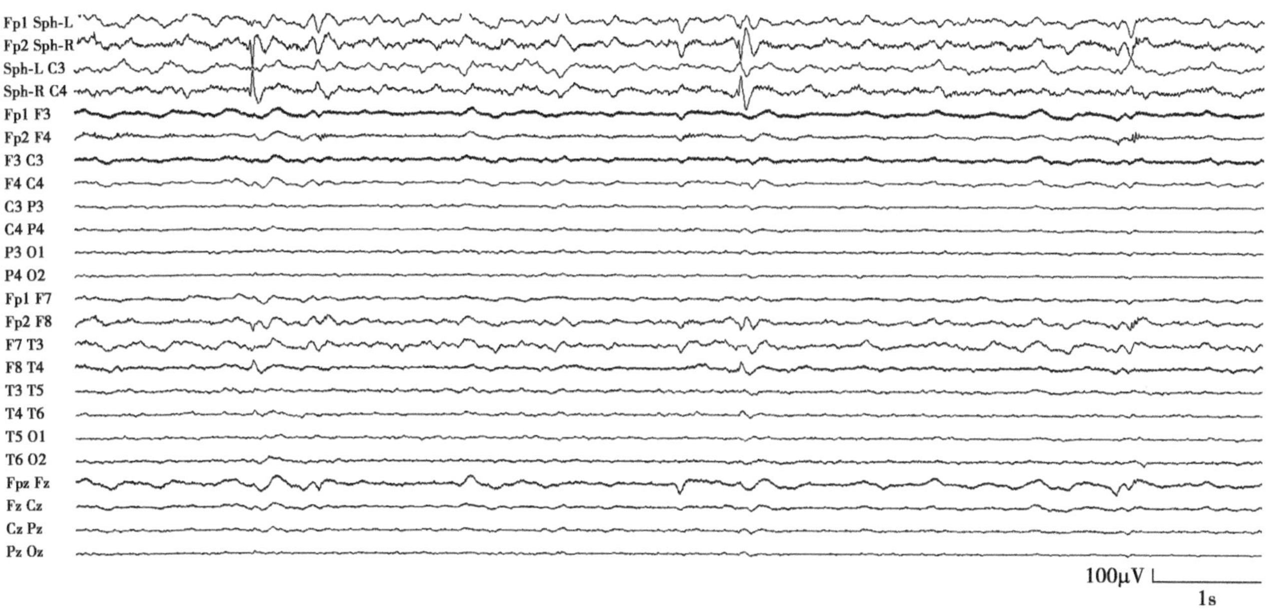

Fig. 3.37 Interictal scalp EEG. (**a**) The background EEG during wakefulness had a basic rhythm of 9.0–11.0 Hz. (**b**) Phase-inverted sharp waves were seen over the bilateral sphenoidal electrode. (**c**) A burst of 3.0–5.0 Hz spike-and-wave complexes and slow waves of medium and high amplitude was seen over the left lead, which occurred simultaneously over the right frontal and central leads. (**d**) The patient was asleep. The EEG showed spike-and-wave complexes over the left lead

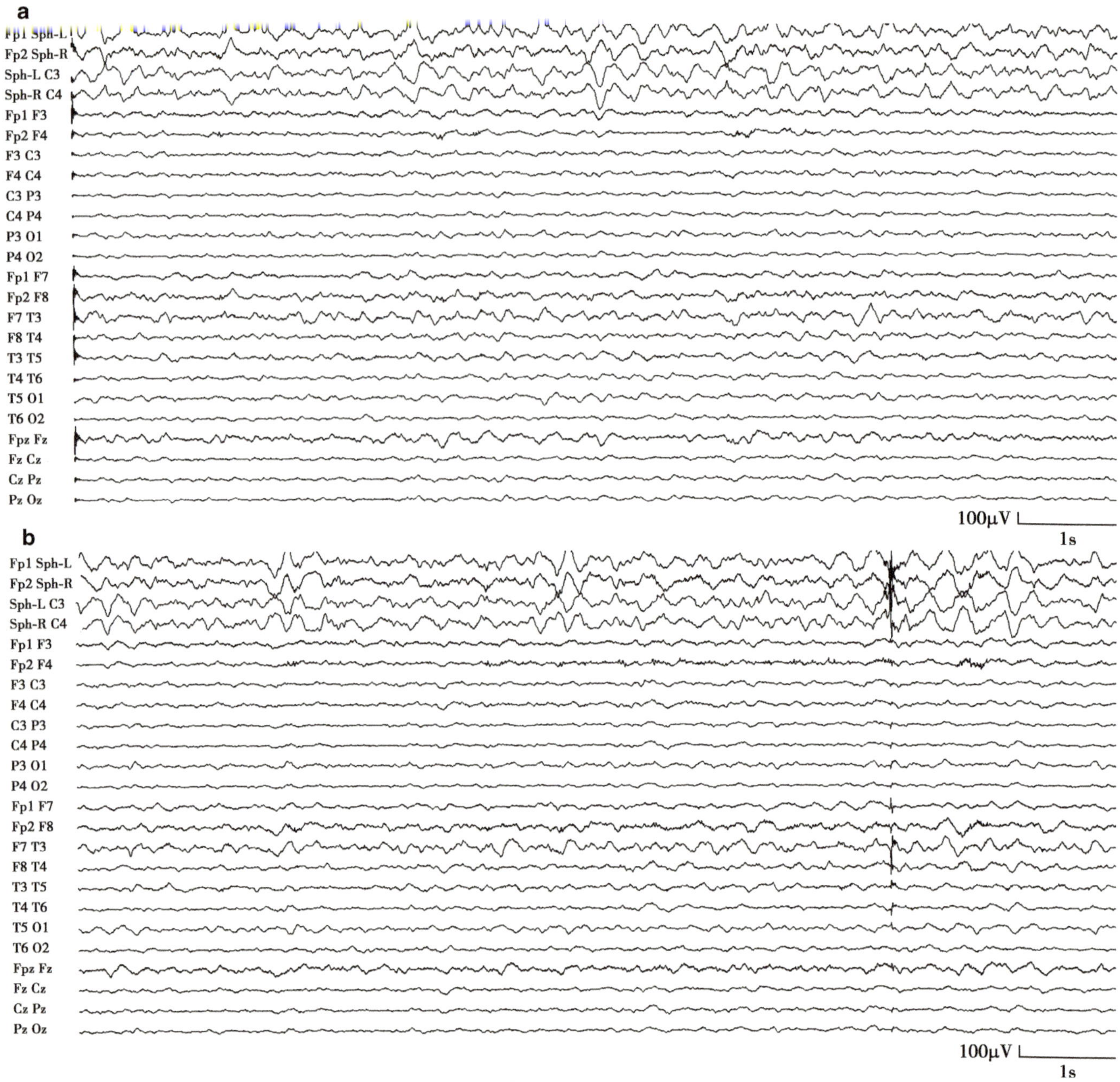

Fig. 3.38 Ictal scalp EEG. (**a**) The patient was asleep on the left side before the seizure. The EEG showed a burst of the rhythm of spikes over the bilateral frontal and temporal regions, followed by a depression in the wave amplitude in all leads, contributing to the formation of the low amplitude fast activities. Later the wave amplitude gradually increased till the rhythm of spikes was formed, followed by the rhythm of spike-and-wave complexes in all leads. (**b**) The patient opened eyes during the seizure, while turning the head to right and then elevating the right limbs. The EEG showed the rhythm of sharp waves, mainly on the left, mixed with EMG artifacts and wobble artifacts. (**c**) The patient opened the mouth to vocalize, with the mouth corners twitched to the right, and the limbs flexed and suffering from tonic clonus. The EEG showed EMG and wobble artifacts. (**d**) The patient had tonicity of limbs, flexion of the left upper limb, and extension of the right upper and the lower limbs, opened mouth to vocalize and tilted the head back, and had clonus 6 s later. The EEG presentation was the basically same as **c**. (**e**, **f**) The patient was tonic with clonus and did not respond to calls. The EEG presentation was the basically same as **c**. (**g**) The patient's clonus gradually slowed down. The seizure ended 9 s later. The EEG showed the rhythm of polyspike and waves complexes with EMG and wobble artifacts

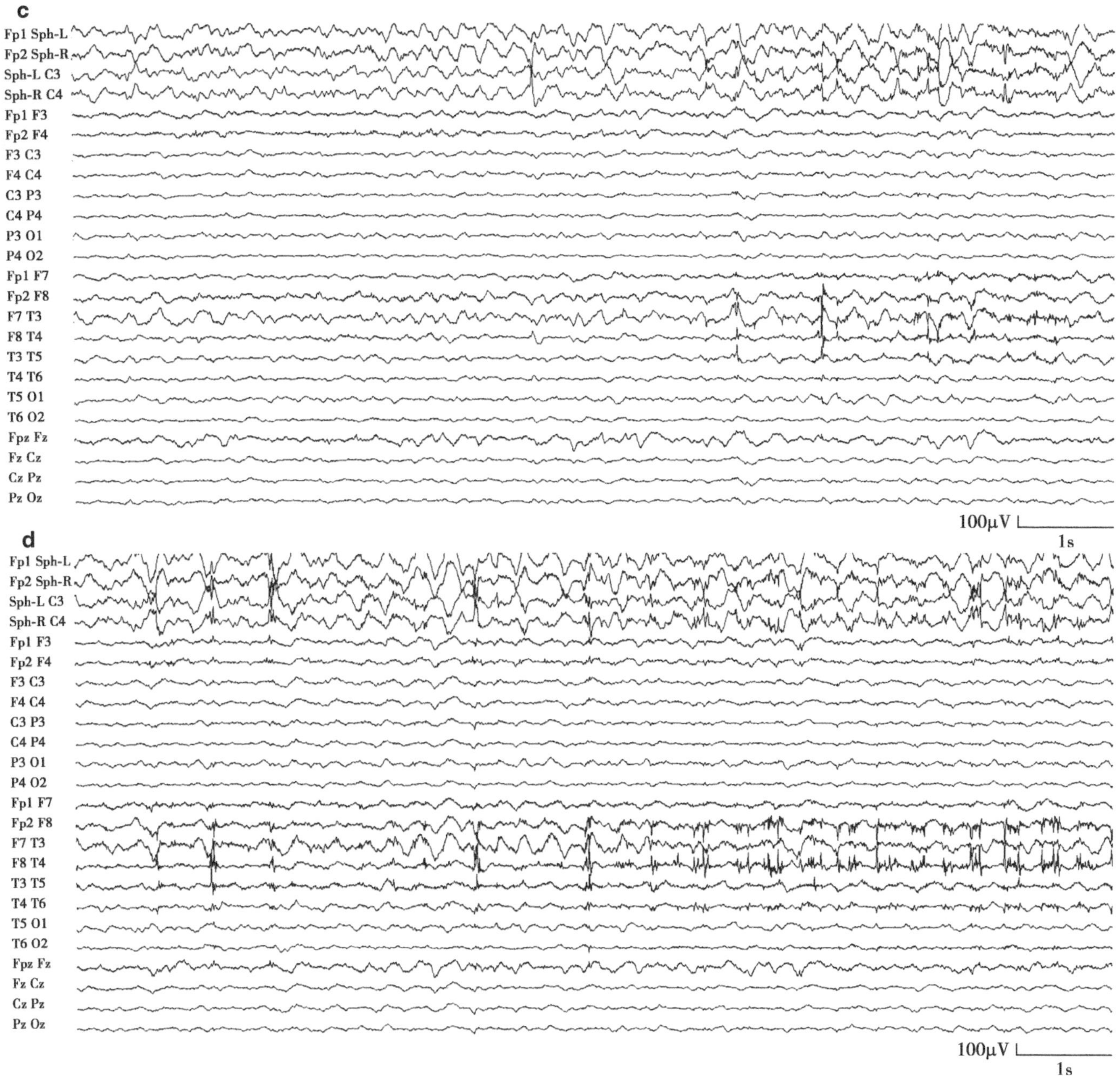

Fig. 3.38 (continued)

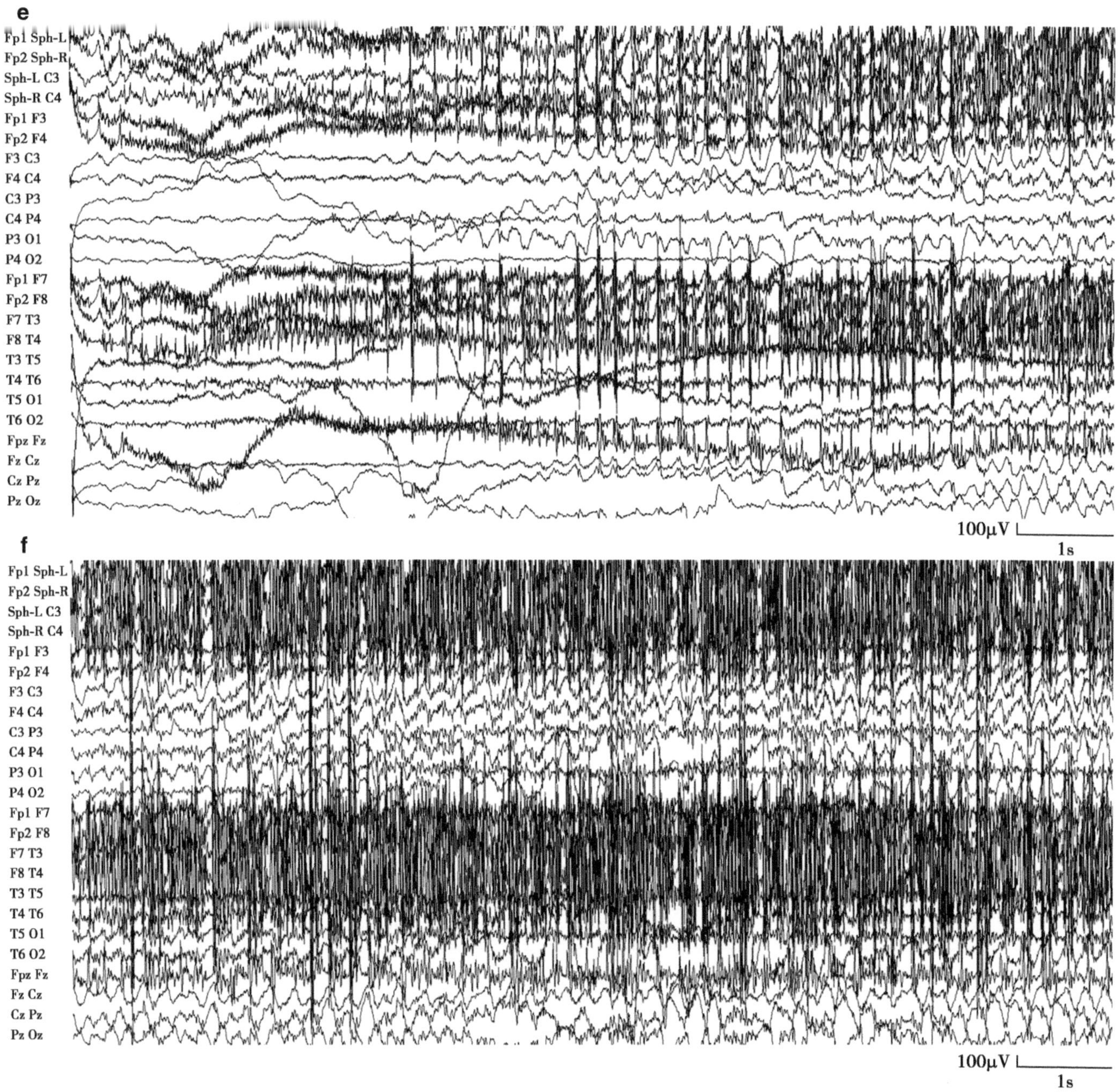

Fig. 3.38 (continued)

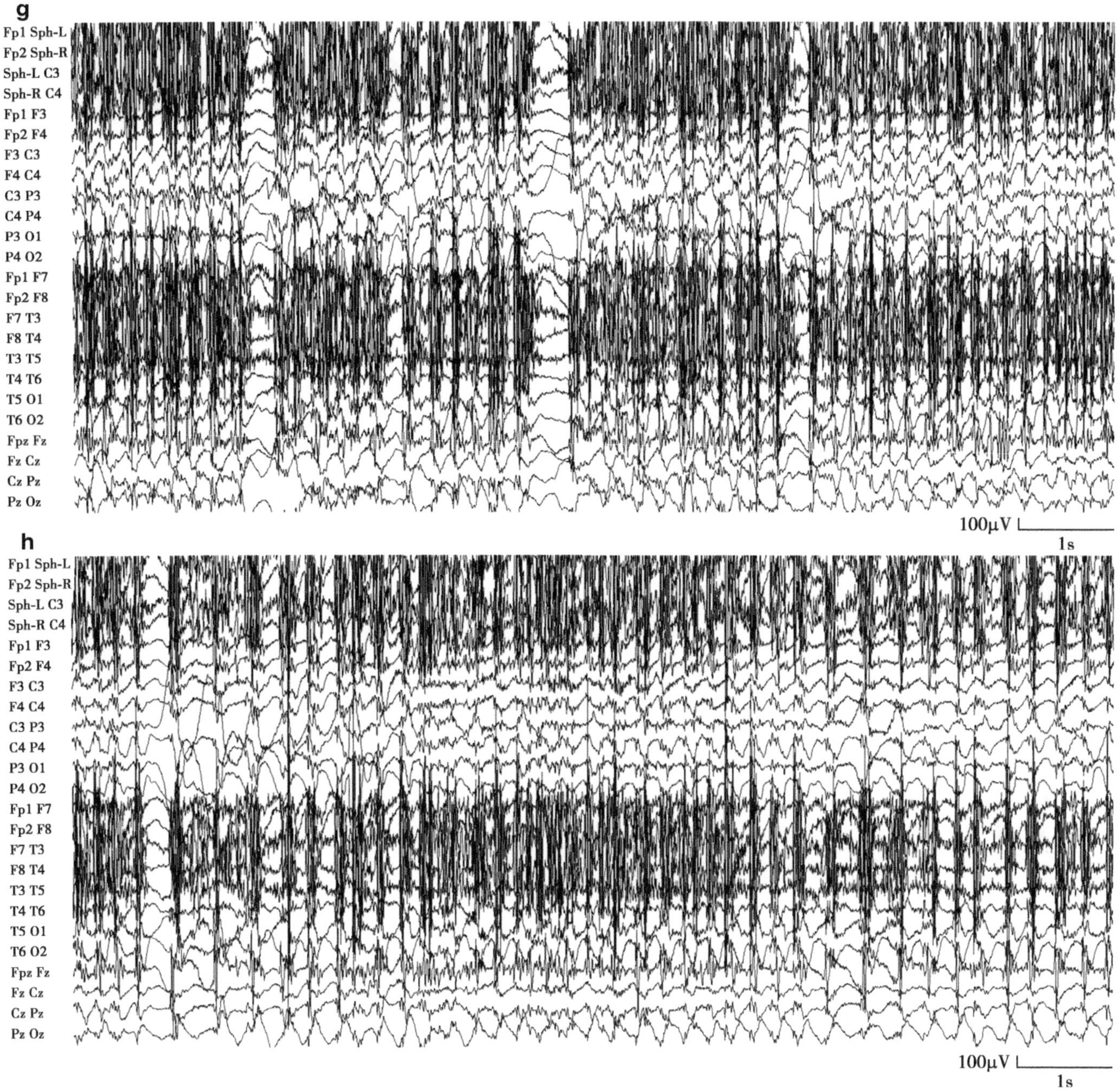

Fig. 3.38 (continued)

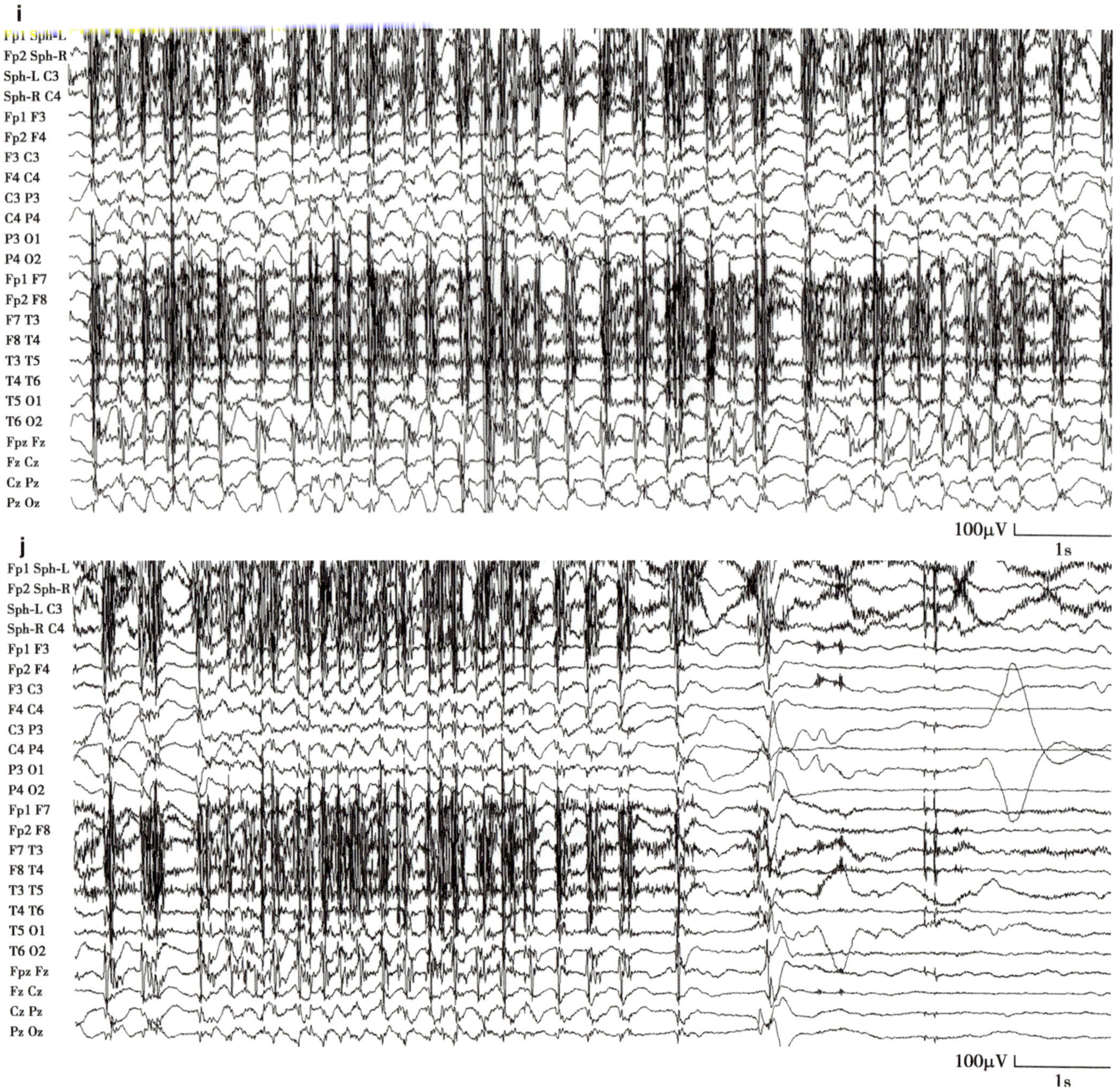

Fig. 3.38 (continued)

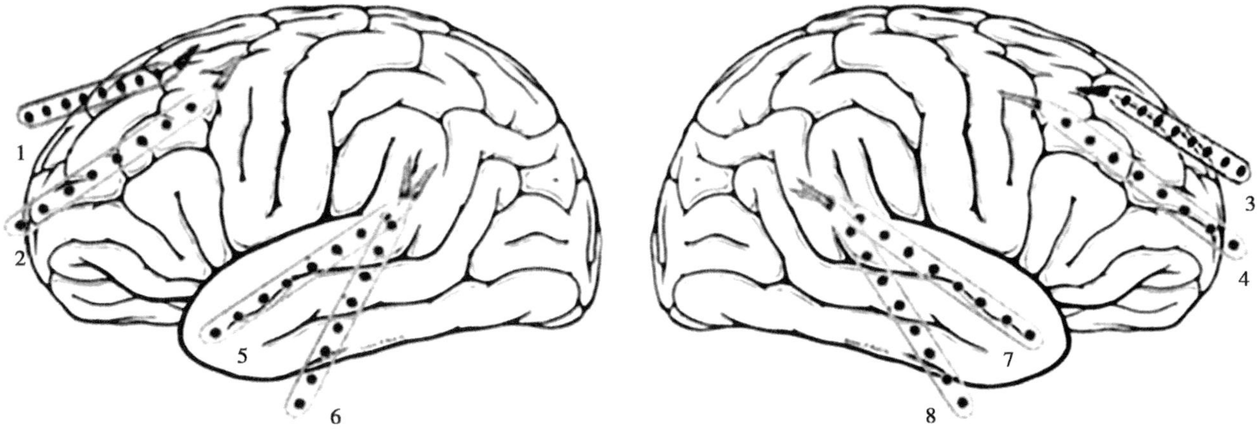

Fig. 3.39 Scheme of intracranial electrodes
Depth electrode 1: the left hippocampus (six contacts); strip electrode 2: the left frontal region (eight contacts); strip electrode 3: the left temporal pole (eight contacts); depth electrode 4: the right hippocampus (six contacts); strip electrode 5: the right frontal region (eight contacts); strip electrode 6: the right temporal pole (eight contacts)

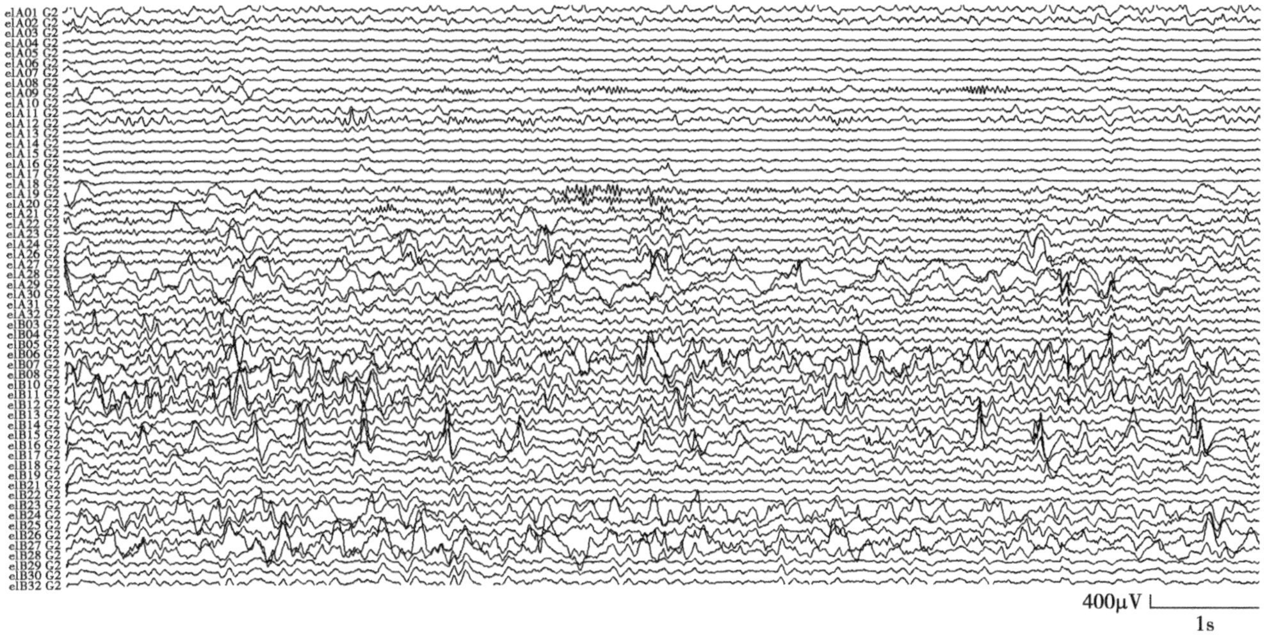

Fig. 3.40 Interictal intracranial EEG
Polyspikes were seen on left frontal (contact numbers el013 and el014); spikes were seen over the left hippocampus (contact number el007); and polyspikes and rhythmic spike-and-wave complexes were seen on the left temporal region (contact numbers el018, el019, el020)

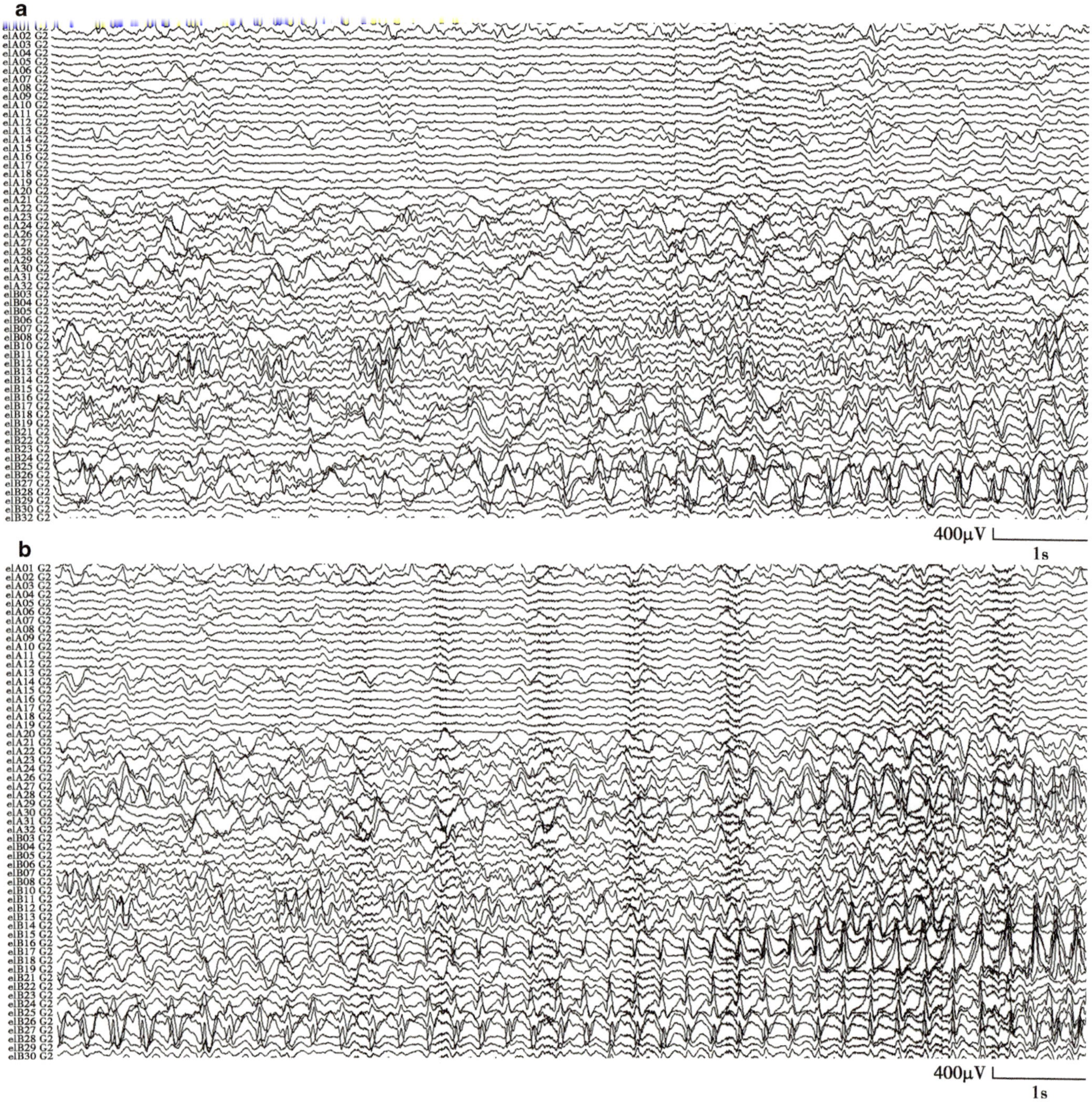

Fig. 3.41 Ictal EEG of intracranial electrodes. (**a**) The patient was asleep and suddenly screamed. The IEEG showed polyspikes on the left frontal and temporal regions (contact numbers el013, el014, el015, el018, el019, el020), followed by the rhythm of spike-and-wave complexes on all leads, after which the rhythm of spikes was seen on the left frontal and temporal regions (contact numbers el013, el014, el015). (**b**) The patient's upper limbs were tonic, and the lower limbs were flexed. The IEEG showed spike rhythm on the left frontal and temporal regions (contact numbers el013, el014, el018, el019, el020), and the rhythm of sharp waves were seen over the remaining leads. (**c**) The patient had seizures with generalized tonic clonus. The IEEG showed the rhythm of spike-and-wave complexes. (**d**) The patient's symptoms and the IEEG presentation were the same as in **c**. (**e**) The patient's clonus gradually slowed down. The IEEG showed the rhythms of spike-and-wave complexes and polyspikes. (**f**) The patient's clonus gradually slowed down. The IEEG showed the rhythm of paroxysmal polyspikes. (**g**) The patient's clonus gradually slowed down till it ended. The IEEG showed the rhythm of paroxysmal polyspikes

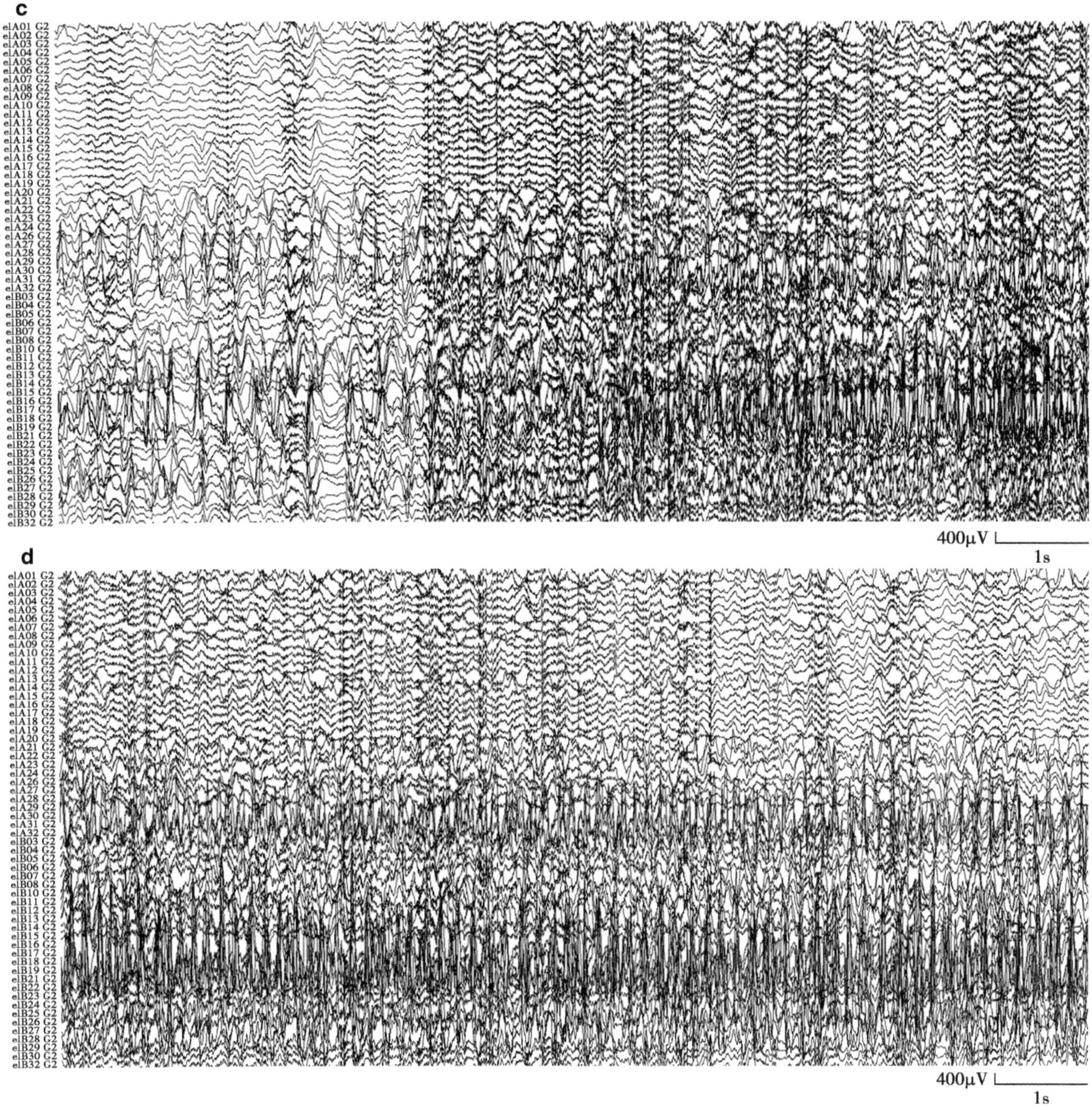

Fig. 3.41 (continued)

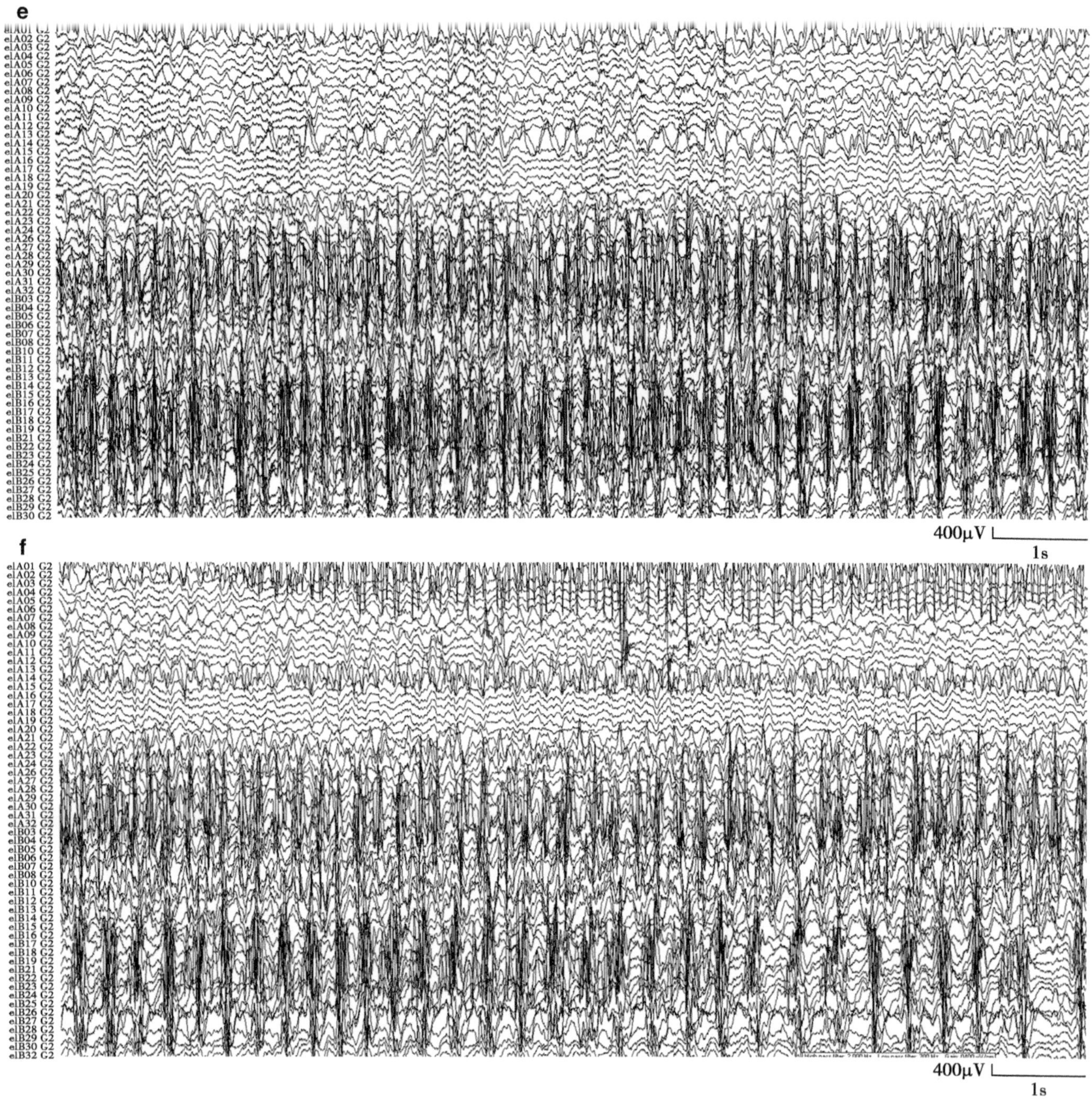

Fig. 3.41 (continued)

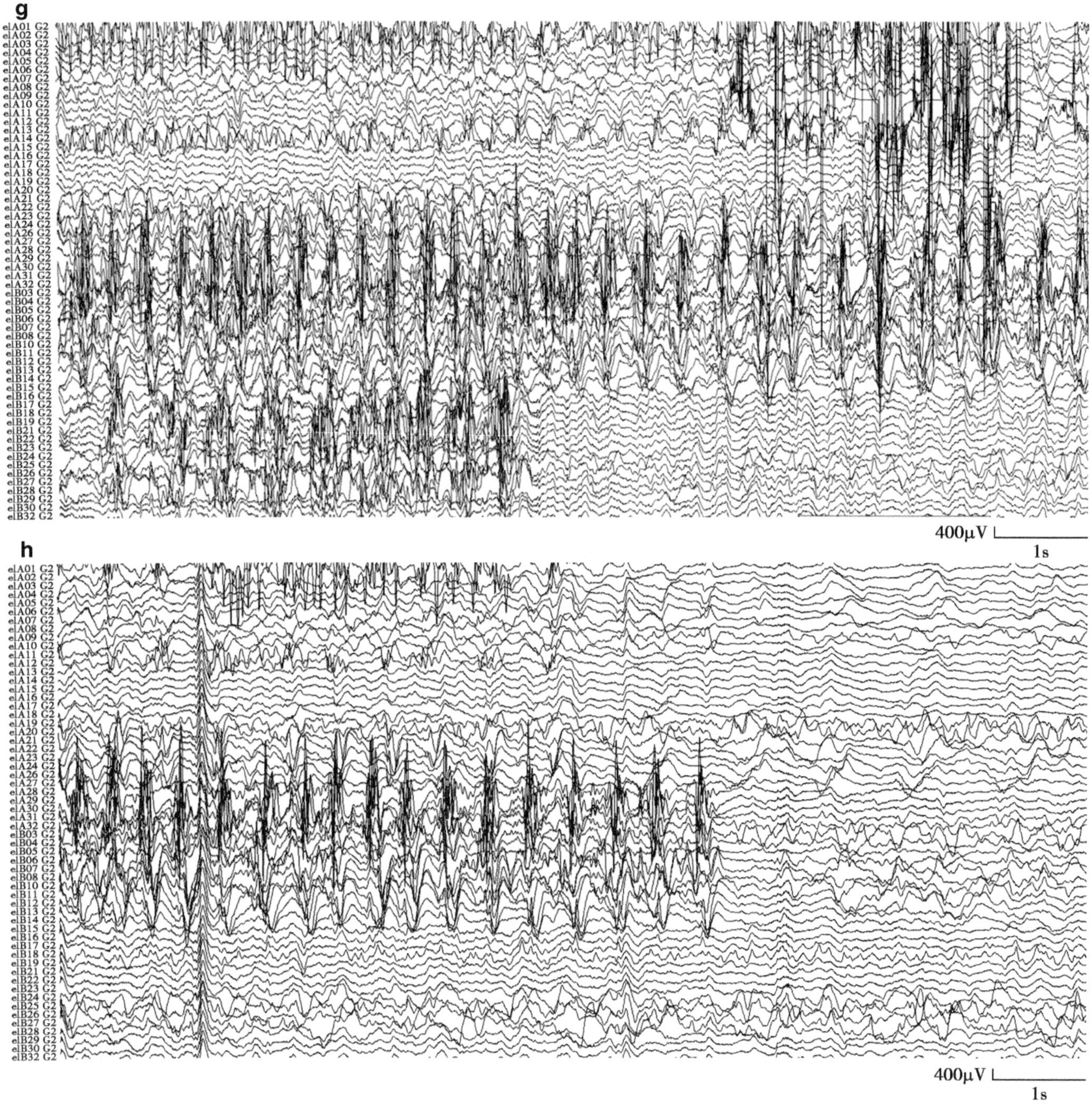

Fig. 3.41 (continued)

[Case Review]

The patient's interictal EEG showed a burst of slow waves and spike-and-wave complexes of high amplitude over the left anterior head; the interictal EEG also showed a burst of the rhythm of spikes, followed by low-amplitude fast activity in all leads and the rhythm of sharp waves mainly over the anterior head. In comprehensive consideration, the epileptic foci were judged to be more likely located over the left frontal and temporal regions, different from seizures purely originating from the temporal lobe cortex. After the implantation of intracranial electrodes, the interictal IEEG recorded revealed synchronous onset over the left frontal and temporal regions. The surgical resection of epileptic foci over the left frontal and temporal was performed. The patient remained seizure-free during a 3-year follow-up after surgery.

Cases of Parietal Lobe Epilepsy

4

Xu Cuiping, Zhang Shouwen, and Huang Zhaoyang

Overview of Parietal Lobe Epilepsy

Anatomy of Parietal Lobe

Parietal lobe is located between frontal lobe and occipital lobe, behind the central sulcus and in front of the connection line of parieto-occipital fissure and preoccipital notch. Postcentral gyrus is located between the central sulcus and postcentral sulcus. The interparietal sulcus divides the parietal lobe into superior parietal lobules and inferior parietal lobules, and the inferior parietal lobules consists of supramarginal gyrus and angular gyrus. The parietal lobe is mainly related to feeling, spatial perception, calculation, vision, and speech functions, etc.

Clinical Manifestations

Parietal lobe epilepsy is relatively rare, accounting for about 5% of drug-refractory focal epileptic patients who need surgical treatment. Patients with parietal lobe epilepsy might experience paraesthesia, including local numbness, tightness, tingling, pain, formication or itching in one lateral limb, prior to a seizure; and the paraesthesia might propagate from distal end to proximal end in a limb. A few patients might experience apraxia or unilateral limb neglect after the seizure. A number of auras provide an important basis for the diagnosis of parietal lobe epilepsy.

EEG Characteristics

Interictal EEGs showed sharp waves and/or spikes limited to the central and/or parietal lead(s), or posterior temporal and/or parietal lead(s). Some patients may present interictal multi-focal epileptiform discharge, such as sharp waves and/or spikes over the temporoparietal occipital, temporal central parietal, and/or frontal central temporal region(s). Very few patients may have interictal background EEG with slow wave activity or without epileptiform discharge. It is noteworthy that one should differentiate the paroxysmal low-amplitude fast activity over the central and/or parietal lead(s) from the normal β wave activities over the central region. Generally, the normal β activities over the central region are well-regulated and have proper amplitude modulation; in contrast, abnormal low-amplitude fast activities have irregular rhythm and phase. Regions with abnormal low-amplitude fast activities may also show mixed low-amplitude sharp waves and irregular slow waves.

Ictal EEGs may start with rhythmic activities over the central and/or parietal lead(s) on one side, which are followed by paroxysmal low-amplitude fast activities over the central, parietal, and/or posterior temporal region(s) and the activities gradually propagate towards other leads of the hemisphere, giving rise to rhythmic discharges in the hemisphere. Some patients' ictal EEGs present weakened background electrical activities or paroxysmal low-amplitude fast activities, and these activities have notable lateral dominance.

X. Cuiping (✉) · H. Zhaoyang
Department of Neurosurgery, Beijing, China

Z. Shouwen
Department of Neurology, Beijing, China

Y. Wang (ed.), *Electroencephalogram for Presurgical Epilepsy Evaluation*, https://doi.org/10.1007/978-981-95-8003-3_4

Cases of Postcentral Gyrus Epilepsy

Case 4.1 Postcentral Gyrus Epilepsy

[Abstract of Medical Records]
Male, 17 years old.

1. *Chief complaint*: Paroxysmal numbness and tonic spasm in right hands and/or forearms for 9 years.
2. *History of present illness*: Nine years ago, the patient fell on the ground with tonic spasms of limbs and loss of consciousness, and the symptoms lasted 1–2 minutes. In the days that followed, the patient experienced paroxysmal numbness of right upper extremities, which spontaneously resolved seconds later. Occasionally, secondary generalized convulsive seizures occurred. The patient was prescribed carbamazepine, sodium valproate, topiramate, etc.; all showed efficacy in the beginning, but the efficacy became poor 2–3 years later. The patient felt numb in the right hands upon the onset of the seizures, and shortly afterwards numbness and tonicity of right forearm appeared, and the patient's body tilted rightwards. In the meantime, blinking and twitching of the right mouth corner were observed. The patient remained conscious during the seizure and was free of any discomfort after the seizure. Each episode lasted more than 10 seconds and mostly occurred at night. Currently the patient is treated with carbamazepine 1100 mg/d, topiramate 200 mg/d, and experiences 3–5 episodes a day.
3. *Past history*: The patient was delivered at full term, with normal motor, language and intellectual development.
4. *Physical examination*: He had slightly decreased memory and calculation ability. Other physical examinations were normal.
5. *Imaging examination*:
   (a) MRI revealed no significant abnormalities.
   (b) SPECT indicated that during interictal phase, the patient's blood perfusion to cerebral cortex was slightly lower in the left side than in the right side; the blood perfusion to the left temporal, parietal, and right frontal regions was decreased. Ictal phase: the patient's left temporal region, where the blood perfusion was decreased originally, regains normal perfusion notably; the originally decreased blood perfusion in the left parietal and right frontal regions have partially alleviated.
6. *EEG*: For details, see Figs. 4.1, 4.2, 4.3, 4.4, and 4.5.

[Case Review]

1. *Case Characteristics*
   (a) *Seizure characteristics*: 1. Prior to the onset of the seizure, the patient felt numb in right hand; the numbness gradually propagated to right forearm, then tonicity of right forearm and twitches of right mouth corner; 2. No loss of consciousness during seizure. 3. Most seizures occurred at night. 4. The patient experienced 3–5 episodes a day.
   (b) *Imaging characteristics*: 1. MRI revealed no notable abnormal change. 2. SPECT findings during interictal phase: blood perfusion to cerebral cortex was slightly lower on left side than on right side; blood perfusion to left temporal region, parietal region, and right frontal region was decreased; findings during ictal phase: the left temporal region where the blood perfusion was decreased had notably regained normal blood perfusion, the original blood perfusion decreased area in the left parietal region, and right temporal region slightly elevated than ictal phase image.
   (c) *EEG characteristics*: Spikes were seen and localized to the left central region during interictal phase; low-amplitude spikes were seen over the left central region, and temporal region during ictal phase.
2. *Diagnosis and treatment strategies and follow-up results*: The patient had stereotyped seizure symptoms manifested as tonic right forearm, twitching of right mouth corner, with definite auras. Prior to each episode, the patient would feel numb in the right hand and the numbness would propagate to right forearm; both interictal and ictal EEG abnormal discharges were located in C3. In light of the seizure symptoms and EEG findings, it was considered that the epileptic focus was located at left postcentral gyrus. In order to determine the relationship between sensorimotor area and speech region, intracranial electrodes were implanted in left posterior frontal region and parietal region. Postoperative monitoring of seizures and electrical stimulation of cortex were performed to determine the sensory-motor cortex and speech region. Interictal IEEG showed that the abnormal discharge was limited to middle and upper parts of left central region; the postcentral gyrus cortex was surgically resected in part, and the part of precentral gyrus focus was resected. In the 1-year followed-up period, the frequency of seizure was decreased significantly. IEEG demonstrated that the epileptic focus was definite but extensive and involving the precentral gyrus. In order to prevent adverse impact on motor function, the epileptic focus was not completely resected by surgical operation. Therefore, the patient still suffered from occasional seizures after the operation.

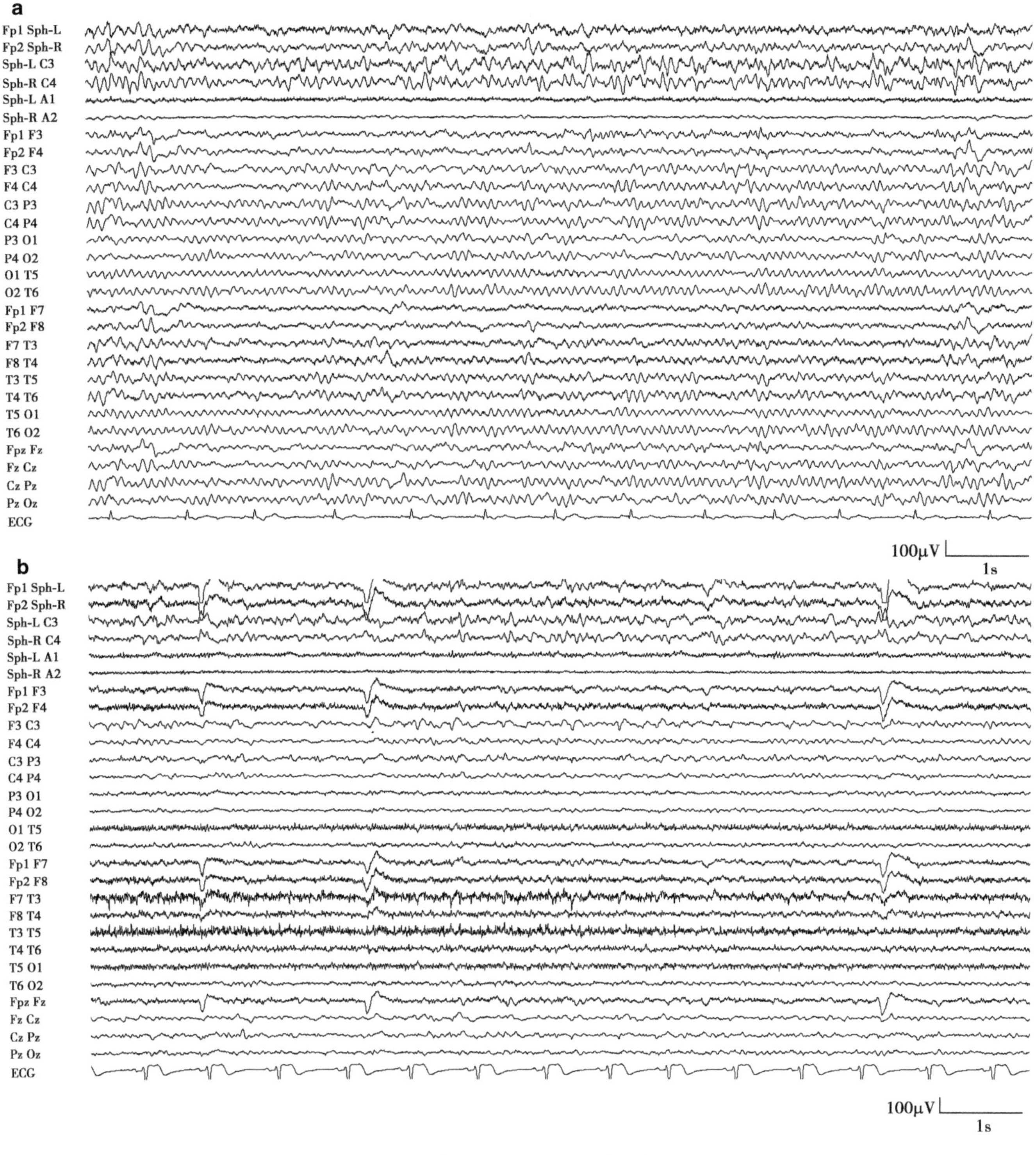

Fig. 4.1 Interictal scalp EEG. (**a**) The patient was awake. EEG background rhythm: 9.0–10.0 Hz. (**b**) Rhythmic low-amplitude spikes over the left central region (C3)

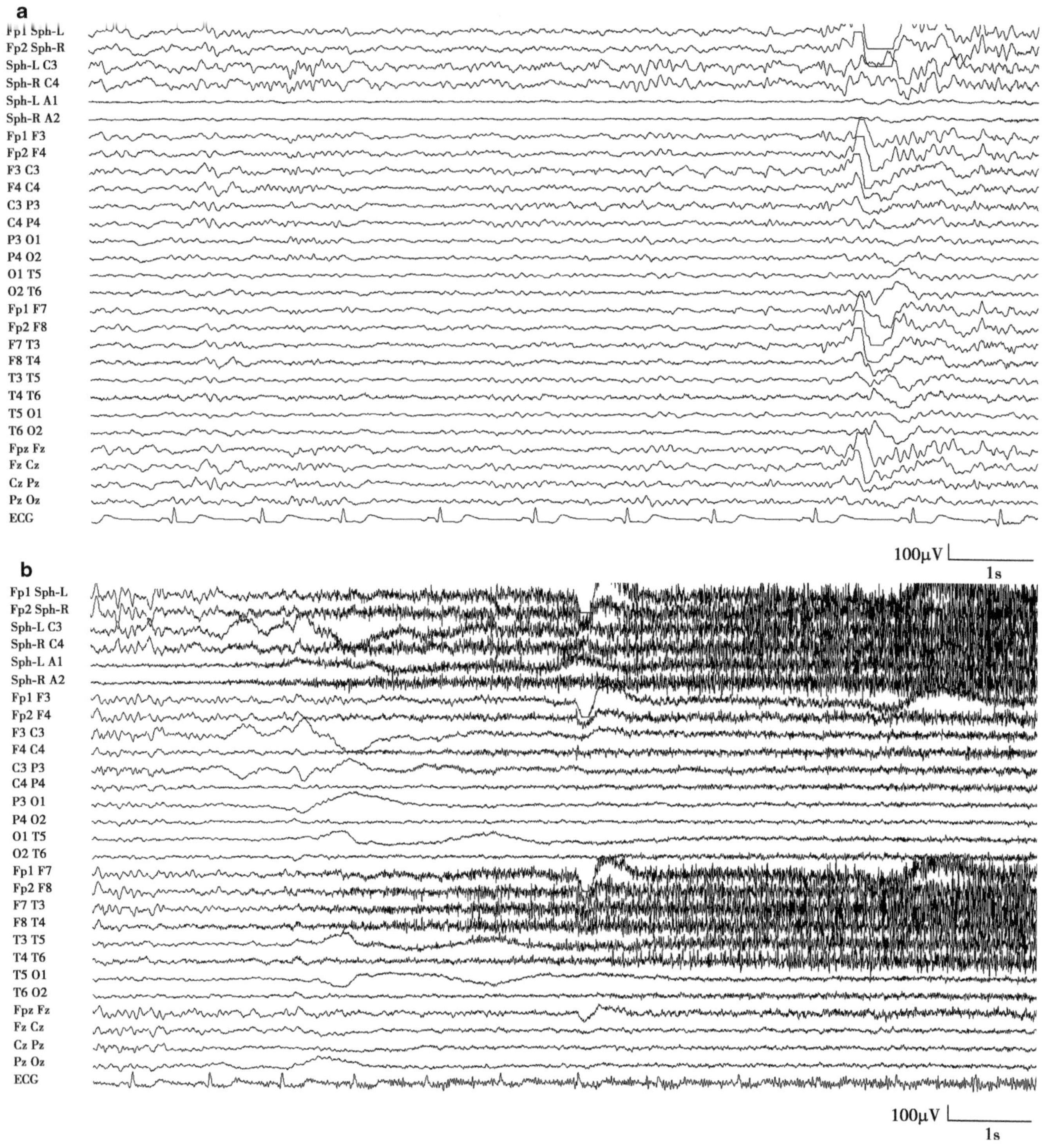

Fig. 4.2 Ictal scalp EEG. (**a**) The patient was asleep. Low-amplitude spikes over the left central region (C3) and anterior temporal region (F7) leads. (**b**) After regaining consciousness, the patient raised his right upper limb with slightly tonic right hand and then slightly raised head. The EEG showed mixed EMG artifacts over the bilateral frontal and temporal regions. (**c**) At the end of the seizure, the patient's right hand was on the belly and head on pillow. The EEG showed mixed EMG artifacts over the bilateral frontal and temporal regions; at the end of the seizure, EEG restored to background EEG of wakefulness

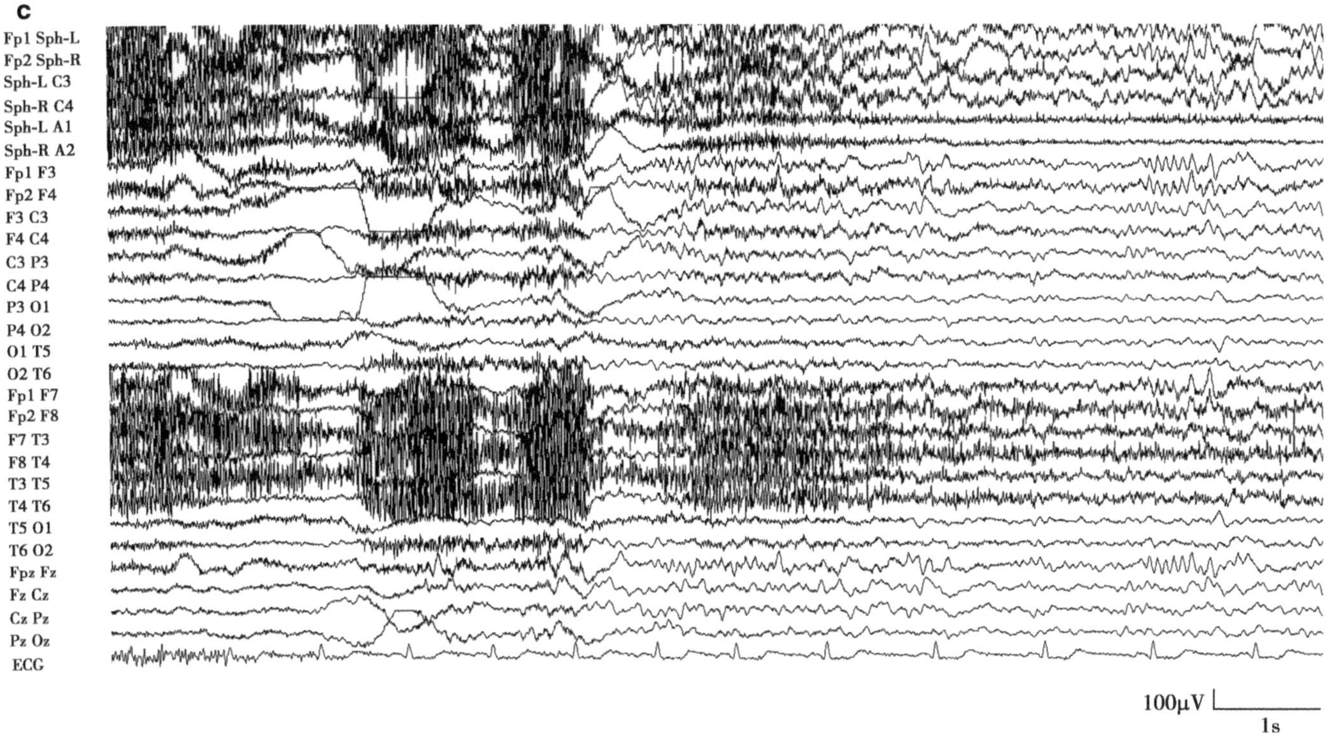

Fig. 4.2 (continued)

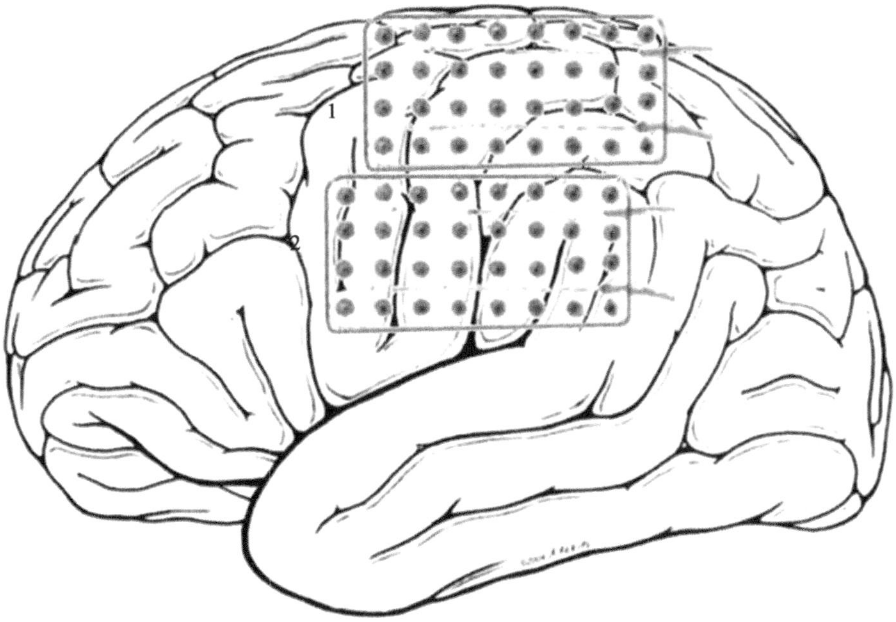

Fig. 4.3 Scheme of intracranial electrodes
Grid electrode 1: 32 contacts upper part over the left central parietal focus; grid electrode 2: 32 contacts lower part over the left central parietal focus

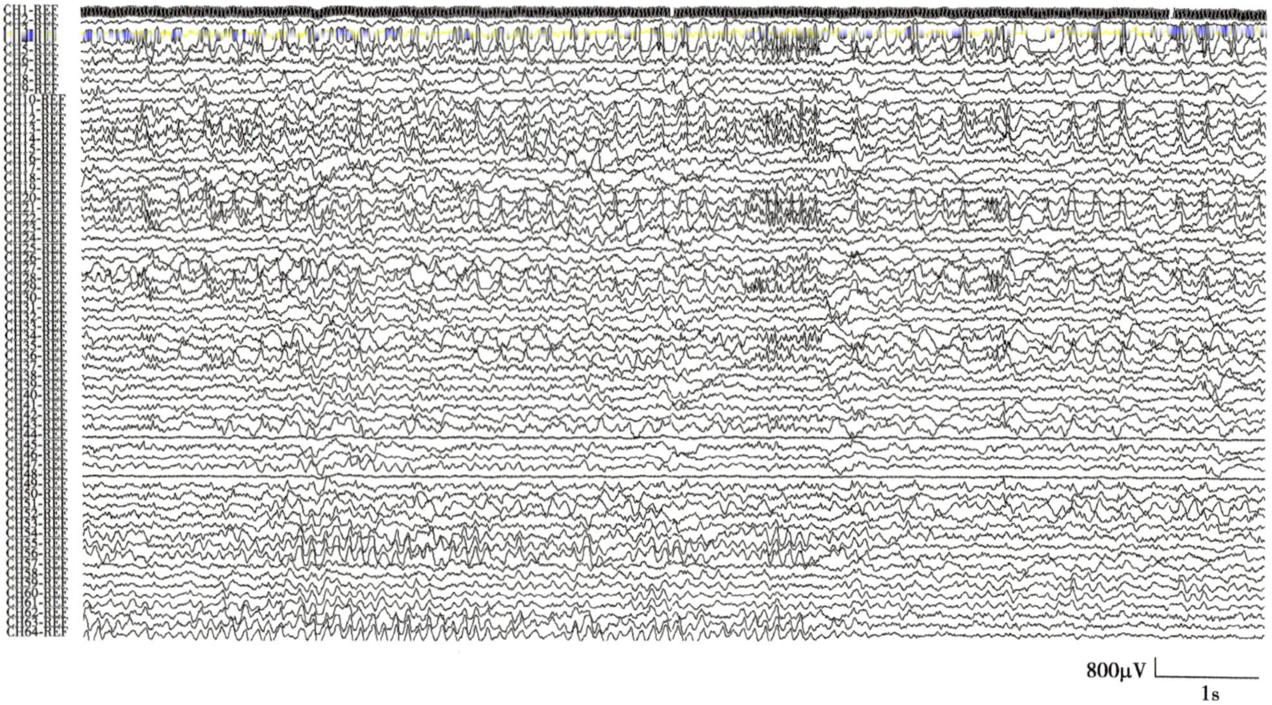

Fig. 4.4 Interictal intracranial EEG
Findings: rhythmic spike slow waves (contact numbers CH3, CH4, CH5), sharp waves (contact numbers CH8, CH11, CH12, CH13, CH14, CH20, CH21, CH22), spike rhythm (contact numbers CH3, CH4, CH5, CH11, CH12, CH13, CH14, CH20, CH21, CH22) over the left central parietal upper region; low amplitude fast activities over left central parietal upper region (contact numbers CH26, CH27, CH28, CH29) and left central parietal lower region (contact numbers CH34, CH35, CH36)

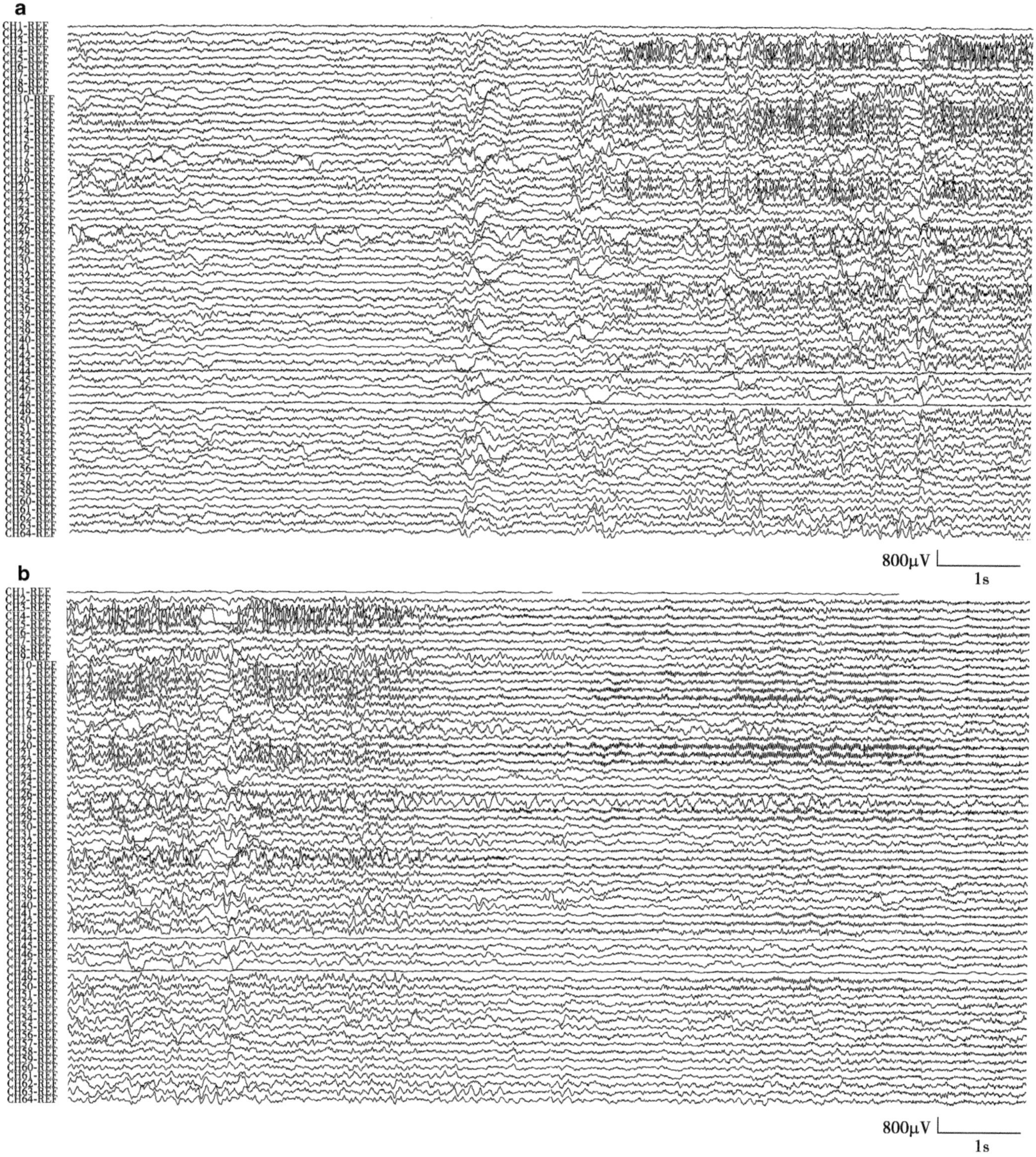

Fig. 4.5 Ictal intracranial EEG. (**a**) The patient was asleep. IEEG was the pre-seizure background EEG; then low amplitude fast activities appeared in left central parietal upper region (contact numbers CH4, CH5, CH11, CH12, CH13, CH20, CH21, CH22, CH26, CH27, CH28, CH29) and left central parietal lower region (contact numbers CH34, CH35); the wave amplitude gradually increased to form spike rhythm and propagated to adjacent cortex. (**b**) The patient's right upper limb was slowly raised, and right hand was making a fist and slightly stiff. IEEG findings: spike rhythm over the left central parietal upper region (contact numbers CH4, CH5, CH11, CH12, CH13, CH14, CH19, CH20, CH21, CH22, CH26, CH27, CH28, CH29), low amplitude fast activities over the left central parietal upper region (contact numbers CH11, CH12, CH13, CH14, CH20, CH21, CH22, CH26, CH27, CH28, CH29), and left central parietal lower region (contact numbers CH34, CH35), gradually propagating to adjacent cortex. (**c**) The patient's right upper limb showed slight clonus. IEEG manifestations: slow wave rhythm over the left central parietal upper region (contact numbers CH3, CH4, CH5, CH8, CH11, CH12, CH13, CH14, CH15, CH19, CH20, CH21, CH22, CH23, CH26, CH27, CH28, CH29) and left central parietal lower region (contact numbers CH36, CH37, CH41, CH42, CH43, CH48, CH49, CH50, CH51, CH57, CH58, CH59)

c

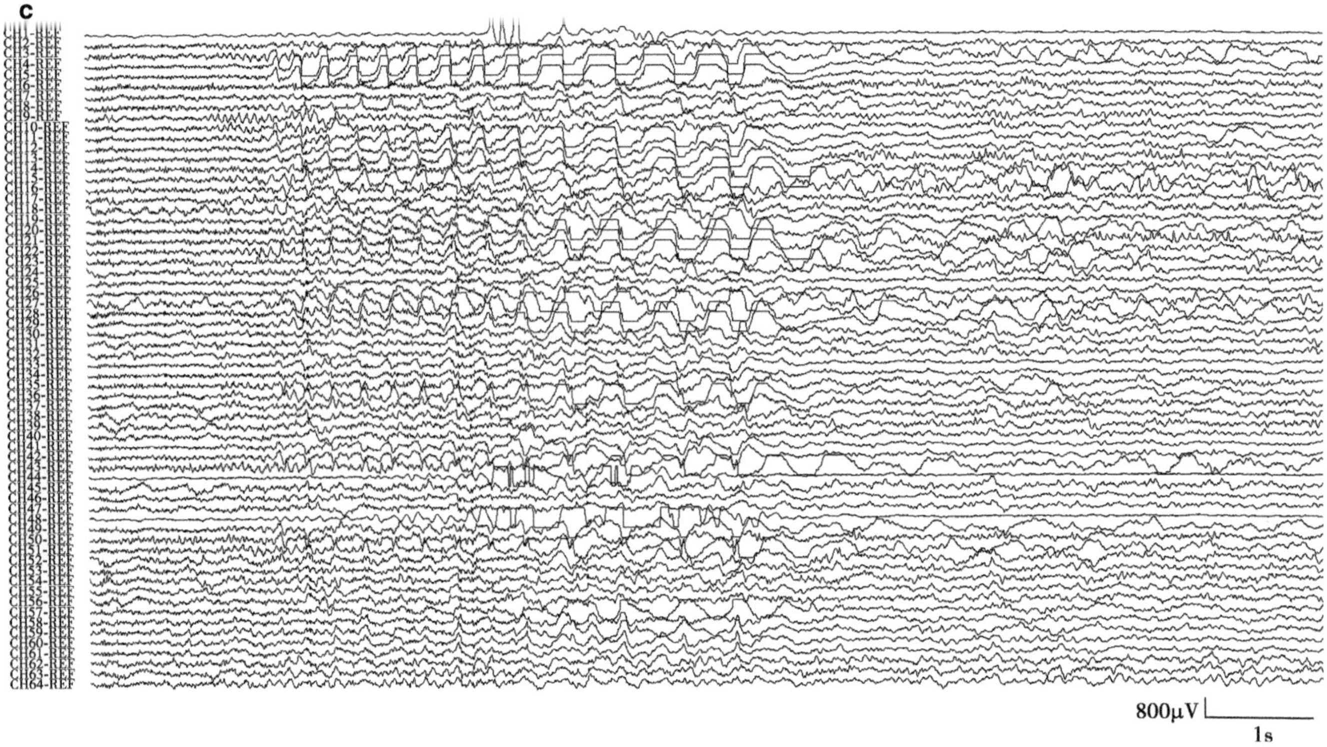

Fig. 4.5 (continued)

Case 4.2 Postcentral Gyrus Epilepsy

[Abstract of Medical Records]
Male, 24 years old.

1. *Chief complaint*: The patient had suffered from paroxysmal numbness of left little finger and secondary tonic-clonic seizure for 17 years.
2. *History of present illness*: The patient experienced confusion and tonic-clonic seizure 17 years ago without apparent predisposing cause; the symptoms lasted about 2 min. The patient was diagnosed with "epilepsy" in a local hospital and administered sodium phenytoin, sodium valproate, and DIANXIANLING (a TCM preparation). No improvement was achieved. Eight years ago, gamma knife radiosurgery was performed and also failed to achieve improvement. The patient is now on oral oxcarbazepine, 450 mg/dose, tid, and lamotrigine, 100 mg/dose, bid, for treatment. Current seizure type: paroxysmal numbness in left little fingertip, propagating along left forearm up to shoulder, giving rise to tonic left forearm, which lasts 3–5 s; according to the patient, no loss of consciousness occurs during the seizure. Sometimes there was secondary numbness and tonicity of right little fingertip, which propagate along the right forearm up to right wrist, leading to tonic-clonic seizure of extremities that lasts about 1 minute. The frequency of seizures was 1–2 times/week. All seizures occur when the patient is awake.
3. *Past history*: The patient was delivered at full term. He underwent surgical resection of megacolon and surgical correction of cryptorchidism 21 years ago. Denied any history of drug hypersensitivity, hyperpyrexia, denied hypoxia, trauma, and family history.
4. *Physical examination*: He had slightly decreased memory and calculation ability. Other physical examinations were normal.
5. *Imaging examination*: MRI revealed symmetrically increased strip signal in callosum.
6. *EEG*: For details, see Figs. 4.6, 4.7, 4.8, 4.9, and 4.10.

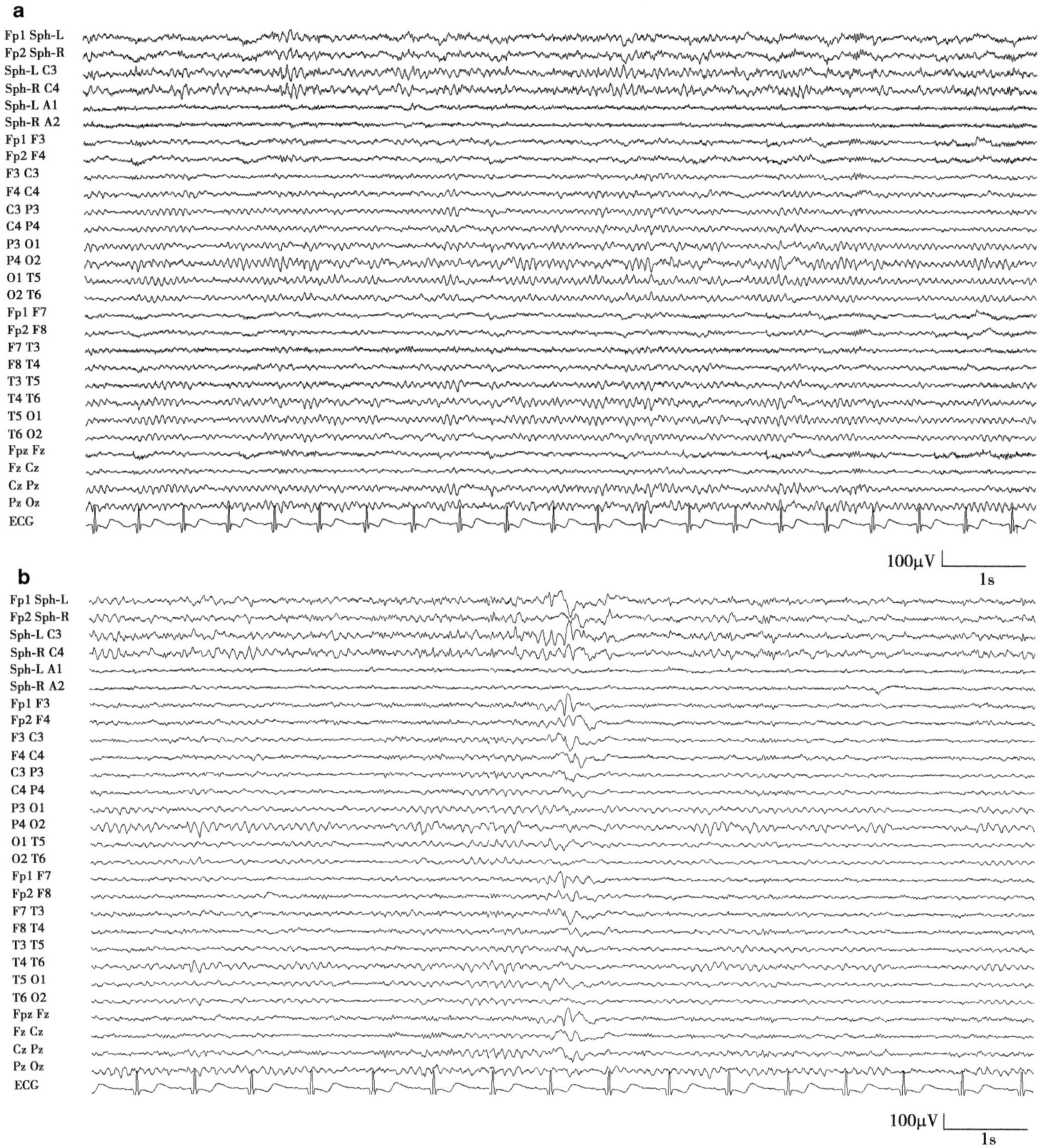

Fig. 4.6 Interictal scalp EEG. (**a**) Background EEG of the patient in conscious state had a rhythm of 9.0–10.0 Hz. (**b**) Sharp waves over the left posterior frontal region (F3) and anterior temporal region (F7) leads. (**c**) The EEG showed sharp waves over the bilateral sphenoidal electrode (Sph-L, Sph-R), mainly the right. (**d**) The EEG showed sharp waves over the right sphenoidal electrode (Sph-R), irregular slow waves over the right frontal region (Fp2, F4), central region (C4), and temporal region (T4)

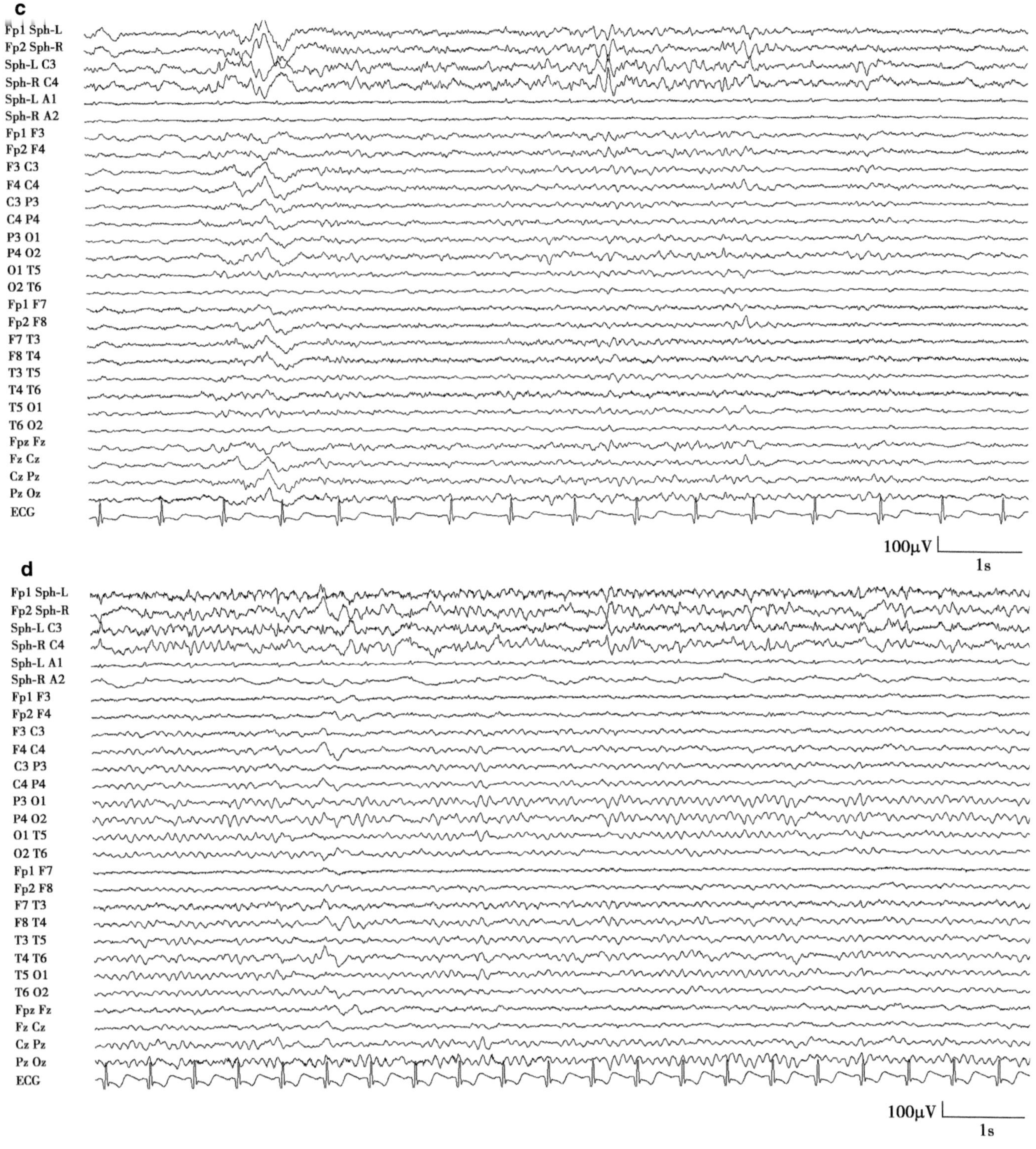

Fig. 4.6 (continued)

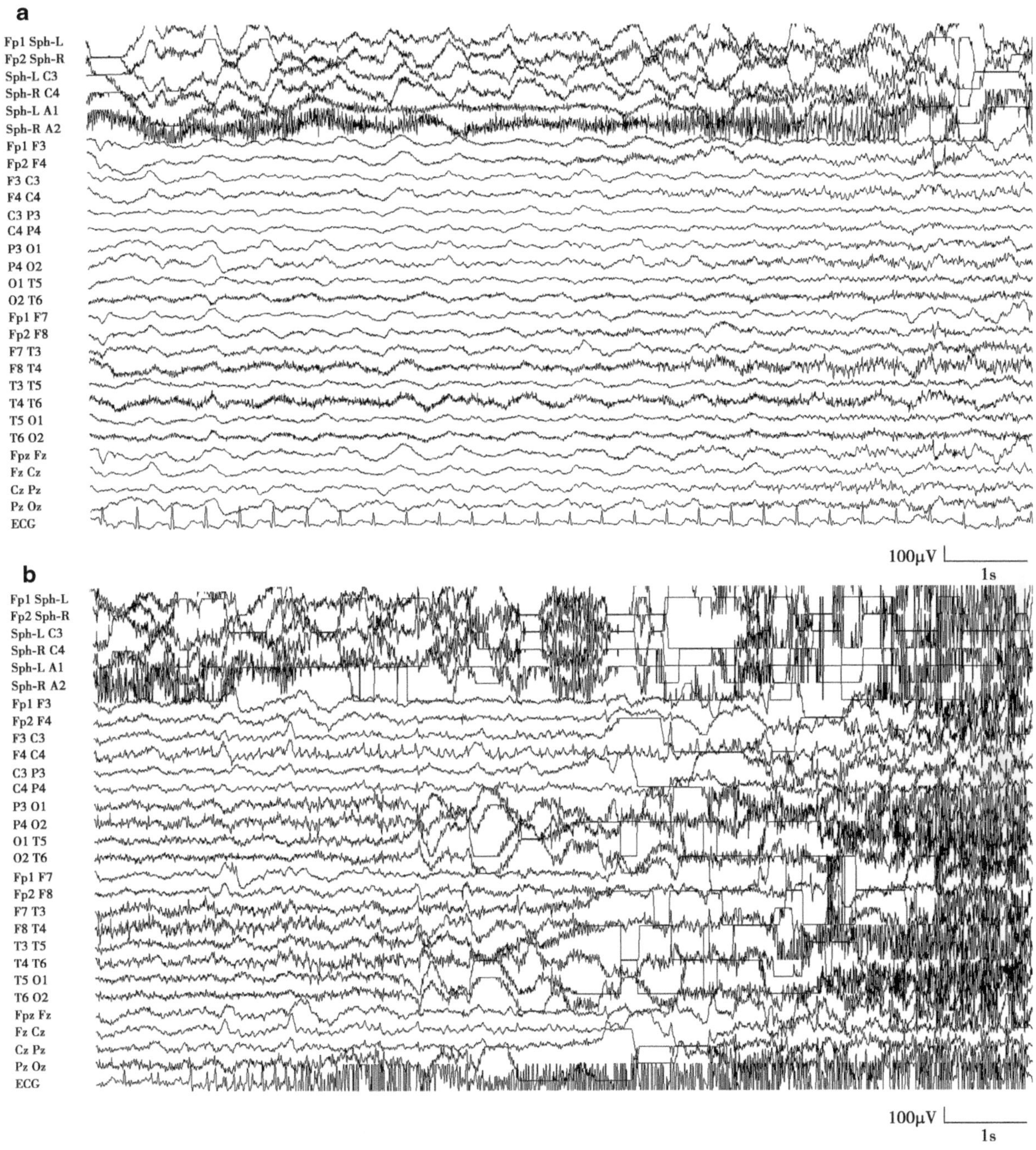

Fig. 4.7 Ictal scalp EEG. (**a**) The patient was awake. After giving an account of numbness in left little finger, he made a fist with left hand and raised the left arm. The patient's EEG was characteristic of pre-seizure slow wave background; during the seizure, low amplitude fast activities was observed in right posterior frontal and central (F4 C4) leads; EMG artifacts were identified in right sphenoidal and mid temporal electrodes. (**b**) The patient's left upper limb was tonic-clonic, with head deflecting to the left and then raised his clonic right arm. The EEG revealed a gradual increase in wave amplitudes of rhythmic sharp waves over the posterior frontal (F4) lead. EMG artifacts were seen in bilateral parietal and temporal regions, which gradually propagated to all leads. (**c**) The patient had clonic right upper limb and bilateral lower extremities and tonic-clinic upper left limb. A large amount of EMG artifacts was seen on the EEG. (**d**) The patient had tonic upper extremities and generalized clonic convulsion. Mixed EMG artifacts were seen on the EEG. (**e**) The patient had tonic-clonic limbs. A large amount of EMG artifacts was seen on the EEG. (**f**) The patient had generalized clonic convulsion and rightward twitching of the mouth corner. EMG artifacts were seen on the EEG. (**g**) The patient's generalized clonic convulsion gradually decreased in frequency. EMG artifacts were seen on the EEG. (**h**) The patient had clonic convulsion in upper right limb and rightward twitching of the mouth corner. The EEG showed generalized rhythm of 2.5–3.0 Hz spike-and-wave complexes, polyspike and wave complexes, the frequency of which gradually slowed down, and was mixed with EMG artifacts. (**i**) The patient's mouth corner twitched rightwards and the clonus in right upper limb gradually stopped. EEG manifestations: extensive rhythm of 1.5–2.0 Hz polyspike and wave complexes, the frequency of which gradually slowed down. (**j**) The patient's twitching of mouth corner gradually discontinued. EEG manifestations: extensive rhythm of 1.0 Hz polyspike and wave complexes. (**k**) At the end of the seizure, the patient failed to respond to calls. The EEG showed extensive decrease in voltage, with EMG artifacts

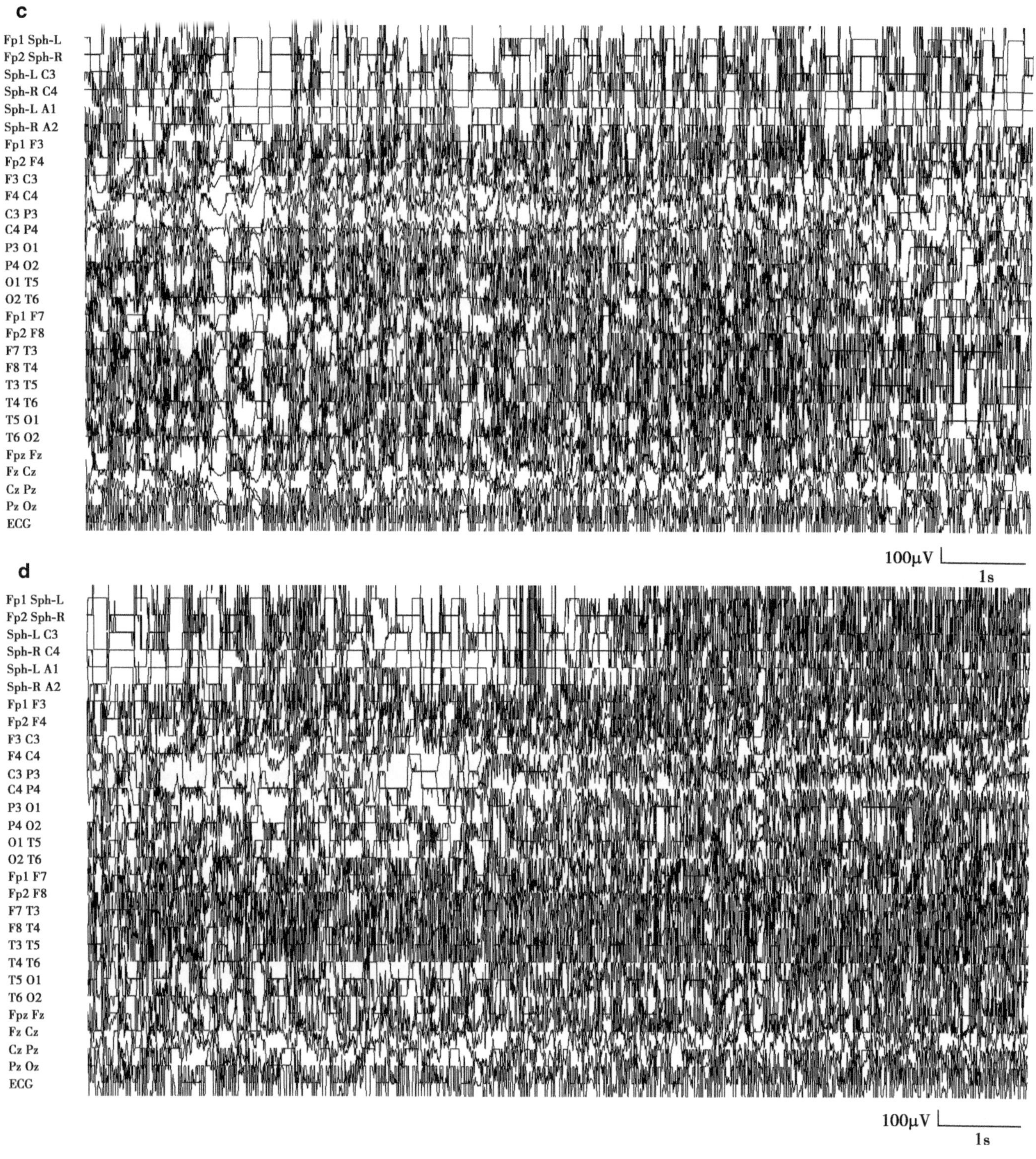

Fig. 4.7 (continued)

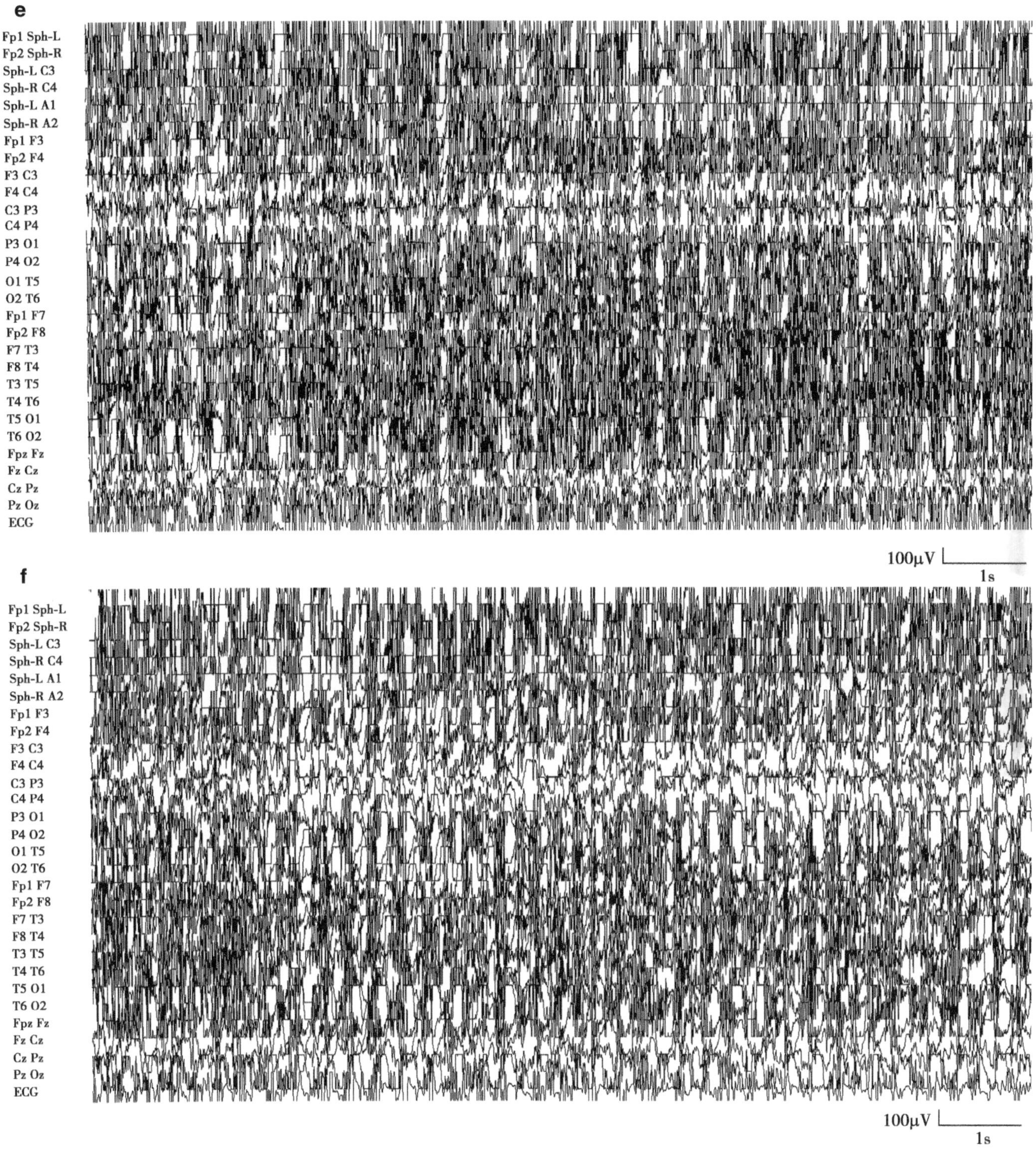

Fig. 4.7 (continued)

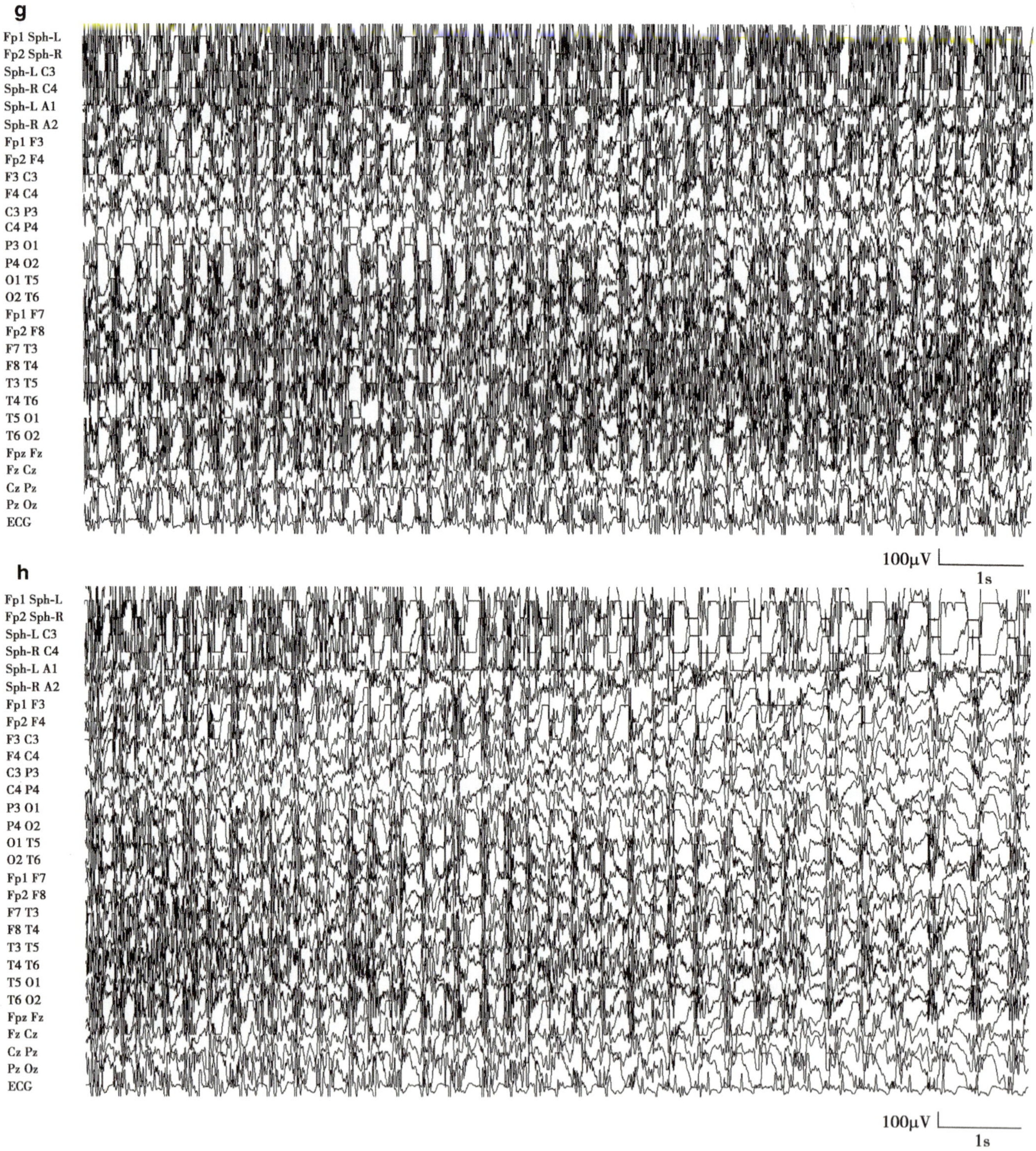

Fig. 4.7 (continued)

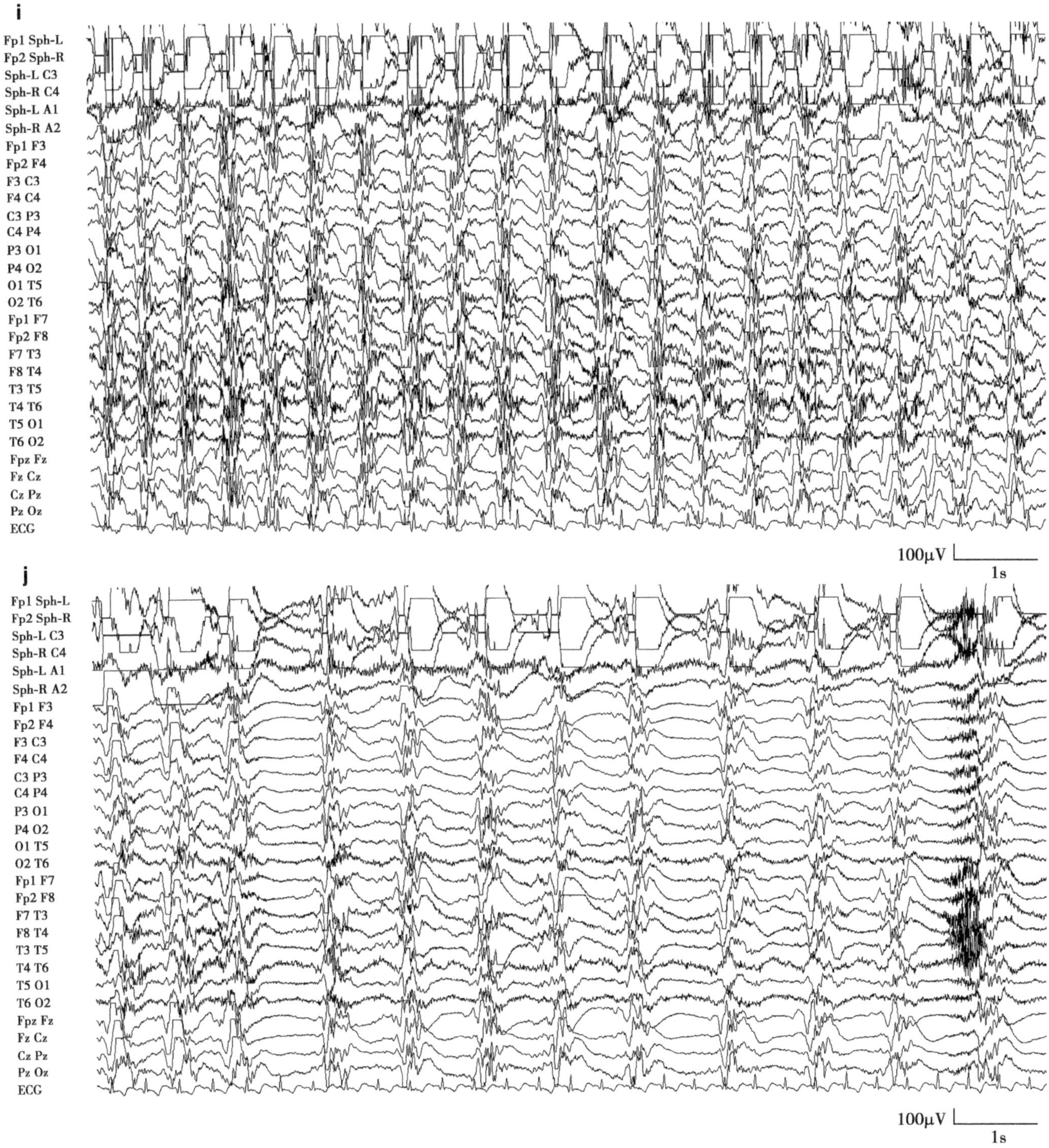

Fig. 4.7 (continued)

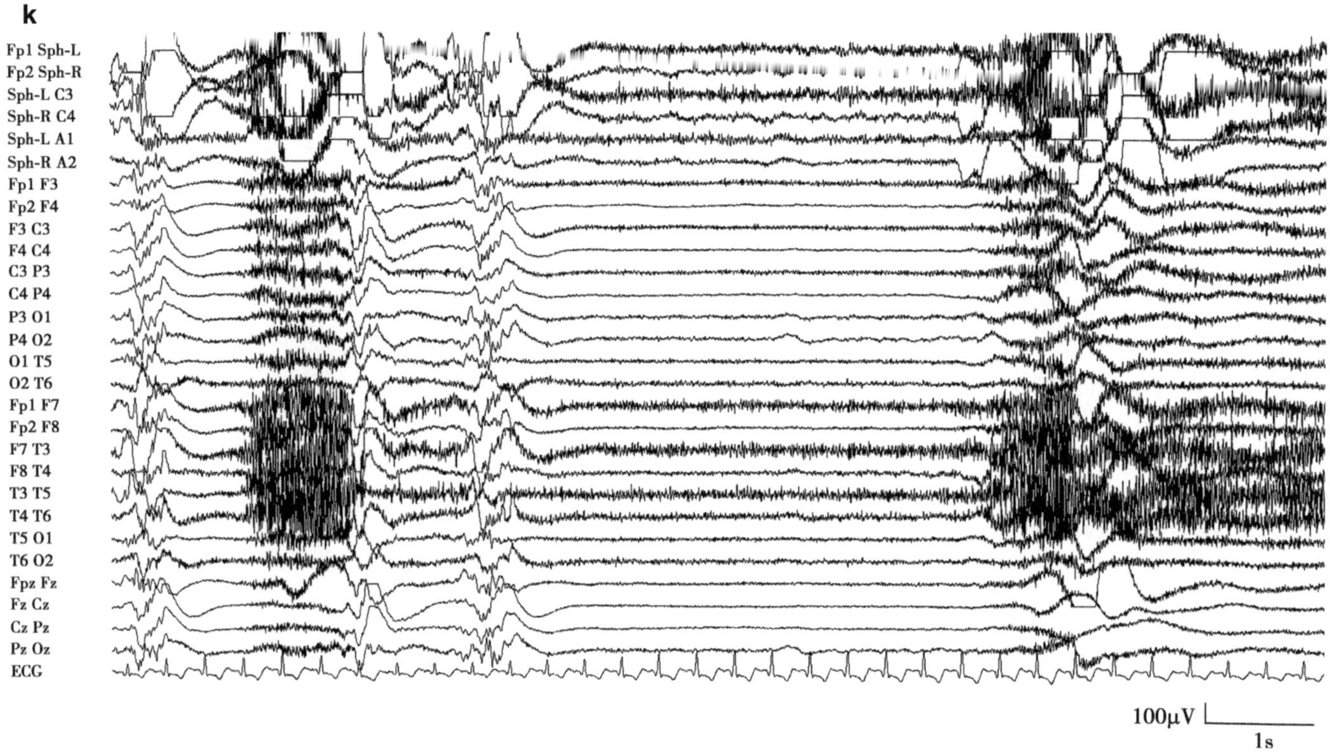

Fig. 4.7 (continued)

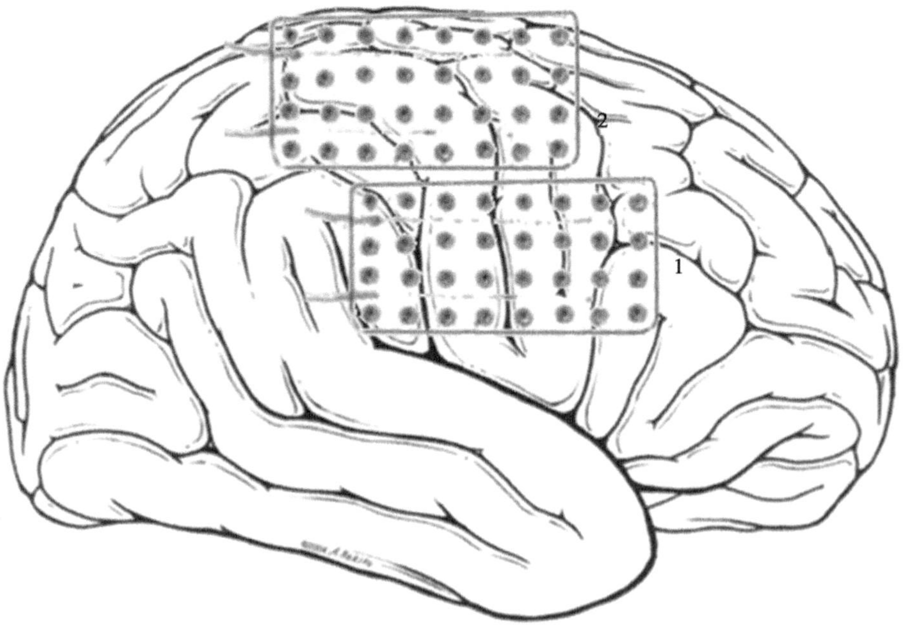

Fig. 4.8 Scheme of intracranial electrodes Grid electrode 1: 32 contacts over the lower part of the right central region; grid electrode 2: 32 contacts over the upper part of the right central region

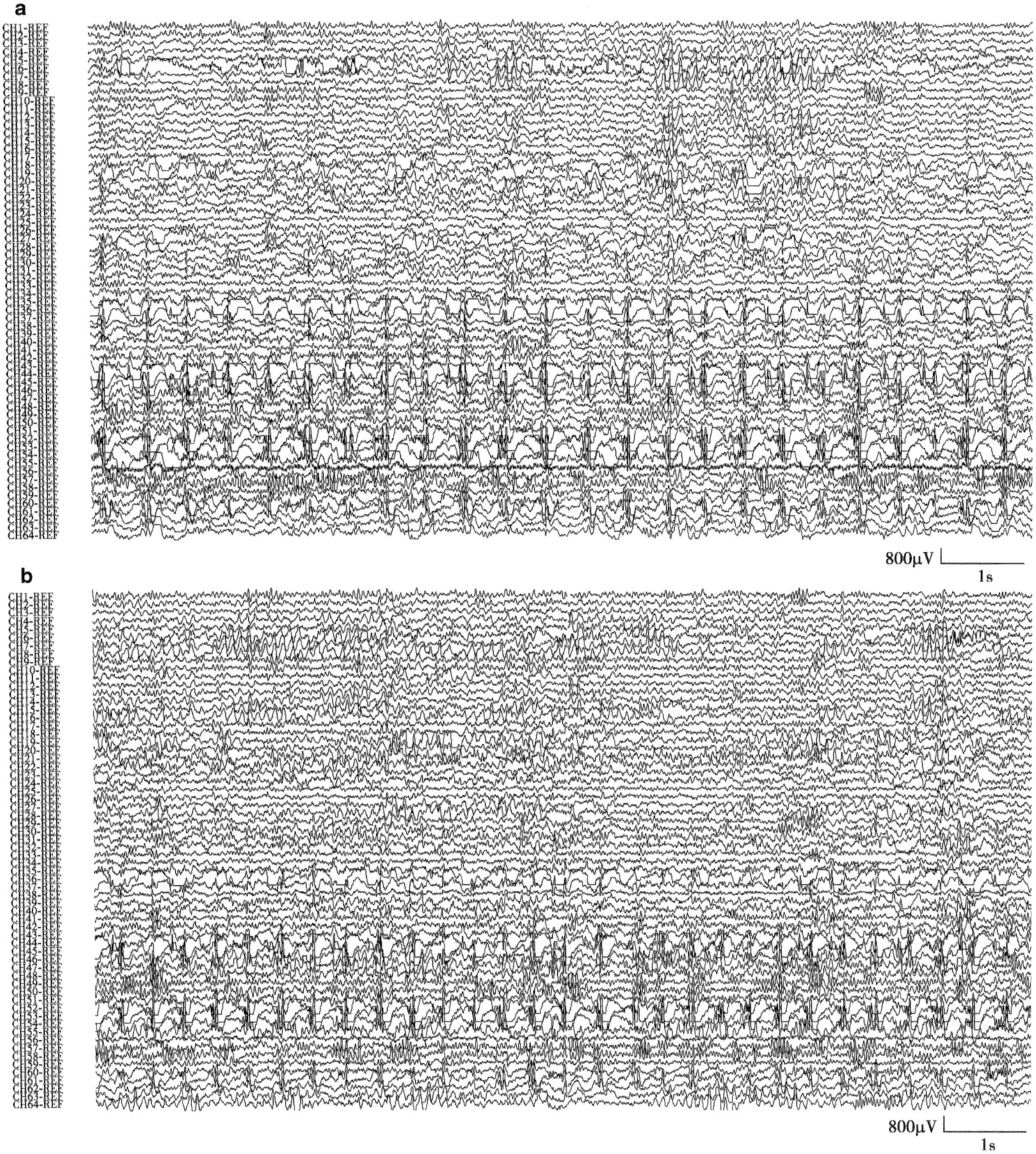

Fig. 4.9 Interictal intracranial EEG. (**a**) IEEG manifestations: rhythmic spike-and-wave complexes, polyspike and wave complexes over the upper right central region (contact numbers CH36, CH37, CH44, CH45, CH46, CH52, CH53, CH54, CH60, CH61, CH62). (**b**) IEEG manifestations: rhythmic spike-and-wave complexes over the upper right central region (contact numbers CH36, CH37, CH44, CH45, CH46, CH52, CH53, CH54, CH60, CH61, CH62)

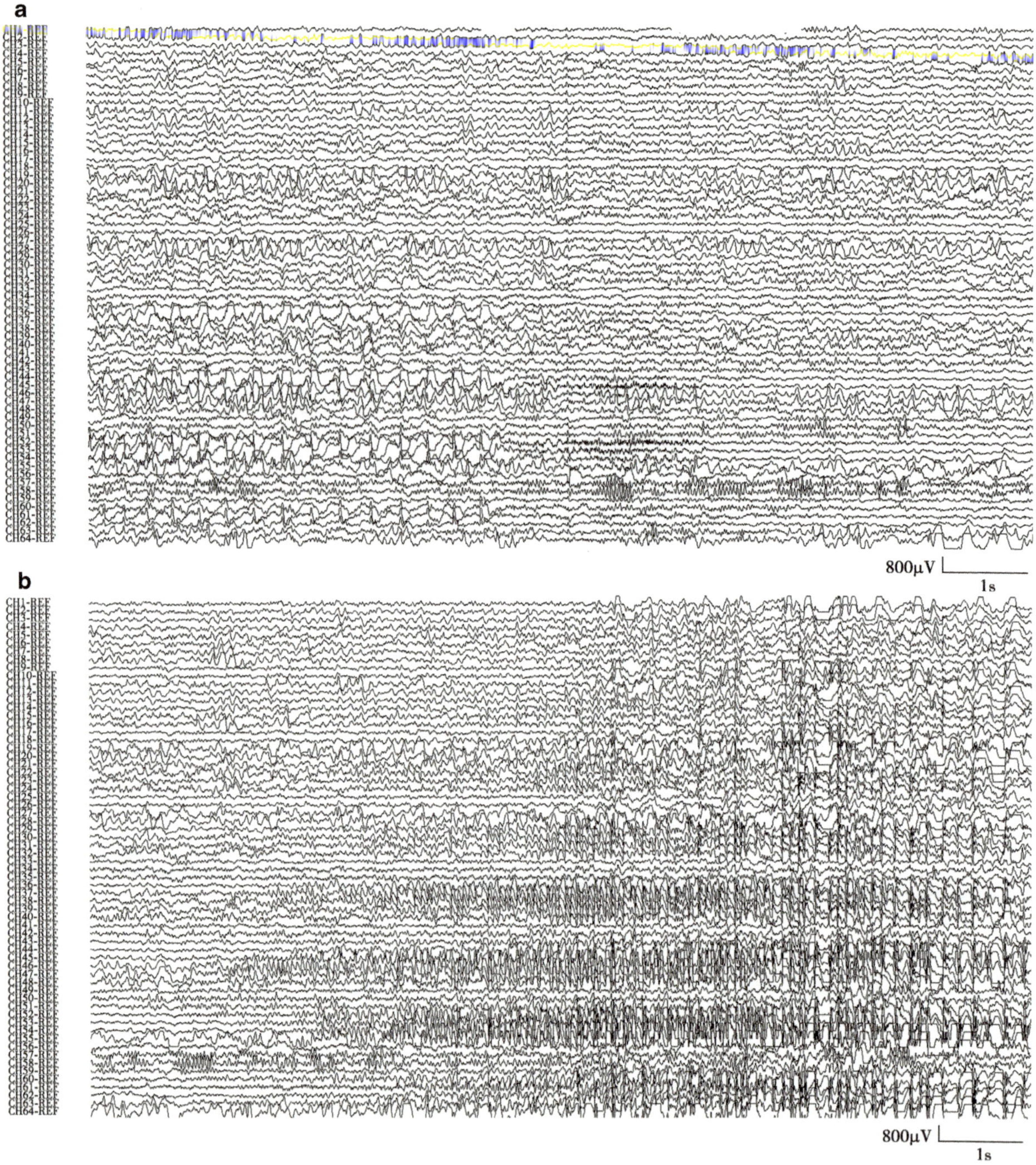

Fig. 4.10 Ictal intracranial EEG. (**a**) The patient was awake. He gave an account of numbness in left little finger and subsequent abduction of left finger. The patient's pre-seizure IEEG was characteristic of a background EEG, manifesting rhythmic spike-and-wave complexes over the upper right central region (contact numbers CH36, CH37, CH44, CH45, CH46, CH52, CH53, CH54, CH60, CH61, CH62) and subsequent low amplitude fast activities over the upper right central region (contact numbers CH45, CH52, CH53, CH54). (**b**) The patient' upper left limb was abducting, raising, clonic, and left hand making a fist. IEEG manifestations: rhythm of spikes in upper right central region (contact numbers CH36, CH37, CH38, CH39, CH44, CH45, CH46, CH47, CH51, CH52, CH53, CH54, CH55, CH60, CH61, CH62, CH63, CH64), involving the lower right central region (contact numbers CH29, CH30, CH31, CH32). (**c**) The patient's upper left limb was tonic-clonic, right upper limb was raised, and head deflecting to the left. IEEG manifestations: rhythm 5.0–6.0 Hz spike-and-wave complexes over the upper right central region (contact numbers CH36, CH37, CH38, CH39, CH44, CH45, CH46, CH47, CH51, CH52, CH53, CH54, CH55, CH60, CH61, CH62, CH63, CH64), involving the lower right central region (contact numbers CH29, CH30, CH31, CH32). (**d**) The patient's upper right limb and bilateral lower extremities were in clonic inflexion state, and upper left limb was tonic-clonic. IEEG manifestations: rhythm of spikes, gradually increasing in wave amplitude and forming rhythm of polyspike and wave complexes. (**e**) The patient had generalized clonic convulsion. IEEG manifestation: persistent rhythm of 2.0–2.5 Hz polyspike and wave complexes. (**f**) The patient had generalized clonic convulsion. IEEG manifestation: rhythm of polyspike and wave complexes. (**g**) The patient had generalized clonus, mainly the lower right limb, at gradually decreased rate. IEEG manifestation: rhythm of polyspike and wave complexes, with gradually slowing down frequency. (**h**) The clonus gradually discontinued and the seizure came to an end. IEEG manifestations: generalized decrease in voltage

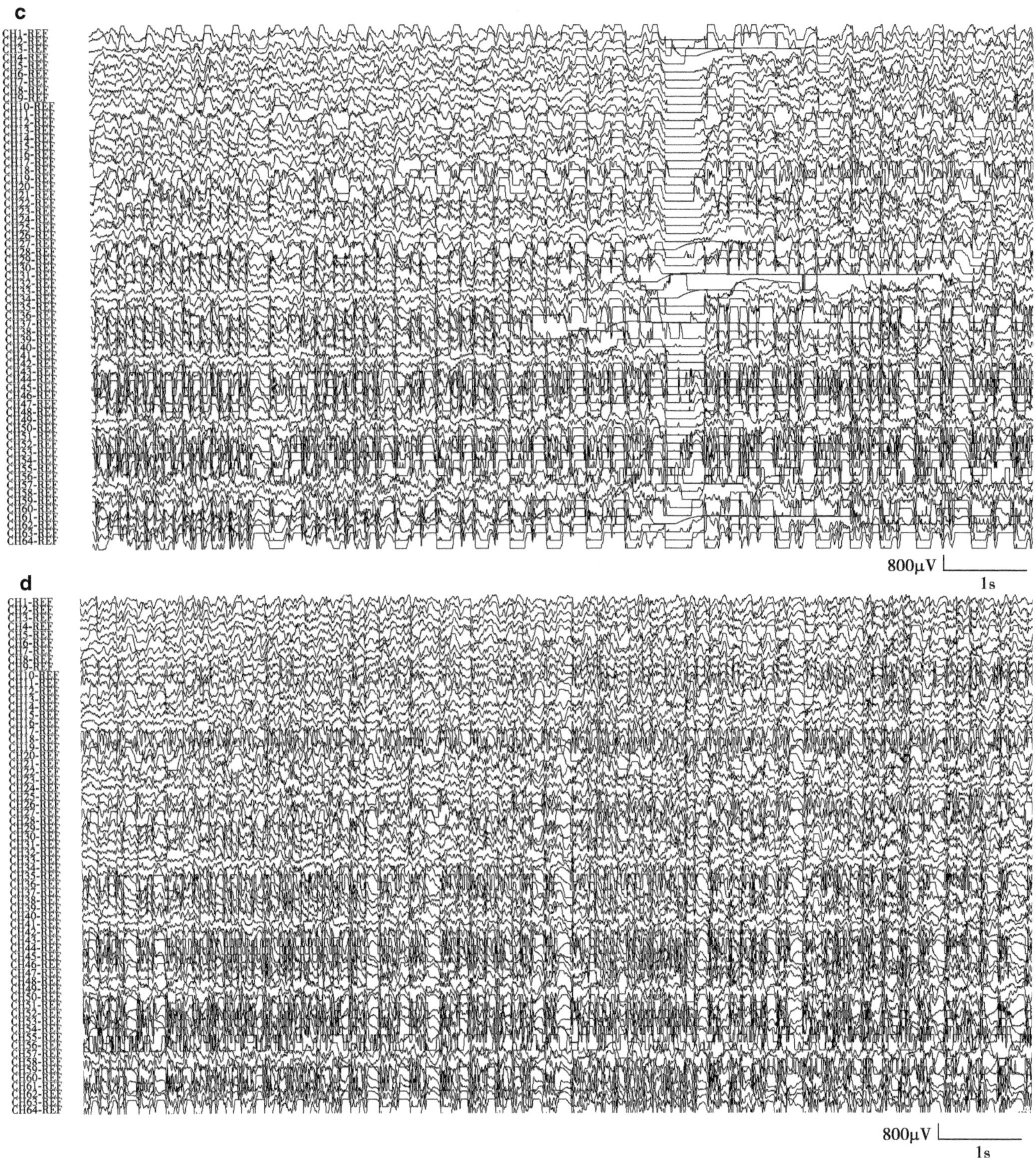

Fig. 4.10 (continued)

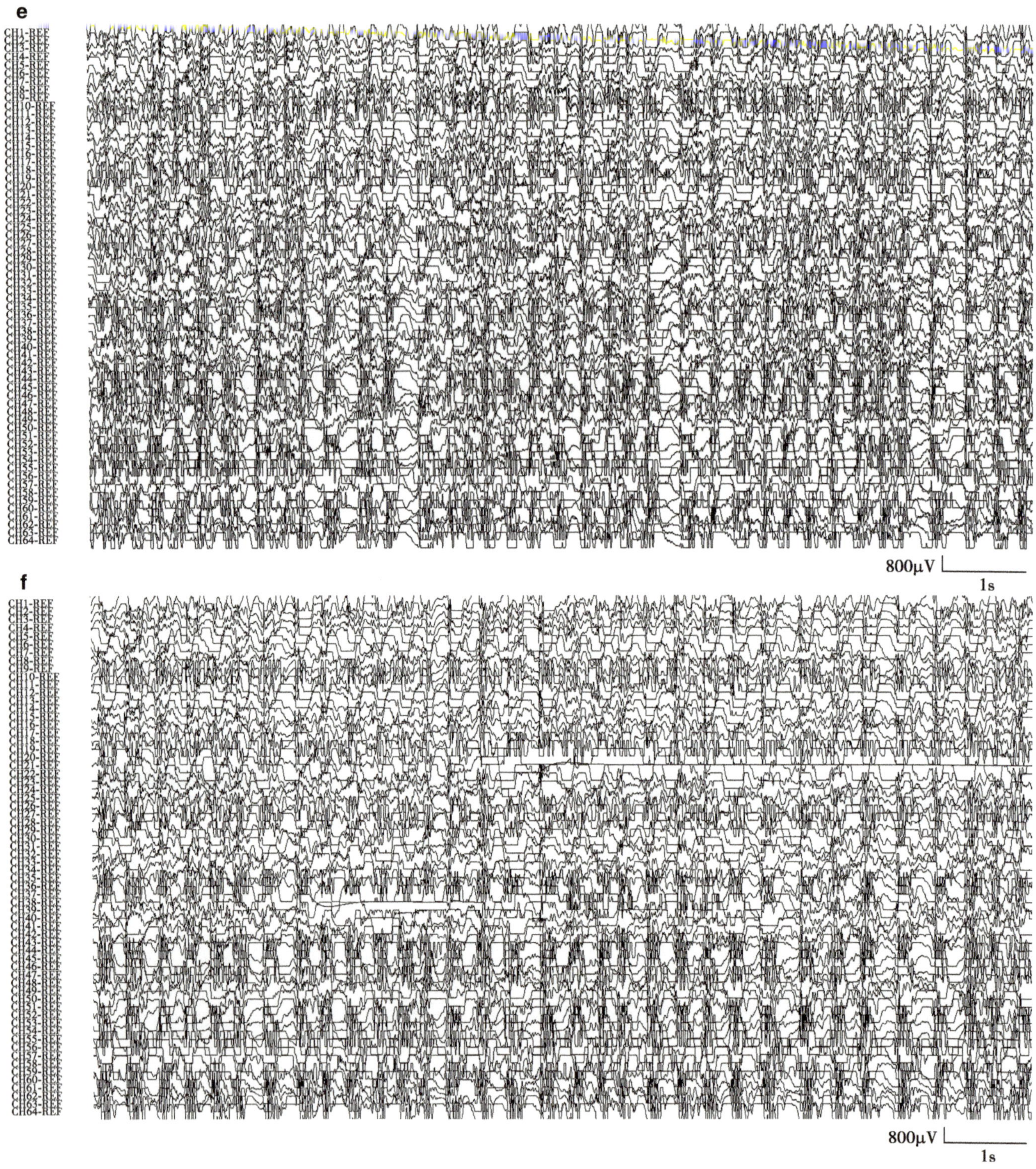

Fig. 4.10 (continued)

g

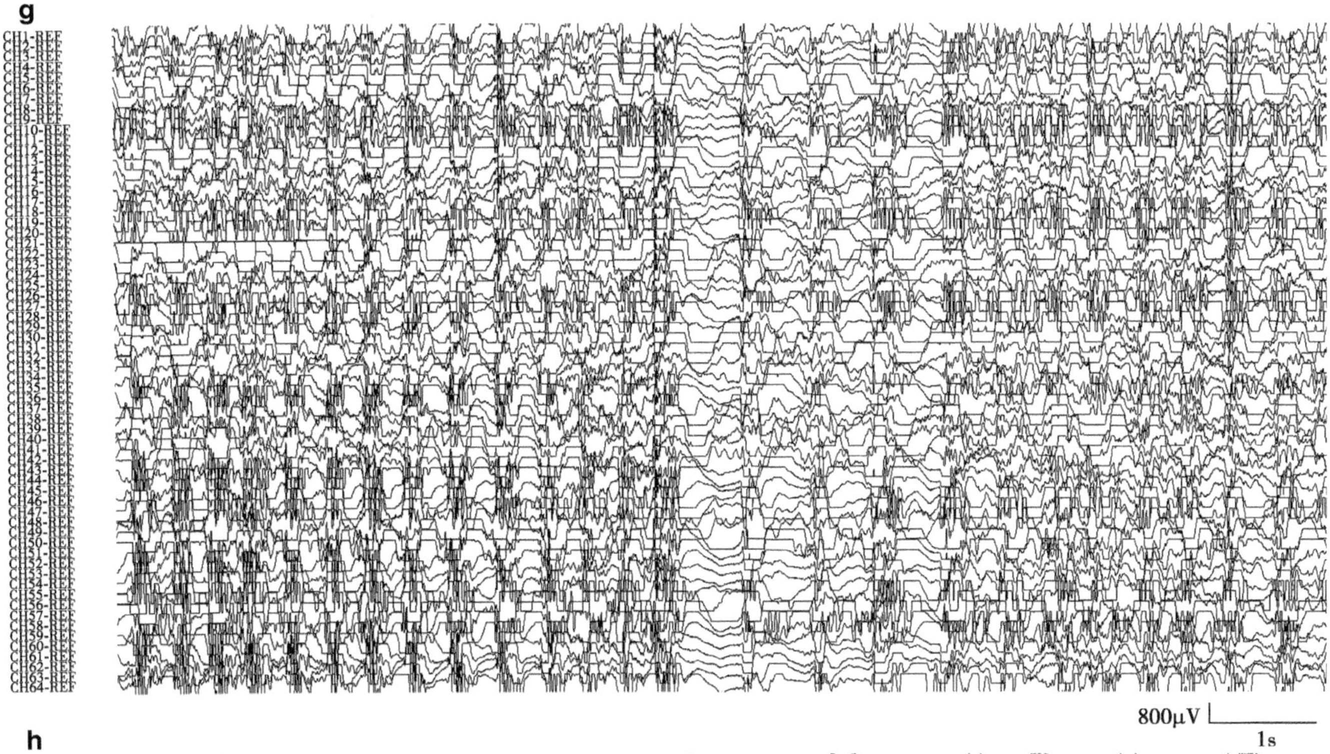

h

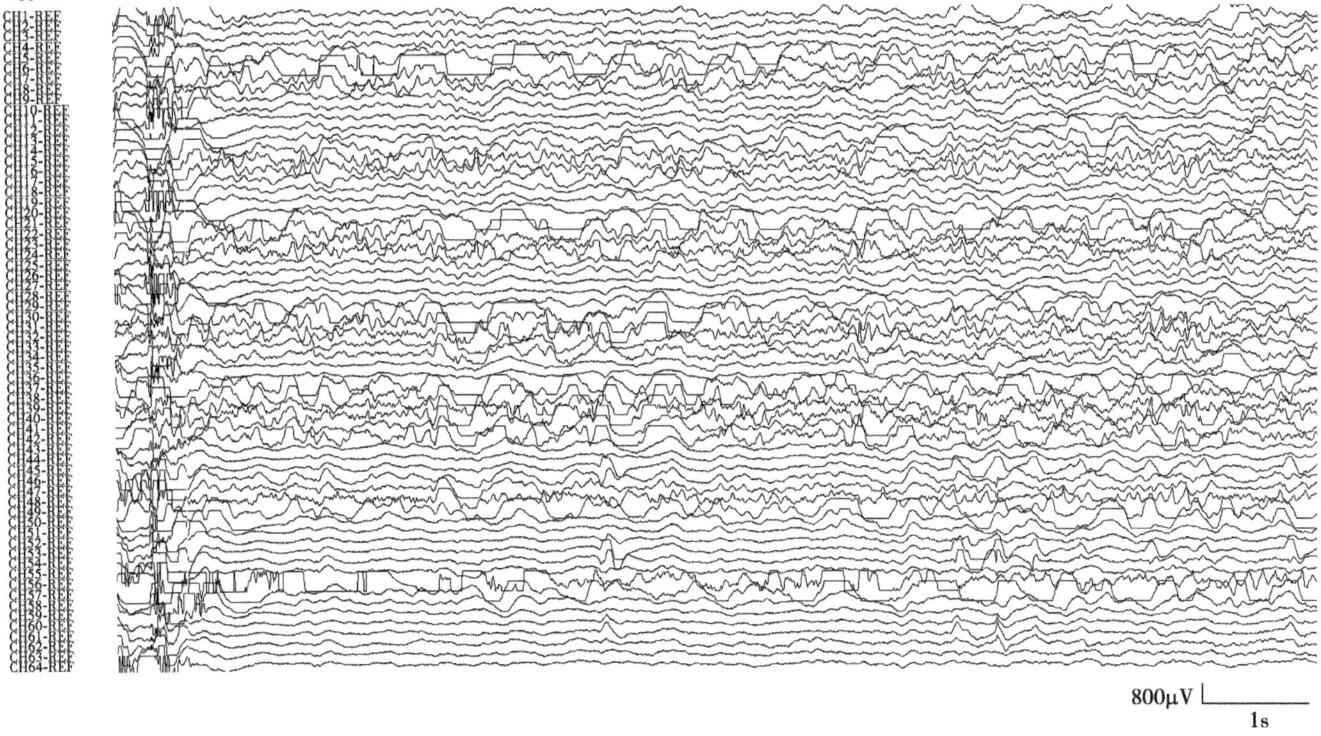

Fig. 4.10 (continued)

[Case Review]

1. *Case Characteristics*
   (a) *Characteristics of seizure*: 1. Episodic numbness of the left pinkie fingertip radiated to the shoulder and followed by tonicity of the left forearm, lasting for 3–5 s; sometimes followed by numbness and tonicity of the right fifth fingertip and upward movement of the right forearm to the right wrist, followed by tonic clonic seizure, lasting about 1 min. 2. Definite aura(s). 3. No loss of consciousness during seizure. 4. 1–2 episodes/week.
   (b) *Imaging characteristics*: MRI revealed symmetrically increased strip signal in callosum, which is not directly related to the positioning of the epileptic focus.
   (c) *EEG characteristics*: The interictal EEG showed sharp waves over the left posterior frontal region, anterior temporal region, and bilateral sphenoidal electrode; slow waves can be identified over the right frontal region, central region, temporal region; the ictal EEG showed low amplitude fast activity over the right posterior frontal region and central region.
2. *Diagnosis and treatment strategies and follow-up results*: The patient had stereotyped seizure symptoms with definite auras; EEG revealed that the interictal abnormal waves were not localized and could be identified in multi-foci in both hemispheres; however, in ictal EEG, the abnormal waves were limited to the central zone of right posterior frontal region. In light of the patient's seizure symptoms and ictal EEG, it was considered that the epileptic focus was located at right postcentral gyrus. In order to determine the relationship between sensorimotor area and epileptic foci, intracranial electrodes were implanted in right posterior frontal region and parietal region. EEG monitoring of seizures and electrical stimulation of cortex were performed to determine the sensory-motor cortex. Interictal IEEG showed that the abnormal discharge was limited to middle and upper parts of right central region; ictal IEEG revealed that the epileptic focus was located at right postcentral gyrus; therefore, the postcentral gyrus cortex was surgically resected in part. The seizures disappeared during a 2-year follow-up after surgery. IEEG demonstrated the origin of seizure was definite and the epileptic focus had been completely resected. Therefore, the patient experiences no seizure after the operation.

Case 4.3 Postcentral Gyrus Epilepsy

[Abstract of Medical Records]
The patient was male and 18 years old.

1. *Chief complaint*: Paroxysmal convulsion of limbs and loss of consciousness for 4 years.
2. *History of present illness*: The patient experienced persistent numbness in right lower limb 4 years ago without apparent predisposing cause, and the numbness was not accompanied by limb twitching. A local hospital considered the patient's condition as "low calcium," but the condition had not resolved after symptomatic treatment. Three months after the onset of the symptom, the patient suddenly experienced convulsion of limbs, foaming at mouth, and loss of consciousness, lasting several minutes. The patient was admitted to the local hospital and diagnosed with epilepsy. His seizure was brought under control after symptomatic treatment. Similar episodes kept emerging intermittently afterwards. Prior to each episode, the patient could feel discomfort in his lower right limb and unexplained numbness followed by twitching of lower right limb, loss of consciousness, and tonic spasm of extremities. Most episodes only had the manifestation of twitching of lower right limb that lasted for several seconds without loss of consciousness. The patient had no weakness and/or numbness of limbs after the end of the episodes. He is now treated with carbamazepine, administered 300 mg in the morning, 300 mg in the afternoon, and 200 mg at night, and clonazepam, 2 mg/dose, b.i.d.
3. *Past history*: The patient was delivered at full term, with normal motor, language and intellectual development.
4. *Physical examination*: No neurological abnormalities were found.
5. *Imaging examination*: MRI revealed no definite pathological change.
6. *EEG*: For details, see Figs. 4.11, 4.12, 4.13, 4.14, and 4.15.

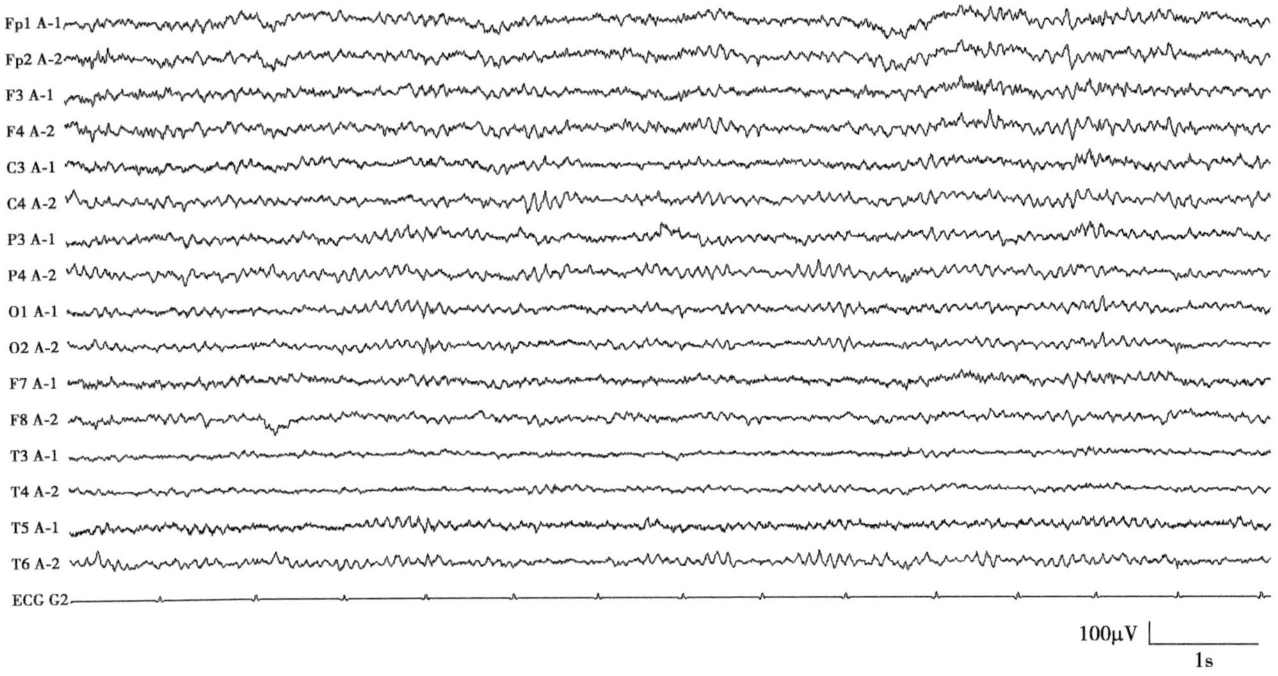

Fig. 4.11 Interictal scalp EEG
Basic rhythm 10.0 Hz, no epileptiform abnormal discharge was observed

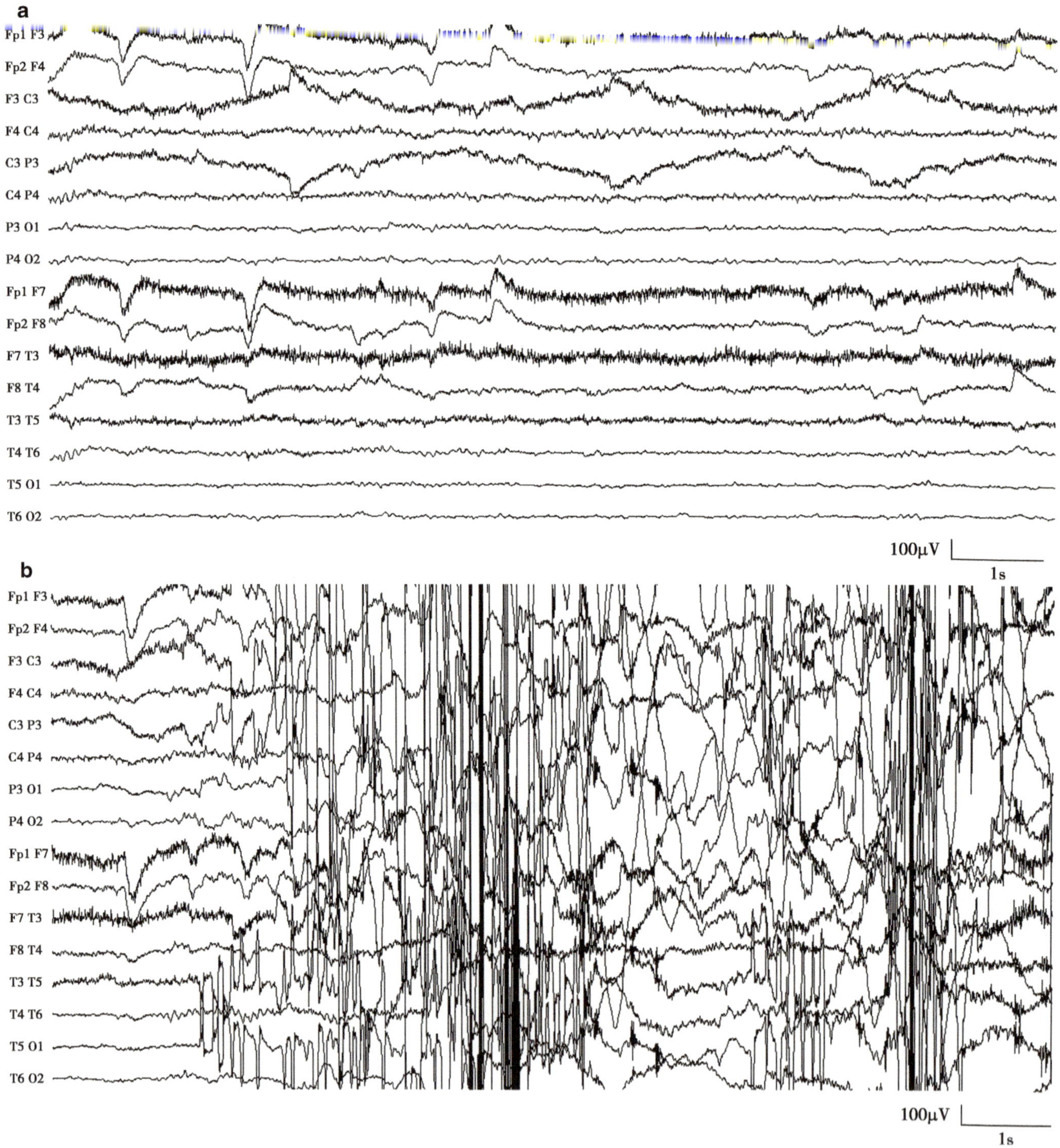

Fig. 4.12 Ictal scalp EEG. (**a**) Prior to the seizure, the patient was clear-minded. The EEG during wakefulness showed eye movement artifacts over the bilateral frontal (Fp1-F3, Fp2-F4, Fp1-F7, Fp2-F8) leads. (**b**) The patient's bilateral lower extremities were inflecting and twitching involuntarily, especially the right side. EEG showed some EMG artifacts and electrode wobble artifacts. (**c**) The patient's symptoms and EEG manifestations are presented in **b**. (**d**) He was wheezing coarsely, pressing his right thigh with his right hand. The EEG presentation was the same as **b**. (**e**) The patient's seizure ended. His EEG gradually regressed to background pattern

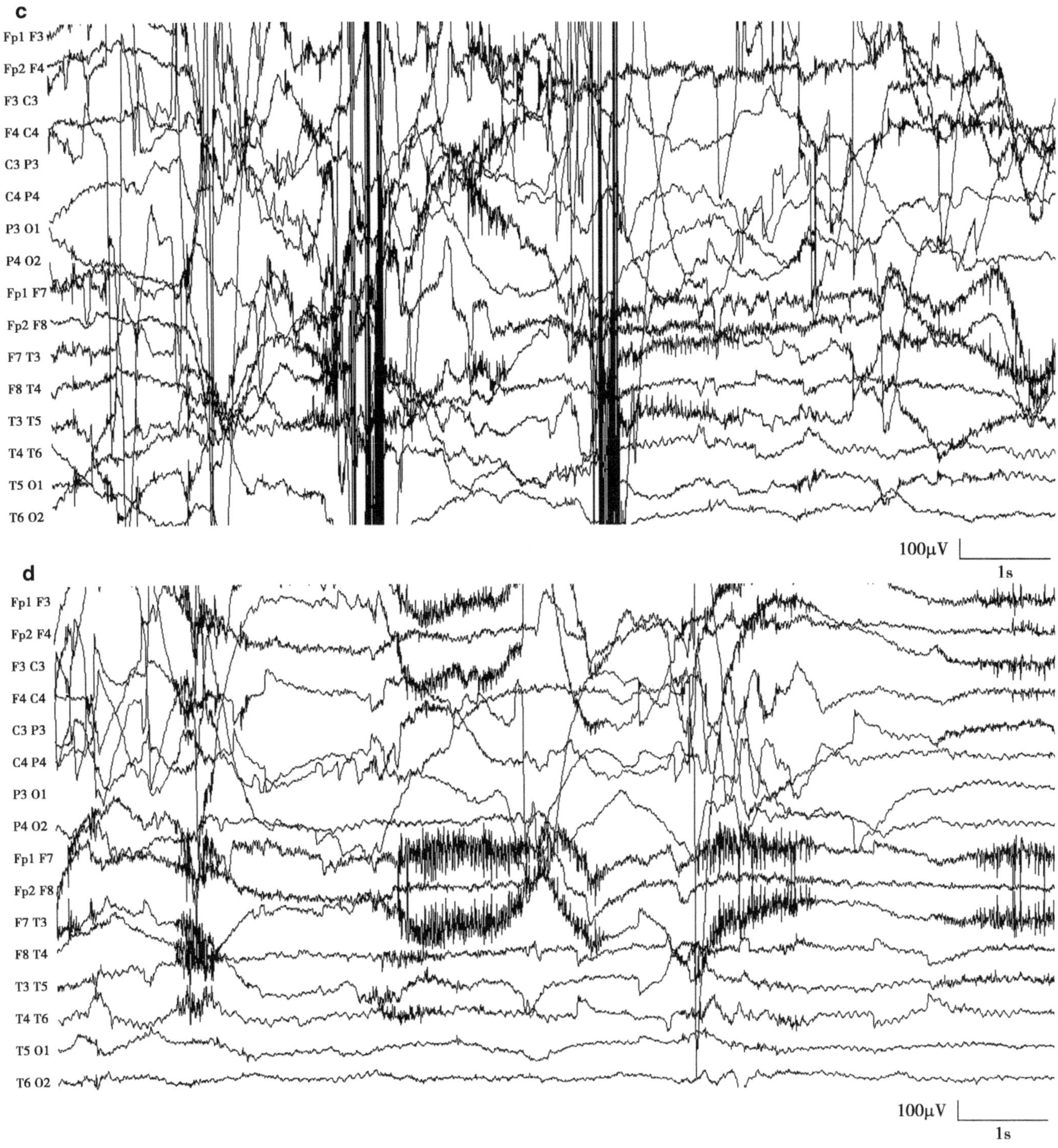

Fig. 4.12 (continued)

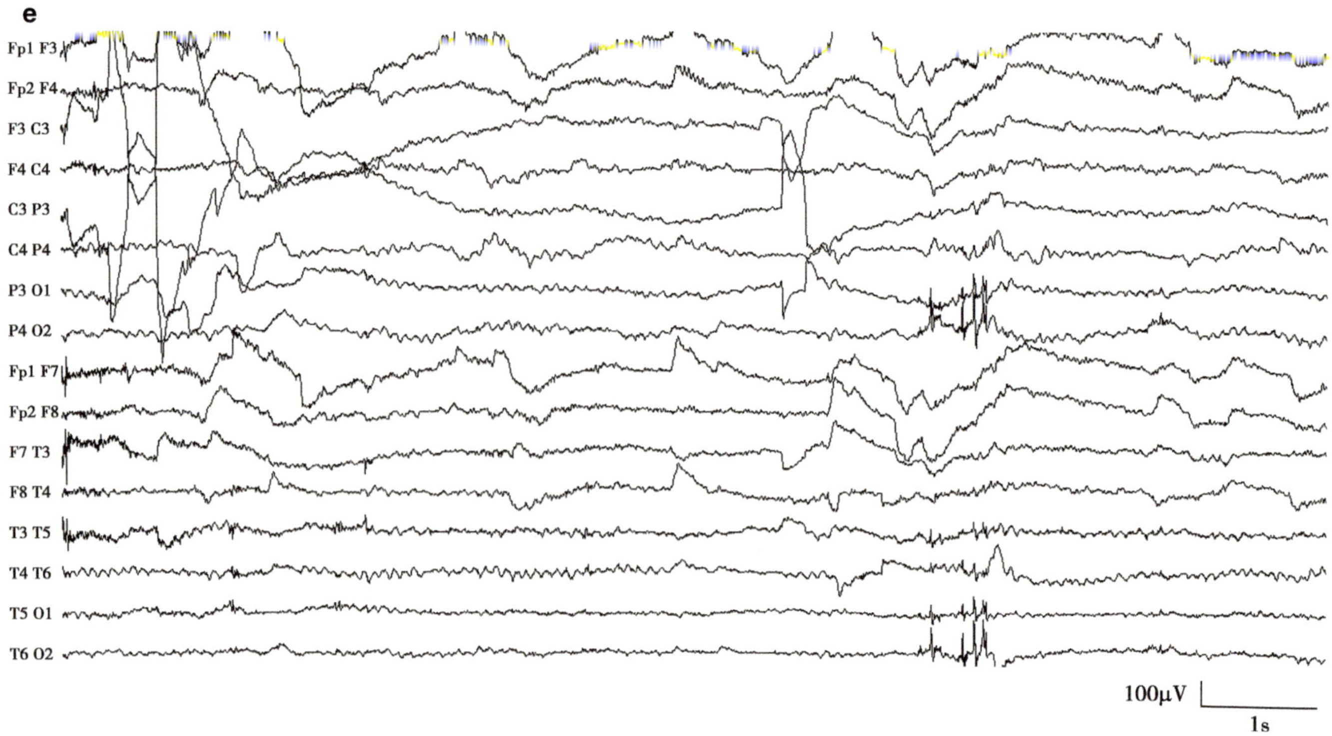

Fig. 4.12 (continued)

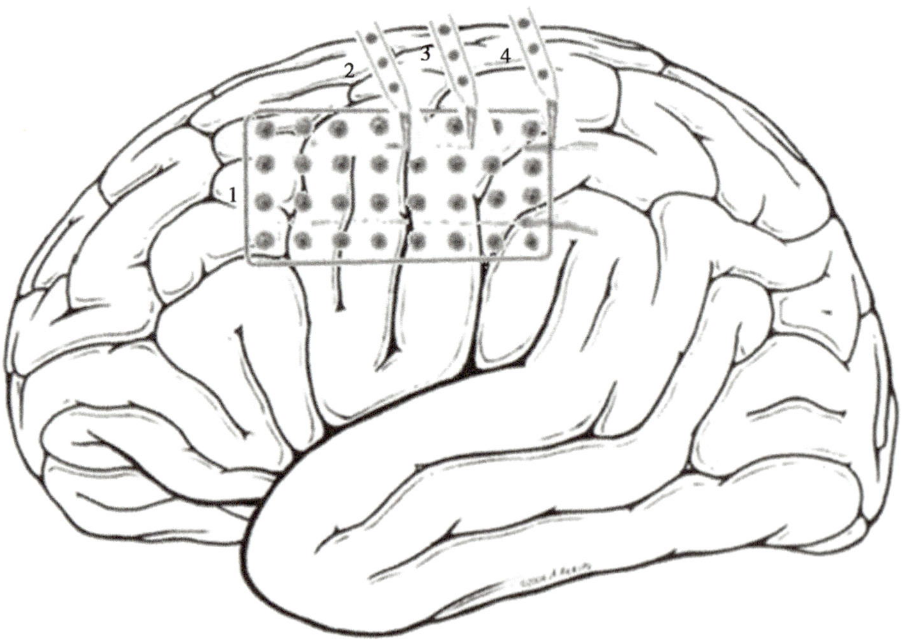

Fig. 4.13 Scheme of intracranial electrodes Grid electrode 1: the left central region (32 contacts); strip electrode 2: the left anterior central interhemispheric fissure (8 contacts); strip electrode 3: the middle of left central interhemispheric fissure (8 contacts); strip electrode 4: the left posterior central interhemispheric fissure (8 contacts)

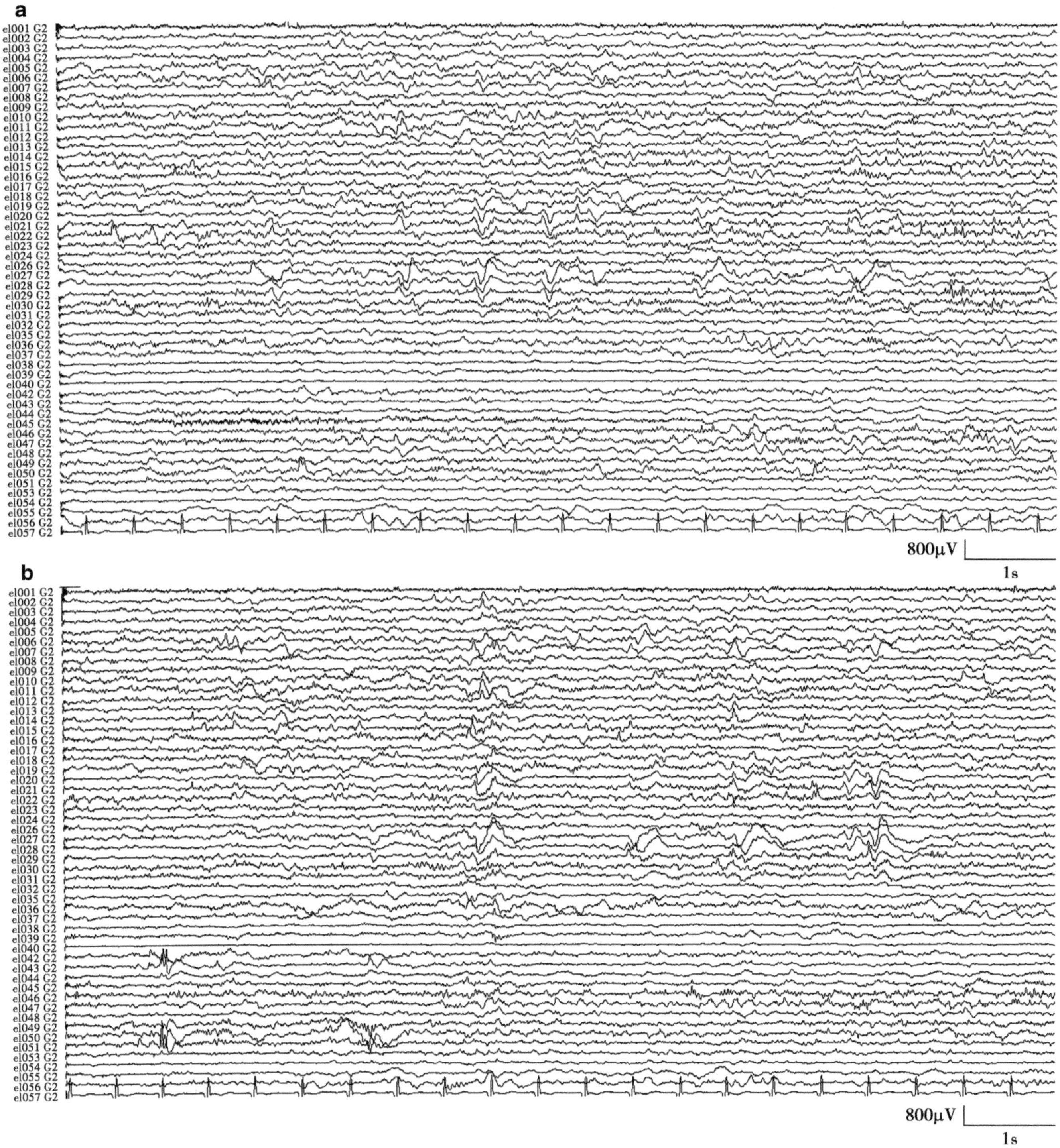

Fig. 4.14 Interictal intracranial EEG. (**a**) The IEEG showed paroxysmal medium-to-high amplitude sharpened slow waves over the left central region (contact numbers el019, el020, el021, el022, el027, el028, el029), low amplitude fast activities over the middle of the left central region of interhemispheric fissure (contact numbers el044, el045, el046, el047). (**b**) The IEEG showed sharp waves and slow waves over the left central region (contact numbers el006, el007, el015, el016, el020, el021, el027, el028, el029); spikes and spike-and-wave complexes were seen on the electrodes of the middle and posterior part of the left central region in interhemispheric fissure (contact numbers el043, el050, el051)

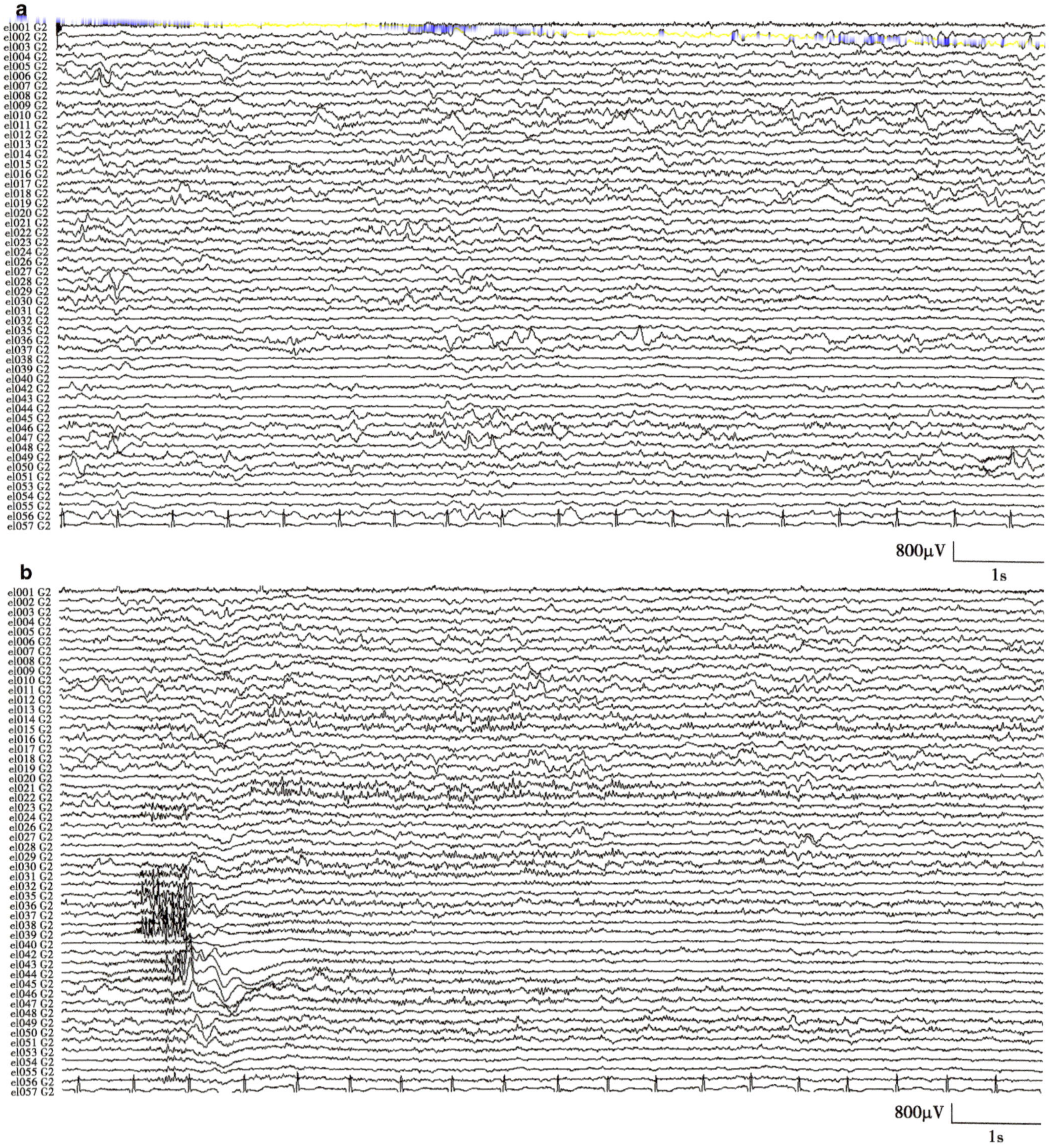

Fig. 4.15 Intracranial electrode EEG—ictal. (**a**) The patient was supine with eyes closed before the seizure. The IEEG showed paroxysmal localized slow waves and sporadic sharp waves over the left posterior central region (contact numbers el010, el011, el017, el018), and irregular sharp waves with low amplitude fast activities were seen over the left central region of interhemispheric fissure (contact numbers el036, el045, el046, el047, el048, el049, el050). (**b**) The patient's right lower extremities twitched several times. The IEEG showed low amplitude fast activities over the anterior and middle parts of left central region electrode (contact numbers el014, el015, el021, el022, el023, el024, el029, el030, el031, el032), and high-amplitude spike rhythm and subsequent low amplitude fast activities were seen on the anterior central region of interhemispheric fissure (contact numbers el35, el36, el37, el038, el039, el043, el044, el045, el046, el047). (**c**) The patient's seizure ended. The IEEG recovered the original background EEG

c

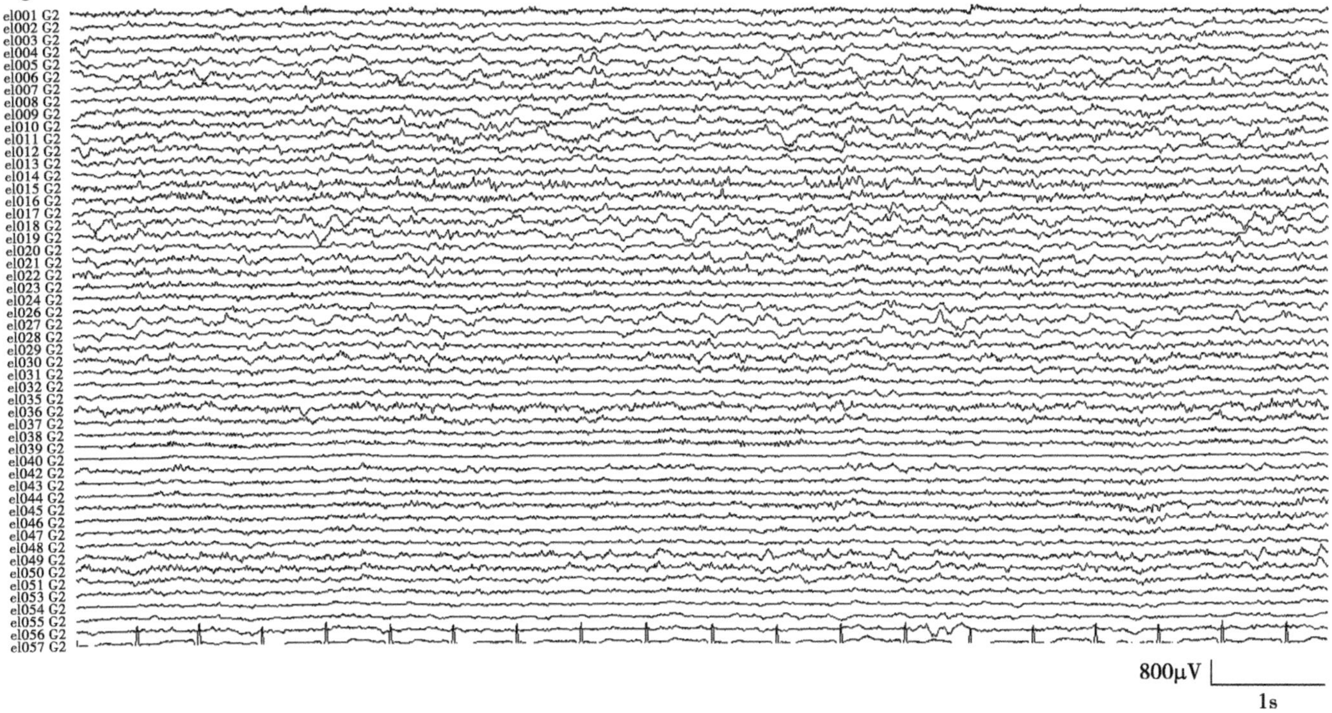

Fig. 4.15 (continued)

[Case Review]

1. *Case Characteristics*
   (a) *Seizure characteristics*: 1. The manifestations of this episode in the patient were involuntarily flexing and twitching of bilateral lower extremities, especially in the right side. 2. The auras were discomfort or unexplained numbness in right lower extremities.
   (b) *Imaging characteristics*: MRI revealed no definite pathological change.
   (c) *EEG characteristics*: No notable epileptiform abnormal discharge was observed in interictal phase; EMG artifacts and electrode wobbling artifacts were observed in ictal phase.
2. *Diagnosis and treatment strategies and follow-up results*: Ictal EEG and MRI revealed no definite information, but the patient had stereotyped seizure symptoms, mainly including numbness and discomfort in right lower limb and twitching of right lower limb. In light of the seizure symptoms, it was considered that the epileptic focus was located in left central region of interhemispheric fissure. In order to define the relationship between the epileptic foci and motor cortex, intracranial electrodes were implanted in left central region and interhemispheric fissure region. Interictal IEEG showed low amplitude fast activity over left central region of interhemispheric fissure; ictal IEEG revealed that the origin of seizure was located in central region and the nearby interhemispheric fissure region, covering a wide range. Through electrical stimulation of cortex, the location of motor cortex had been identified. The cortex in left postcentral gyrus and part of the cortex in left anterior central region of interhemispheric fissure had been surgically resected. After the surgery, the patient was seizure-free during a 1-year follow-up. The good results of the surgical treatment might be attributable to definite identification of origin of seizure and complete resection of epileptic focus.

Case 4.4 Postcentral Gyrus Epilepsy

[Abstract of Medical Records]
Female, 28 years old.

1. *Chief complaint*: Paroxysmal aphasia, weakness of left limbs, sometimes with tonic-clonic seizure for 15 years.
2. *History of present illness*: Fifteen years ago (approximately 13 years old), the patient experienced episode of seizure, initially unable to speak without obvious inducement, then the strength of left limb was weak, and after a few seconds, she became unconscious with twitching limbs. She was diagnosed with epilepsy in a local hospital and received drug therapy; no more details are available. Each seizure is now preceded by an aura that cannot be accurately described, followed by an inability to speak, but she could understand the speech of others, accompanied by weakness of the left limb that lasts for several seconds followed by numbness of the left limb, and clear consciousness throughout the seizure. Sometimes the patient experiences loss of consciousness, with both eyes staring at left side and leftward distortion of mouth corner and tonic-clonic seizure of extremities. The conditions are more severe in left side than in right side and last dozens of seconds before resolution. Seizure occurred several times a day. No obvious circadian pattern was observed. The patient took TCM preparations, but the efficacy was unsatisfactory.
3. *Past history*: The patient experienced jerk of limbs after hyperpyrexia at 4 years old.
4. *Physical examination*: No neurological abnormalities were found.
5. *Imaging examination*: MRI showed no obvious abnormalities.
6. *EEG*: For details, see Figs. 4.16, 4.17, 4.18, 4.19, and 4.20.

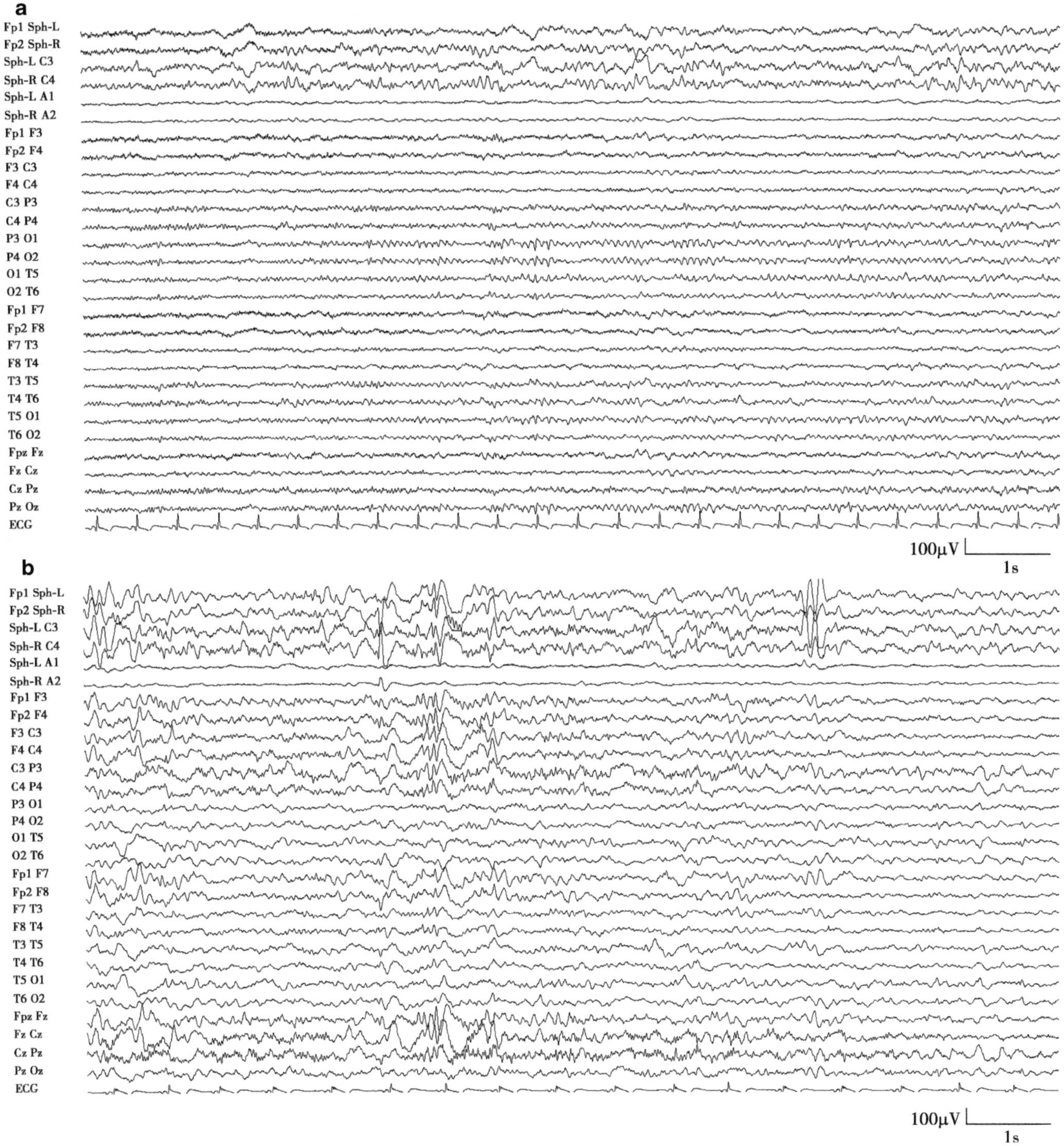

Fig. 4.16 Interictal scalp EEG. (**a**) The patient was awake. EEG background rhythm: 9–10 Hz. (**b**) The EEG showed independent sharp waves over the bilateral sphenoidal electrodes, spike-and-wave complexes over the bilateral frontal regions, and sharp waves over the right temporal region

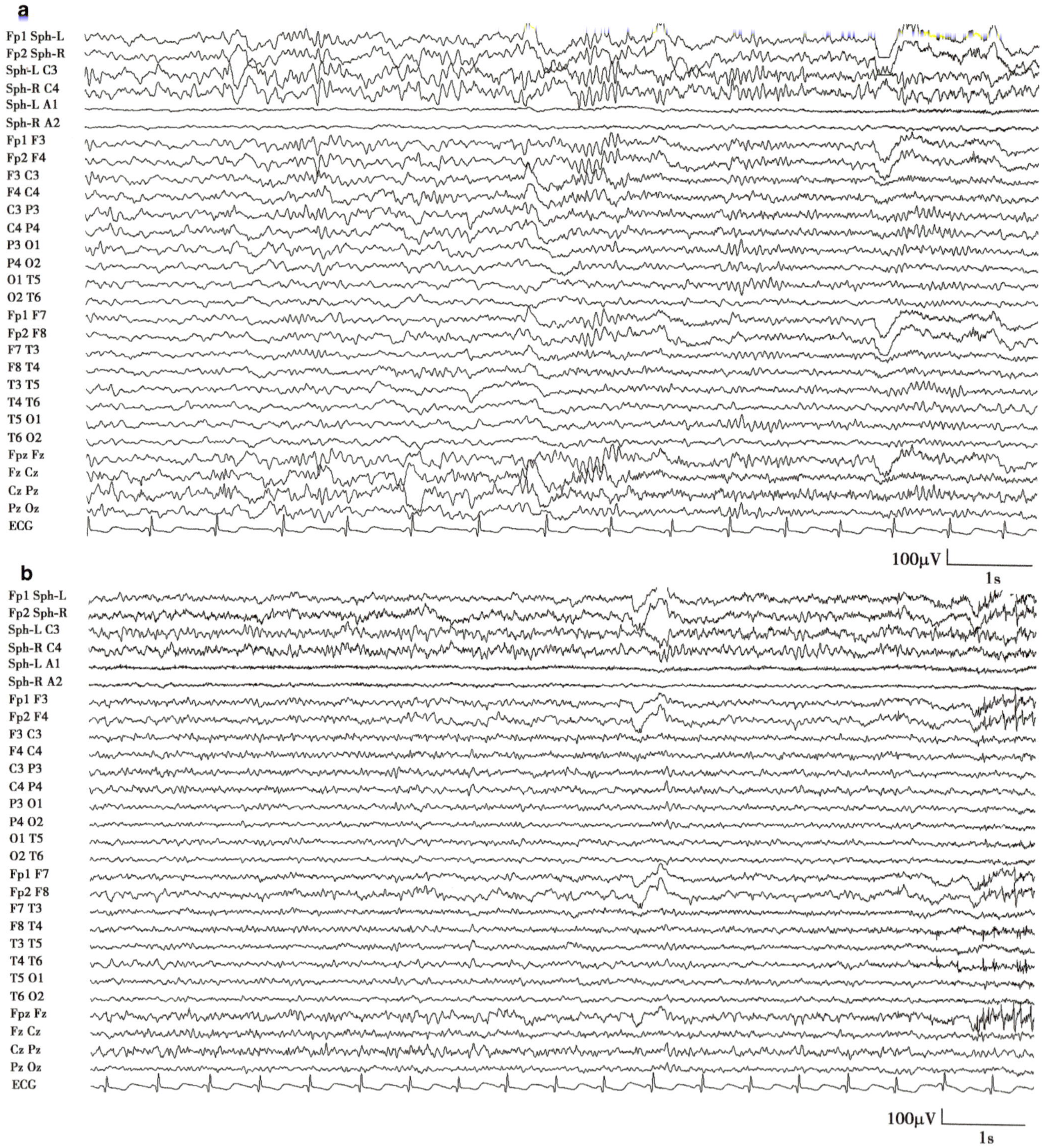

Fig. 4.17 Ictal scalp EEG. (**a**) The patient had vacant look in both eyes when waking up from sleep. EEG revealed the patient has electroencephalogram characteristic of Phase II sleep prior to a seizure. (**b**) The patient would become dialeptic and have vacant look in both eyes and then the patient's left upper limb lifted up. The EEG showed low-amplitude sharp waves over the right temporal region with left-right asymmetry. (**c**) The patient's mouth corners twitched to the left. The EEG showed mixed EMG artifacts. (**d**) The patient had twitching of the corners of the mouth to the left side, head clonus, followed by slight clonus of the upper left limb. The EEG showed mixed EMG artifacts. (**e**) Persistent clonus in the head and upper left limb and subsequent clonic and tonic activities of upper right limb are observed in the patient. The EEG showed mixed EMG artifacts. (**f**) Persistent clonus of upper body at increasing frequency is also observed in the patient. The EEG presentation was the same as **e**. (**g**) When the patient's upper body clonus gradually discontinues, the seizure come to an end. Mixed EMG artifacts (4 s) were observed; there were rhythm of fast activity over the right sphenoidal electrode, and wobbling artifacts occurred at the end of the seizure

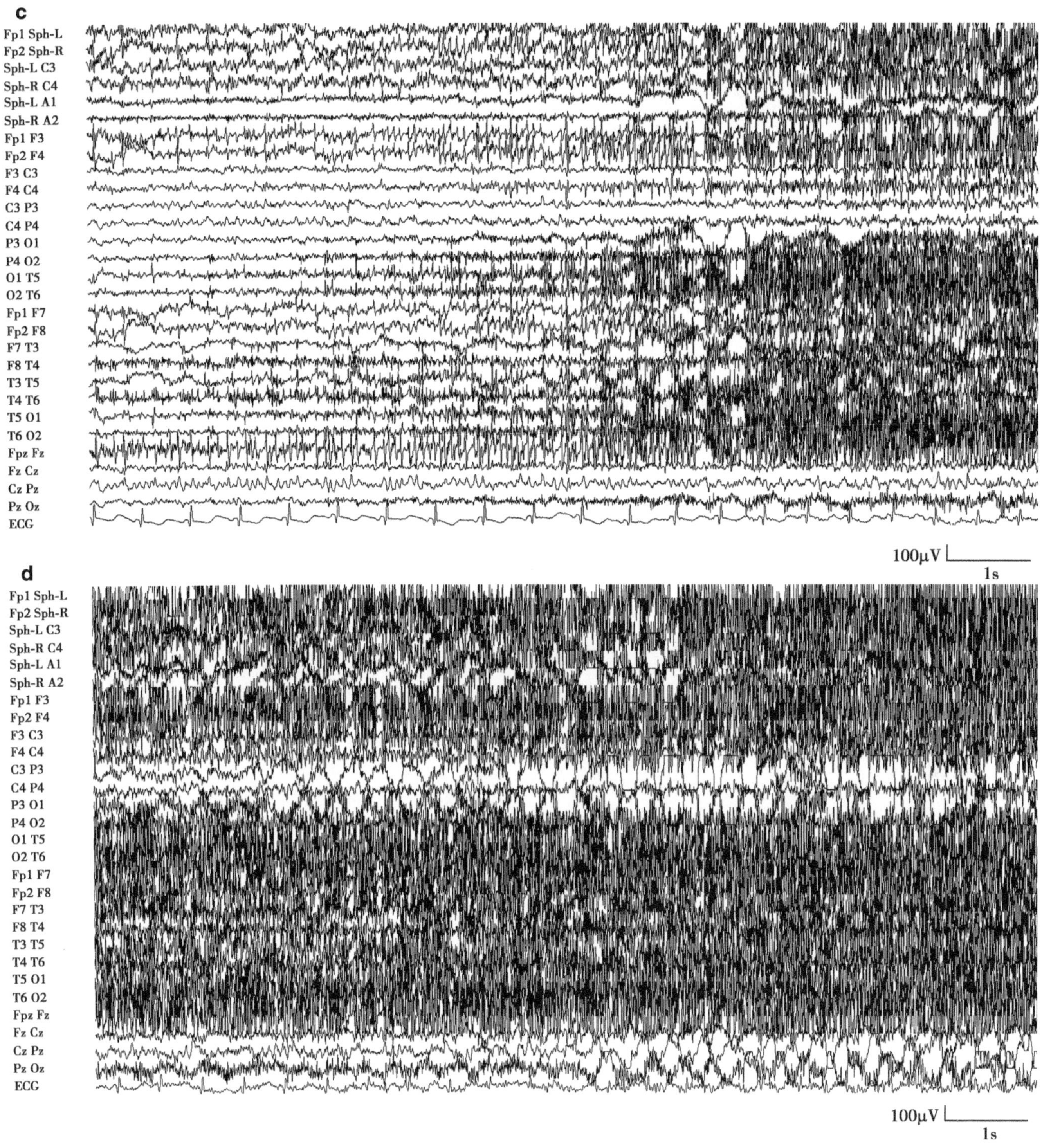

Fig. 4.17 (continued)

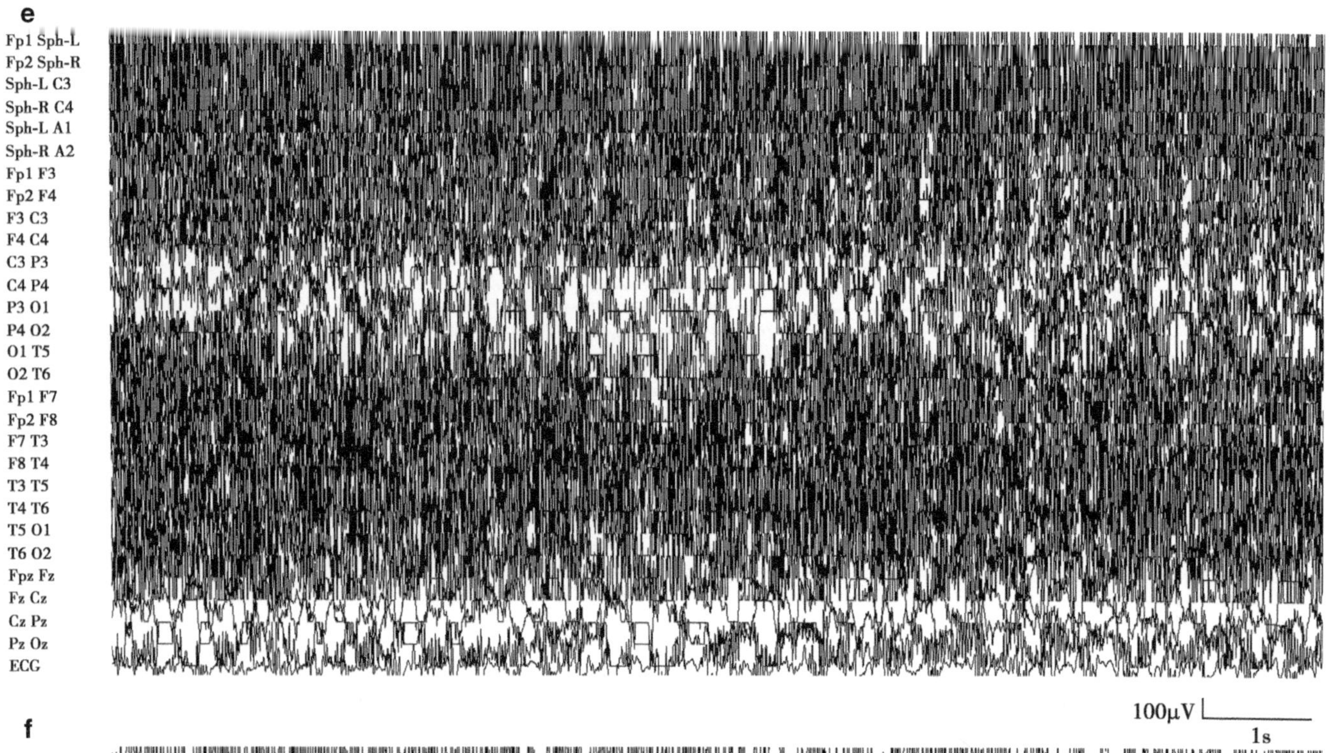

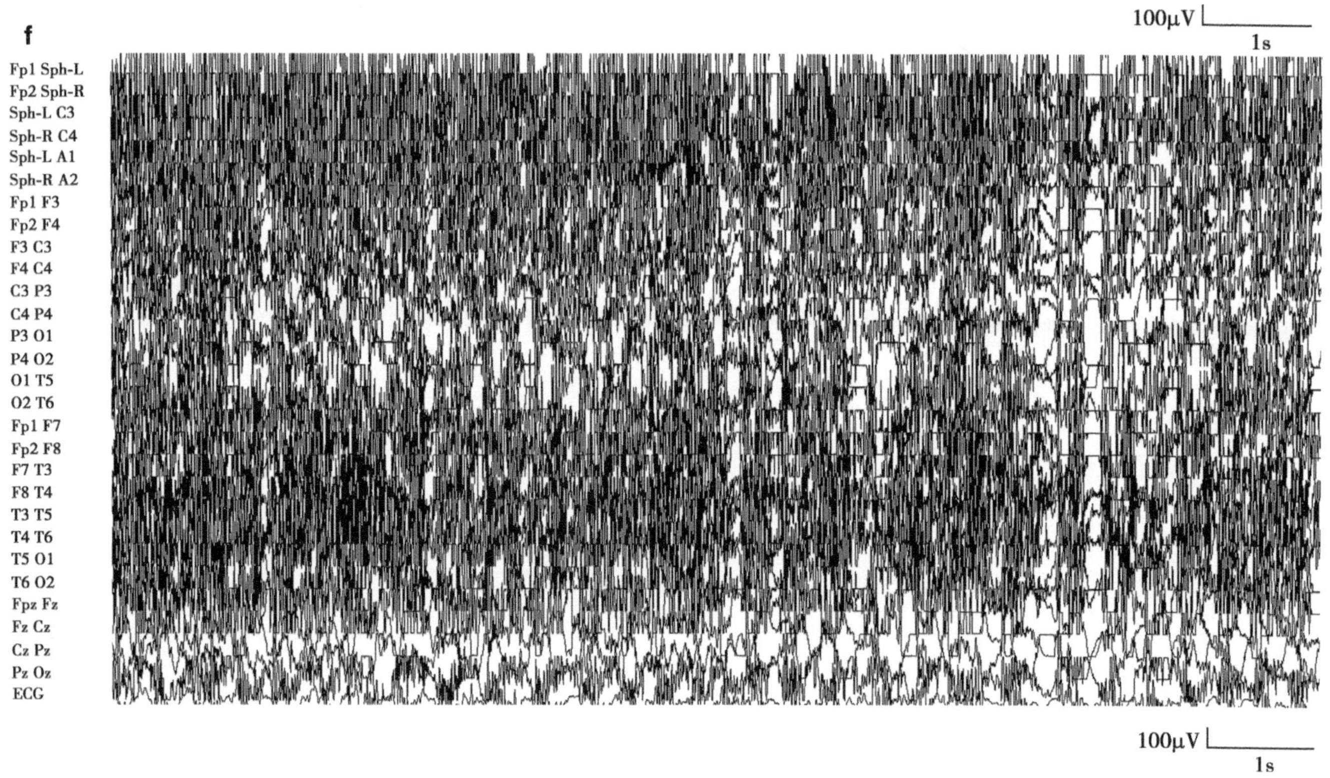

Fig. 4.17 (continued)

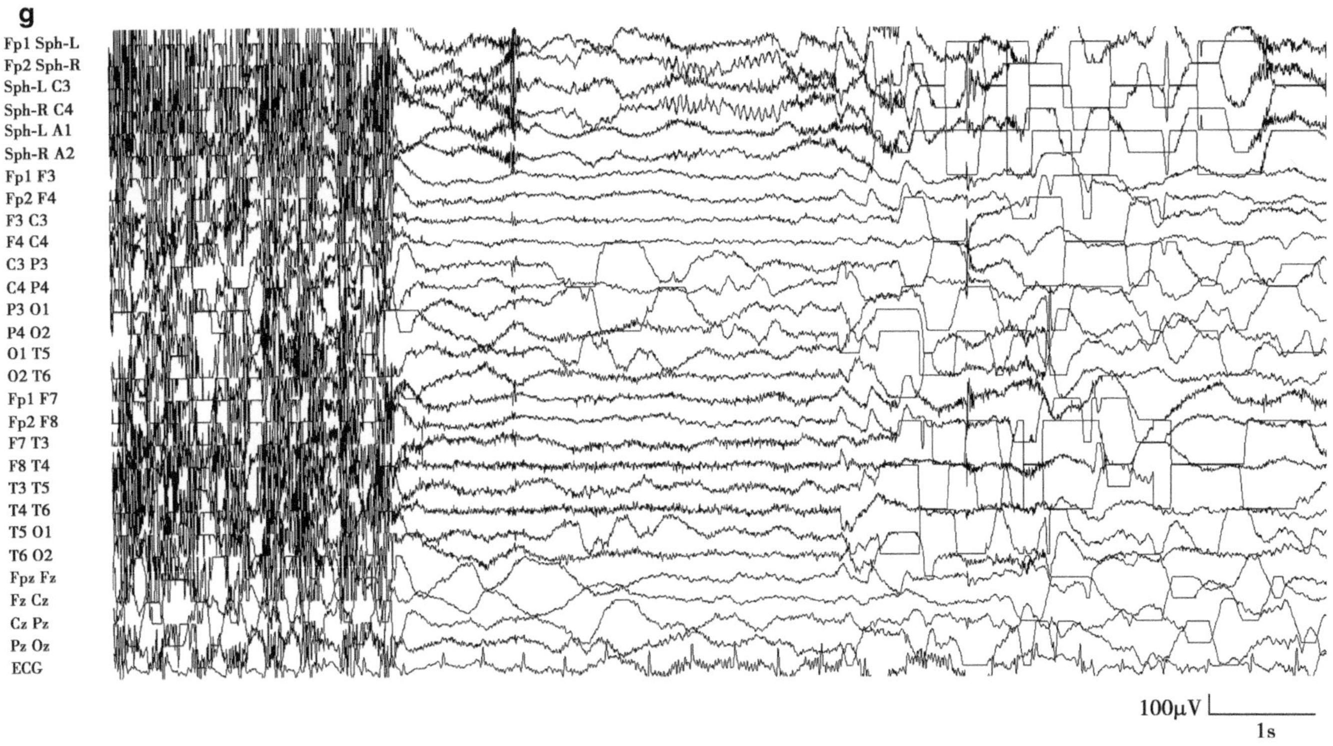

Fig. 4.17 (continued)

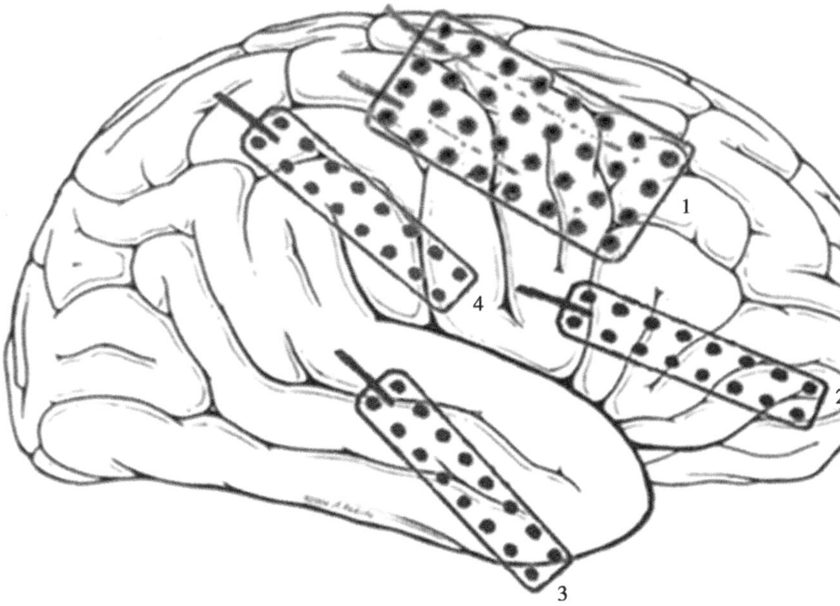

Fig. 4.18 Scheme of intracranial electrodes
Grid electrode 1: the central zone of right posterior frontal region (32 contacts); grid electrode 2: the inferior frontal gyrus (16 contacts); grid electrode 3: the right middle temporal to temporal base regions (16 contacts); grid electrode 4: the right parietal region (16 contacts)

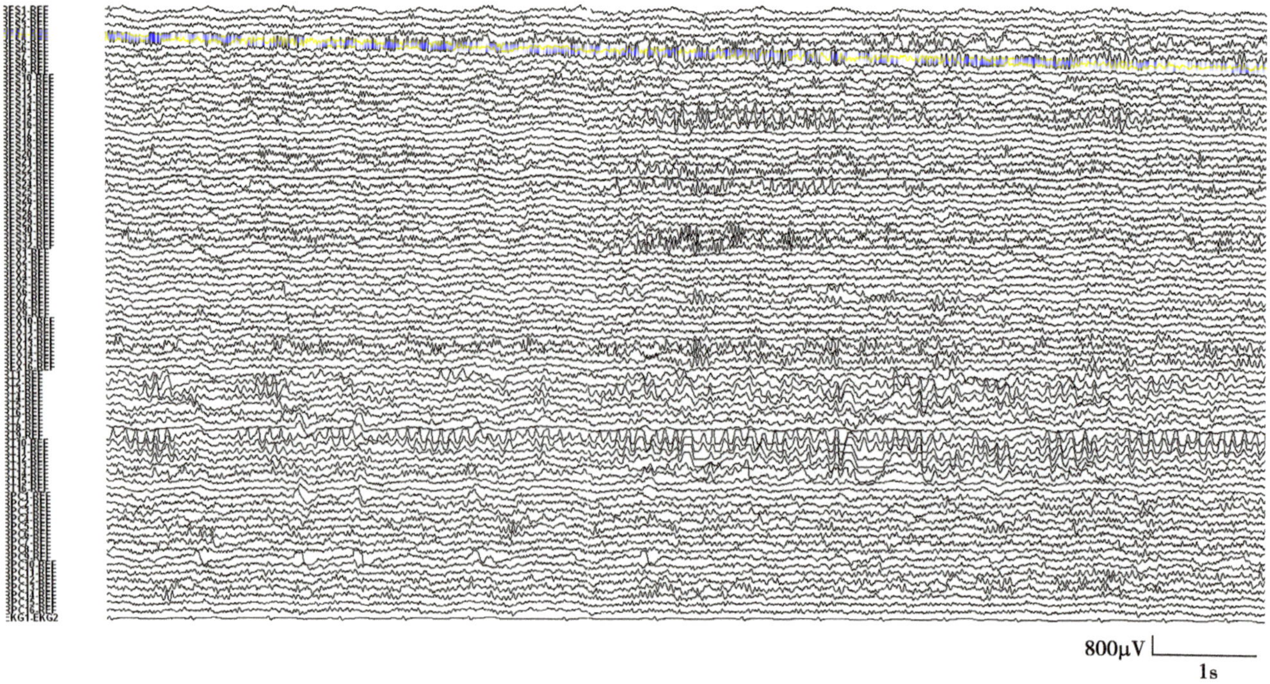

Fig. 4.19 Interictal intracranial EEG
Low-amplitude sharp waves over the right posterior frontal central region (contact numbers CH7, CH14, CH15, CH16, CH24), right posterior frontal region central region (contact numbers CH5, CH6, CH21, CH22, CH30, CH31, CH32), and low amplitude fast activities over the right inferior frontal gyrus (contact numbers CH45, CH46, CH47)

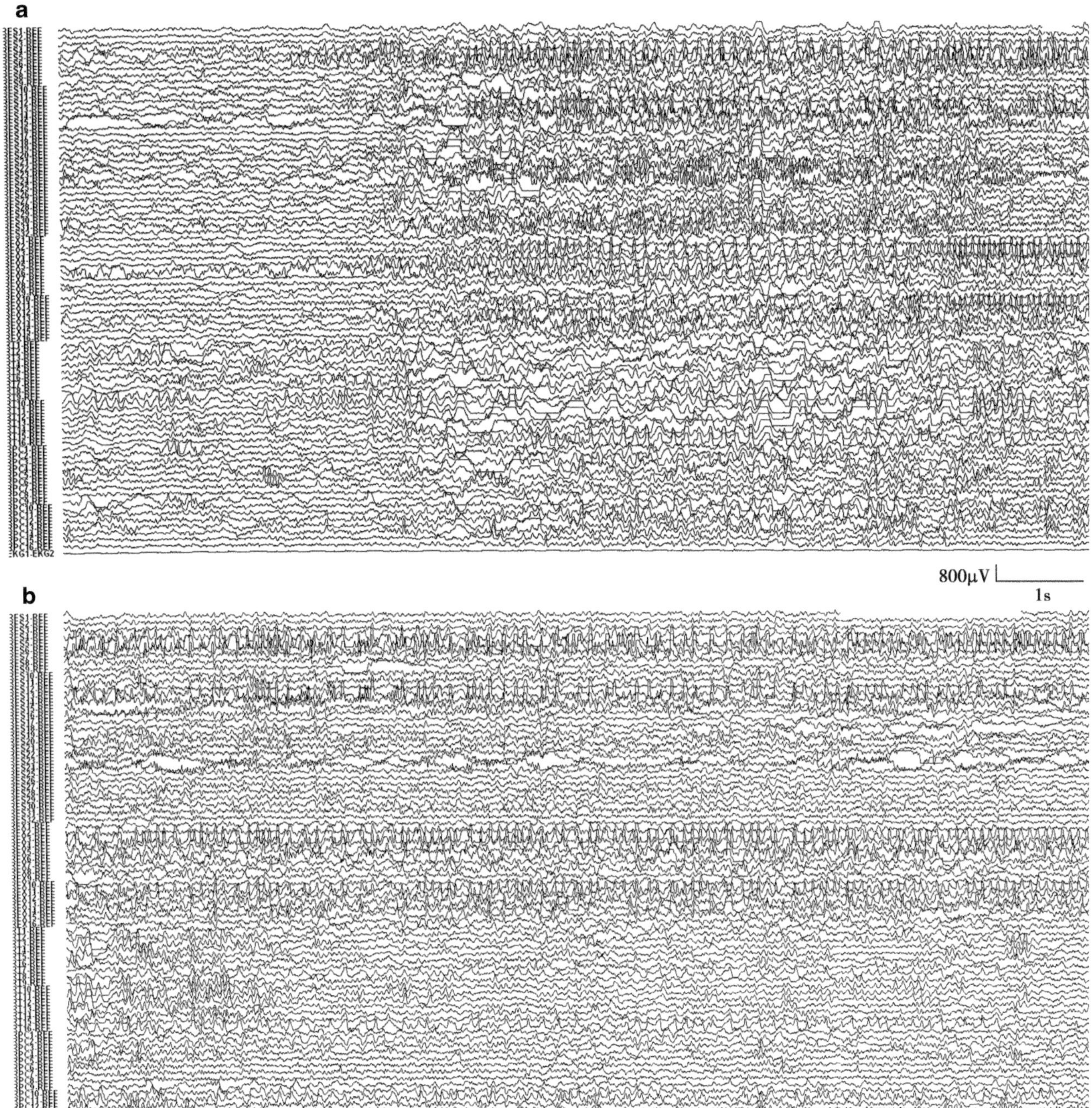

Fig. 4.20 Ictal intracranial EEG. (**a**) The patient was asleep. The IEEG showed sharp wave rhythm over the right posterior frontal central region (contact numbers CH4, CH5, CH6, CH13), right inferior frontal gyrus (contact numbers CH34, CH35, CH36, CH43, CH44, CH45), right middle temporal region (contact numbers CH56, CH63, CH64), right parietal region (contact numbers CH74, CH75); low amplitude fast activities were seen over the right posterior middle frontal and central regions (contact numbers CH22, CH23, CH24, CH30, CH31, CH32). (**b**) The patient's eyes are open and have a vacant look. The IEEG showed sharp wave rhythm over the right posterior frontal and central region (contact numbers CH5, CH6, CH13, CH14), right inferior frontal gyrus (contact numbers CH34, CH35, CH43), and right middle temporal region (contact numbers CH64). (**c**) The patient has jerks of left mouth corner and deviation of head leftwards. The IEEG showed sharp wave rhythm over the right posterior frontal central region (contact numbers CH5, CH6, CH12–CH14), right inferior frontal gyrus (contact numbers CH34, CH35, CH43), and right middle temporal region (contact numbers CH64). (**d**) The patient has clonic movements in her head and left limbs. The IEEG showed sharp wave rhythm over the right posterior frontal and central region (contact numbers CH5, CH6, CH13, CH14, CH15, CH21, CH22, CH30, CH31) and right inferior frontal gyrus (contact numbers CH36, CH37, CH38, CH45, CH46, CH47). (**e**) The patient had generalized clonus and tonicity of left limbs. The IEEG showed sharp wave rhythm over the right posterior frontal central region (contact numbers CH5, CH6, CH7, CH13, CH14, CH15, CH16, CH22, CH23, CH24, CH30, CH31, CH32), right inferior frontal gyrus (contact numbers CH36, CH37, CH38, CH39, CH45, CH46, CH47), right middle temporal region (contact numbers CH63, CH64), and right parietal region (contact numbers CH72).

c

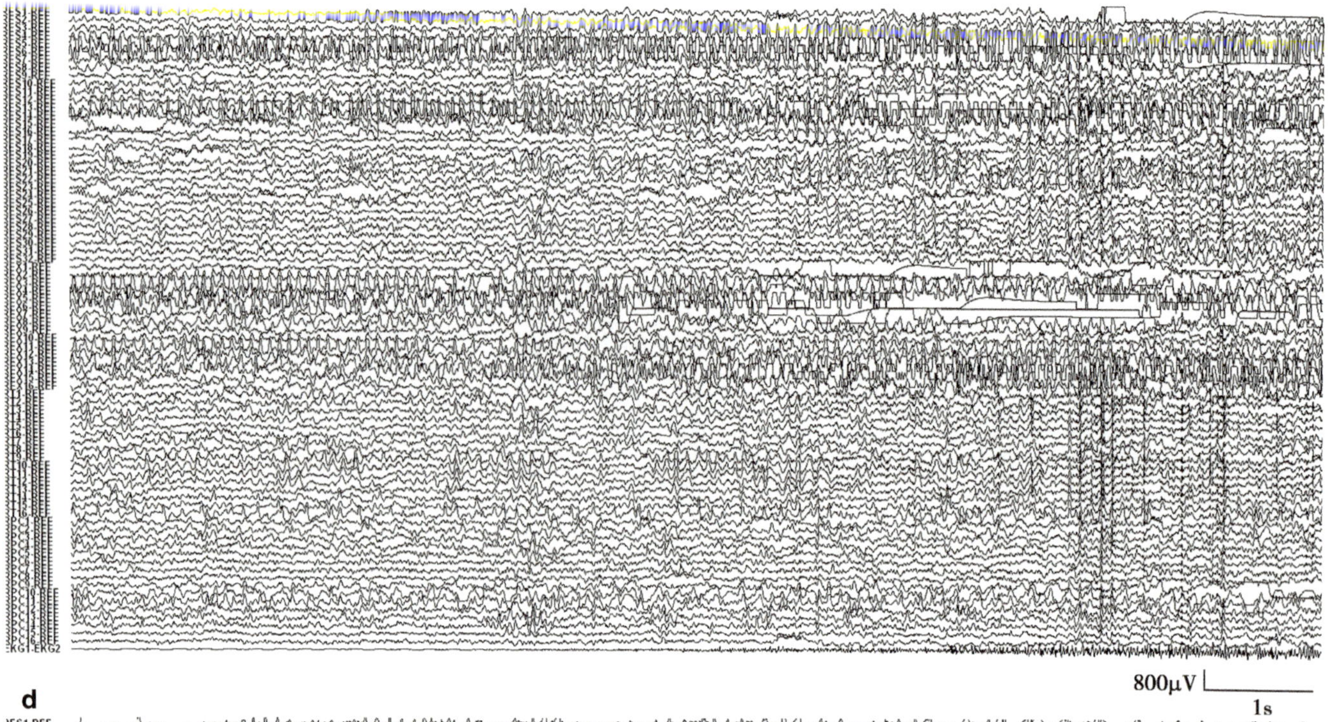

d

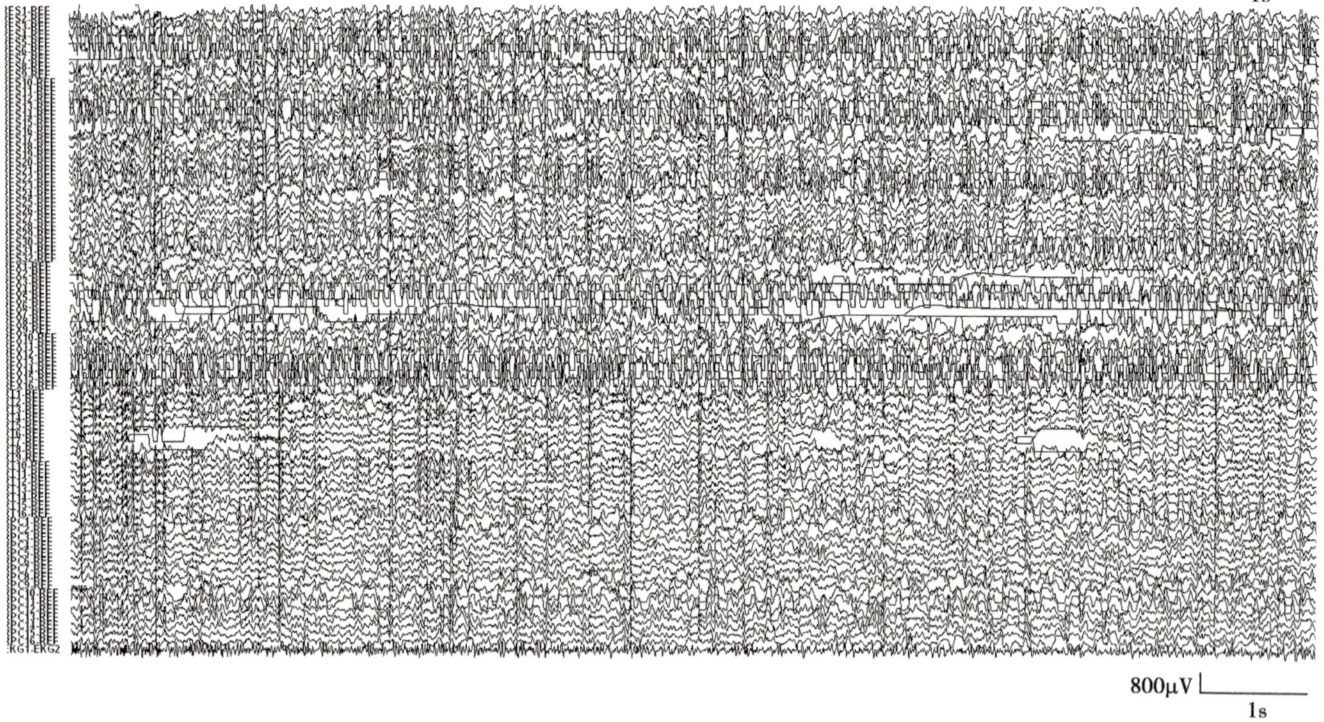

Fig. 4.20 (continued) (**f**) The patient had tonic clonus in left limbs and flexion clonus in right limbs. The IEEG showed the rhythm of spike-and-wave complexes. (**g**) The patient had generalized tonic clonus. The IEEG presentation was the same as **f**. (**h**) The patient had generalized tonic clonus. The IEEG presentation was the same as **f**. (**i**) The patient had generalized clonic convulsion. Rhythm of 2.0–3.0 Hz polyspike and wave complexes were seen.Fig. 4.20 (continued) (**j**) The patient has bilateral clonus in her upper extremities at gradually decreasing frequency. Rhythms of 2.0 Hz polyspike and wave complexes were seen. (**k**) The patient has persistent clonus in bilateral upper extremities. Rhythms of 1.5–2.0 Hz polyspike and wave complexes were seen. (**l**) The patient has clonus in upper right limb. Rhythms of 1.5–2.0 Hz polyspike and wave complexes were seen. (**m**) The patient's clonus in upper right limb discontinues. Rhythms of 1.0 Hz polyspike and wave complexes were seen. (**n**) The patient gasps coarsely. Rhythms of 1.0 Hz polyspike and wave complexes were seen. (**o**) At the end of the seizure, the patient becomes unconscious and fails to respond to calls. Rhythm of 1.0 Hz polyspike and wave complexes were seen; at the end of the seizure, the voltage is extremely depressed

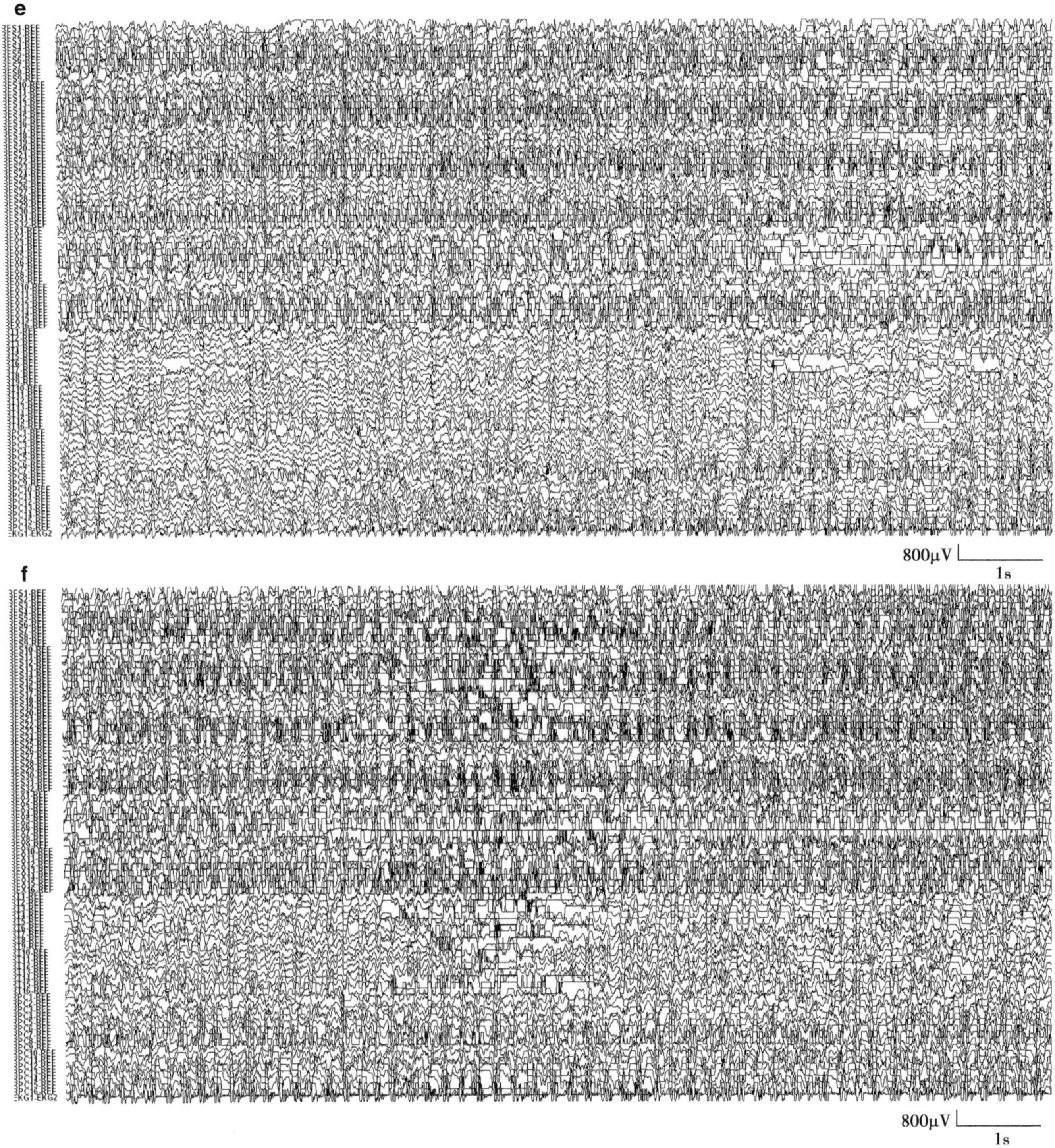

Fig. 4.20 (continued)

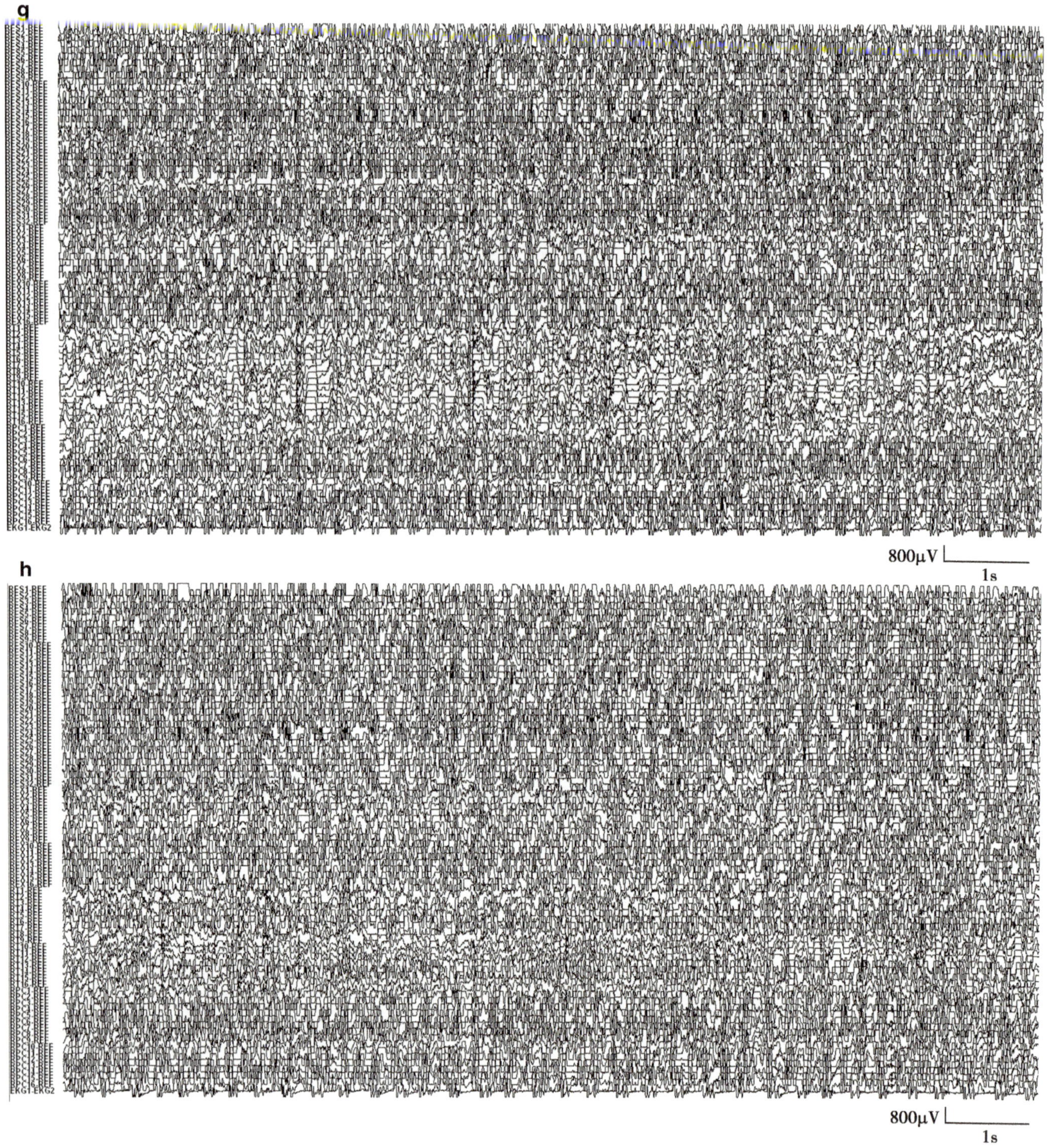

Fig. 4.20 (continued)

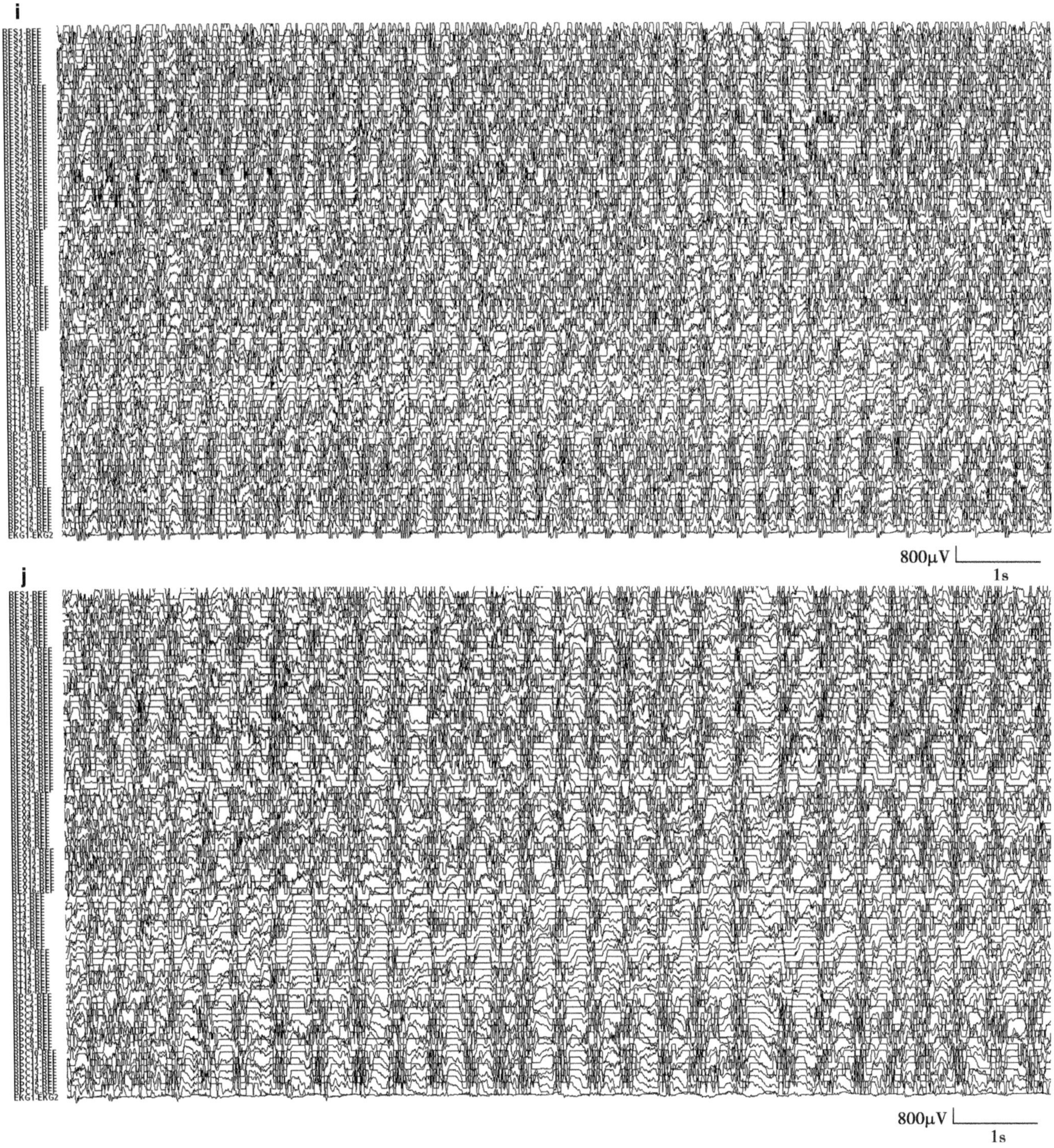

Fig. 4.20 (continued)

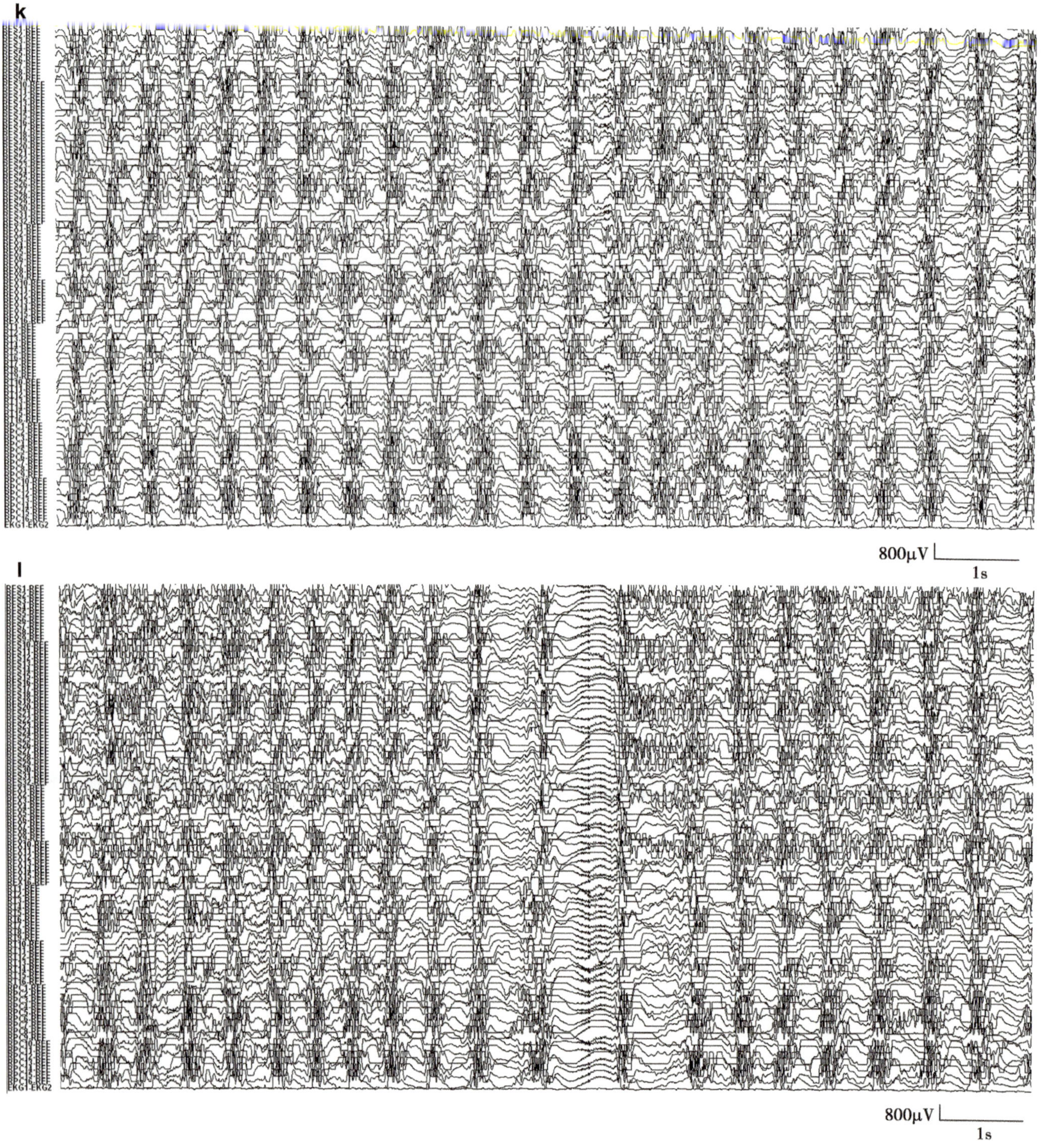

Fig. 4.20 (continued)

m

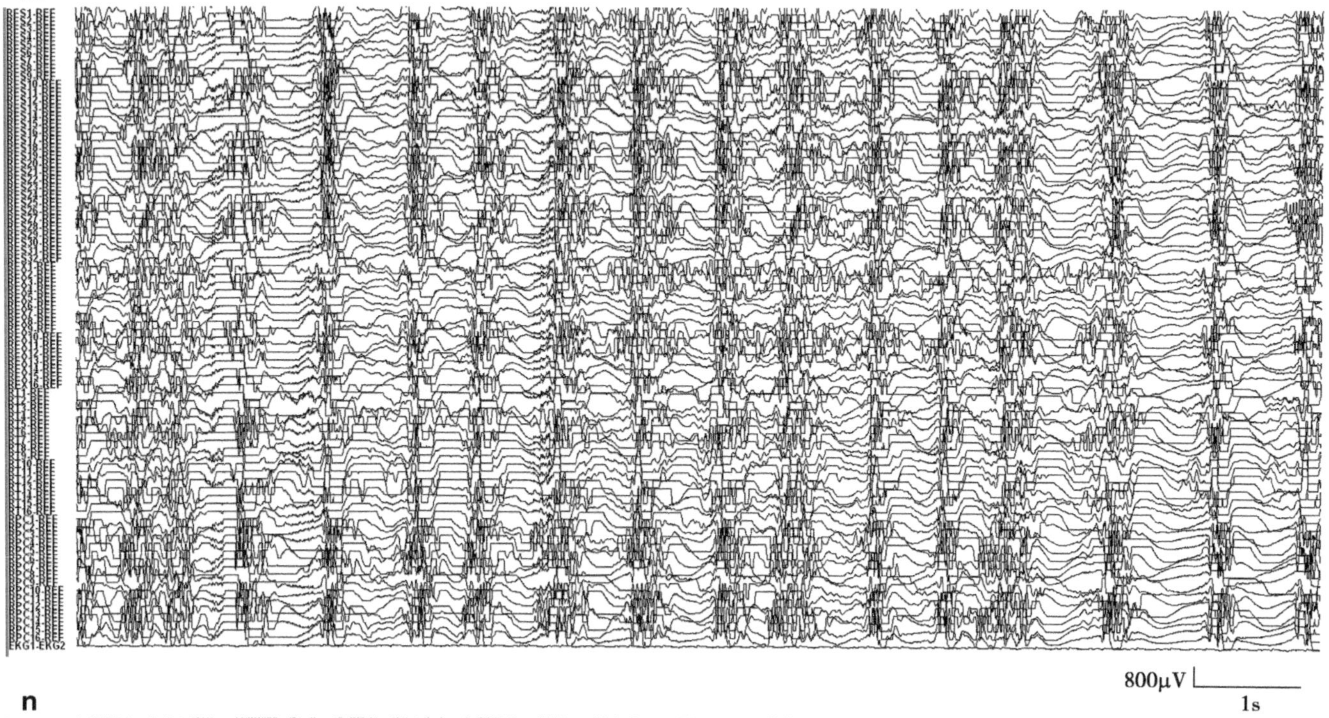

n

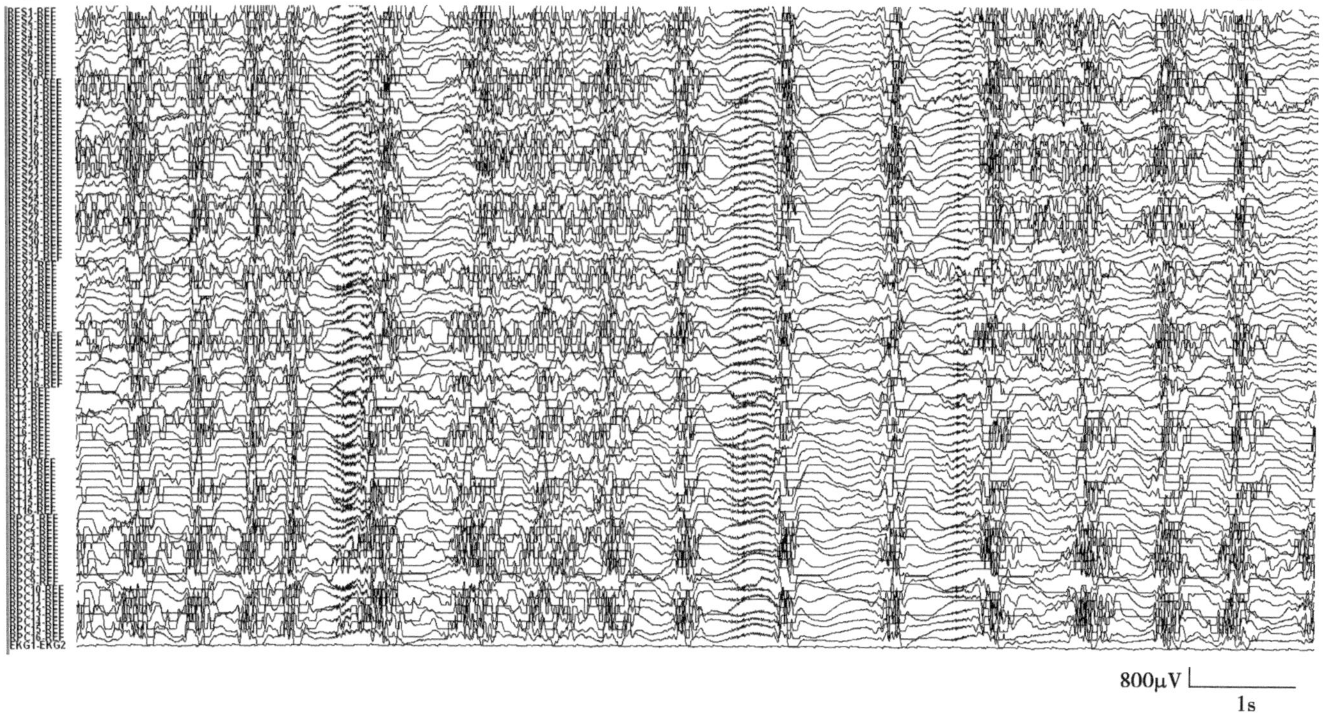

Fig. 4.20 (continued)

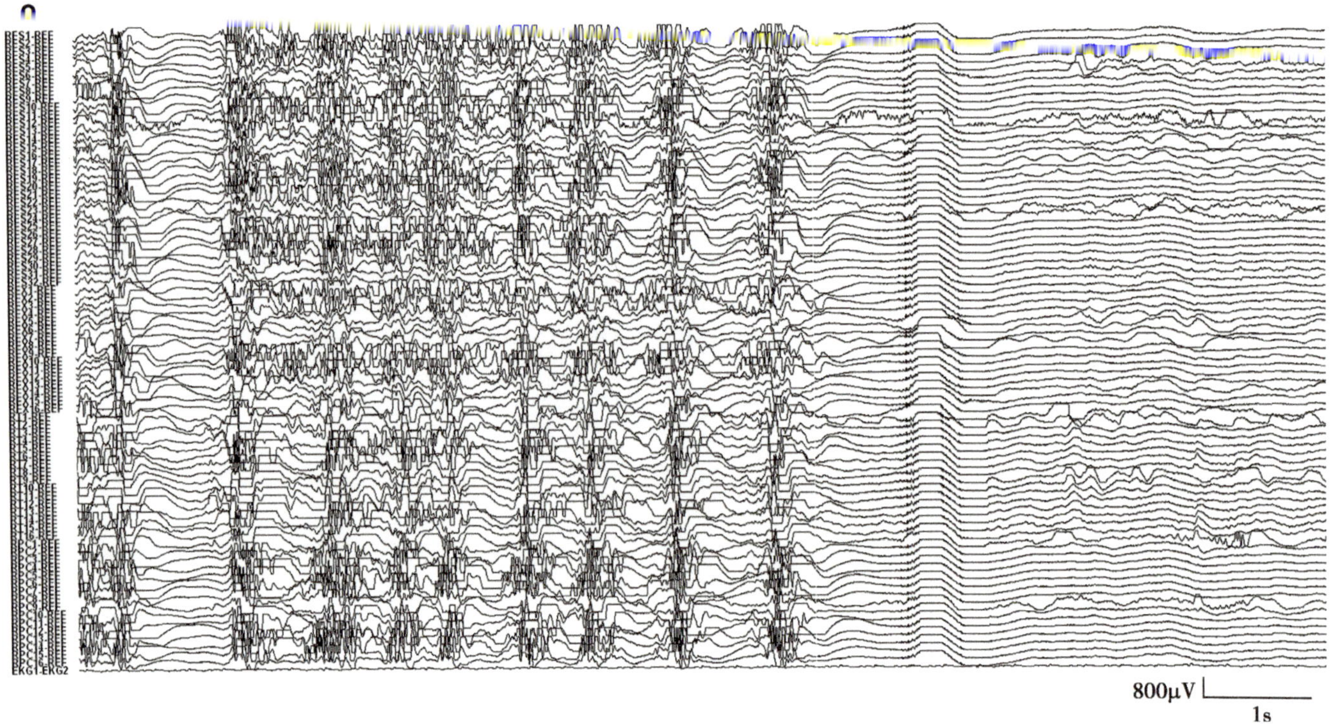

Fig. 4.20 (continued)

[Case Review]

1. *Case Characteristics*
   (a) *Seizure characteristics*: 1. In ictal phase, the patient had aphasia with weakness of left limbs but could understand others speech; afterwards, the patient would experience numbness in left limbs. Sometimes, the patient had two eyes staring leftwards and leftward distortion of mouth corner and secondary generalized tonic-clonic seizures. 2. The patient had definite aura(s), which could not be described clearly by the patient. 3. The patient suffered from several seizures a day.
   (b) *Imaging characteristics*: MRI showed no obvious abnormalities.
   (c) *EEG characteristics*: The interictal EEG showed sharp waves over the bilateral sphenoidal electrode, a few spike-and-wave complexes were observed over the bilateral frontal region, and sharp waves were identified over the right temporal region; ictal EEG showed sharp waves over the right temporal region.
2. *Diagnosis and treatment strategies and follow-up results*: The patient's seizure symptoms included weakness and subsequent numbness of left limbs and, occasionally leftward distortion of mouth corner and secondary generalized tonic-clonic seizures; the patient had paraesthesia but could not explain it clearly; MRI revealed no significant abnormality; ictal EEG was recorded in right temporal region. At first, the epileptic foci were considered to be located in right posterior frontal region or parietal region in light of the seizure symptoms; however, ictal EEG revealed that the focus was in right temporal region; therefore, intracranial electrodes were implanted in right posterior frontal region, parietal region, and temporal region. EEG monitoring of seizures and electrical stimulation of cortex were performed to determine the sensory-motor cortex. Interictal IEEG revealed that abnormal discharge was localized in central zone of the right posterior frontal region; ictal IEEG revealed that the focus was in right posterior frontal and central regions. In light of this, the postcentral gyrus cortex was surgically resected. In the 2-year follow-up period, the frequency of seizures was decreased significantly. IEEG demonstrated that the origin of seizure was definite but extended to the motor cortex; as a result, the resection of the epileptic focus was incomplete. In spite of this, after the surgical operation, the patient achieved good results because the epileptic network had been partially destructed.

Cases of Posterior Parietal Epilepsy

Case 4.5 Left Posterior Parietal Epilepsy

[Abstract of Medical Records]
Male, 21 years old.

1. *Chief complaint*: Paroxysmal numbness of right hand and twitch of right limbs for 15 years.
2. *History of present illness*: The patient experienced febrile convulsion (39.4 °C) and subsequent convulsion of limbs, head tilt back and loss of consciousness 15 years ago (at 6 years old); the symptoms lasted for about 30 min. The patient's seizure frequency has been 5–6 episodes a year since then. Oral sodium valproate shows no notable efficacy. In 1997, the patient was diagnosed with epilepsy by a local hospital and treated with oral TCM preparation(s). The patient's seizures gradually disappeared. The patient discontinued the antiseizure medication in 2000; in autumn of 2004, the patient's seizure recurred. The patient told the family that he experienced the numbness in his right hand and had subsequent jerks of the right arm, right leg and left limbs. The patient was conscious, able to open mouth but incapable of talking. The symptoms lasted 2–3 min. The patient went to hospital again and was prescribed carbamazepine, 300 mg/dose, tid., for treatment. The seizure frequency was decreased to 1–2 episodes a year, mostly occurred at 5 a.m. The seizure types were the same as before. At present, the patient is on oral carbamazepine, 200 mg/dose, tid.
3. *Personal history*: Obstructed labor at birth.
4. *Physical examination*: The patient had poor memory. No other neurological abnormalities were found.
5. *Imaging examination*: MRI revealed large patch of irregular low T1 and high T2 signals of ambiguous boundary in left frontal-parietal lobe and right temporal lobe; the heterogeneous signal intensity within the lesion. The cerebral surface gyrus was structurally disorder.
6. *EEG*: For details, see Figs. 4.21 and 4.22.

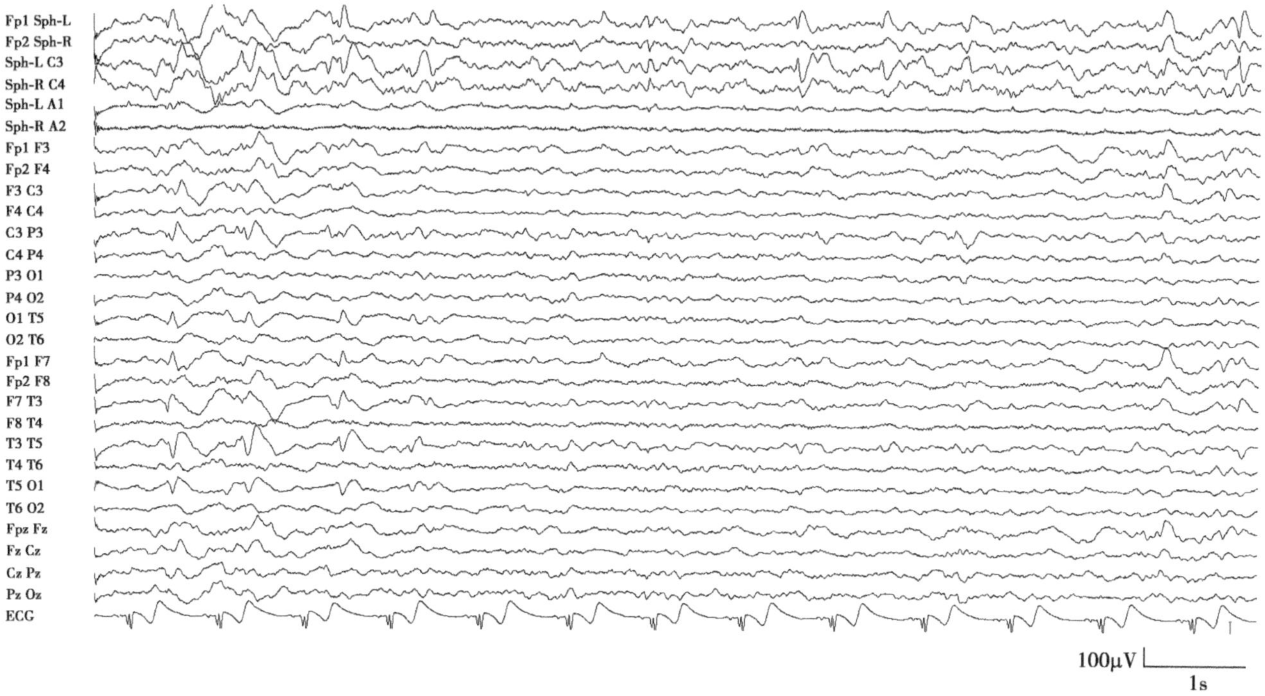

Fig. 4.21 Interictal scalp EEG
Sharp waves and sharp-and-wave complexes were seen over the left temporal (T3, T5), central (C3), frontal (Fp1, F3), and occipital (O1) regions; sharp waves were seen over the left sphenoidal electrode (Sph-L)

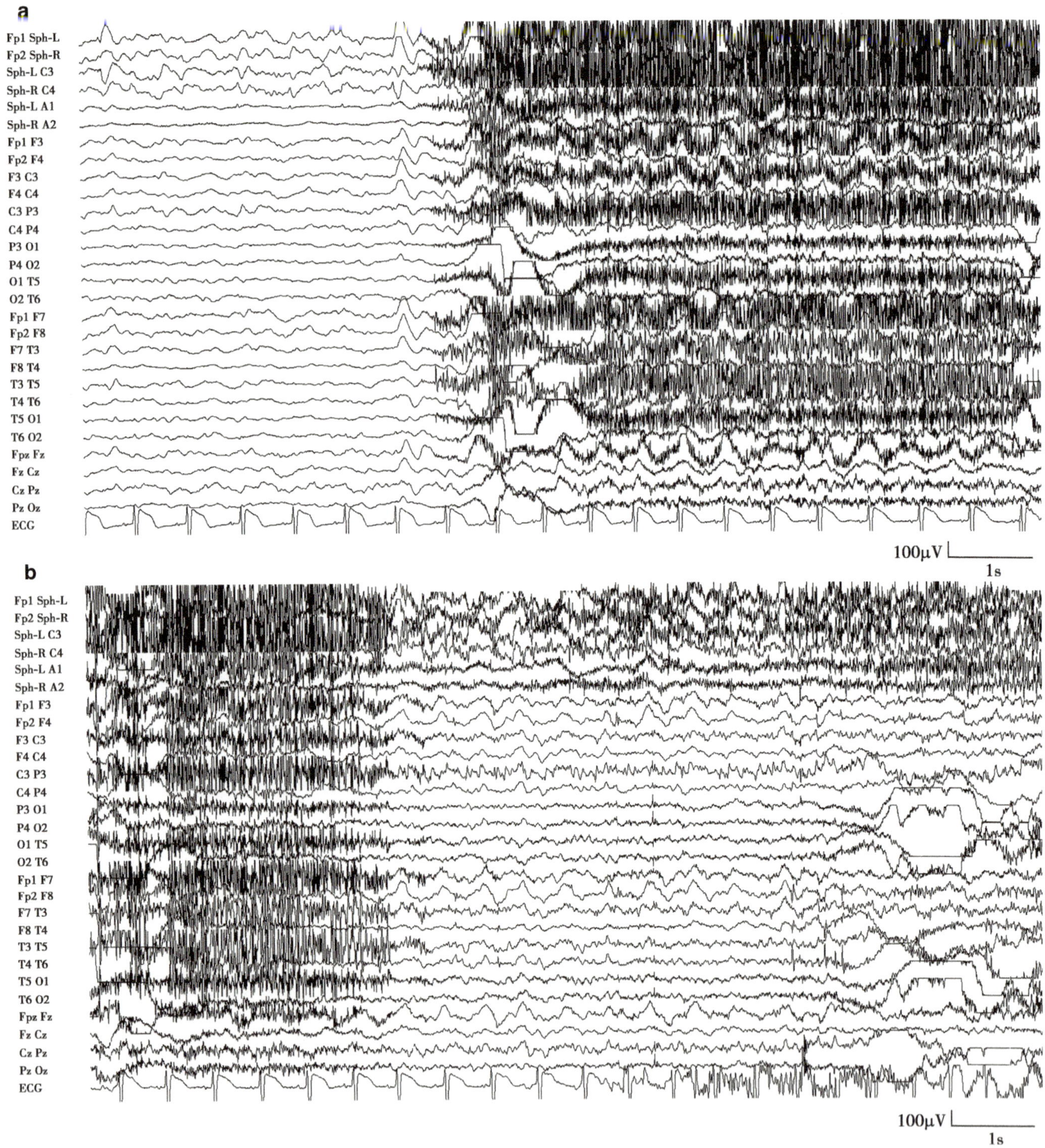

Fig. 4.22 Ictal scalp EEG. (**a**) The patient woke up from sleep. The Phase I sleep EEG showed mixed EMG artifacts after the patient woke up and slow wave rhythm. (**b**) The patient called "papa," then tonic-clonic seizure appeared in the patient's right hand, followed by superducting of upper left limb. EEG manifestations: slow waves over the bilateral frontal (Fp1-F3, Fp2-F4, Fp1-F7, Fp2-F8) regions; sharp waves, low amplitude fast activities over the left central (C3-P3) regions. (**c**) The patient's body deflected rightwards with tonic clonus in right limbs. Mixed EMG artifacts were seen. (**d**) The patient had generalized tonic clonus. The patient's EEG manifestations were the same as shown in **c**. (**e**) The patient had generalized tonic clonus. The patient's EEG manifestations were the same as shown in **c**. (**f**) The patient had generalized tonic clonus. The patient's EEG manifestations were the same as shown in **c**. (**g**) The patient experienced generalized clonus at gradually decreasing frequency. The EEG showed rhythms of generalized spike-and-wave complexes and polyspike and wave complexes, mixed with EMG artifacts. (**h**) The patient had clonus in the head and upper left limb at gradually decreasing frequency. The EEG showed generalized rhythms of 2.5–3.0 Hz polyspike and wave complexes, mixed with EMG artifacts. (**i**) The patient had minimal clonus in the head and upper left limb and the clonus gradually discontinued. The EEG showed rhythms of generalized 2.0–2.5 Hz polyspike and wave complexes, mixed with EMG artifacts. (**j**) The clonus discontinued and the patient kept gasping coarsely. The EEG showed rhythms of generalized 1.0–2.0 Hz polyspike and wave complexes, mixed with EMG artifacts. (**k**) The patient gasps coarsely. High-amplitude slow waves mixed with spikes and EMG artifacts were observed

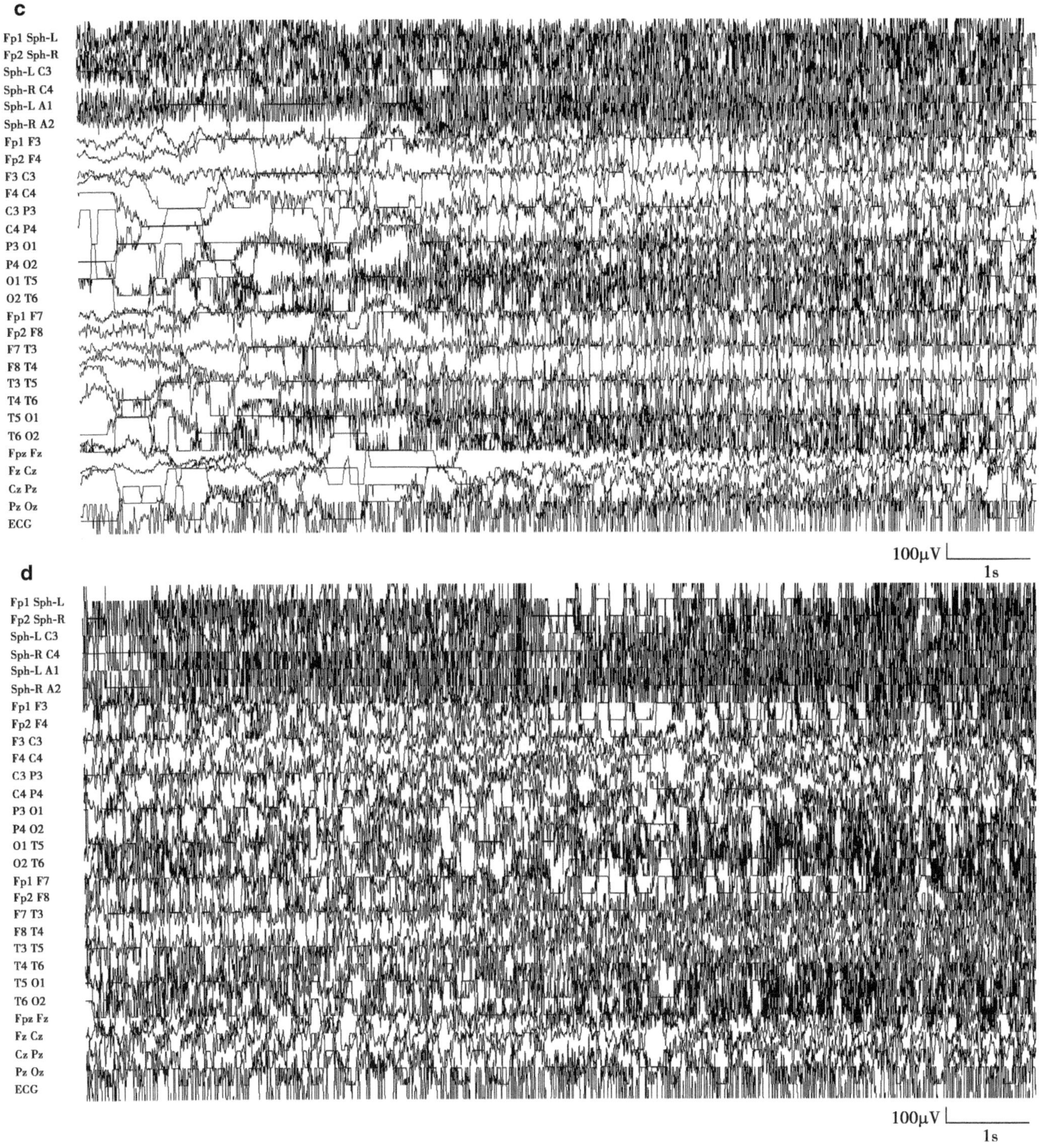

Fig. 4.22 (continued)

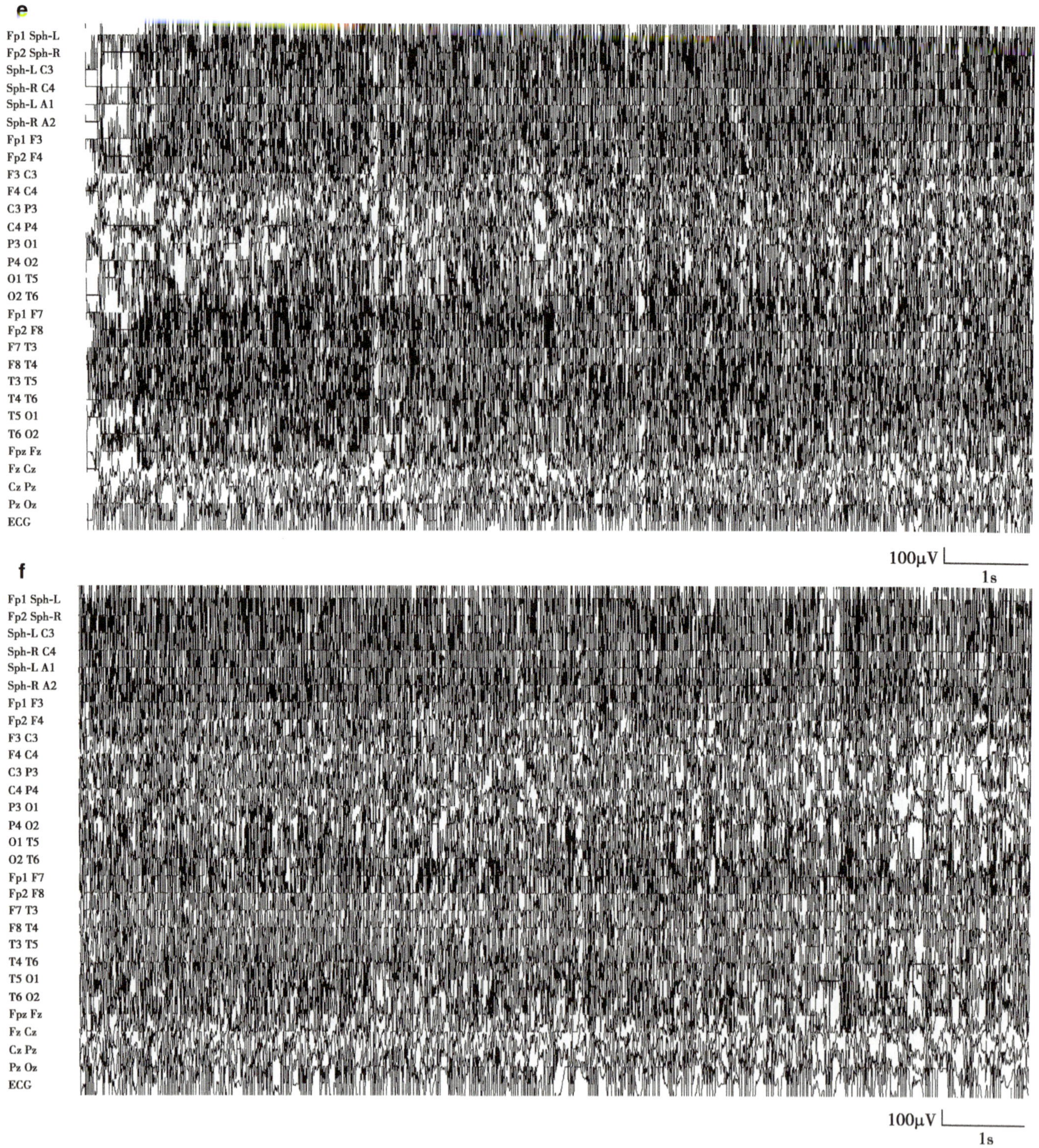

Fig. 4.22 (continued)

g

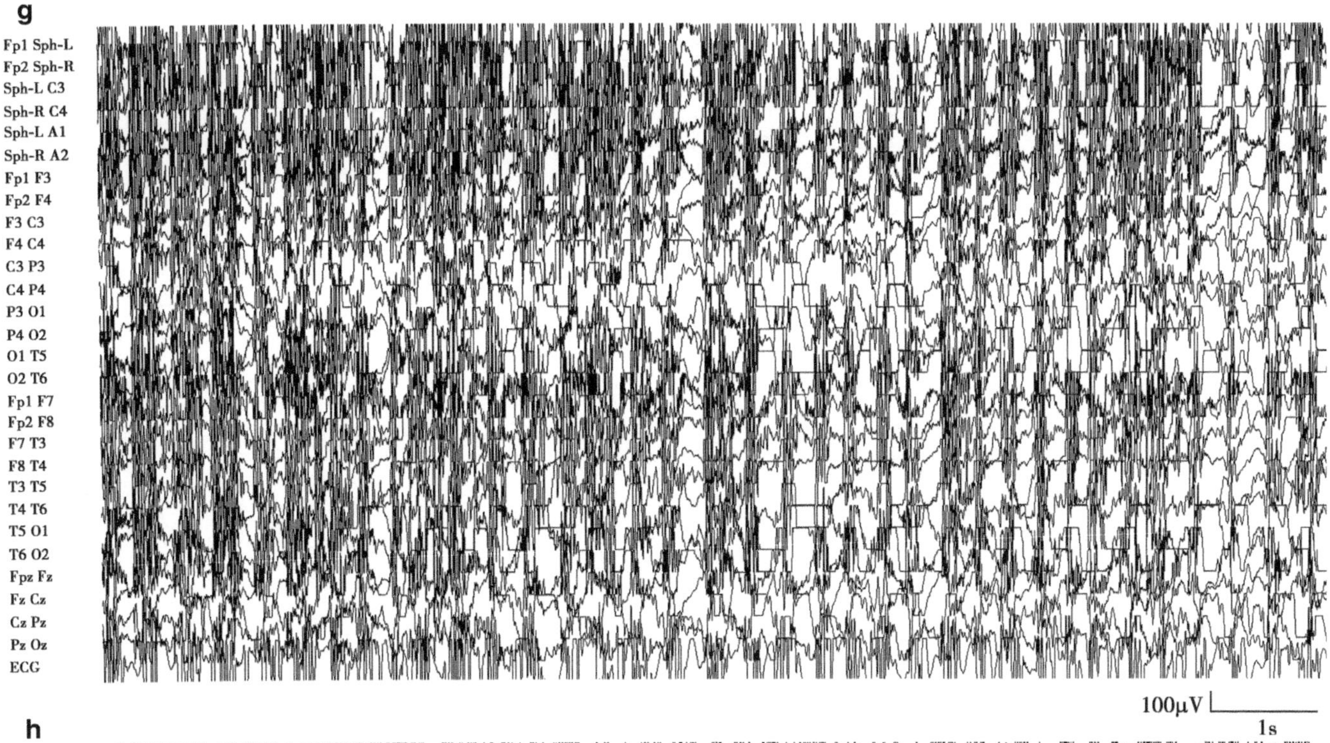

h

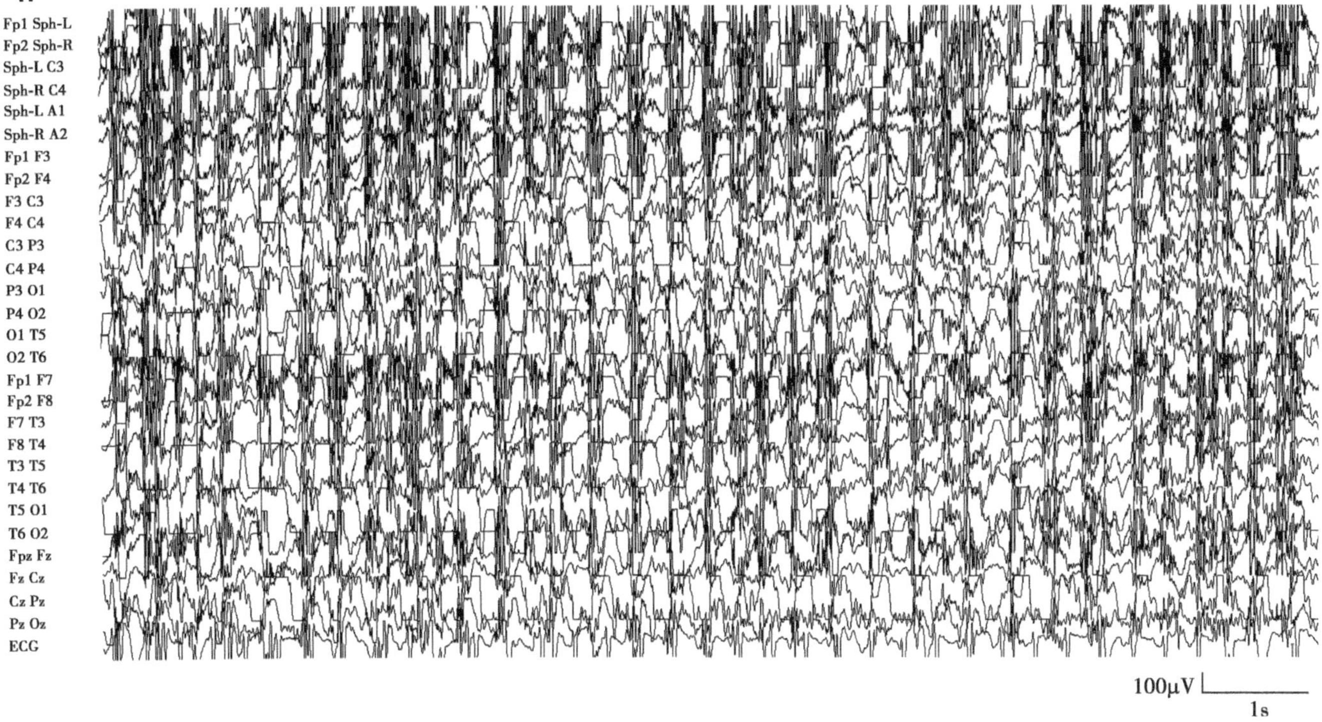

Fig. 4.22 (continued)

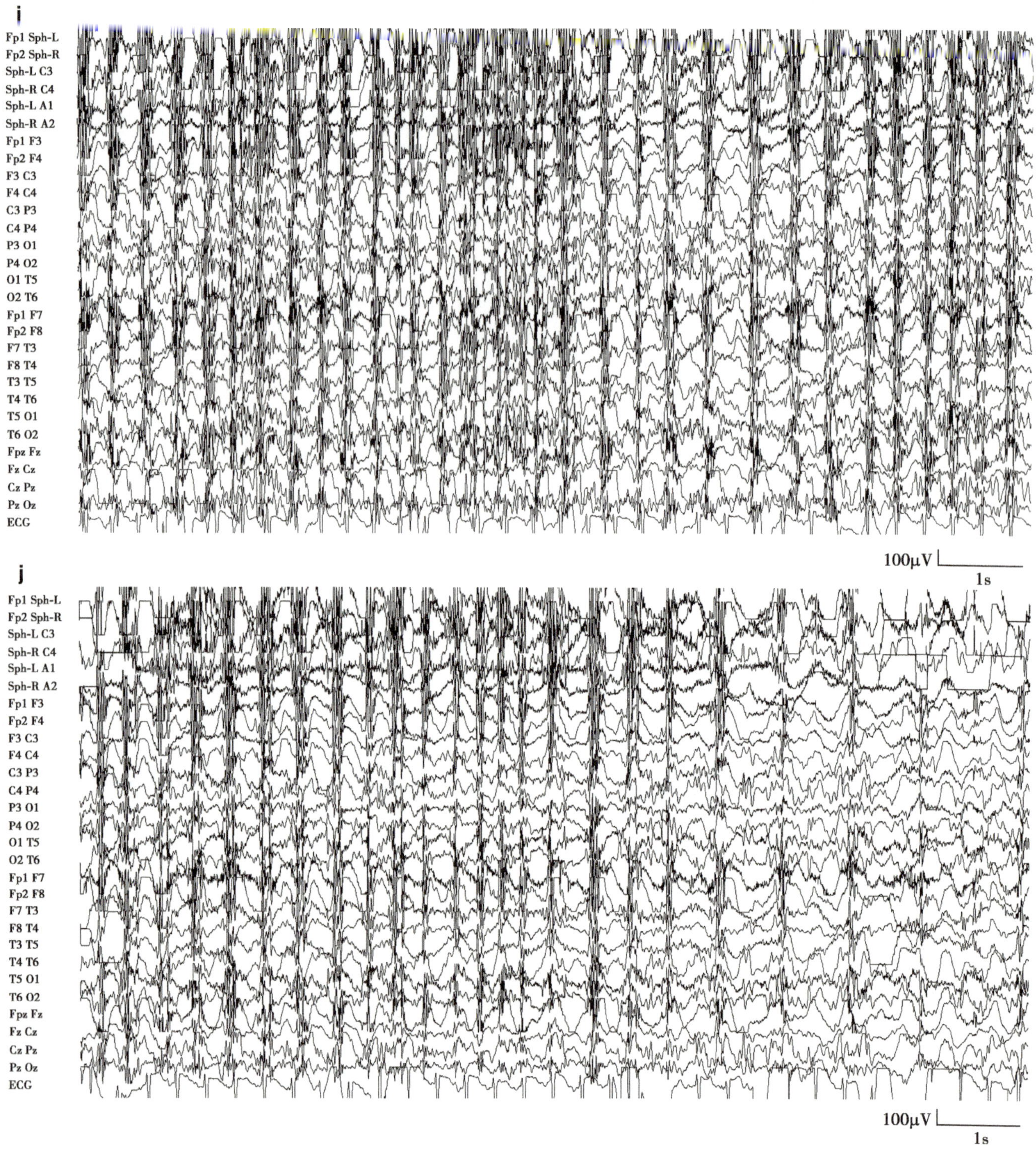

Fig. 4.22 (continued)

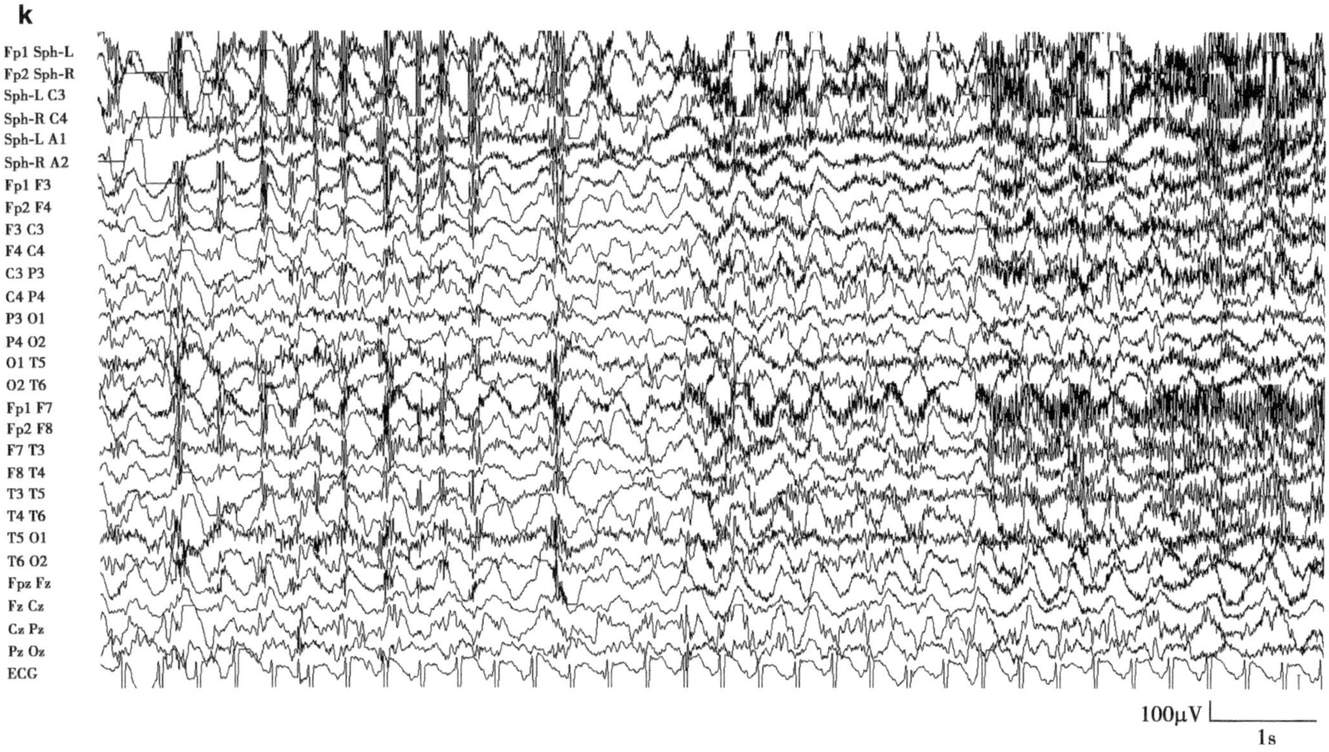

Fig. 4.22 (continued)

[Case Review]

1. *Case Characteristics*
   (a) *Seizure characteristics*: 1. The patient had numbness of right hand and gradually developed convulsion in right arm and right leg. 2. Definite aura (numbness of right hand). 3. 1–2 episodes a year.
   (b) *Imaging characteristics*: MRI revealed a large patch of irregular low T1 and high T2 signals in left frontal-parietal lobe and right temporal lobe; the boundary was ambiguous.
   (c) *EEG characteristics*: The interictal EEG showed sharp waves over the left sphenoidal electrode, central and temporal region; sharp-and-wave complexes were observed over the left frontal region, central, and temporal region; the interictal EEG showed slow waves over the bilateral frontal region.
2. *Diagnosis and treatment strategies and follow-up results*: The patient had definite seizure aura—numbness of right hand; MRI revealed abnormal signals in left frontal-parietal lobe and right temporal lobe; interictal EEG manifestations included multi-focal spikes in left side, and ictal EEG revealed slow waves in bilateral frontal regions. In the beginning, the epileptic focus was considered to be located in the left postcentral gyrus; in light of the abnormality found by MRI in left frontal-parietal lobe, the focus in parietal lobe and the peripheral epileptic focus could be directly resected. The inferior parietal lobules were partially resected. The seizures disappeared during a 1-year follow-up after surgery. The patient's seizure symptoms were in agreement with MRI suggestions. Therefore, the patient's lesions and epileptic focus were completely resected. After the operation, the patient achieved good results.

Case 4.6 Epilepsy in Right Posterior Parietal Cortices

[Abstract of Medical Records]
Male, 13 years old.

1. *Chief complaint*: The patient had paroxysmal loss of consciousness and twitch of four extremities for more than 9 years.
2. *History of present illness*: The patient was unconscious for several days after a fall from a height 9 years ago (at 4 years old), and when waking up, he had weakness in his left limb and sometimes episodic falls, which were not treated. After 1 year, the patient experienced involuntary swaying of left upper limb several times a day and received carbamazepine therapy. He had aura, which could not be accurately expressed, followed by tonicity of the left limbs, and to a greater extent by strong bilateral convulsion of the limbs, with head and eyes deflected, and the seizure lasted for several minutes; the mental state was poor at the end of the seizure, and the seizure occurred more often during sleep at night. Seizure frequency: 3–5 episodes/day. The patient visited a local hospital where carbamazepine therapy was administered but the therapeutic efficacy was poor. The patient is now on oral carbamazepine regimen, 100 mg/dose, bid. The number of daily seizure frequency varies.
3. *Personal and family history*: No history of associated diseases.
4. *Physical examination*: The patient was conscious and had decreased memory and poor intelligence. The patient has Grade 5 muscle strength in proximal end, Grade 3 muscle strength in distal end of left limbs, and Grade 5 muscle strength in right limb. The Babinski sign on the left side was positive.
5. *Imaging examination*: MRI revealed softening lesion(s) in right central parietal region.
6. *EEG*: For details, see Figs. 4.23, 4.24, 4.25, 4.26, and 4.27.

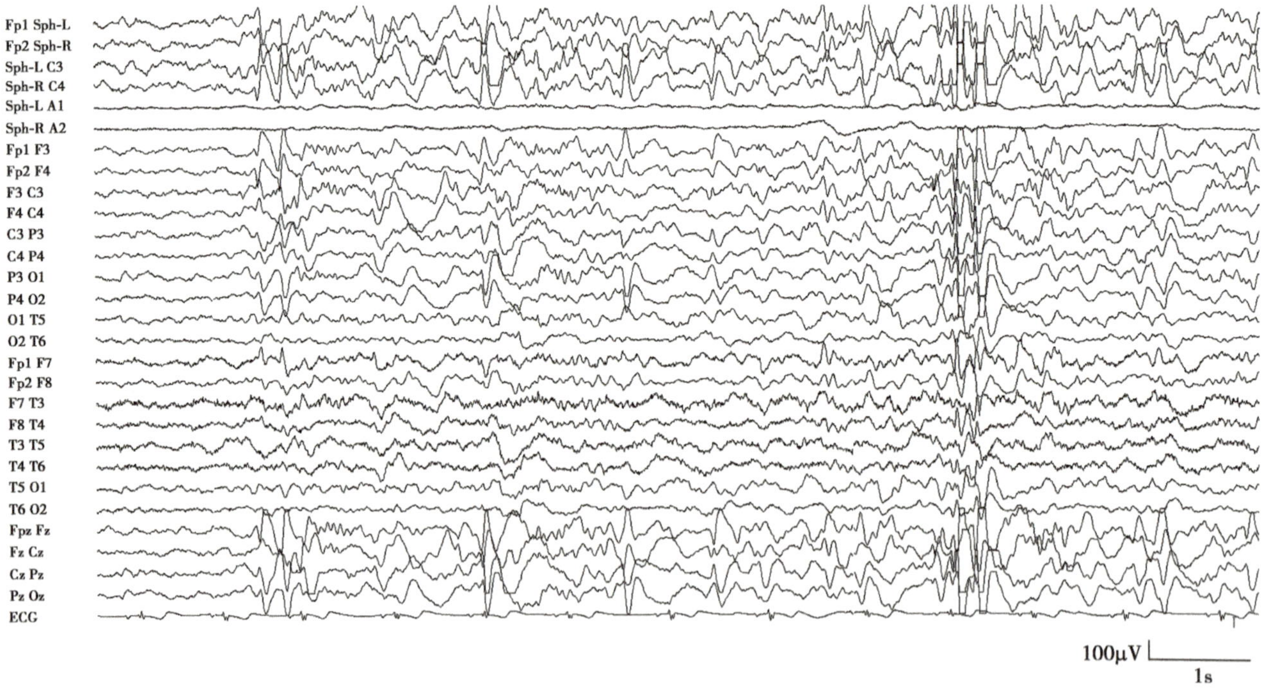

Fig. 4.23 Interictal scalp EEG
Sharp-and-wave complexes were observed over the bilateral posterior frontal, central, parietal, right temporal, midline leads; sharp waves were observed over the bilateral sphenoidal electrodes

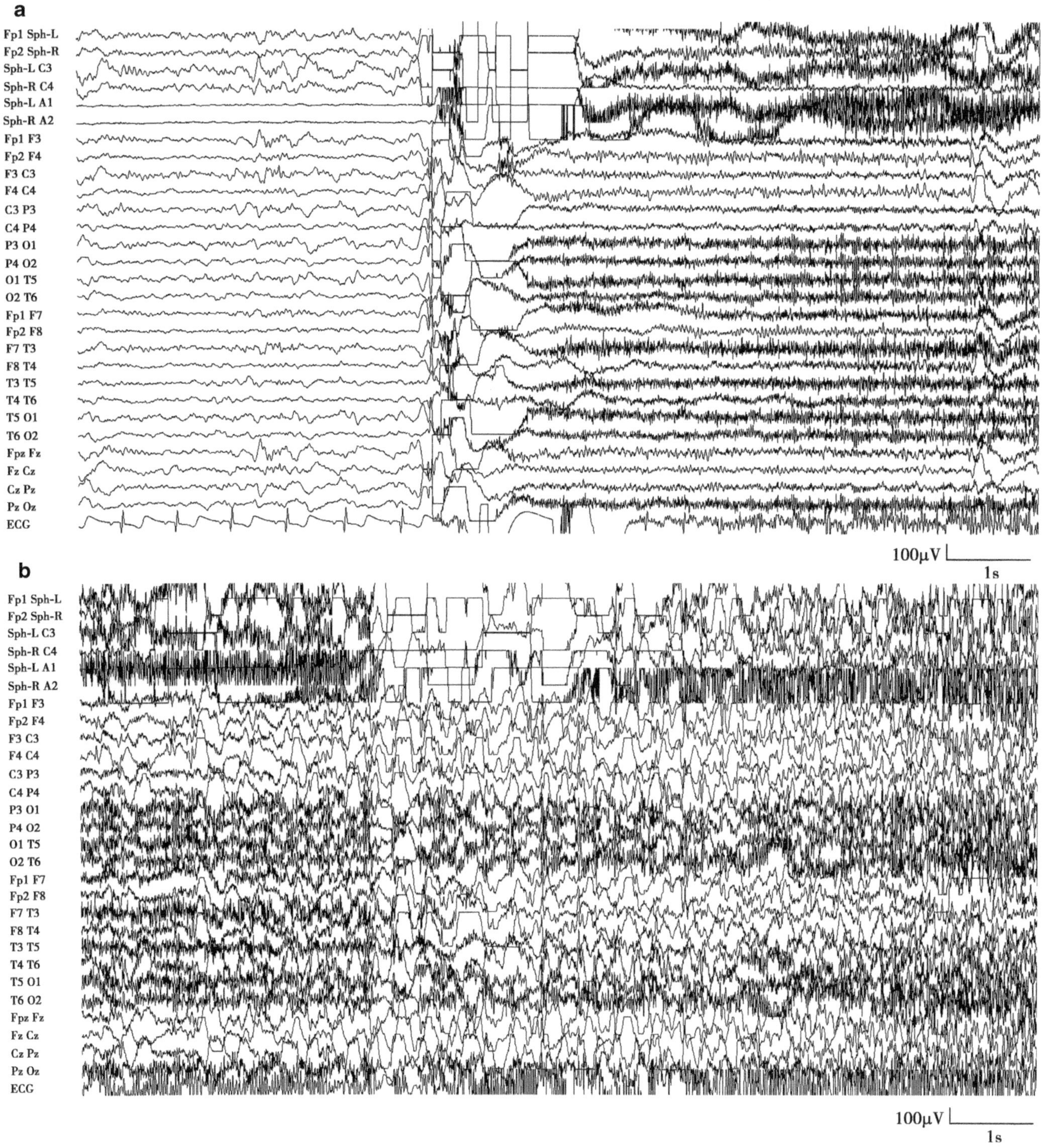

Fig. 4.24 Ictal scalp EEG. (**a**) The patient while sleeping abruptly raises both upper limbs in tonic state, then both lower limbs become tonic. EEG manifestations: the patient had characteristic of Phase II sleep background EEG. In ictal phase, spike-and-wave complexes were observed; afterwards, the electric deflection followed by low amplitude fast activity appeared, especially evident over the right posterior frontal region. (**b**) The patient had tonic-clonic limbs. Rhythms of spike-and-wave complexes were observed in EEG, especially over the right side. (**c**) The patient had tonic-clonic limbs. Rhythm of spikes mixed with EMG artifacts was observed. (**d**) The patient had tonic-clonic limbs. The patient's EEG manifestations were the same as shown in **c**. (**e**) The patient had inflexed and clonic extremities and significantly clonic upper left limb. Rhythm of spikes was observed. (**f**) The patient had mild clonus in both upper limbs. Spike rhythm was observed. (**g**) The patient's right upper limb was slightly clonic. Rhythm of spike-and-wave complexes were observed at gradually decreasing frequency. (**h**) The patient presented left upper limb jerks and bilateral lower extremities. The EEG showed extensive polyspike and wave complexes with artifacts; at the end of the seizure, the generalized voltage was lowered with artifacts

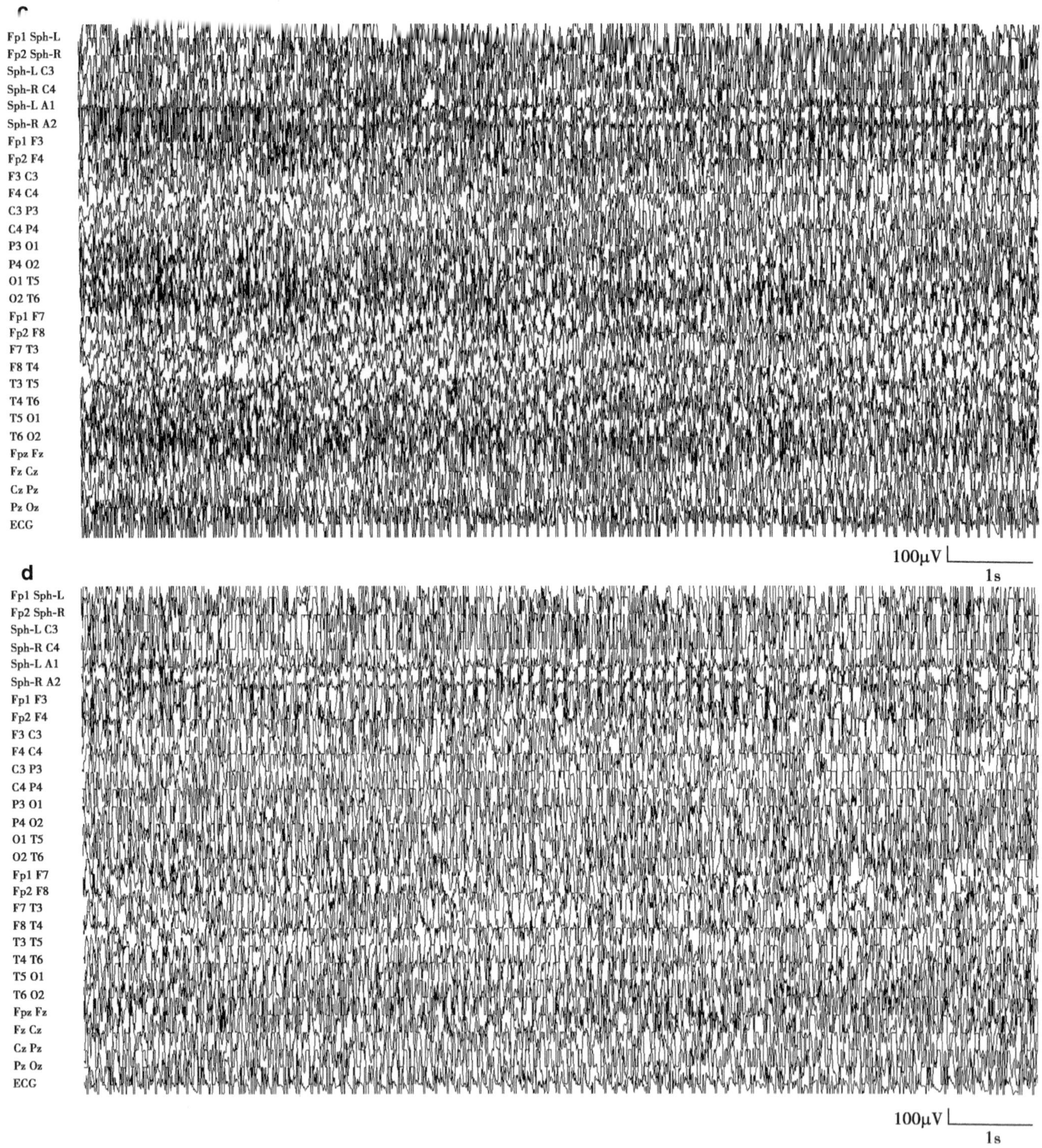

Fig. 4.24 (continued)

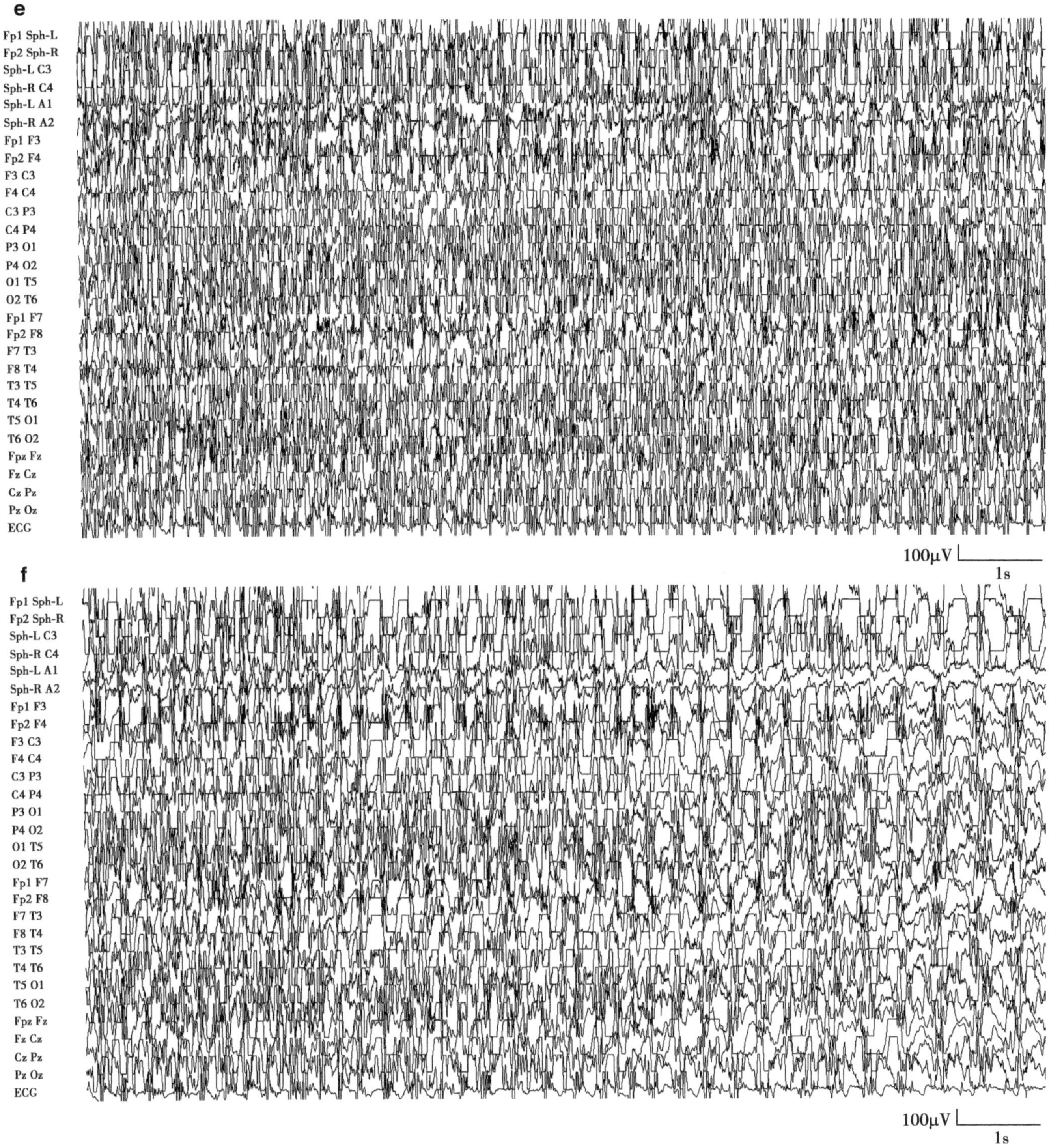

Fig. 4.24 (continued)

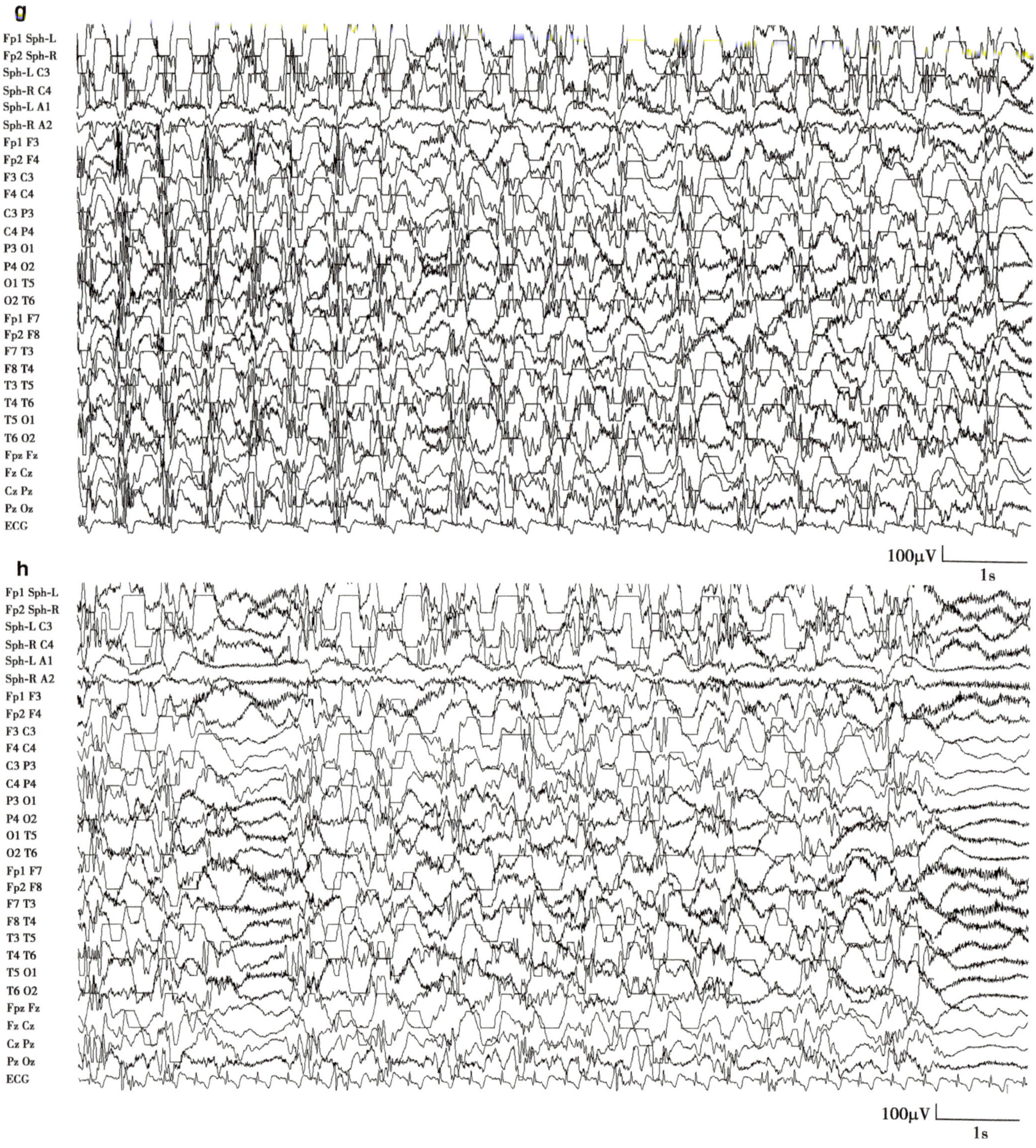

Fig. 4.24 (continued)

Fig. 4.25 Scheme of intracranial electrodes
Grid electrode 1: the central zone of right posterior frontal and central region (32 contacts); Grid electrode 2: the right posterior middle temporal region (32 contacts); Grid electrode 3: the right parieto-occipital region (32 contacts)

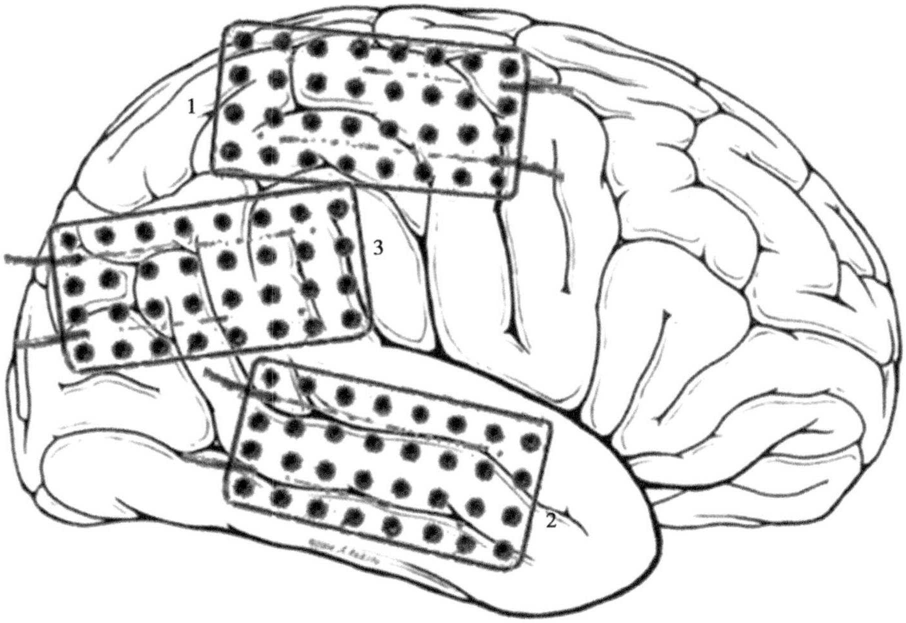

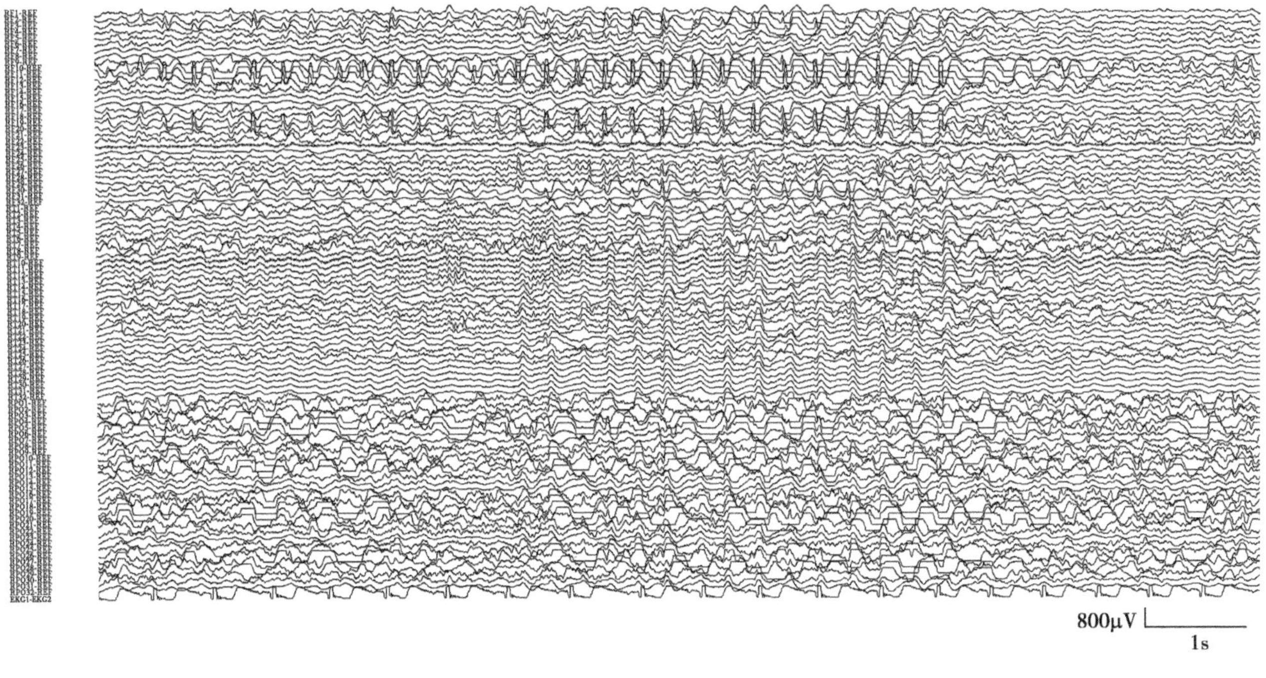

Fig. 4.26 Interictal intracranial EEG
Rhythms of sharp-and-wave complexes were observed over the right posterior frontal central region (contact numbers CH2, CH3, CH9, CH10, CH11, CH12, CH17, CH18, CH19, CH20, CH26, CH27, CH28, CH30, CH31)

a

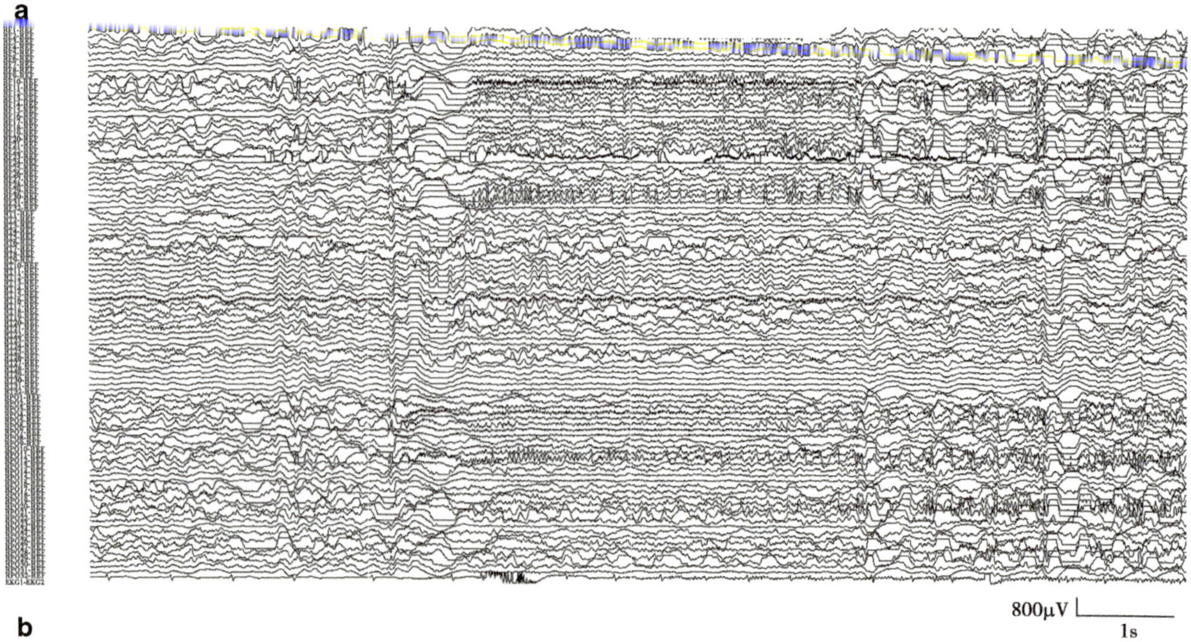

b

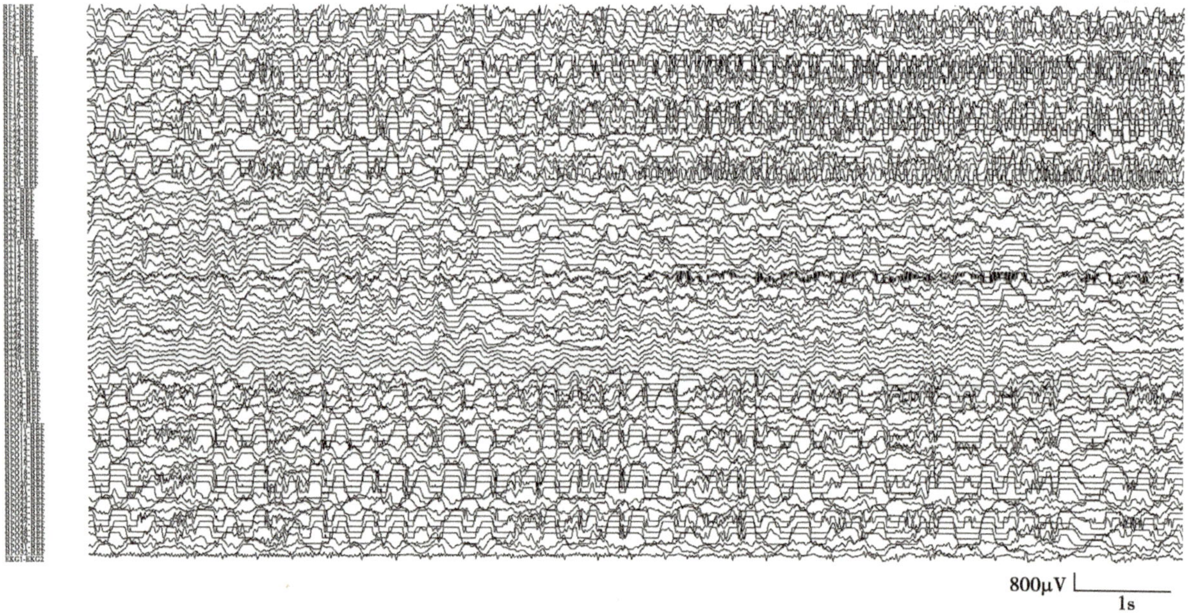

Fig. 4.27 Ictal intracranial EEG. (**a**) The patient while sleeping abruptly raises both upper limbs in tonic state, then both lower limbs become tonic. IEEG manifestations: low-amplitude fast rhythms were identified over the right parieto-occipital region (contact numbers CH67, CH68, CH75, CH76), right posterior frontal central region (contact numbers CH9, CH10, CH11, CH12, CH13, CH14); low-amplitude sharp wave rhythms were observed over the central region of right posterior frontal region (contact numbers CH29, CH30, CH31). (**b**) The patient had tonic-clonic limbs. The IEEG showed spike rhythms over the right posterior frontal, central region (contact numbers CH2, CH3, CH4, CH10, CH11, CH12, CH13, CH14, CH18, CH19, CH20, CH21, CH22, CH30), and rhythm of spike-and-wave complexes were observed over the right parieto-occipital region (contact numbers CH69, CH70, CH76, CH77, CH83, CH84, CH85, CH91, CH92, CH93). (**c**) The clonus of limbs in the patient gradually discontinued. The IEEG showed spike rhythm of gradually increasing amplitude over the right posterior frontal, central region (contact numbers CH2, CH3, CH4, CH10, CH11, CH12, CH13, CH14, CH18, CH19, CH20, CH21, CH22, CH30), and the rhythm of spike-and-wave complexes of gradually increasing amplitude were seen over the right parieto-occipital region (contact numbers CH69, CH70, CH76, CH77, CH83, CH84, CH85, CH91, CH92, CH93). (**d**) The patient showed clonus of limbs and made sounds from mouth. The IEEG showed spike rhythms over the right posterior frontal, central region (contact numbers CH2, CH3, CH4, CH10, CH11, CH12, CH13, CH14, CH18, CH19, CH20, CH21, CH22, CH30), and rhythms of spike-and-wave complexes were observed over the right parieto-occipital region (contact numbers CH69, CH70, CH76, CH77, CH83, CH84, CH85, CH91, CH92, CH93). (**e**) The patient showed clonus of limbs and made sounds from mouth. The IEEG showed rhythm of spike-and-wave complexes over the right posterior frontal, central region (contact numbers CH2, CH3, CH4, CH10, CH11, CH12, CH13, CH14, CH18, CH19, CH20, CH21, CH22, CH30), and right parieto-occipital region (contact numbers CH69, CH70, CH76, CH77, CH83, CH84, CH85, CH91, CH92, CH93). (**f**) The clonus of upper limbs in the patient gradually discontinued. The IEEG showed rhythm of spike-and-wave complexes over the right posterior frontal, central region (contact numbers CH2, CH3, CH4, CH10, CH11, CH12, CH13, CH14, CH18, CH19, CH20, CH21, CH22, CH30), and slow wave rhythms were observed over the rest remaining leads

c

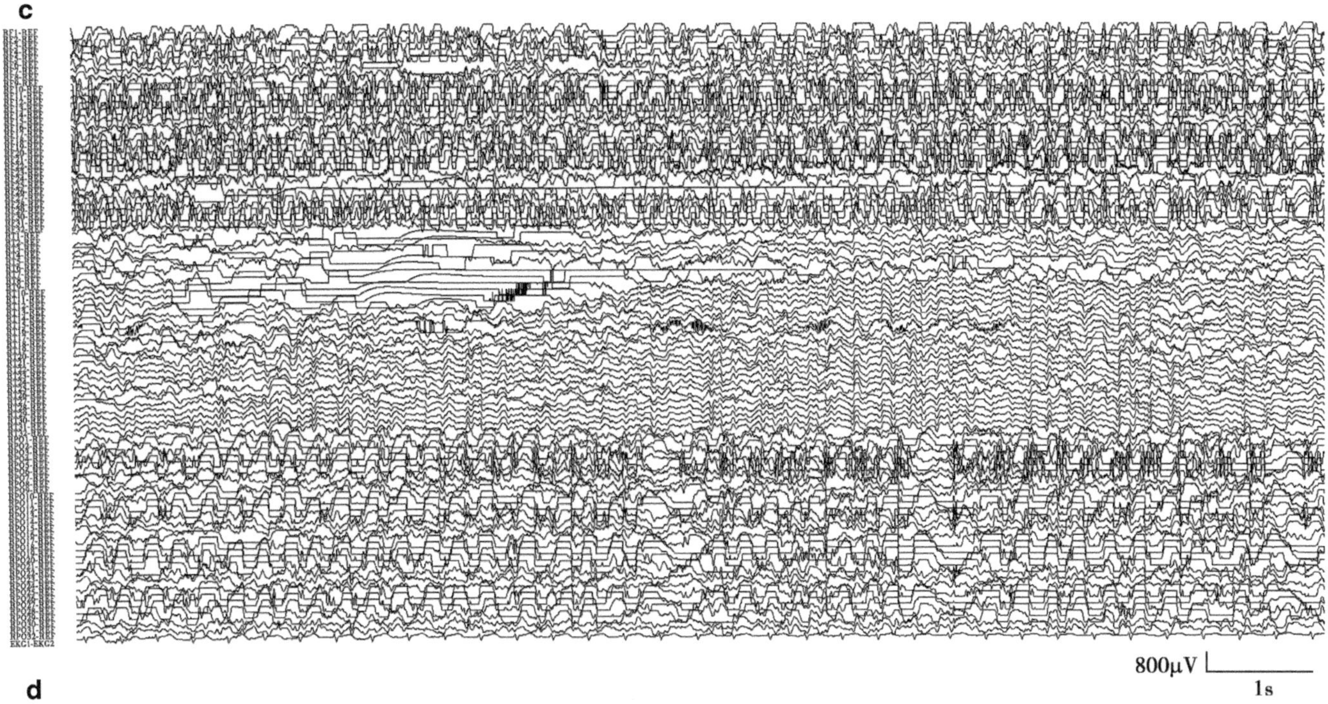

d

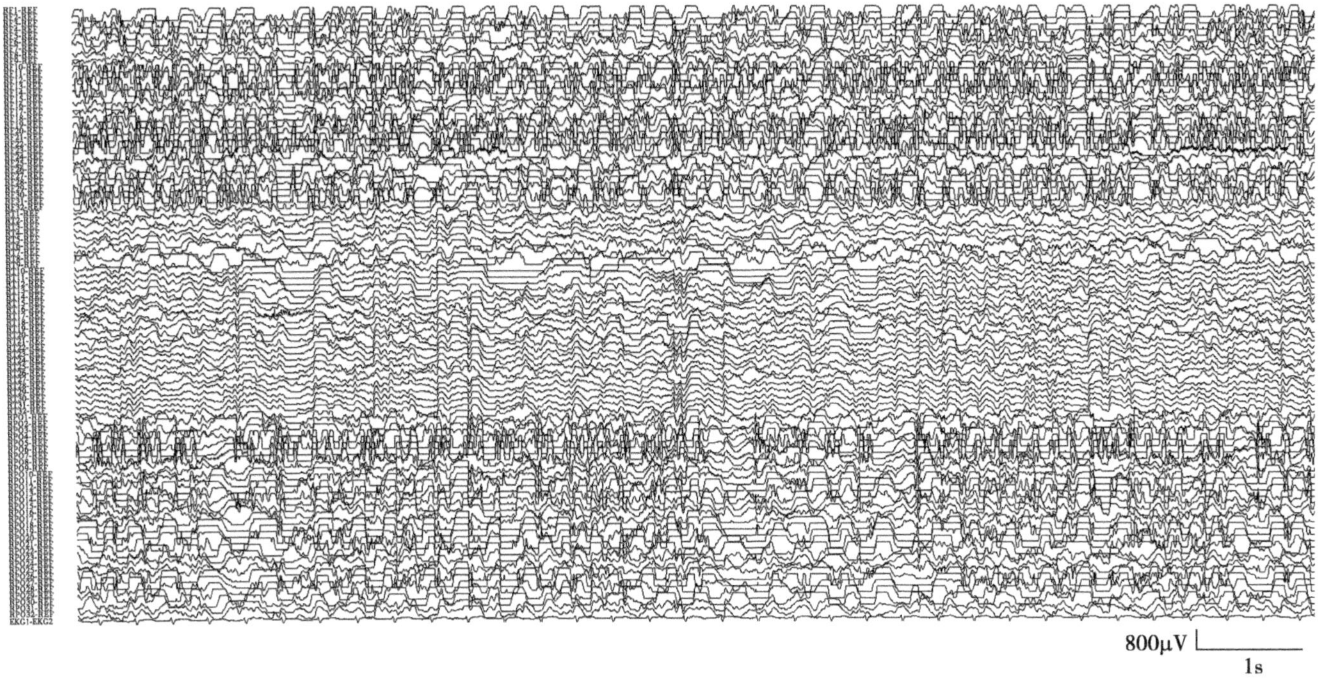

Fig. 4.27 (continued)

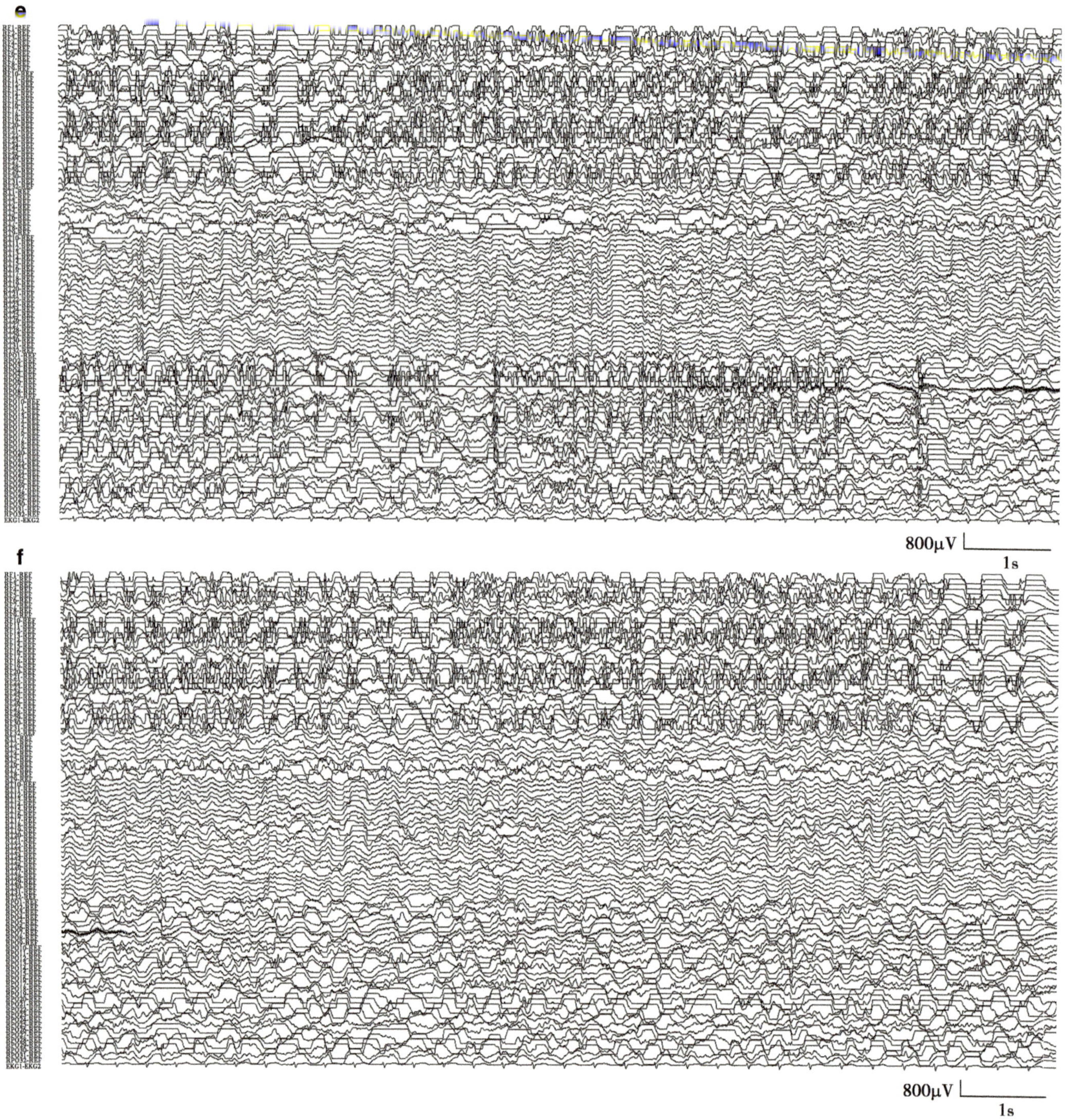

Fig. 4.27 (continued)

[Case Review]

1. *Case Characteristics*
   (a) *Seizure characteristics*: 1. Tonic-clonic seizure in left limbs, and secondary generalized tonic-clonic seizure, manifested as involuntary left upper limb jerks at early onset. 2. Aura(s) present, but the patient failed to give a clear description. 3. The patient had a history of head trauma at 4 years old. Since then, the patient has suffered from 3 to 5 episodes a day, mostly at night.
   (b) *Imaging characteristics*: MRI revealed softening lesion(s) in right central and parietal region.
   (c) *EEG characteristics*: Sharp-and-wave complexes were observed in the sleeping EEG of the patient over the bilateral frontal, central, parietal, right temporal, and midline region, especially the right side; during the ictal phase, sharp-and-wave complexes were observed; afterwards, low amplitude fast activity was observed, especially the right posterior frontal region.
2. *Diagnosis and treatment strategies and follow-up results*: The patient had stereotyped seizure symptoms, with tonic-clonic left limbs secondary to generalized clonic seizure; MRI revealed the presence of softening focus in right central parietal region, and the focus did not contradict the seizure symptoms. In light of the interictal and ictal EEGs, intracranial electrodes were implanted in right posterior frontal, parietal, temporal, parieto-occipital regions. Ictal IEEG manifestations: starting from right parietal region and rapidly involving the right frontal region. The right inferior parietal lobules and superior parietal lobules were partially resected. The seizures disappeared during a 1-year follow-up after surgery. As the patient's MRI revealed the lesion(s) and IEEG identified the origin of seizure definitely, the lesion(s) and the epileptic focus was completely resected by surgical operations. After the operation, the patient achieved good treatment results.

Cases of Occipital Lobe Epilepsy

5

Du Wei, Zhang Xiating, Yu Tao, Wang Li, and Yang Yingxue

Overview of Occipital Lobe Epilepsy

Anatomy of Occipital Lobe

Occipital lobe is located at posterior cerebral hemisphere. It is of triangular shape, with a blunted round tip called the occipital pole. In the medial surface of cerebral cortex, the boundary between the parietal lobe and occipital lobe is the parieto-occipital sulcus; the calcarine fissure that runs horizontally towards the occipital pole can be seen posterior to the posterior edge of corpus callosum; the calcarine fissure divides the occipital lobe into the dorsal cuneus and the ventral lingualis gyrus. According to the Brodmann areas, the occipital lobe consists of Areas 17, 18, and 19. The occipital lobe connects to other cerebral regions through many nerve tracts, including the superior longitudinal fasciculus, which runs above the insula, and the inferior longitudinal fasciculus, which runs shallowly between the lateral surface and the ventral surface of the occipital and temporal lobes; superior occipito-frontalis fasciculus is located deep in the hemisphere and surrounded by corpus callosum, capsula interna, cauda nuclei caudati, and lateral ventricle; inferior occipito-frontalis fasciculus is located at the root of temporal lobe below the insula and caudate nucleus and connects the basal surface of the frontal lobe and parietal occipital cortex; these fasciculi provide channels for rapid connections between the occipital lobe and frontal, temporal, and parietal cortex. Therefore, seizures that originated from the occipital lobe can easily spread to the ipsilateral frontal, temporal and parietal lobe, and even the contralateral lobe. Therefore, the characteristics of occipital lobe epilepsy are closely related to the anatomic structure and physiological functions of the occipital lobe.

D. Wei · Y. Tao (✉)
Department of Neurosurgery, Beijing, China
e-mail: Yutao@xwhosp.org

Z. Xiating · W. Li · Y. Yingxue
Department of Neurology, Beijing, China

Clinical Manifestations

The major clinical manifestations of occipital lobe seizure include various visual symptoms, including simple optical illusion, complicated optical illusion, loss of vision and visual illusion, etc. Simple optical illusion refers to the movement of monochromatic or colorful round spots or circles of varied quantity and size from one side to the other side of the field of vision; complicated optical illusion refers to the seeing of people, animals, objects, or scenarios that actually do not exist; loss of vision refers to transient partial or complete loss of vision; visual illusion means misinterpretation of the objects seen, such as magnification, shrinkage, zooming out, zooming in, or distortion. Some basic visual phenomena, such as flashing lights, amaurosis, etc., are probably originated from the visual cortex of occipital lobe; more complicated optical illusions are probably originated from the lateral occipital cortex. Other common symptoms of occipital seizure include paroxysmal rapid blinking, spasm of eyelid, staring, and palinopsia.

In patients who do not manifest aura(s), symptomatological localization would be in a dilemma. A seizure may propagate forwards by route above the lateral fissure, giving rise to localized motor symptoms similar to those in frontal lobe seizures; or propagate forwards via a route below the lateral fissure, giving rise to automatism, which suggests the propagation to the medial temporal lobe; however, these automatic symptoms are not specific, rather, they are similar to those that are a part of a psychomotor seizure. In multiple epileptic seizures of some patients, the propagations along above or below the lateral fissure may even coexist.

Occipital lobe epilepsy in childhood may even have digestive tract symptoms such as paroxysmal abdominal pain or vomiting, etc. Generally, drug therapies have good efficacy in such patients and there is no need to consider surgical treatment. Differentiation of seizures from such epilepsy syndrome is important.

Y. Wang (ed.), *Electroencephalogram for Presurgical Epilepsy Evaluation*, https://doi.org/10.1007/978-981-95-8003-3_5

EEG Characteristics

In interictal EEG of patients with occipital lobe epilepsy, unilateral or bilateral discharge of spikes/sharp waves, spike-and-wave complexes/sharp-and-wave complexes can be seen in occipital region and may propagate to ipsilateral posterior temporal region or parietal region, sometimes with the highest amplitude in the posterior temporal region, or separate or synchronous discharge of spikes, spike-and-wave complexes are seen only in temporal lobe. Ictal manifestations are mainly 10–20 Hz low-amplitude fast activity or spike rhythm originated from unilateral occipital region or posterior temporal region quickly spread to the ipsilateral parietal region, and the wave amplitude gradually increases and propagates to the contralateral posterior head or ipsilateral anterior head.

Cases of Occipital Lobe Epilepsy

Case 5.1 Occipital Lobe Epilepsy

[Abstract of Medical Records]
Male, 12 years old.

1. *History of present illness*: At 6 months after birth, the patient's parents noticed that the patient showed such symptoms as nodding and staring downwards, which lasted for seconds. No treatment was performed and no recurrence was observed later. Then 7 years ago (at 5 years old), the patient experienced paroxysmal loss of consciousness and limb jerks (the specific form is unknown), accompanied by urinary incontinence and upward deviation of eyes, without apparent predisposing cause(s); the symptoms lasted for about 2 hours and relieved after rescue in a hospital. The patient was prescribed oral phenobarbital but still experienced seizures occasionally (at interval of several months). 5 years ago (at 7 years old), the patient had seizures at increased frequency in the same form as before, due to fever and rashes. After switching to sodium valproate and sodium phenytoin, the patient's seizure frequency decreased. Later, the patient's seizure frequency increased after discontinuation of sodium phenytoin on his own; the patient's seizure was mainly manifested as loss of consciousness, lifting up of upper extremities, extension of lower extremities, stiffness of limbs, twitching for a few minutes, which lasted for several hours in severe cases. At the end of a seizure, the patient would feel weakness of left limbs, which could last for hours. Sometimes, the patient's only manifestation of seizure is dialeptic without jerks; the symptom would last for seconds before relief. According to an account in the patient's own words, the patient would have red or black vision before the onset of most seizures but have no palpitation, rising epigastric sensation, dizziness, etc. The patient shows no signs of automatism during and after a seizure. Currently, the patient is on oral oxcarbazepine, 450 mg/dose, bid; sodium valproate, 100 mg/dose, bid, but the seizure still occurs several times a week.
2. *Past history*: The patient was born postmaturely after a spontaneous labor and had a history of postnatal hypoxia. Motor, speech, and intelligence development were normal.
3. *Personal and family history*: No history of associated diseases.
4. *Physical examination*: Visual acuity: 0.5 in left eye, 0.4 in right eye. Examination of visual field (less reliable due to the poor cooperation of the patient): left eye nasal visual field defect was identified; paracentral scotoma was found in right eye. No abnormality was identified in sensory, motor, physiological, and pathological reflex examinations.
5. Imaging examination:
   (a) MRI revealed no notable abnormal change.
   (b) MRS revealed that NAA concentration level was slightly lower in left hippocampus (NAA/Cr: 1.09) than in right hippocampus (NAA/Cr: 1.25). Cho concentration level was slightly lower in left hippocampus (Cho/Cr: 1.23) than in right hippocampus (Cho/Cr: 1.36).
6. *EEG*: For details, see Figs. 5.1, 5.2, 5.3, 5.4, and 5.5.

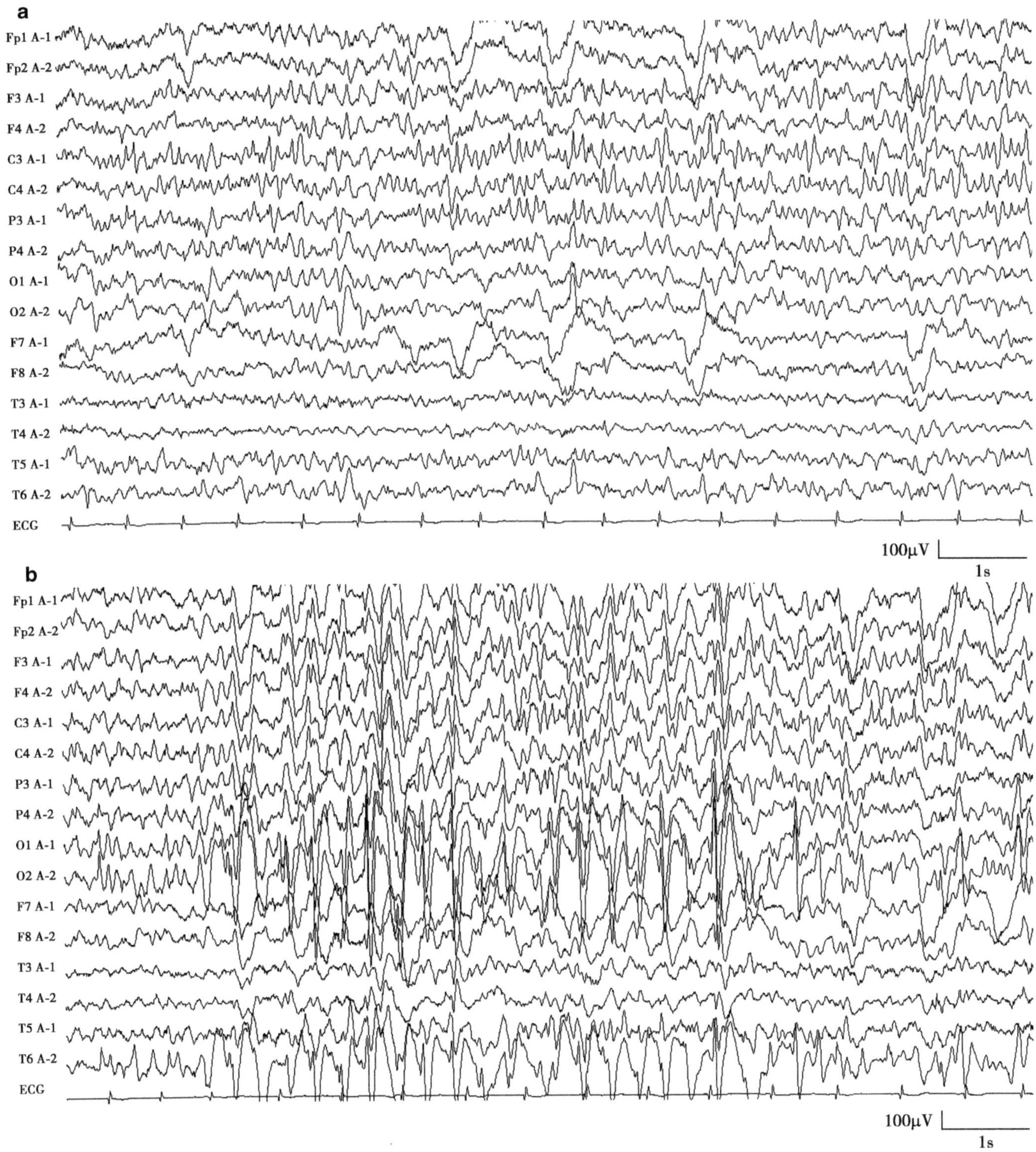

Fig. 5.1 Interictal scalp EEG. (**a**) Basic rhythm 8 Hz; poor α wave form over the occipital region, the high-amplitude 5.0–6.0 Hz slow waves mixed in the signal of all leads were slightly excessive. Sporadic high-amplitude sharp waves were seen over the right posterior temporal region (T6), occipital region (O2) leads. (**b**) The patient was awake. In EEG, sporadic rhythms of high-amplitude spike-and-wave complexes were identified in the bilateral occipital region (O1, O2), right posterior temporal region (T6) leads, involving bilateral frontal region (Fp1, Fp2, F3, F4), parietal region (P3, P4), anterior temporal region (F7, F8) leads, especially over the leads on the right side. (**c**) EEG manifestations: multiple high-amplitude spikes and spike-and-wave complexes were seen over the bilateral occipital region (O1, O2), right posterior temporal region (T6) in Phase II sleep background electroencephalogram (EEG)

c

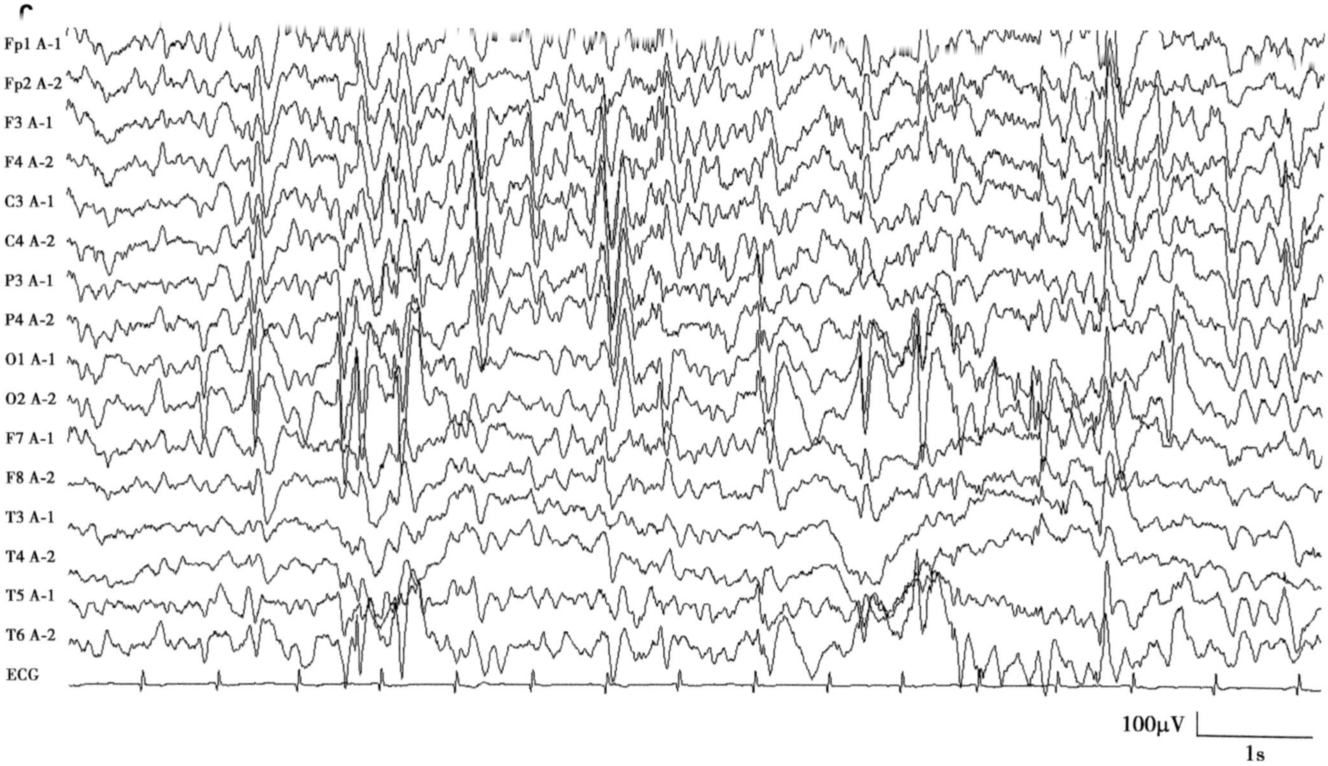

Fig. 5.1 (continued)

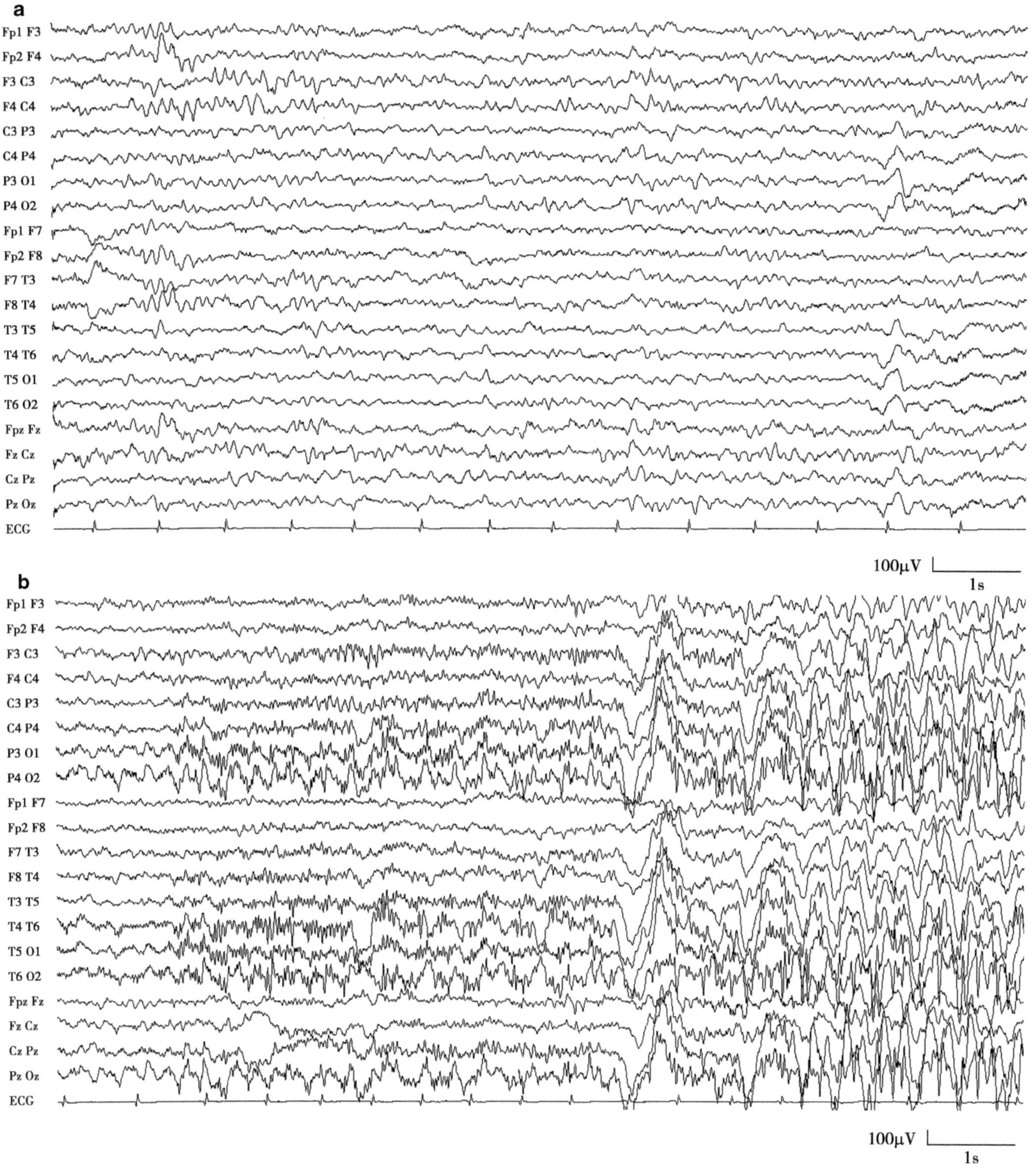

Fig. 5.2 Ictal scalp EEG. (**a**) The patient was in supine position, resting with eyes closed before the seizure. The patient's EEG was in Phase I sleep, with disintegrated α rhythms in occipital region. (**b**) Upon the onset of seizure, the patient opened his eyes to indicate that he had the feeling of seizure. EEG manifestations: Low to mid amplitude fast rhythm over the bilateral occipital region (P3 O1, P4 O2), the middle and posterior temporal region (T3 T5, T4 T6, T5 O1, T6 O2), parieto-occipital midline (Pz Oz) leads; the amplitude gradually increased to form spikes; about 6 s later, the wave involved the entire posterior head and presented a rhythm of 3.0–4.0 Hz spike or spike-and-wave complexes. (**c**) The patient remained supine with eyes closed. The EEG showed high-amplitude spike rhythm over the bilateral parietal region (C3, P3, C4, P4), occipital region (P3, O1, P4, O2), posterior temporal region (T4, T6, T5, O1, T6, O2), and parieto-occipital midline (Cz, Pz, Pz, Oz) leads, especially over the leads on the right side. (**d**) The patient's symptoms and EEG manifestations were the same with those presented in **c**. (**e**) The patient's symptoms were basically the same with those presented in **c**. The discharge frequency of spike-and-wave complexes gradually decreased. (**f**) The patient's seizure ended. The EEG gradually recovered to the background EEG manifestations

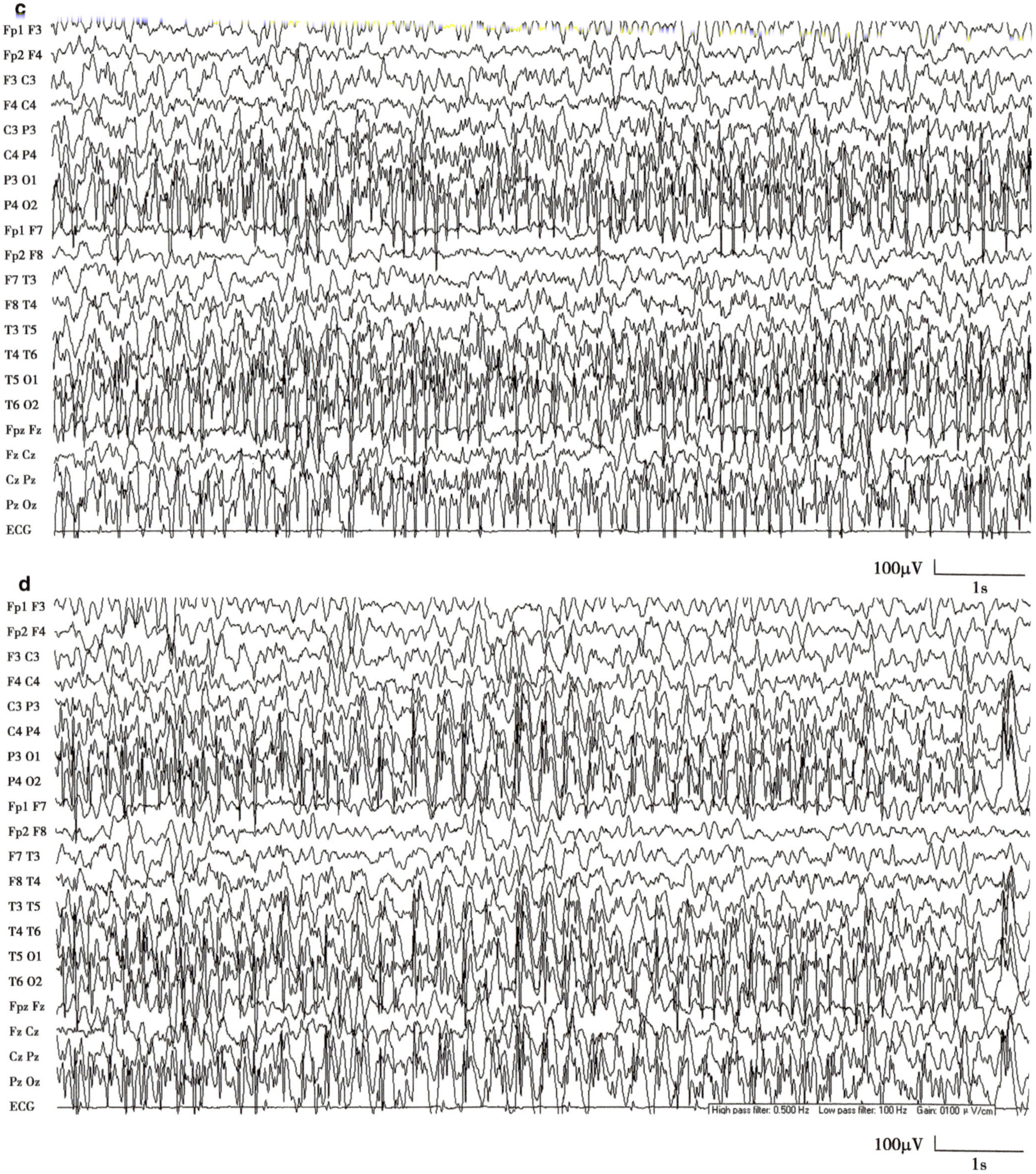

Fig. 5.2 (continued)

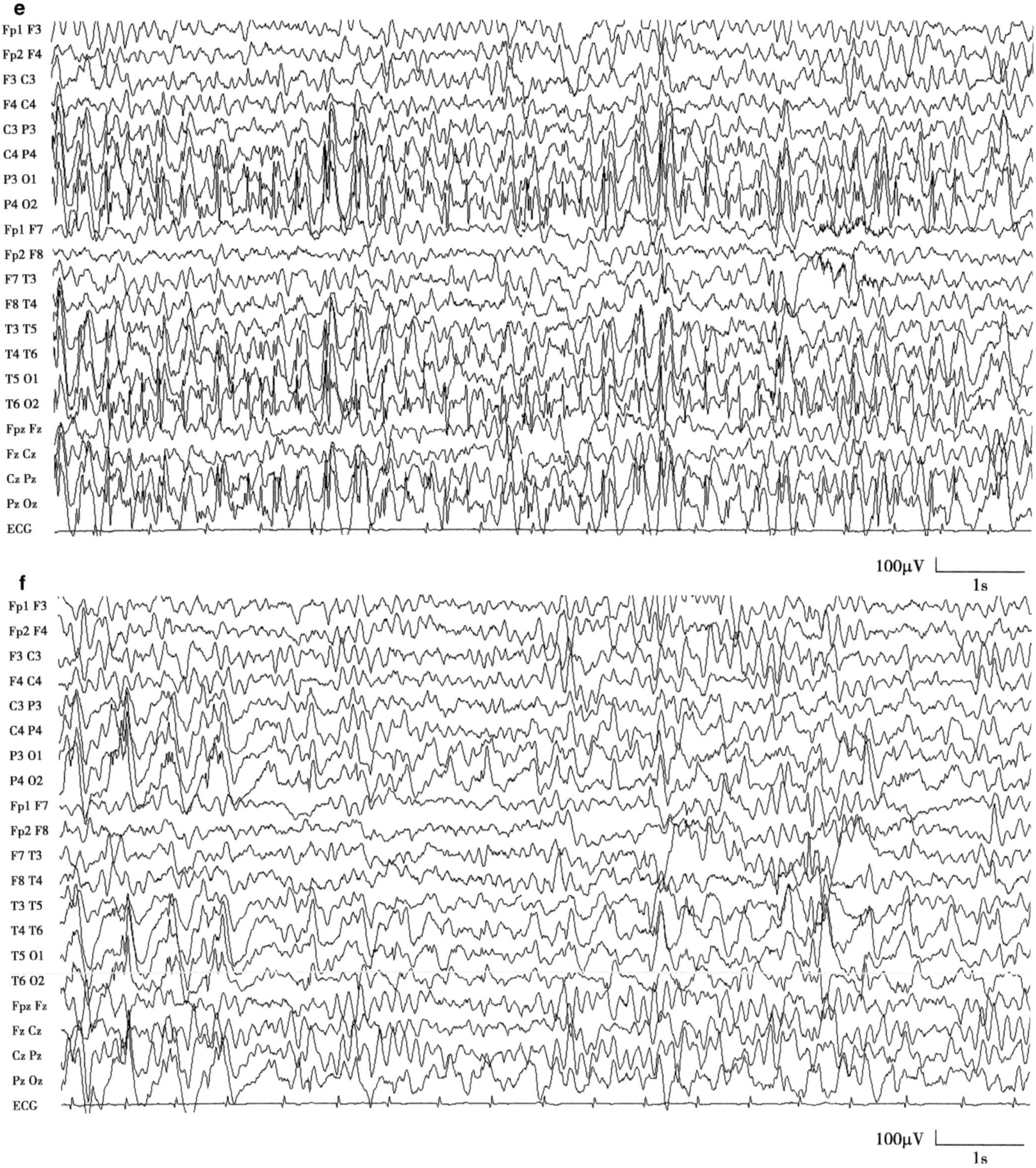

Fig. 5.2 (continued)

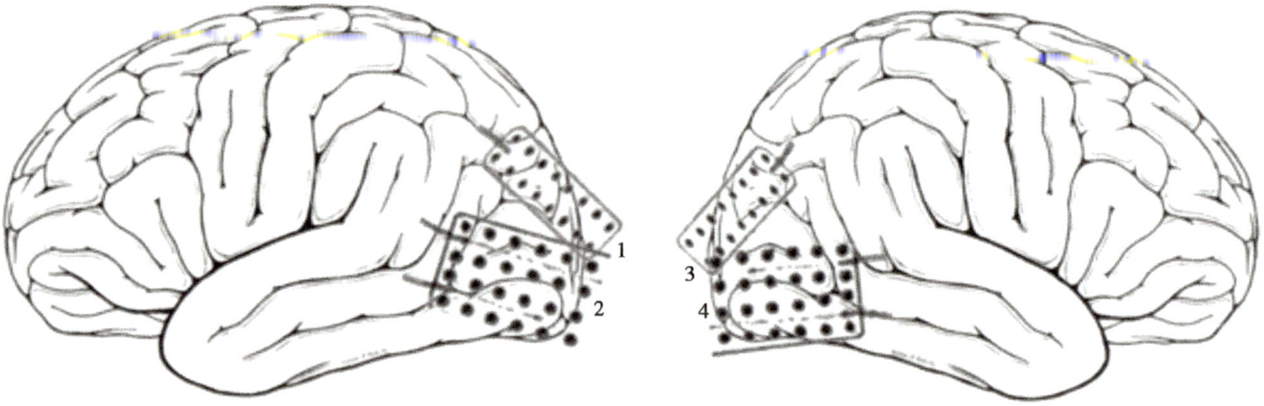

Fig. 5.3 Scheme of intracranial electrodes
Grid electrode 1: the left occipital region of interhemispheric fissure (16 contacts); Grid electrode 2: the left occipital pole (24 contacts); Grid electrode 3: the right occipital region of interhemispheric fissure (16 contacts); Grid electrode 4: the right occipital pole (24 contacts)

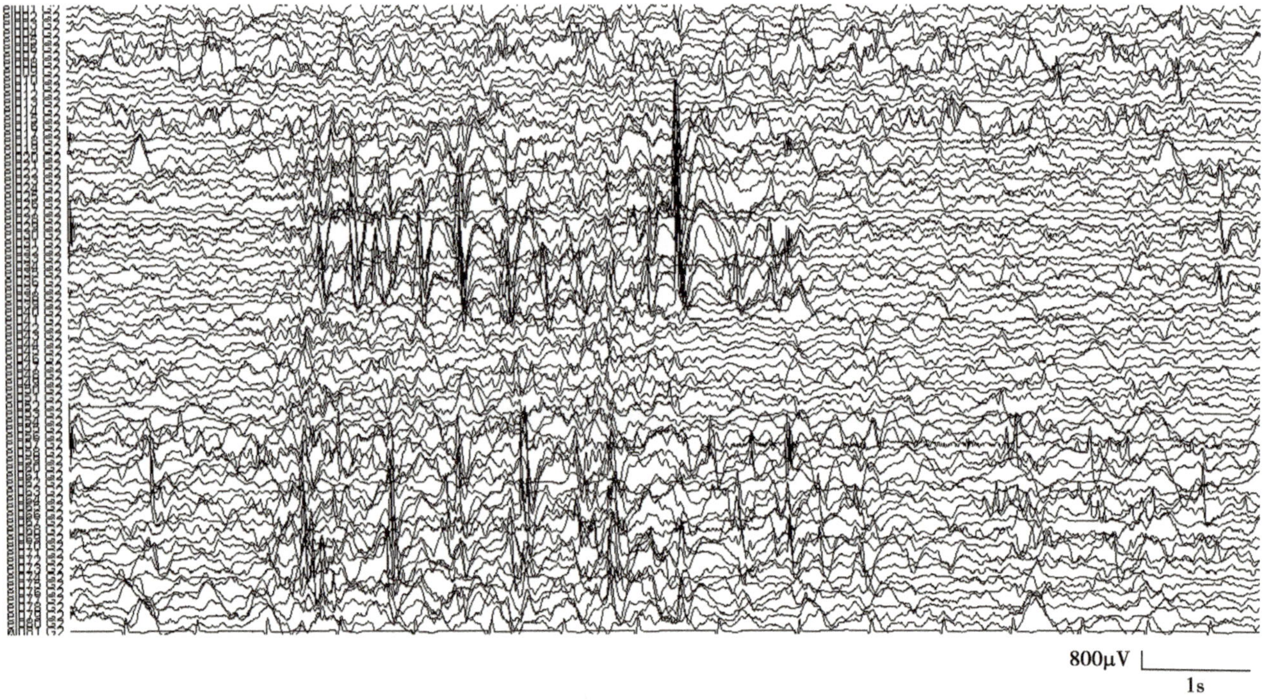

Fig. 5.4 Interictal intracranial EEG
Paroxysmal rhythm of high-amplitude spike-and-wave complexes over the bilateral occipital regions (contact numbers el023, el024, el025, el026, el029, el030, el031, el032, el035, el036, el037, el038, el057, el058, el059, el060, el063, el064, el065, el066, el069, el070, el071, el072, el075, el076, el077, el078), especially on the left side (contact numbers el023, el024, el025, el026, el029, el030, el031, el032, el035, el036, el037, el038)

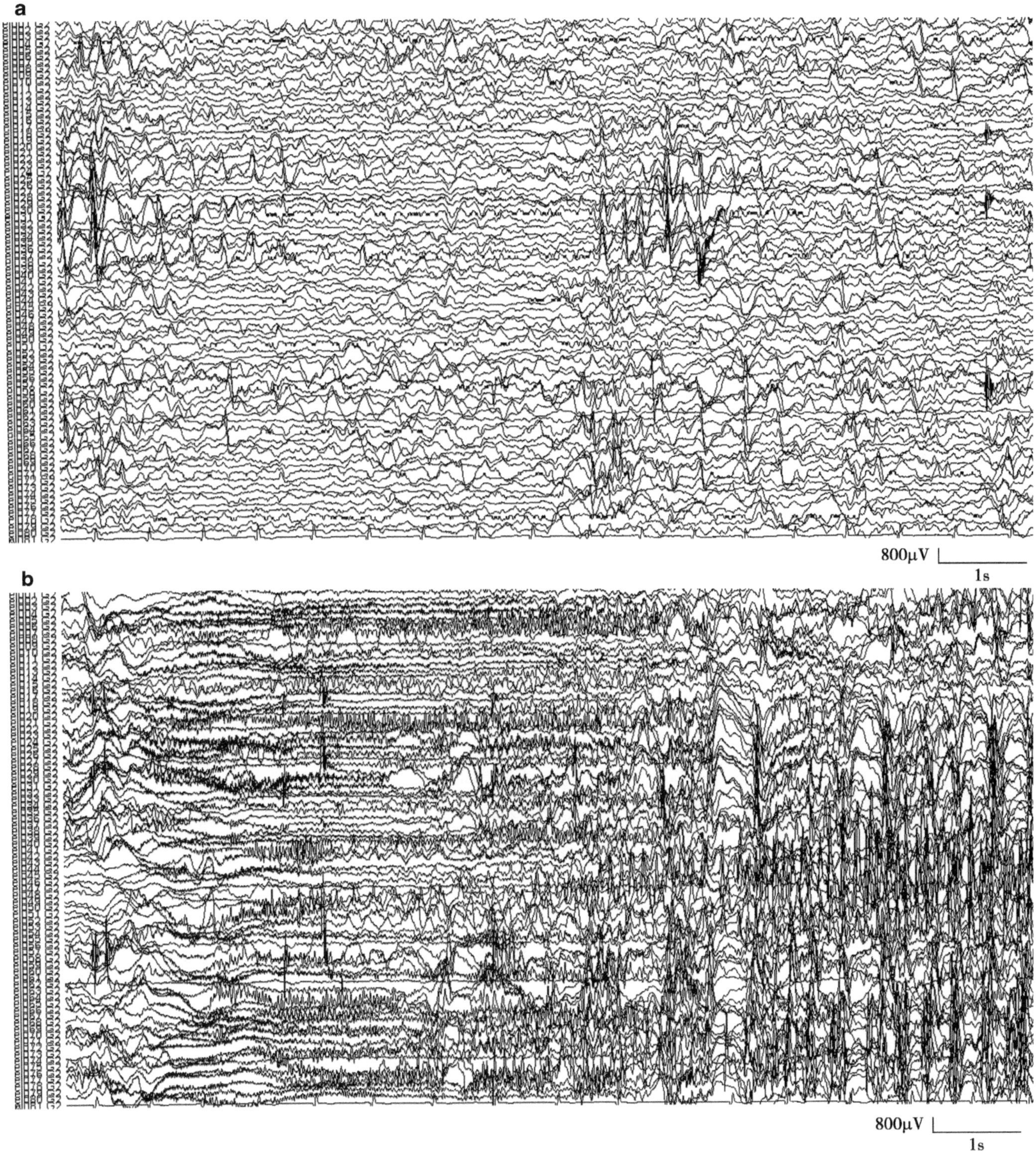

Fig. 5.5 Ictal intracranial EEG. (**a**) Prior to the onset of seizure, the patient was in supine position; ready to tell relatives of his feeling of the seizure. No significant change was observed. (**b**) The patient was resting in bed, with both eyes gazing in upper left direction without such symptoms as jerks of limbs. Low amplitude fast activity was observed; the amplitude gradually increased and later took on the pattern of spike rhythm; abnormal discharges appeared early and most evident over the left occipital region (contact numbers el017, el018, el019, el020, el023, el024, el025, el029, el030, el031). (**c**, **d**) During the seizure process, rhythms of extremely high-amplitude spike-and-wave complexes, polyspike, and wave complexes appeared and lasted for about 40 s. (**e**, **f**) During the seizure process, rhythms of extremely high-amplitude spike-and-wave complexes, polyspike, and wave complexes appeared and lasted for about 40 s. (**g**) The patient's seizure ended. Rhythms of spike-and-wave complexes were seen over the left occipital region (contact numbers el023, el024, el025, el029, el030, el031, el035, el036, el037), right occipital region of interhemispheric fissure (contact numbers el043, el044, el045, el052, el053, el054, el055)

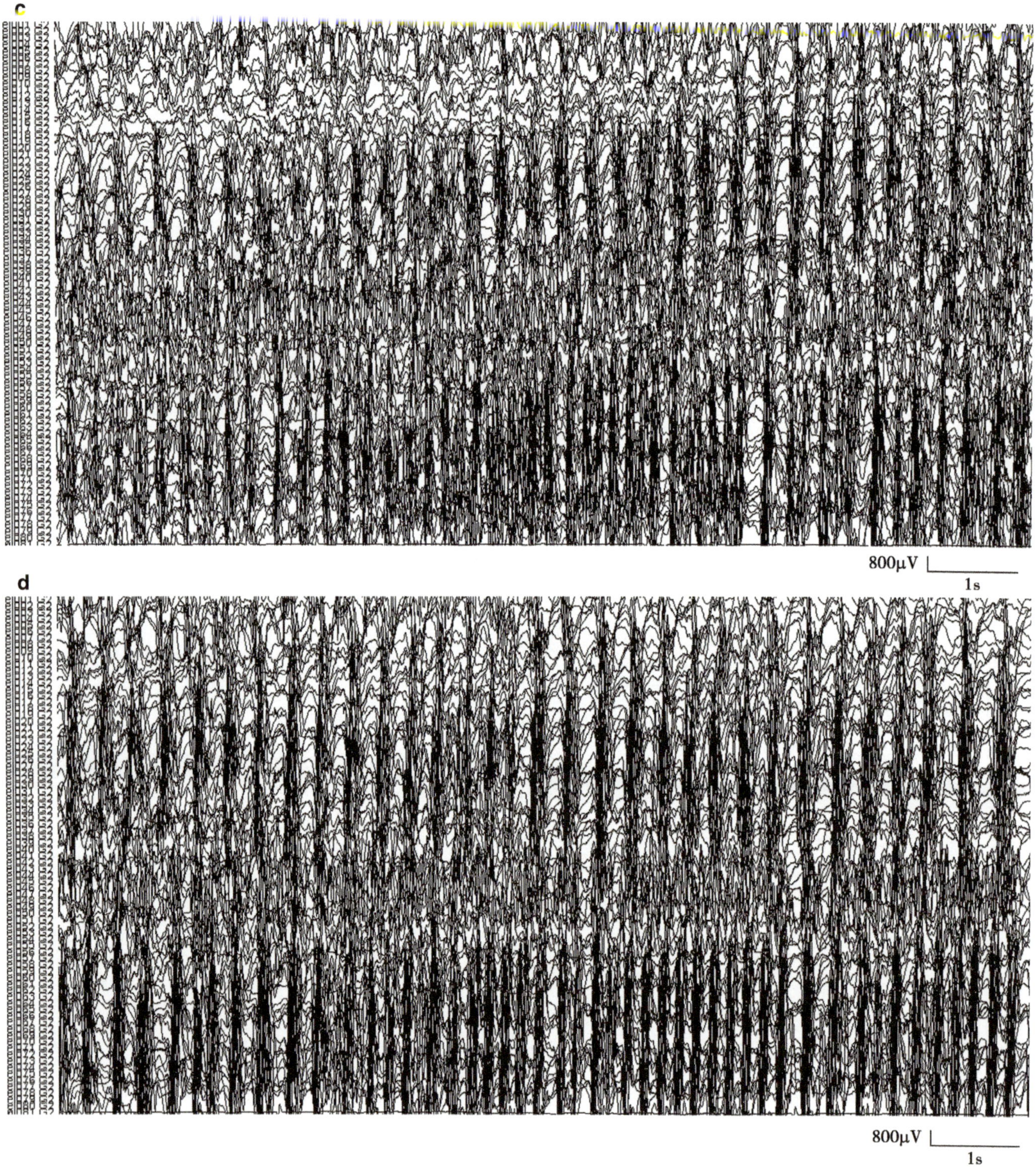

Fig. 5.5 (continued)

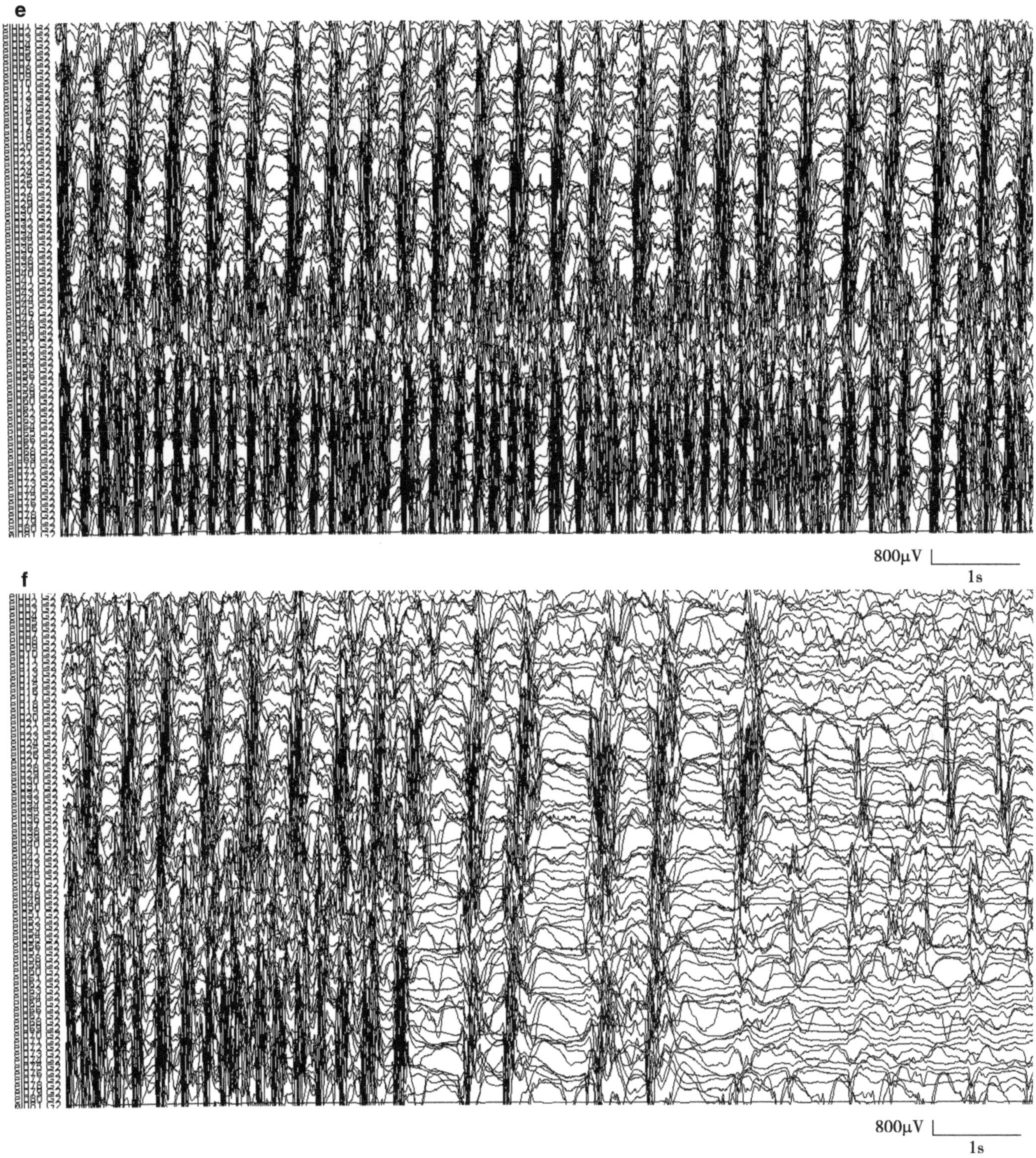

Fig. 5.5 (continued)

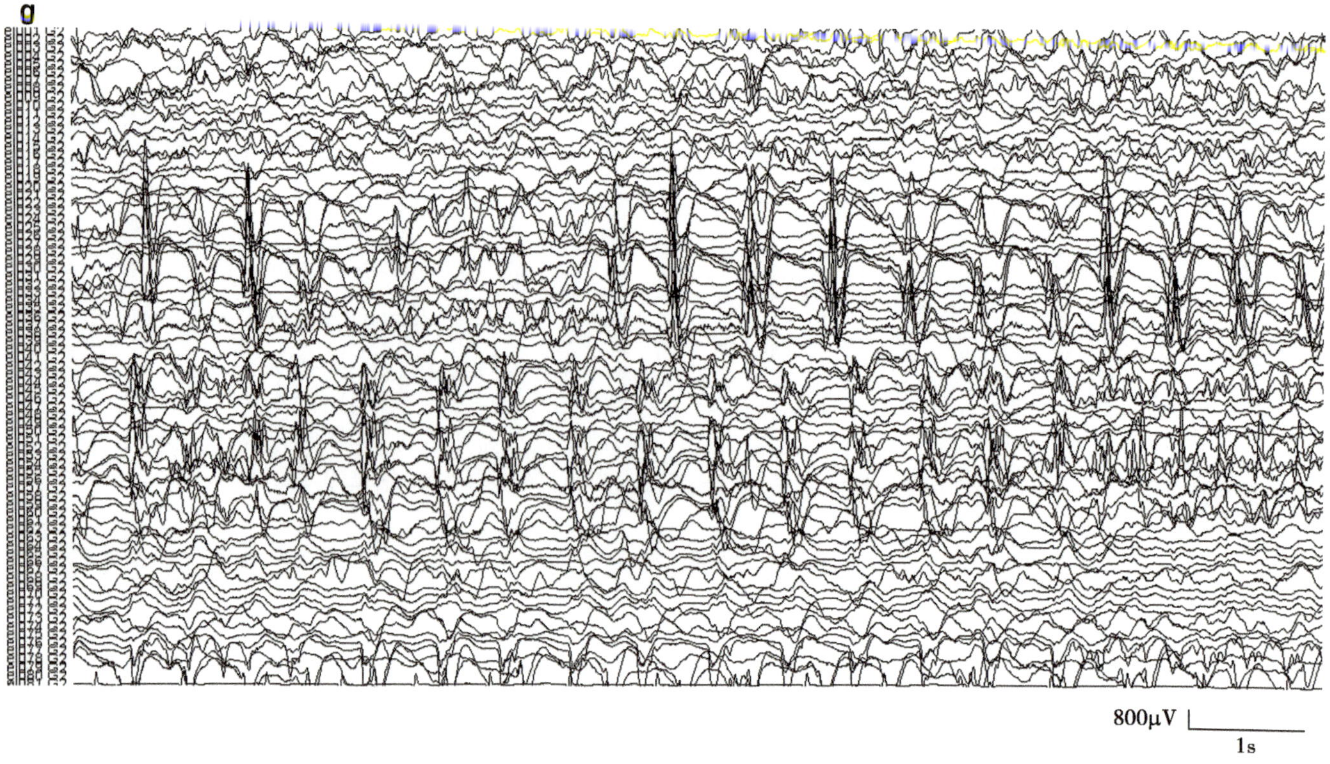

Fig. 5.5 (continued)

[Case Review]

Both interictal and ictal scalp EEG showed the abnormalities were more evident on the right side; in ictal phase, initial intracranial electrode signals were most evident on the left side, while scalp EEG would cause a false impression. The patient was preliminarily diagnosed with occipital lobe epilepsy, but the affected side could not be determined. However, both the interictal and ictal scalp EEG manifestations showed the abnormal discharges were more significant on the right side. Intracranial cortex electrodes were implanted symmetrically in bilateral occipital regions. A subtle difference between the left and right side in terms of burst rhythmic activities at the initial stage of the seizure was found: the left side had burst rhythmic activities 200 ms earlier than the right side. It was thus determined that the epileptic foci were in the left occipital lobe. The left occipital cortex was surgically resected and a 1.5 × 1.5 cm focus in right occipital region was also resected. The patient experienced a seizure 1 year after the surgical operation. No more seizures were observed after adjustment of the antiseizure medication. In this case, it would be hard to lateralize the epileptogenic focus without the application of intracranial electrodes; the lateralization could have been wrong had it not been for the intracranial electrodes.

Case 5.2 Occipital Lobe Epilepsy

[Abstract of Medical Records]
Male, 17 years old.

1. *Chief complaint*: Paroxysmal deviation of the head to the right, with loss of consciousness and jerks of limbs for more than 3 years.
2. *History of present illness*: The patient experienced an episode 3 years ago on his way to school: his head deflected rightwards without apparent predisposing cause, with both eyes gazing rightwards and rightward distortion of mouth corner. Afterwards, the patient became unconscious, presenting jerks of limbs, accompanied by urinary incontinence, odaxesmus, and no foaming at mouth. After about 2 min, the jerks stopped and the patient lapsed into a confusional state, with both hands involuntarily groping, unbuttoning, and even wandering. About 2–3 min later, the patient regained complete consciousness. There was no obvious aura before the attack. The above symptoms occurred repeatedly, and sometimes he only had rightward deflection of head, distortion of right mouth corner, and unresponsiveness; the symptoms lasted for about 1 min and then alleviated. The seizure occurred 4–5

times per month. Diurnal seizures were more than nocturnal ones. The patient went to a local hospital and received medication treatment, but the conditions were not resolved. He received treatment with gamma knife surgery and carbamazepine therapy (100 mg/dose, b.i.d.) 2 years ago, but the conditions aggravated and the seizure occurred more than 10 times per month. His dose regimen was adjusted 5 months before to carbamazepine, 600 mg/dose, bid.; lamotrigine, 100 mg/dose, bid; sodium valproate, 400 mg/dose, bid, but no significant improvement had been observed.

3. *Physical examination*: His memory and computing capability had deteriorated recently. No pathological signs were induced.
4. *Imaging examination*:
   (a) MRI showed ambiguous boundary of grey and white matter, and local high signal in the right anterior temporal lobe.
   (b) SPECT showed decreased blood flow over the right frontal, temporal, parietal, medial temporal lobe, occipital cortex and basal ganglia, and decreased blood flow near the midline of the left frontal cortex.
   (c) MRS showed that the NAA concentration in the right hippocampus was lower than that in the left hippocampus. The ChO concentration in the right hippocampus was higher than that in the left hippocampus.
5. *EEG*: For details, see Figs. 5.6, 5.7, 5.8, 5.9, and 5.10.

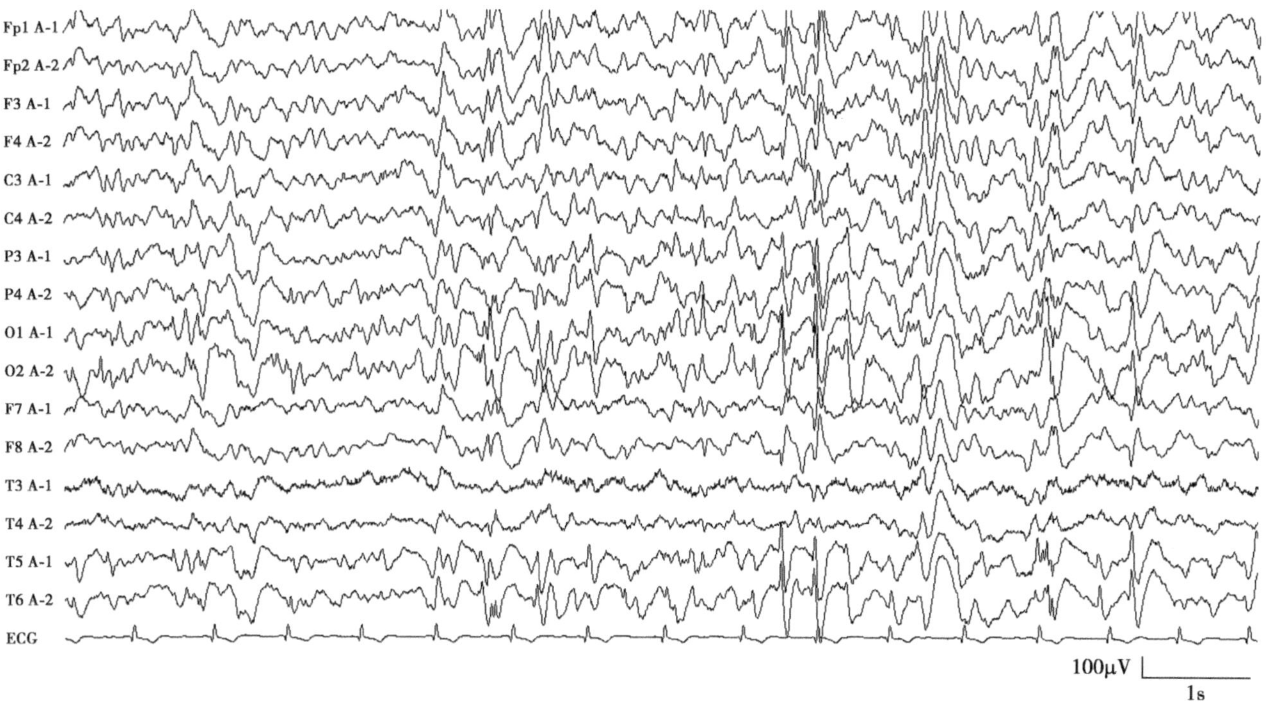

Fig. 5.6 Interictal scalp EEG
The basic rhythm is 9.0 Hz; middle and high amplitude 4.0–5.0 Hz slow waves were mixed in all leads. The discharges of high amplitude spike-and-wave complexes were observed over the leads in bilateral parietal regions (P3, P4), occipital regions (O1, O2) and posterior temporal regions (T5, T6), sometimes appearing as 2.0–3.0 Hz rhythm, spreading to bilateral anterior regions of the head

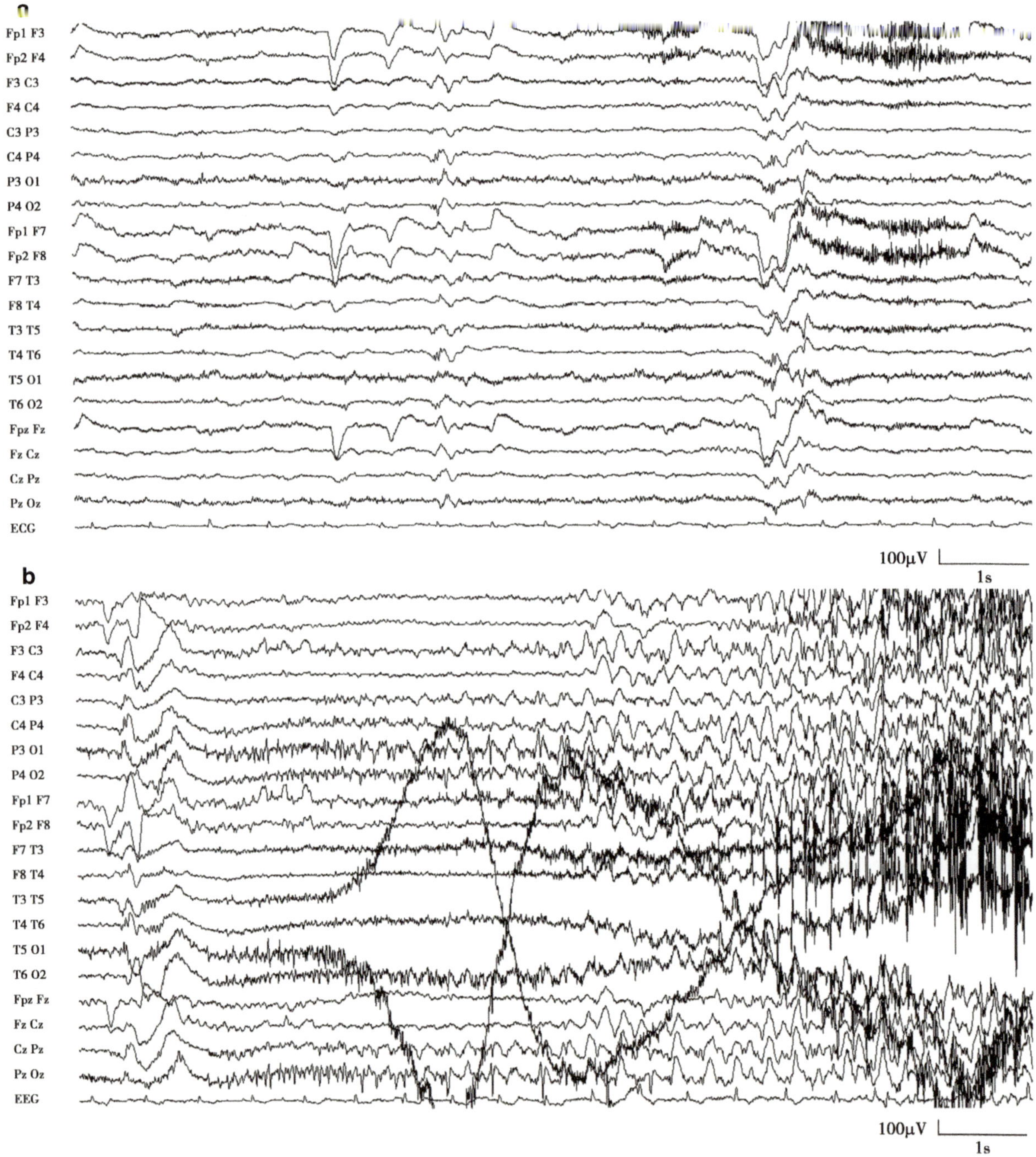

Fig. 5.7 Ictal scalp EEG. (**a**) Before the seizure, the patient was sitting in bed and talking to his family. The EEG showed alpha suppression, which was characteristic of a conscious patient with eyes opening. Eyelid movement artifacts caused by blinking were observed over the bilateral frontal regions (Fp1 F3, Fp2 F4, Fp1 F7, Fp2 F8, Fpz Fz). (**b**) During the seizure, the patient's head was bowed and the body was slightly turned to the right and slowly backwards. EEG showed fast activities and spike rhythms over the leads in left frontal region (Fp1 F3, Fp1 F7), central region (F3 C3), parietal region (C3 P3), occipital region (P3 O1), and parieto-occipital midline (Cz Pz, Pz Oz). About 2 s later, low to middle amplitude 4.0–5.0 Hz slow wave rhythms appeared over the leads at the same sites, especially on the left side, and gradually spreaded to the other ipsilateral and counter lateral leads. Electrode wobbling artifacts could be seen over the leads in the left middle temporal region, and a lot of EMG artifacts could be seen over the leads in bilateral frontotemporal regions. (**c**) The patient was in the supine position, with the head turning to the right, both eyes gazing rightwards and the right limbs flexed. The patient became irresponsive to calls when his head and body began swaying slightly. EMG artifacts and electrode wobbling artifacts could be seen. (**d**) The patient's limbs became flexed and clonic. About 5 s later, a tonic-clonic seizure started. The patient's EEG manifestations were the same as shown in **c**. (**e**) The patient's limbs remained tonic-clonic. The patient's EEG manifestations were the same as shown in **c**. (**f**) The frequency of clonuses gradually lowered. EEG showed numerous EMG artifacts. (**g**) The clonuses stopped when the seizure ended. At the end of the seizure, all waves had low and flat amplitude. (**h, i**) The patient was wheezing coarsely and drooling. EEG showed low and flat amplitude. A lot of EMG artifacts and electrode wobbling artifacts were seen over the bilateral frontotemporal regions. (**j**) The patient was wheezing coarsely and drooling. EEG showed low and flat amplitude. A lot of EMG artifacts and electrode wobbling artifacts were seen over the bilateral frontotemporal regions

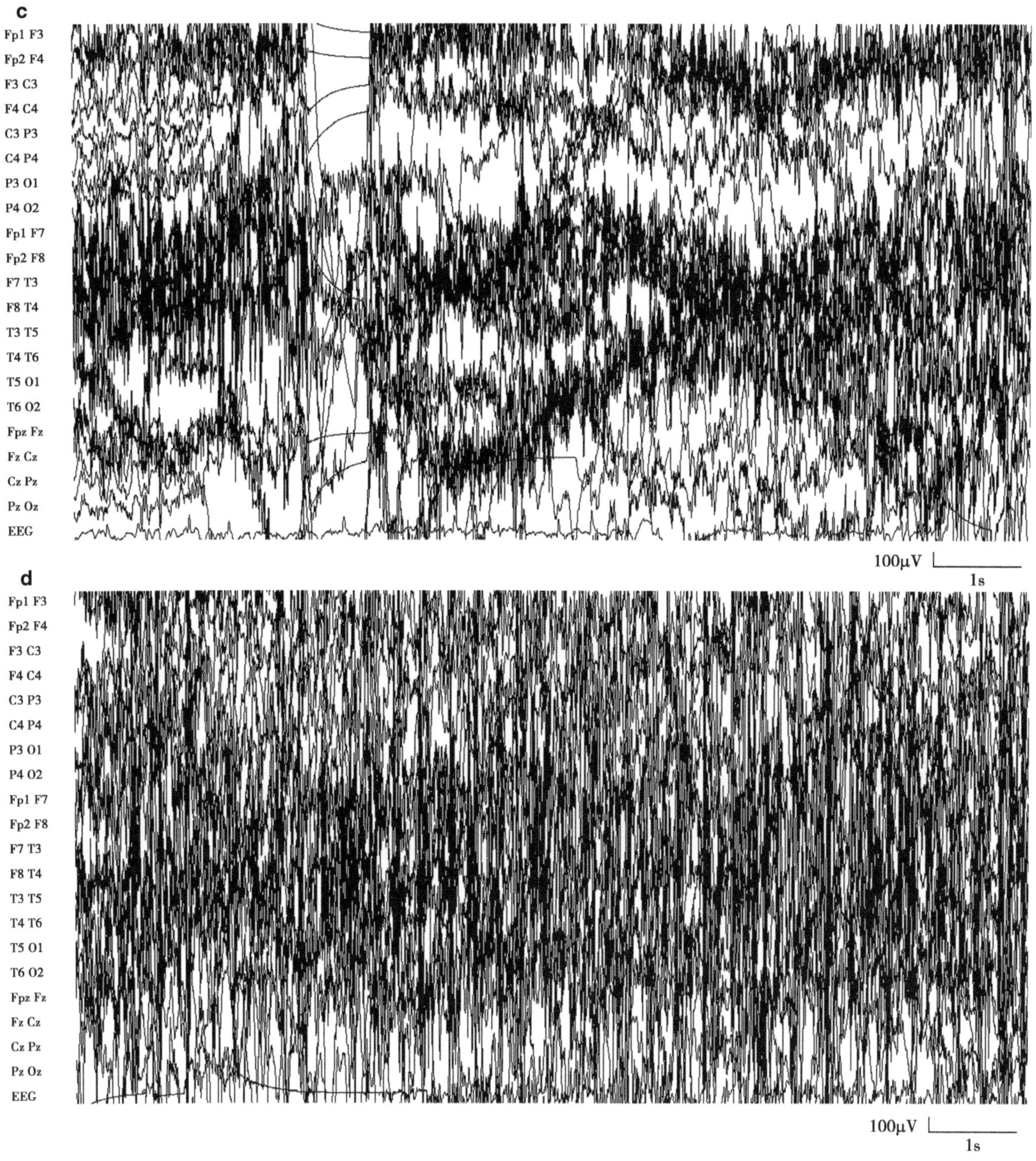

Fig. 5.7 (continued)

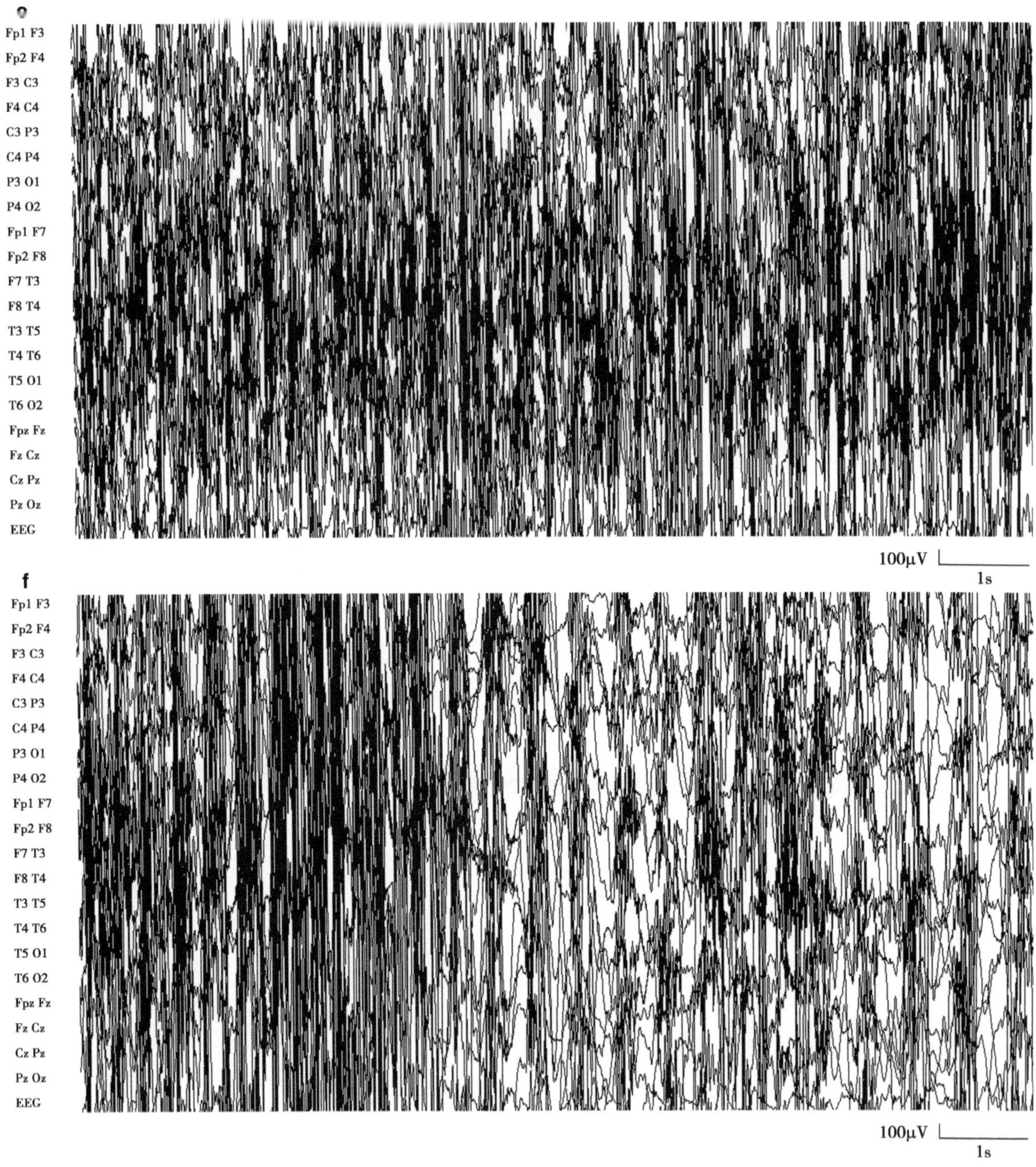

Fig. 5.7 (continued)

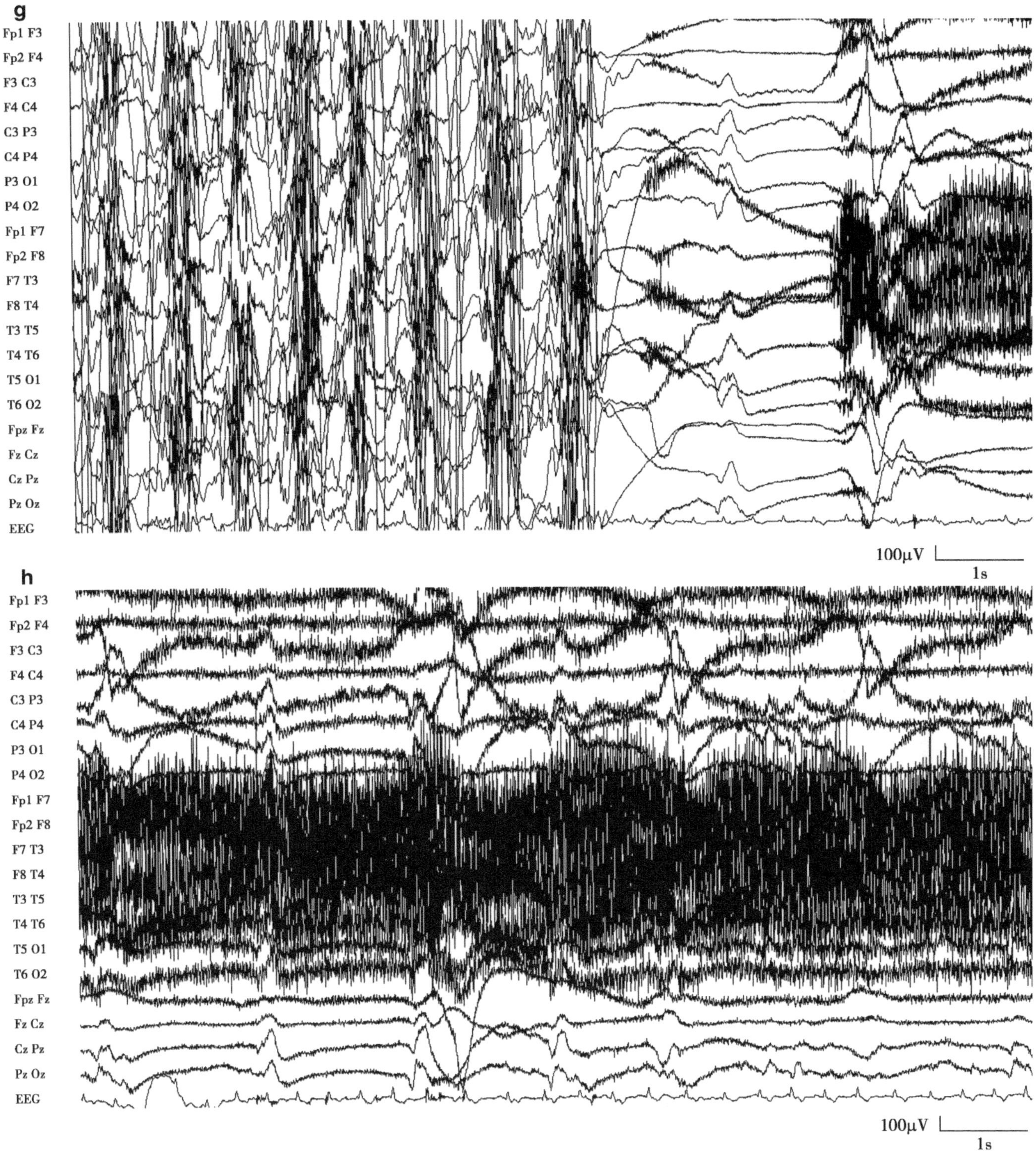

Fig. 5.7 (continued)

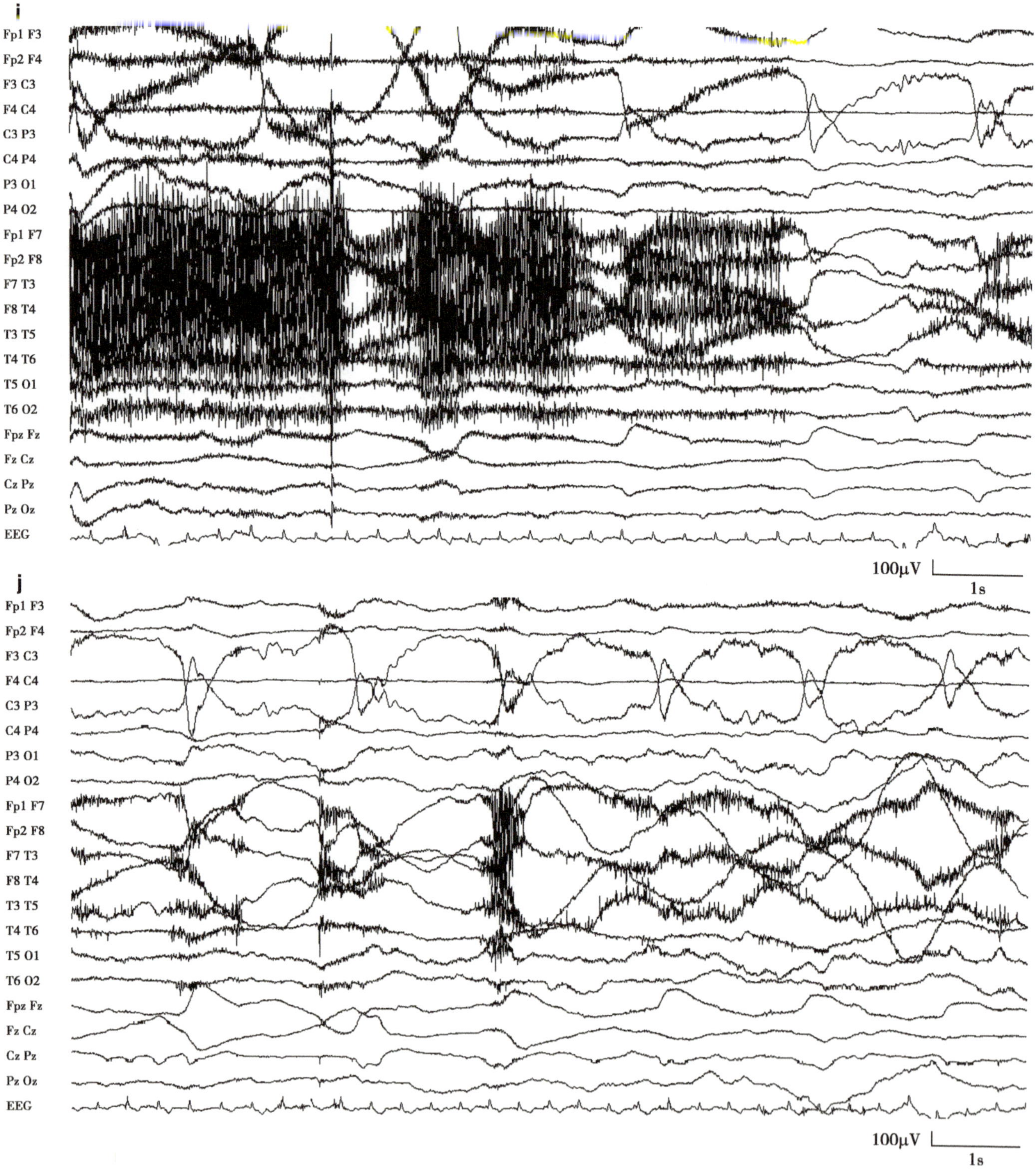

Fig. 5.7 (continued)

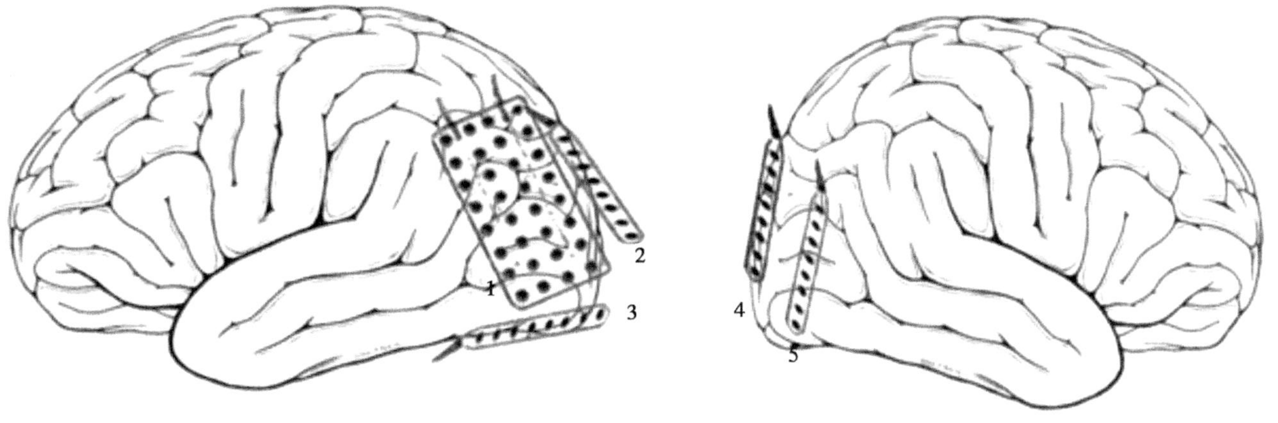

Fig. 5.8 Scheme of intracranial electrodes
Grid electrode 1: the left occipital lateral side (32 contacts); Strip electrode 2: the left posterior occipital region of interhemispheric fissure (8 contacts); Strip electrode 3: the left occipital pole (8 contacts); Strip electrode 4: the right posterior occipital region of interhemispheric fissure (8 contacts); Strip electrode 5: the right occipital lateral side (8 contacts)

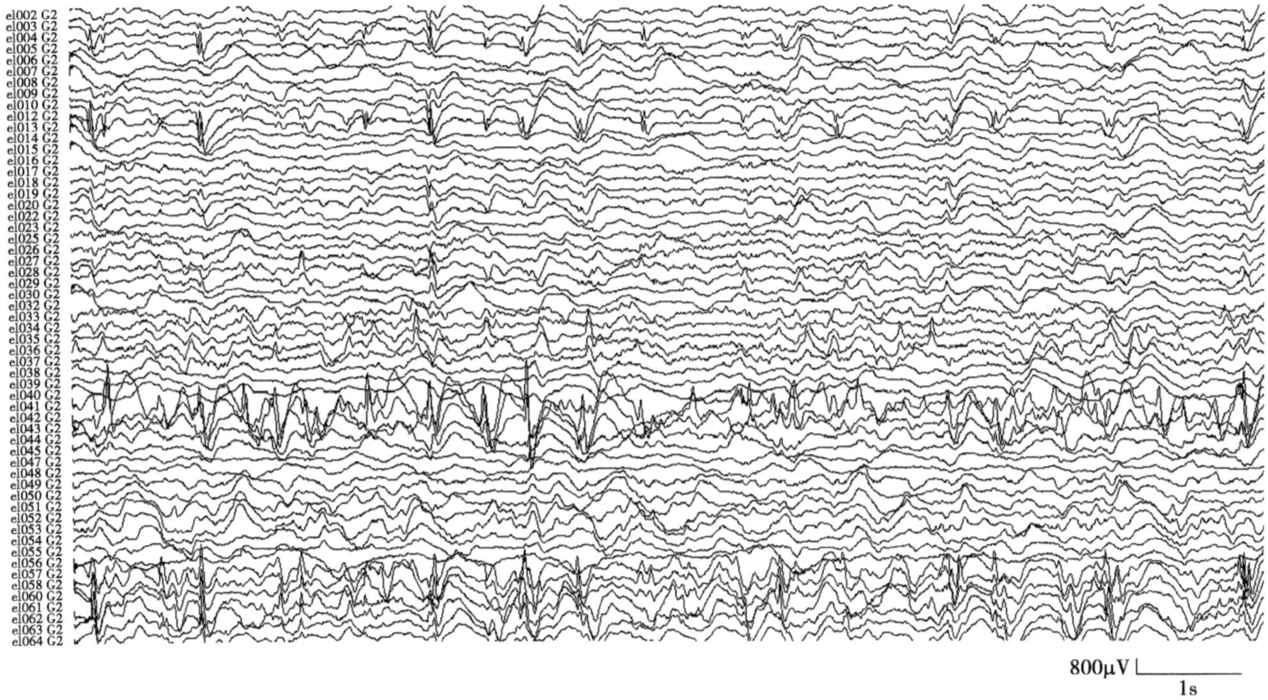

Fig. 5.9 Interictal intracranial EEG
Persistent high-amplitude rhythms of spike-and-wave complexes over the left occipital lateral (contact numbers el004, el005, el012, el013), occipital region (contact numbers el041, el042, el043) especially over the left occipital pole, involving right occipital lateral (contact numbers el057, el058, el060, el061, el062)

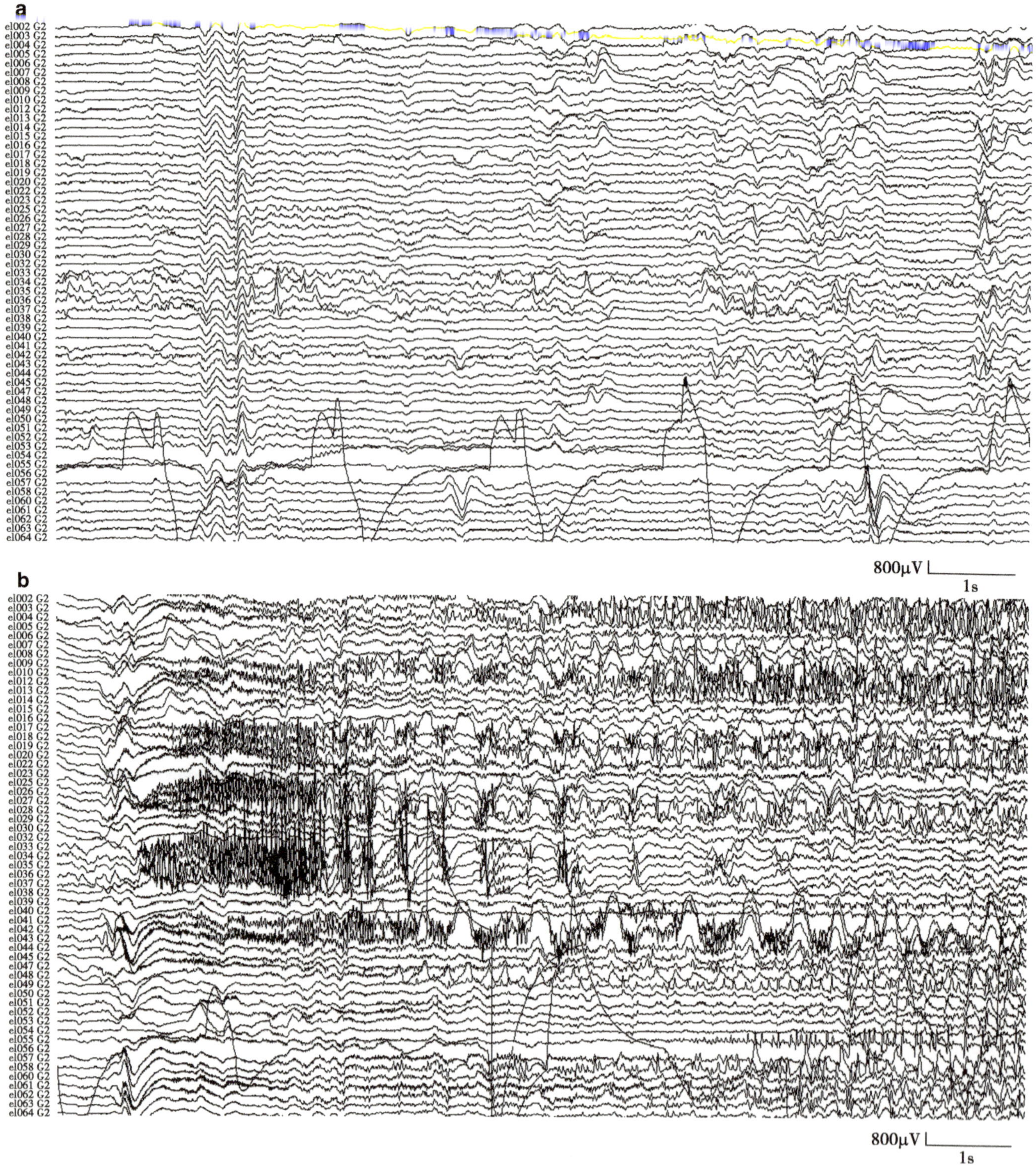

Fig. 5.10 Ictal intracranial EEG. (**a**) Before the onset of the seizure, the patient was sleeping in right lateral decubitus position. IEEG presented the background IEEG. (**b**) At times of the seizure, the patient's upper right limb flexed with clonus and head slightly deflected to the left. IEEG showed low amplitude fast activity over the left lateral occipital region (contact numbers el002, el003, el004, el009, el010, el012, el013, el017, el018, el019, el020, el025, el026, el027, el028), left medial occipital region (contact numbers el033, el034, el035, el036), left occipital region (contact numbers el041, el042, el043); 3 s later, it changed to rhythms of spikes or polyspike and wave complexes; 6 s later, spike rhythms were seen over all the above-mentioned regions. (**c**) The patient's head tilted backward, upper left limb and lower right limb slowly flexed; the patient's both upper limbs were tonic and slightly clonic, and the patient was making a sound "Ah" through throat. Extremely high-amplitude spike rhythm was observed. (**d**) The patient had tonic-clonic limbs. The patient's IEEG manifestations were the same as shown in **c**. (**e**) The patient had tonic-clonic limbs. The patient's IEEG manifestations were the same as shown in **c**. (**f**) The frequency of clonuses gradually lowered. IEEG showed a gradually slowing down rhythm. (**g**) The patient's seizure ended. IEEG showed low-amplitude fast rhythm over the left supraoccipital and medial occipital region of longitudinal fissures (contact numbers el026, el027, el028, el034, el035, el036)

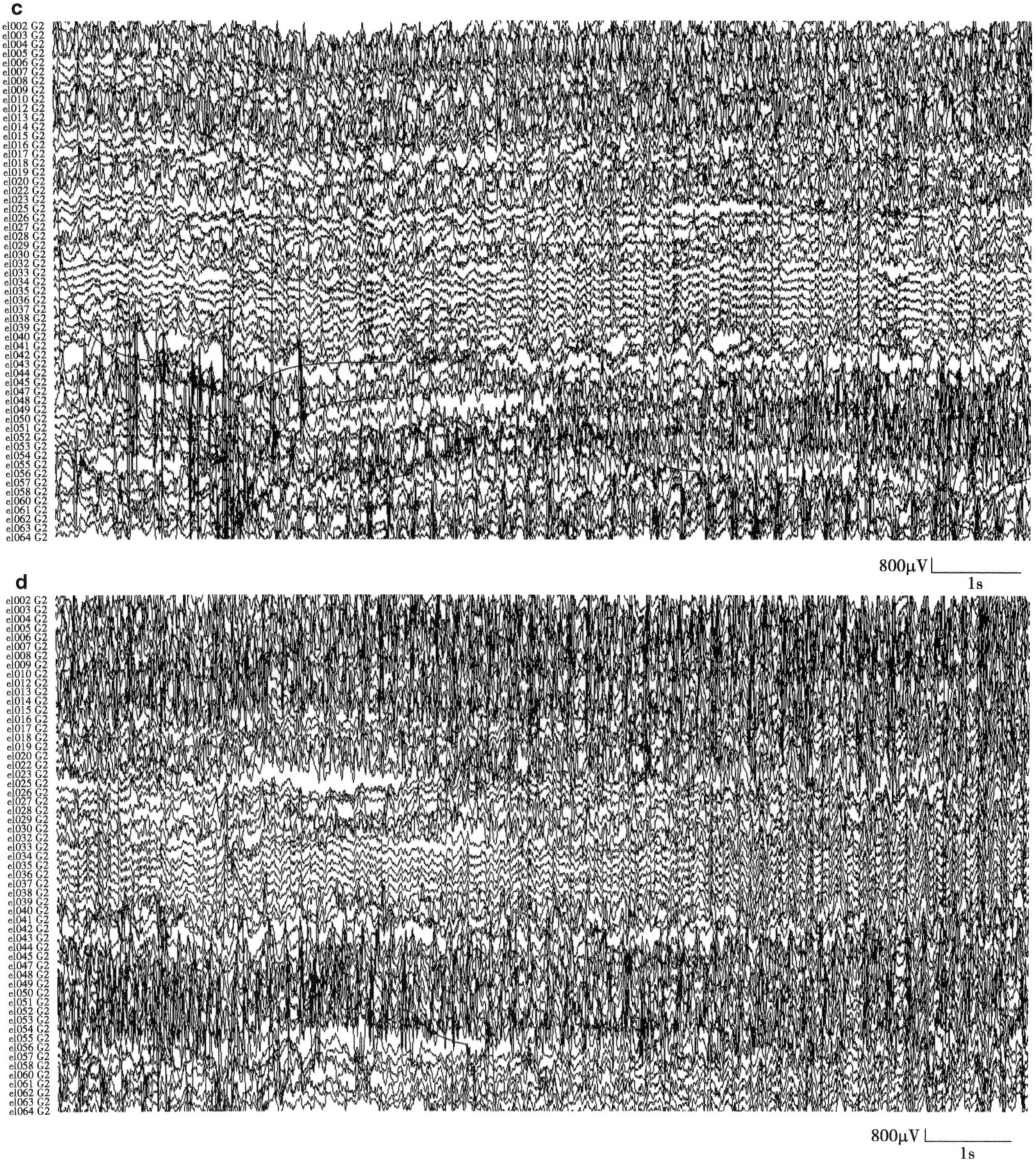

Fig. 5.10 (continued)

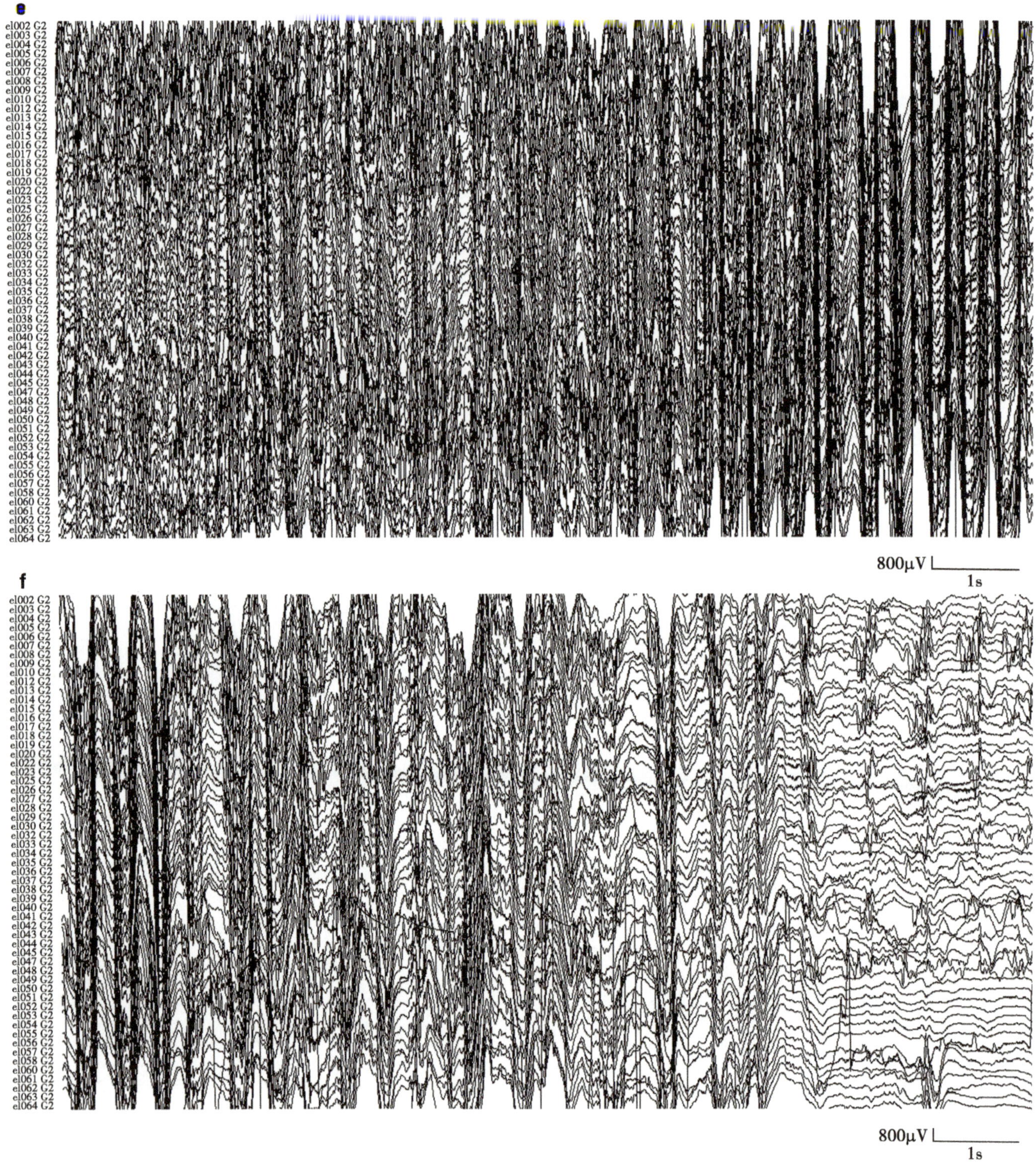

Fig. 5.10 (continued)

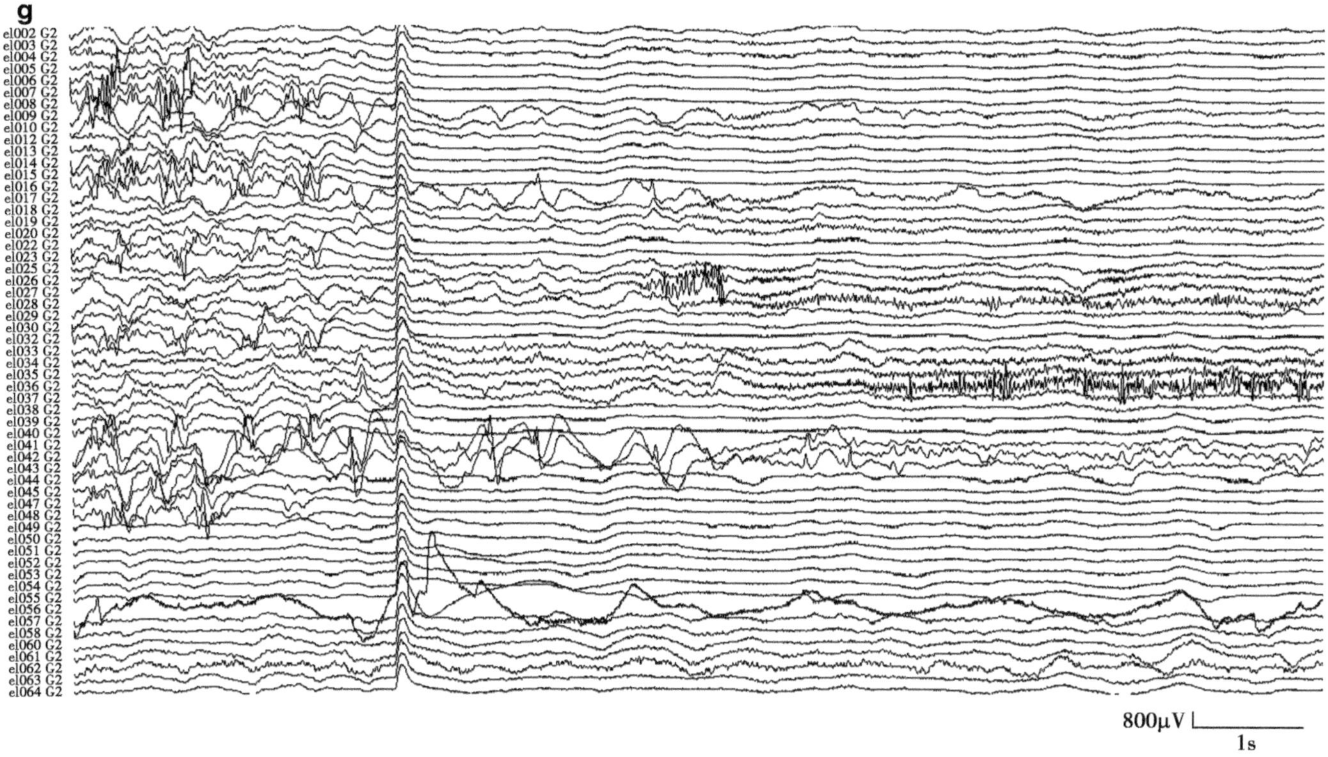

Fig. 5.10 (continued)

[Case Review]

The patient's clinical symptoms originated from left side; ictal scalp EEG revealed the seizure originated from the left side; ictal intracranial electrode EEG originated from the left side; the diagnosis was definite. Occipital lobe epilepsy generally caused synchronous intermittent abnormal electrical activities in bilateral occipital lobe cortices. On the other hand, ictal abnormal electrical activities might involve a wide range and could lead to propagation to temporal lobe, dorsolateral prefrontal cortex, producing corresponding clinical symptoms. In this case, cortical electrodes were implanted in the patient for the purpose of lateralizing the epileptic foci and determining the specific range and early propagation area of the origin of seizure in order to provide a basis for surgical resection of the epileptogenic cortex. The left basioccipital and occipital pole resection was performed. The seizures disappeared during a 1-year follow-up after surgery. The abnormal MRI signals in the patient's right temporal region were not related to the epileptic seizure.

Case 5.3 Occipital Lobe Epilepsy

[Abstract of Medical Records]
Male, 10 years old.

1. *Chief complaint*: Recurrent episodes of blinking, unconsciousness for 3 years.
2. *History of present illness*: The patient experienced several falls to the ground 3 years ago, with limbs jerks and unresponsiveness to calls. He was diagnosed with epilepsy in a local hospital and drug therapies were administered, but the efficacy was unsatisfactory. Thereafter, there was recurrent blinking of both eyes, head turning to the left, left upward squinting of both eyes, slight movements of the left limbs, accompanied by swallowing movements and unconsciousness. He recovered after 1 minute and his hands groped in front of the chest. There were diplopia and amaurosis auras before the seizure. Starting from 5 months ago, the patient showed rightward deviation of head during seizure, rightward gazing of both eyes, and

movement of right limbs. The seizures generally occurred at an interval of 2–3 days, and there could be several seizures in a day.

3. *Past history*: No history of associated diseases.
4. *Personal history*: History of postnatal asphyxia.
5. *Family history*: One of the patient's aunts died early from epilepsy.
6. *Physical examination*: No neurological abnormalities were found.
7. *Imaging examination*:
   (a) MRI revealed pathological changes in white matter of brain, suggesting the possibility of leukodystrophy
   (b) SPECT revealed localized hypoperfusion of blood over the right temporal and occipital lobe.
   (c) MEG revealed the dipole clusters of the abnormal discharges over the bilateral occipital regions, mainly the right side.
8. *EEG*: For details, see Figs. 5.11, 5.12, 5.13, 5.14, and 5.15.

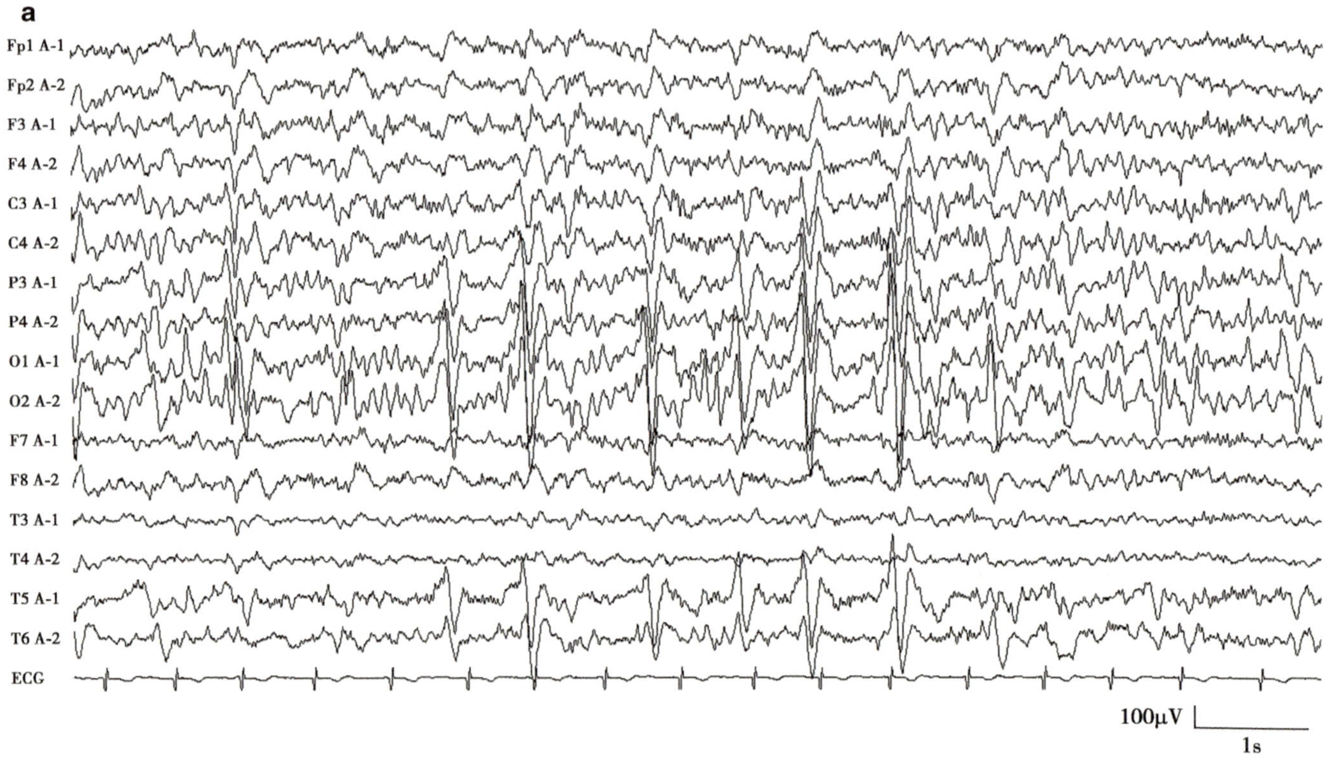

Fig. 5.11 Interictal scalp EEG. (**a**) EEG manifestations: basic rhythm: 8.0 Hz; medium amplitude 5.0 Hz slow waves in anterior region. Extremely high-amplitude rhythmic sharp waves can be seen over the bilateral occipital regions (O1, O2), parietal regions (P3, P4) and posterior temporal regions (T5, T6), mainly the left side, the rhythm was 2.0–3.0 Hz. (**b**) EEG manifestations: Phase II sleep, bilateral spindle waves were basically symmetric; high-amplitude sharp waves, sharp-and-wave complex over the bilateral parietal regions (P3, P4), occipital regions (O1, O2), and posterior temporal regions (T5, T6). (**c**) EEG manifestations: Phase II sleep, sporadic high-amplitude spikes over the right posterior frontal region (F4), central region (C4), parietal region (P4), occipital region (O2), and posterior temporal region (T6)

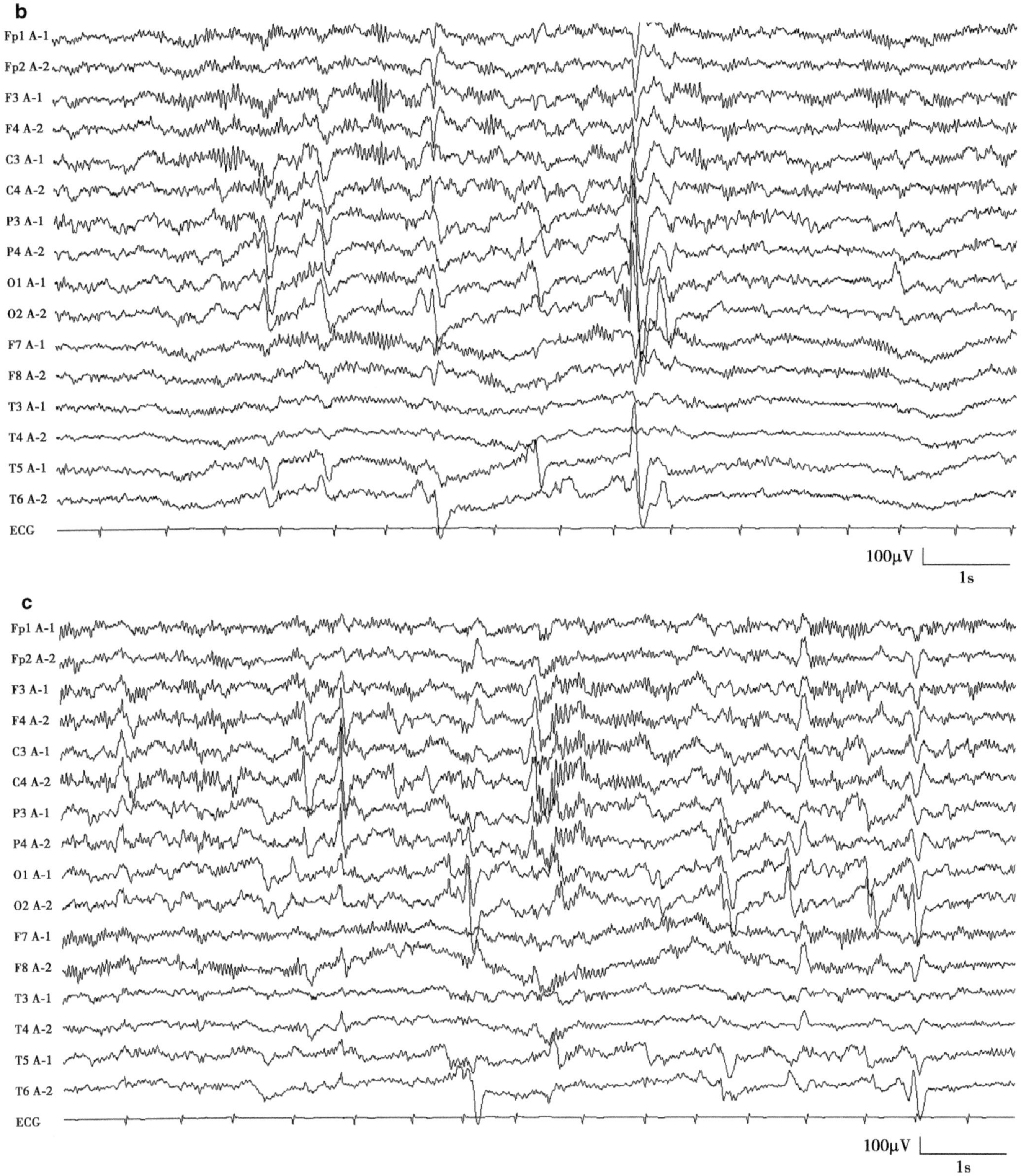

Fig. 5.11 (continued)

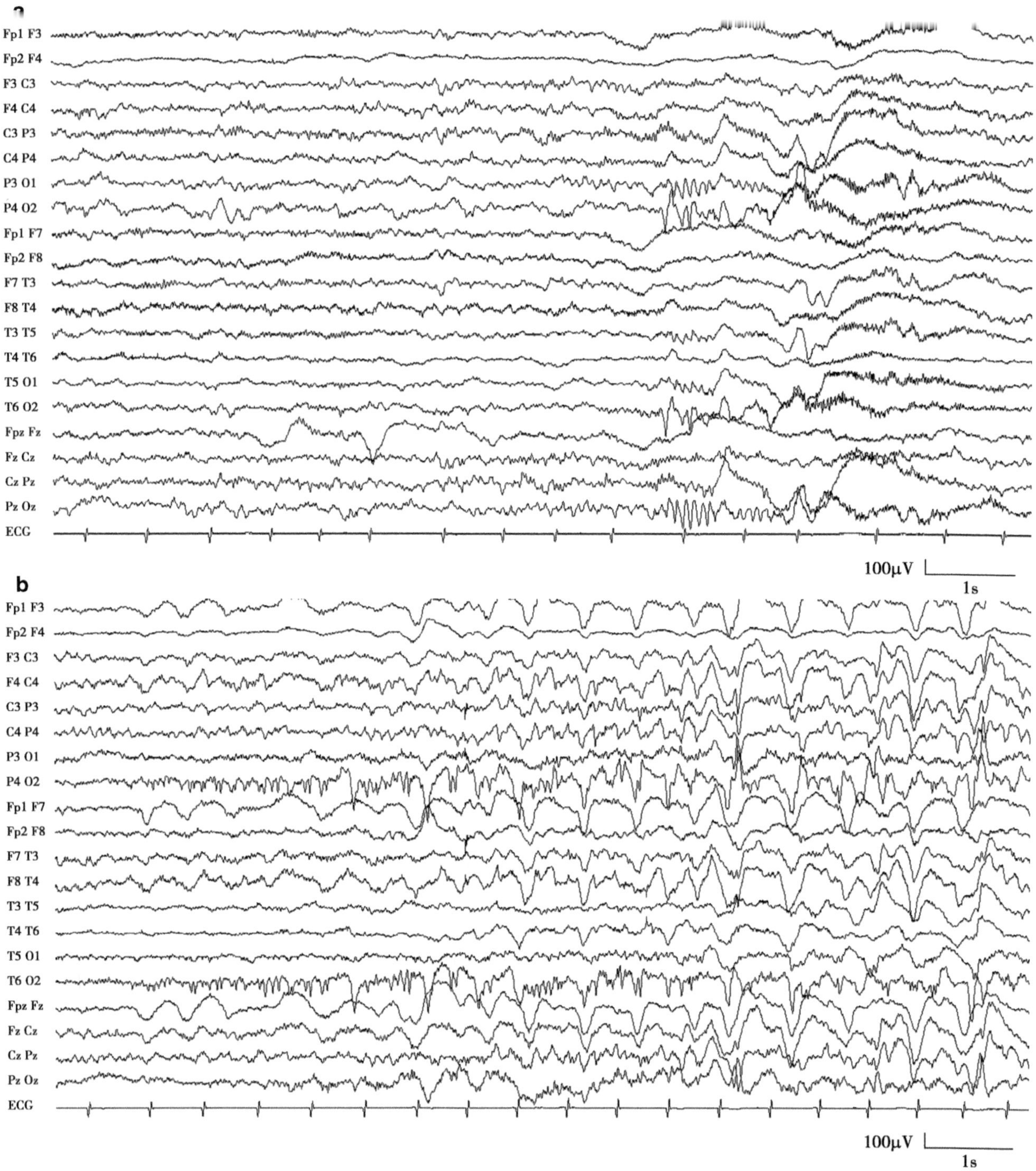

Fig. 5.12 Ictal scalp EEG. (**a**) The patient's right lower extremities were slightly swaying. The EEG showed generalized irregular 2.0–3.0 Hz slow waves of high-amplitude, mainly over the parieto-occipital region; sporadic medium-to high-amplitude spikes were seen over the left central parietal region (F3 C3, C3 P3), mid-temporal region (T3 T5), and right occipital region (P4 O2, T6 O2). (**b**) The patient raised head and wanted to sit up, with vacant look in the eyes. The EEG manifestations were basically the same as in **c**; EMG artifacts were seen over the bilateral temporal regions. (**c**) The patient lay and failed to respond to questions. The EEG showed generalized irregular 3.0–4.0 Hz slow waves. (**d**) The patient had the same symptoms as before. The EEG presentation was the same as **e**. (**e**) The patient remained in supine position but responded to questions. The EEG manifestation was basically the same as in **e**. (**f**) The patient's seizure ended. The EEG gradually restored to the background EEG. (**g**, **h** and **i**) The seizure ended. The EEG gradually restored to the background EEG During the seizure, the patient put his hands down slowly on his forehead, blinked rapidly, looked left with both eyes, and did not respond when asked. The EEG showed low amplitude fast activities over the right occipital region (P4 O2, T6 O2), with amplitude gradually increasing to form low- to mid-amplitude spike rhythms; 3 s later, the amplitude kept increasing and frequency gradually reduced to 10.0–11.0 Hz rhythmic spikes, involving the right central parietal region (F4 C4, C4 P4). Then 4 s later, the frequency gradually decreased to 2.0–3.0 Hz sharp-and-wave complexes; eye movement artifacts were observed over the left frontal region (Fp1 F3, Fp1 F7, Fpz Fz)

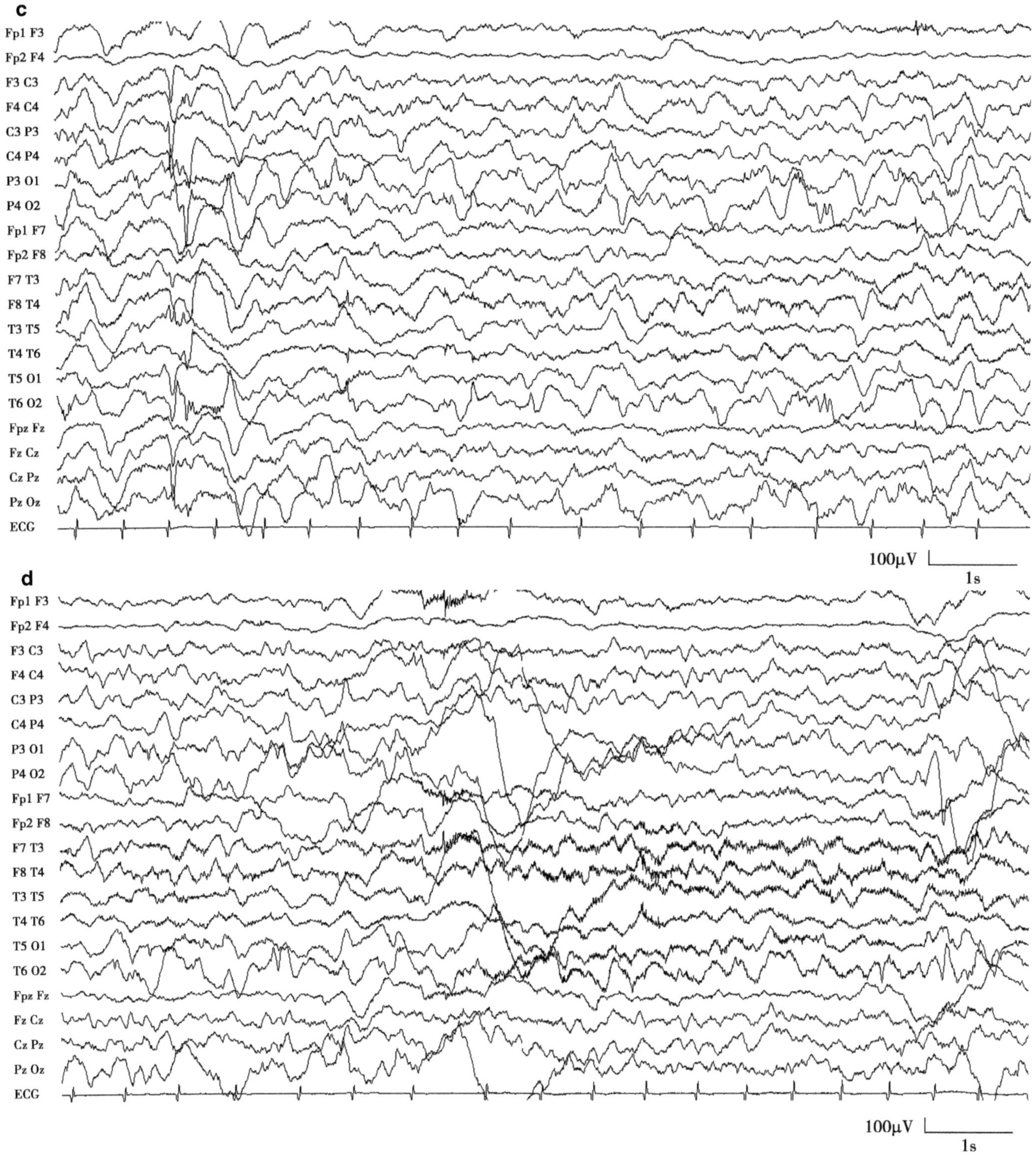

Fig. 5.12 (continued)

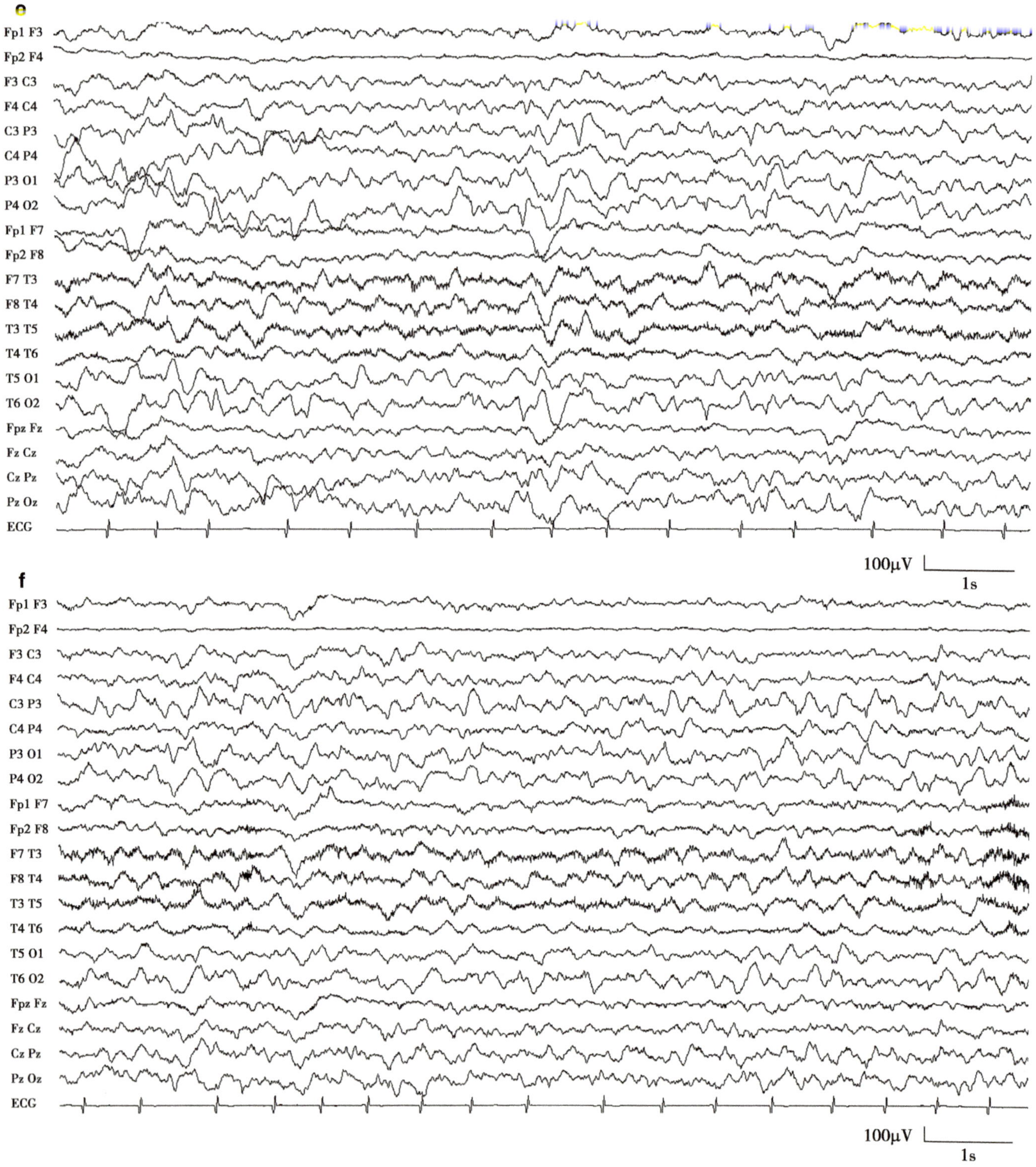

Fig. 5.12 (continued)

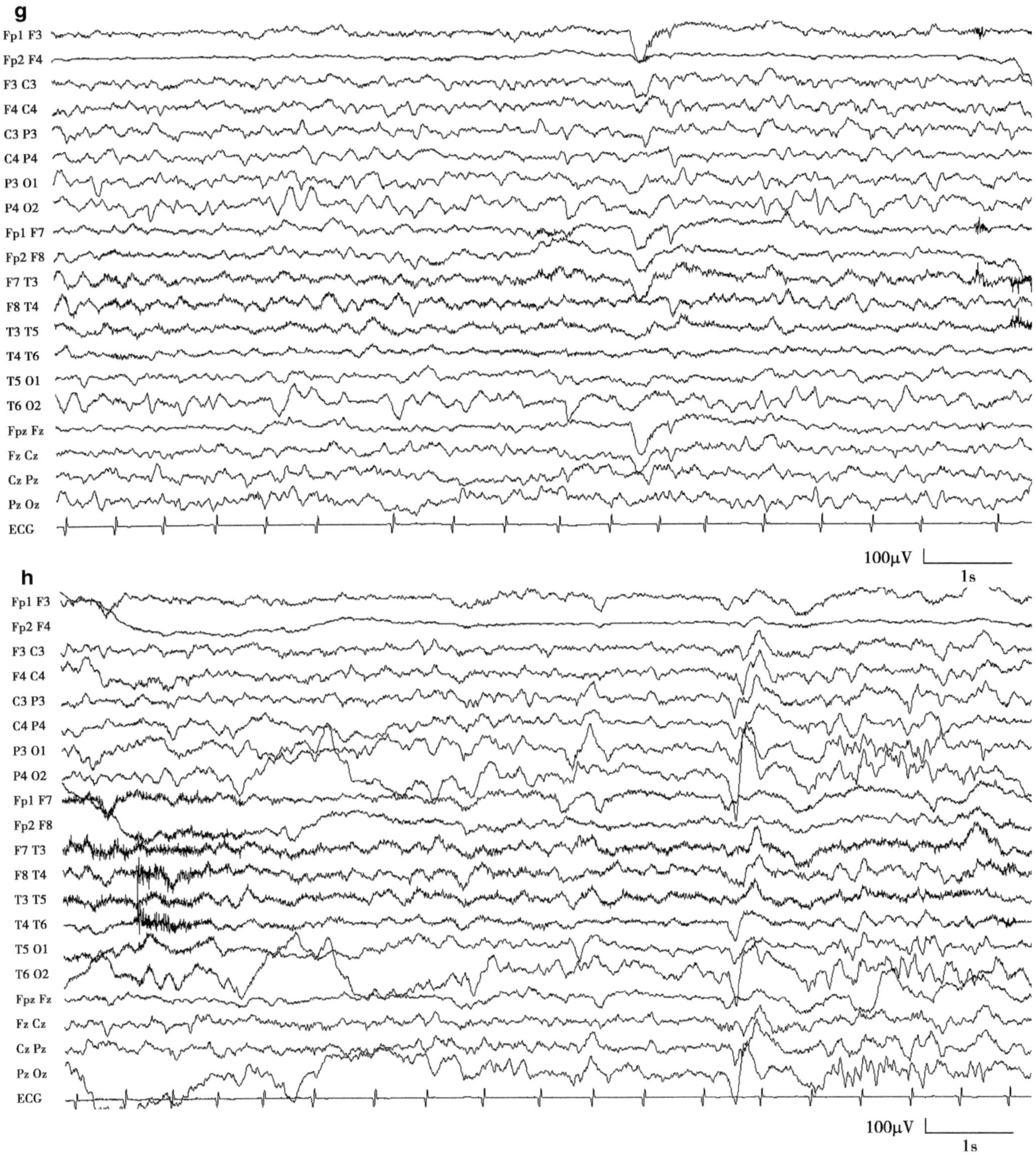

Fig. 5.12 (continued)

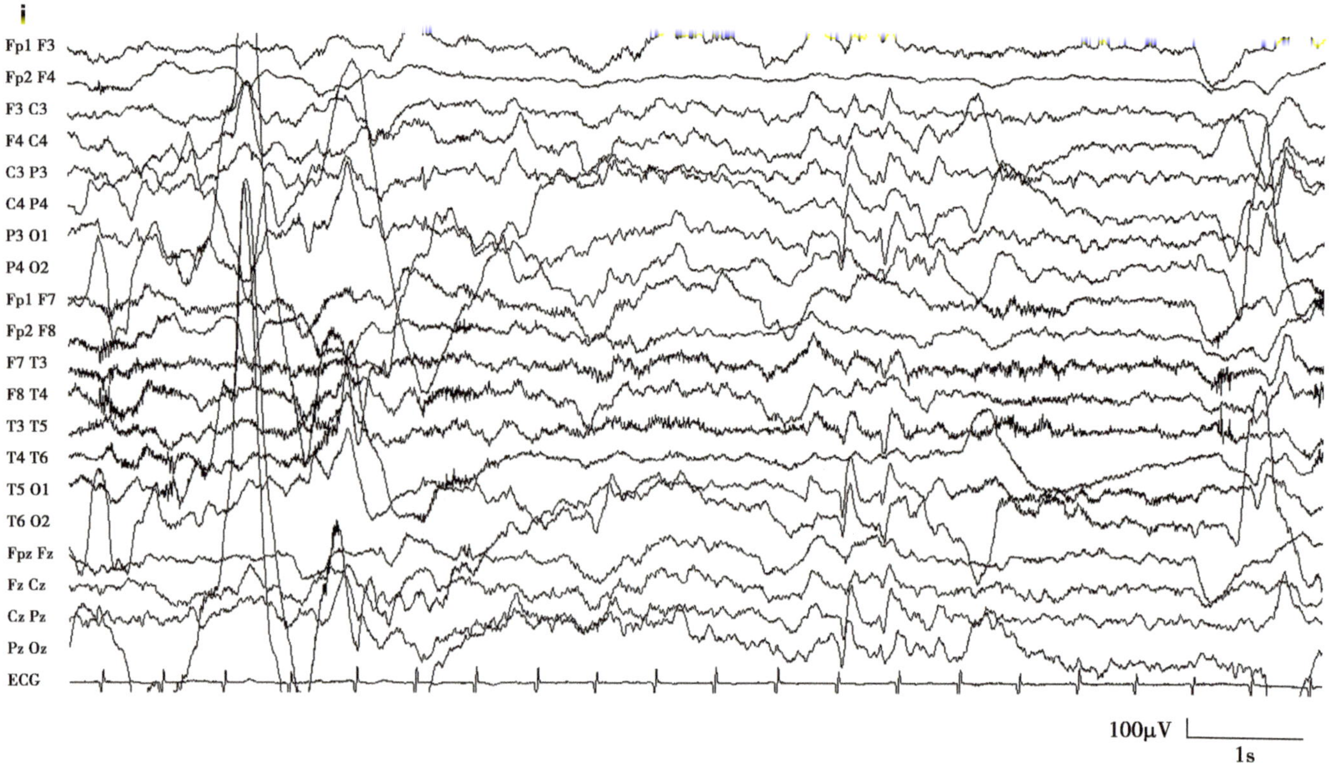

Fig. 5.12 (continued)

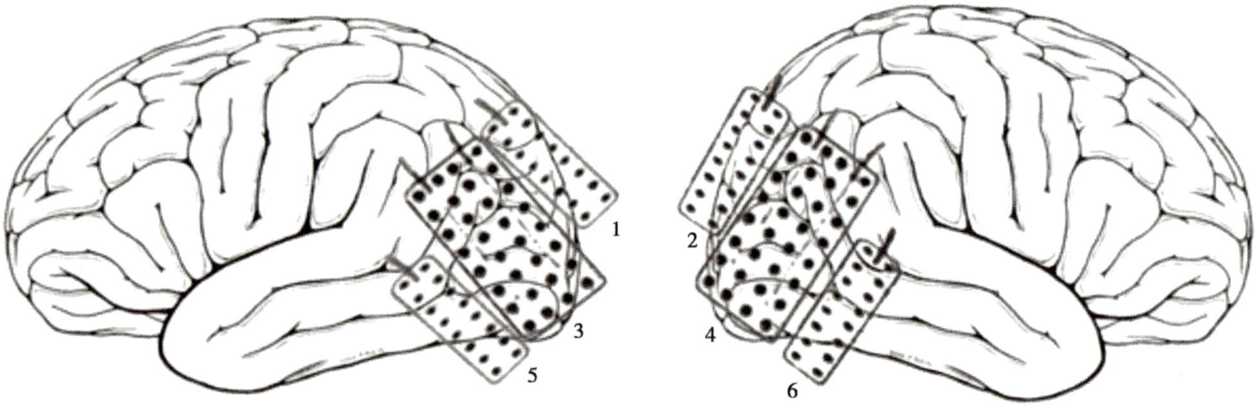

Fig. 5.13 Scheme of intracranial electrodes
Grid electrode 1: the left medial occipital region of interhemispheric fissure (16 contacts); Grid electrode 2: the right medial occipital region of interhemispheric fissure (16 contacts); Grid electrode 3: the left lateral occipital region (32 contacts); Grid electrode 4: the right lateral occipital region (32 contacts); Grid electrode 5: the left basioccipital part (16 contacts); Grid electrode 6: the right basioccipital part (16 contacts)

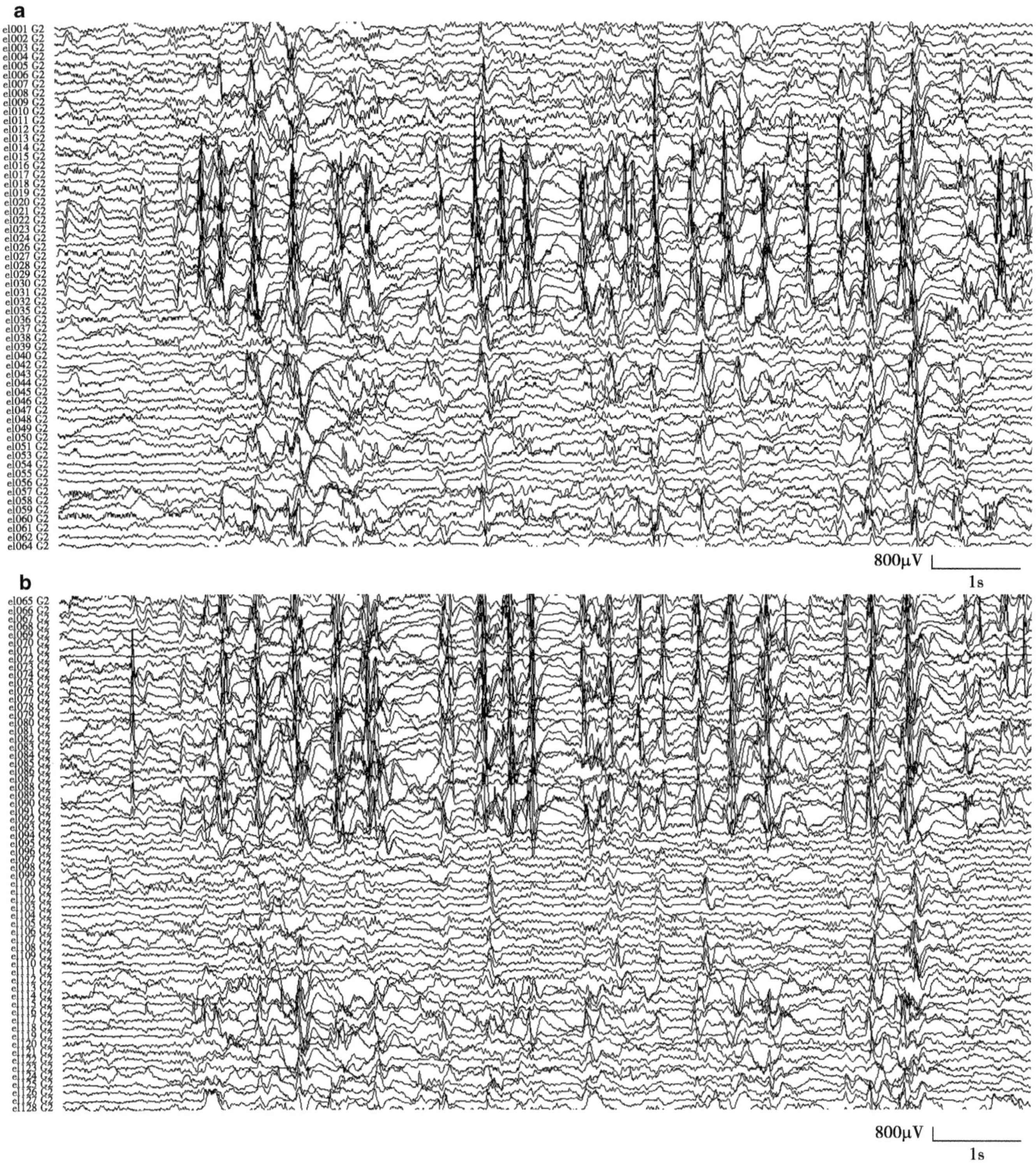

Fig. 5.14 Interictal intracranial EEG. (**a**) Manifestations in the first 64 leads of IEEG. (**b**) Manifestations in the second 64 leads of IEEG. The burst of rhythms of high-amplitude spike-and-wave complexes and polyspike and wave complexes were seen over the right occipital region (contact numbers el019, el020, el021, el022, el023, el028, el029, el030, el031, el066, el067, el068, el069, el073, el074, el075, el076, el077, el078, el081, el082, el083, el084, el085, el089, el090, el091, el092, el093, el113, el114, el115, el116, el117, el118, el119, el125, el126, el127), mainly the medial occipital region of interhemispheric fissure (contact numbers el019, el020, el021, el022, el023, el028, el029, el030, el031)

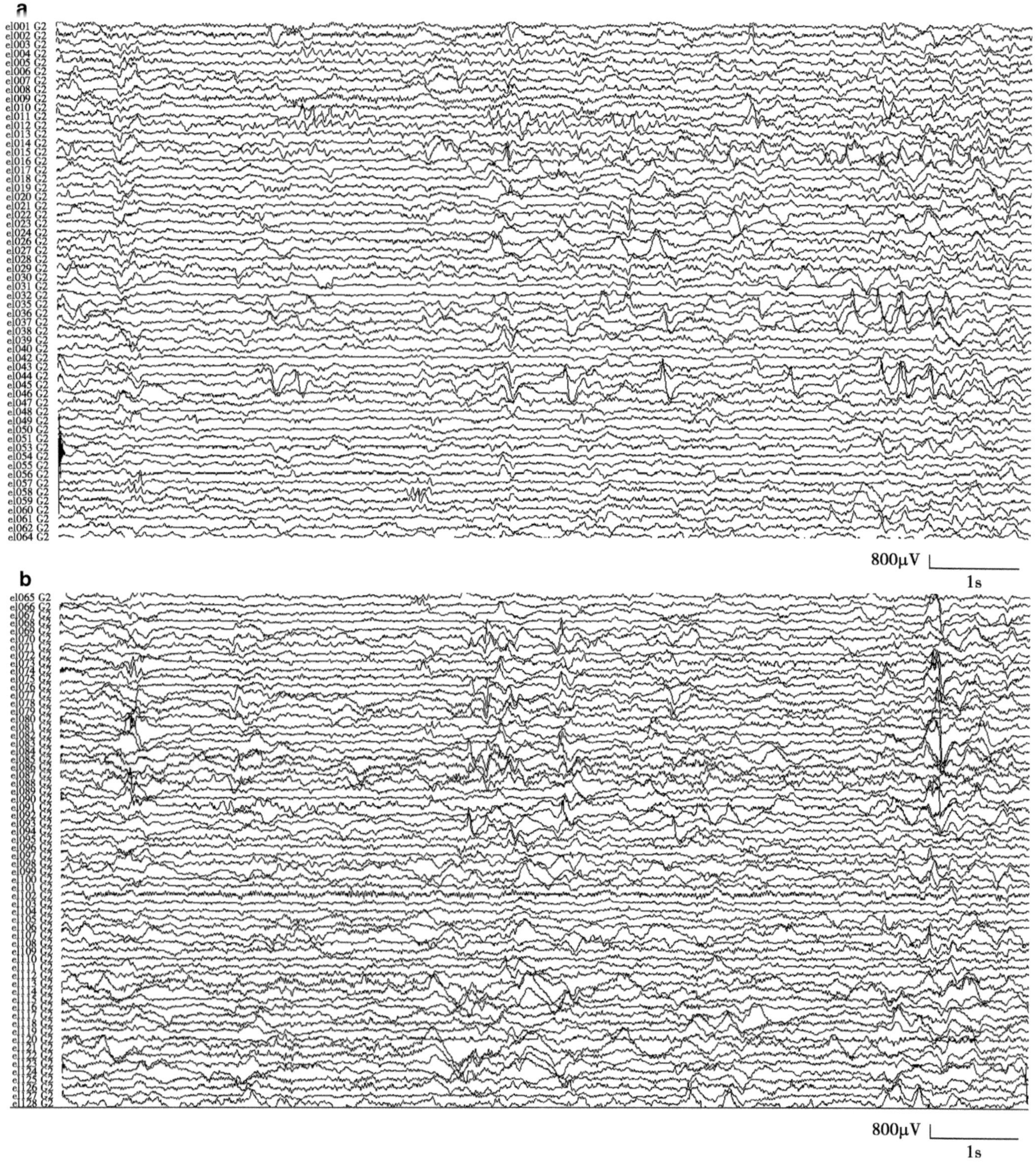

Fig. 5.15 Ictal intracranial EEG. (**a**) Before the seizure, the patient was awake and with bilateral lower extremities flexed. Upper figure shows the first 64 leads; lower figure shows the second 64 leads. The IEEG showed low amplitude fast activities over the anterior right occipital region (contact numbers el077, el078, el079, el086, el087). (**b**) During the seizure, the patient blinked frequently, swept the eyes from side to side, and tilted both lower limbs to the right. Upper figure shows the first 64 leads; lower figure shows the second 64 leads. The low amplitude fast activity propagated to all leads (earlier on right side). (**c**) The patient blinked quickly and failed to respond to calls. Upper figure shows the first 64 leads; lower figure shows the second 64 leads. The IEEG showed low amplitude fast activity, polyspikes, and wave complexes over the right occipital region (contact numbers el077, el078, el079, el085, el086, el091, el092, el093, el117, el118, el119, el123, el124, el125, el126, el127, el128) at mid- and late ictal phase. (**d**) The seizure ended. Upper figure shows the first 64 channels; lower figure shows the second 64 channels. The IEEG recovered to the background activity

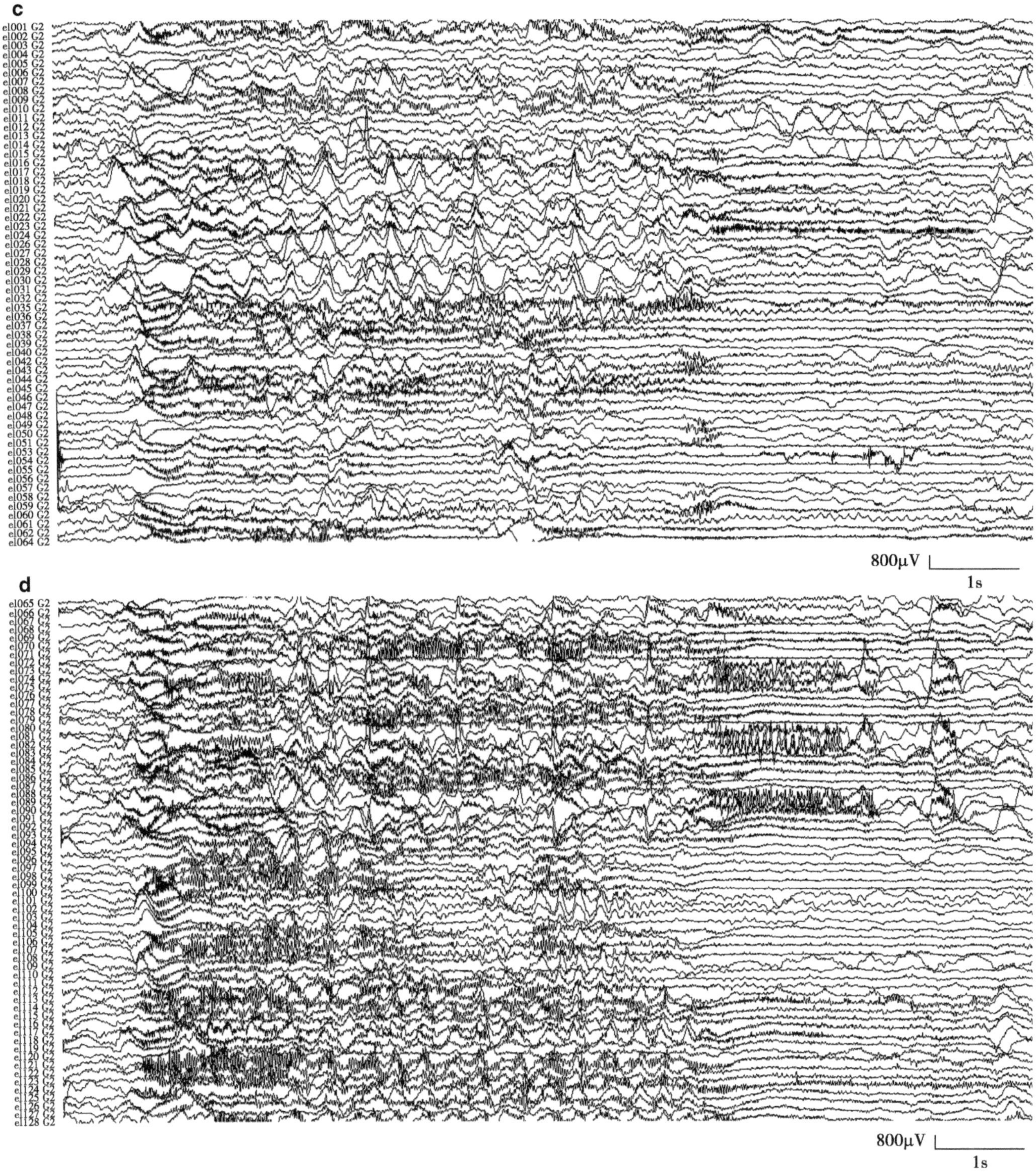

Fig. 5.15 (continued)

[Case Review]

The patient's interictal and ictal scalp EEG manifestations and clinical symptoms could not be definitely localized. Therefore, intracranial electrodes had to be implanted to define the epileptic focus. Occipital lobe epilepsy can easily produce bilateral synchronous abnormal electrical activities. If the origins of the activities could not be determined, the application of intracranial electrodes is acceptable. The determination of the cortical range to be resected on the basis of the lateralization of origins of seizure is also important. The patient underwent right occipital region resection and was followed up for 1 year. He is seizure free.

Case 5.4 Occipital Lobe Epilepsy

[Abstract of Medical Records]
Male, 13 years old.

1. *Chief complaint*: Episodic loss of consciousness for 4 years.
2. *History of present illness*: The patient developed loss of consciousness with limbs tonic-clonic 4 years ago. The symptoms persisted for about half a minute and then spontaneously resolved. He went to a local hospital for consultation and was diagnosed with epilepsy. Topiramate was administered, but the efficacy was unsatisfactory. The patient frequently experienced paroxysmal blurred vision, dialeptic seizure, teichopsia in field of vision up to 10 times a day. During a seizure, the patient had alternative leftward and rightward head deflection, tonic limbs, and in some cases, secondary generalized tonic-clonic seizure. The patient is now taking oral sodium valproate at 1000 mg/d and nitrazepam, 10 mg/d.
3. *Past history*: The patient was born spontaneously after full-term gestation; suffered from intracranial infection at 1 month old (no detailed information available) and had 1 convulsion.
4. *Personal and family history*: No history of associated diseases.
5. *Physical examination*: No neurological abnormalities were found. Psychological assessment: VIQ is 96, PIQ is 83, FIQ is 94.
6. *Imaging examination*:
   (a) MRI revealed the presence of atrophy of left parietal occipital lobe and cerebral softening focus.
   (b) MRS revealed the NAA concentration was slightly higher in left hippocampus than in corresponding right side.
   (c) SPECT revealed the mild low perfusion in left temporal lobe.
7. *EEG*: For details, see Figs. 5.16, 5.17, 5.18, 5.19, and 5.20.

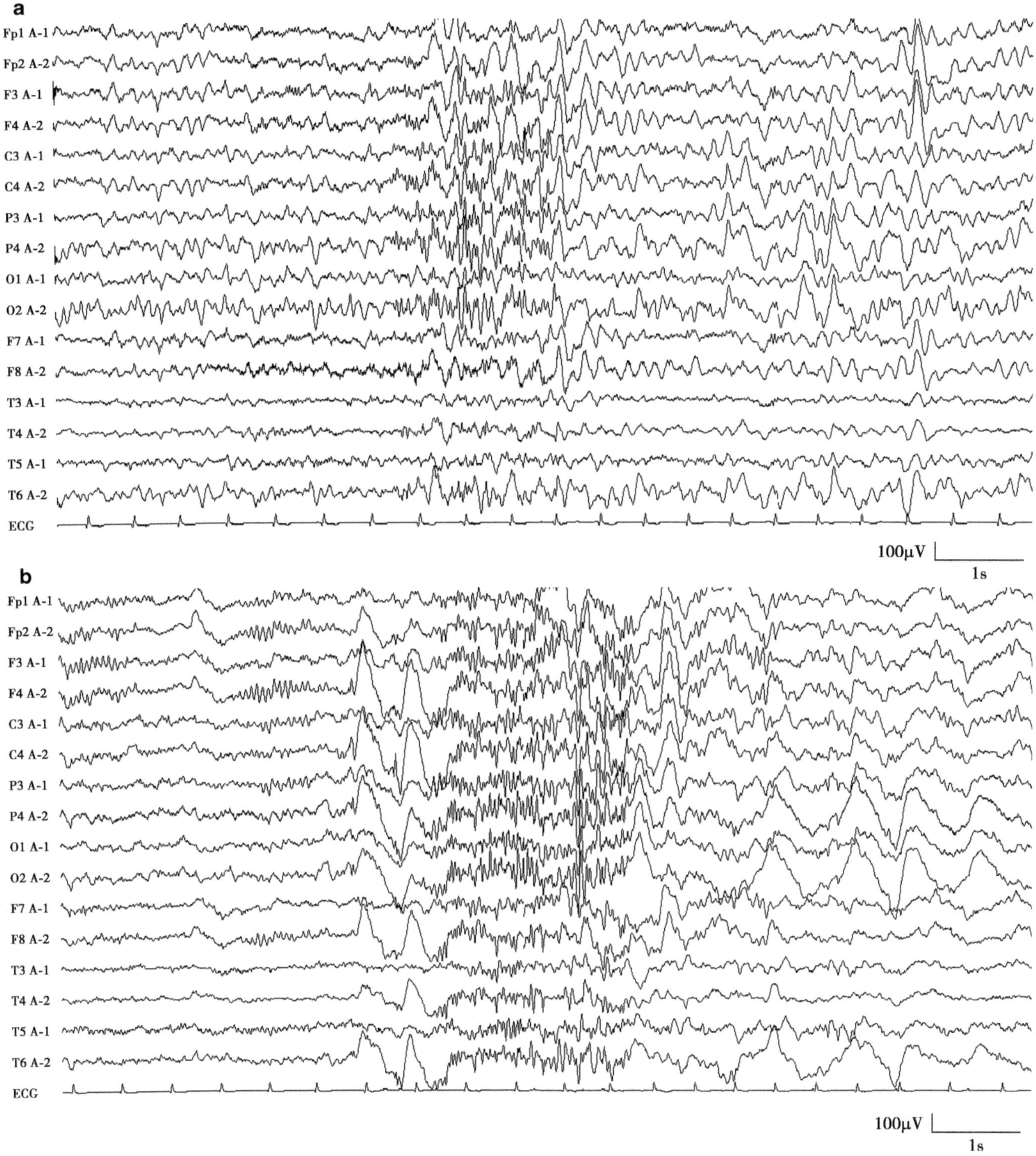

Fig. 5.16 Interictal scalp EEG. (**a**) The background EEG rhythm was 8.0 Hz. Sporadic medium- to high-amplitude 4.0–5.0 Hz slow waves were seen over the bilateral hemispheres. The wave amplitude was slightly higher on the right side than the left, mainly parietal region (P4), occipital region (O2), and posterior temporal region (T6). Paroxysmal spike rhythm occurred over the right central region (C4), parietal region (P4), occipital (O2), and posterior temporal region (T6). (**b**) The EEG showed the Phase II sleep background, medium- to high-amplitude spike rhythm over the bilateral hemispheres, mainly the right central region (C4), parietal region (P4), occipital region (O2), and posterior temporal region (T6). Sporadic high-amplitude spike-and-wave complexes occurred over the right posterior frontal region (F4), central region (C4), parietal region (P4), and occipital region (O2)

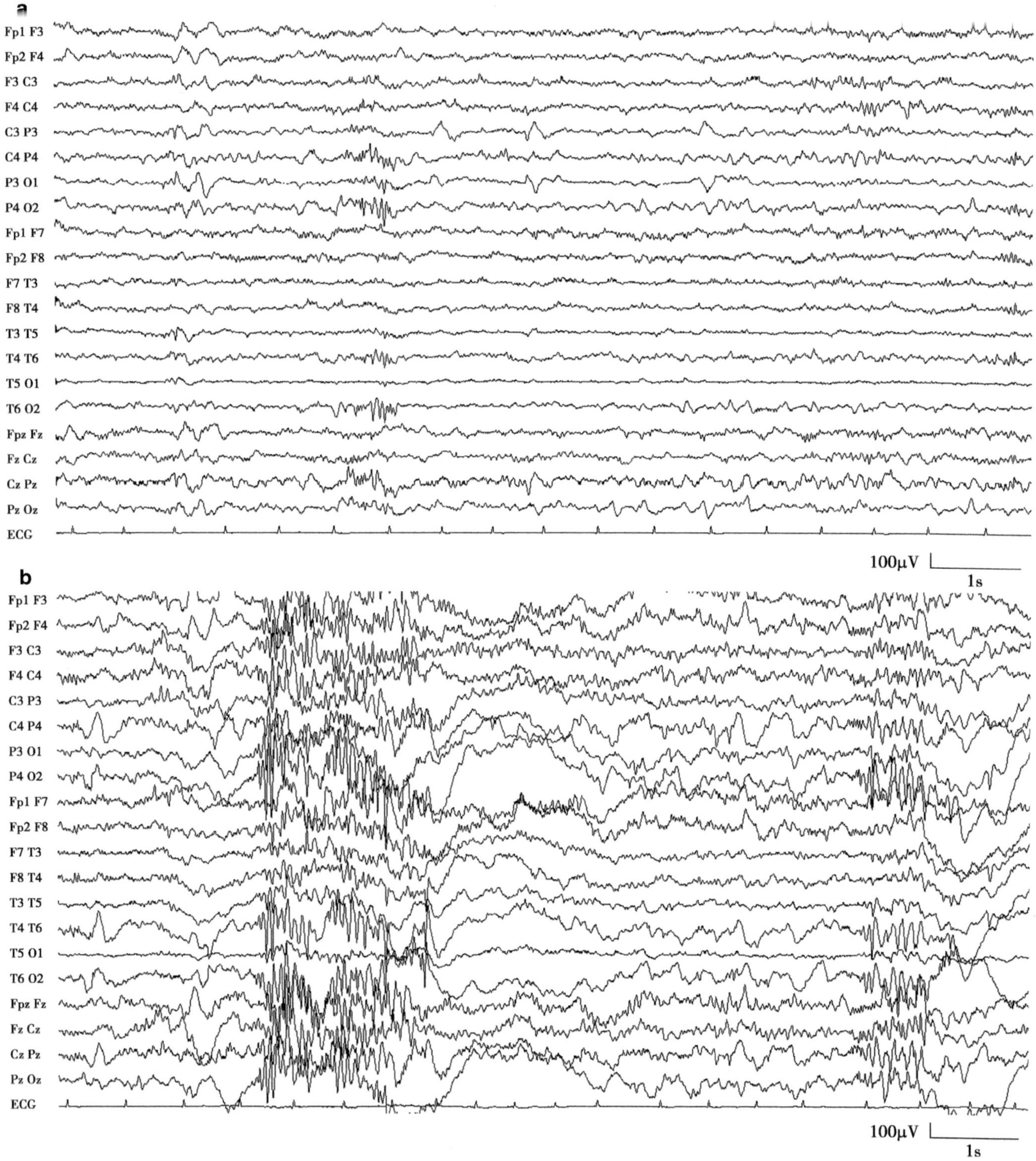

Fig. 5.17 Ictal scalp EEG. (**a**) Before the seizure, the patient was sleeping in a supine position. The EEG showed the Phase II sleep background. The sporadic low to mid amplitude sharp waves were observed over the left temporoparietal region (C3 P3, P3 O1, T3 T5, T5 O1) and midline channels (Cz Pz); low to mid amplitude spike rhythm was observed over the right temporoparietal occipital region (C4 P4, P4 O2, T4 T6, T6 O2) and midline channels (Cz Pz). T5 O1 channel showed signal problem(s). (**b**) During the seizure, the patient's eyes were open for about 3 s before closing, and the patient hinted the relatives to record the seizure. The EEG showed 10.0–11.0 Hz spike rhythm lasting for about 2 s, especially evident in the right parieto-occipital region (P4 O2), posterior temporal region (T4 T6, T6 O2). (**c**) The patient was in supine position with eyes closed. The EEG showed paroxysmal medium-to high-amplitude spike rhythm over the right parieto-occipital region (P4 O2), posterior temporal region (T4 T6, T6 O2), and midline (Pz Oz), with irregular slow waves. (**d**) The seizure ended. The EEG showed sharp waves and irregular slow waves over the right parieto-occipital region (C4 P4, P4 O2), posterior temporal region (T4 T6, T6 O2), and midline channels (Cz Pz, Pz Oz). (**e**) At the end of the seizure, the patient's EEG gradually recovered to background EEG

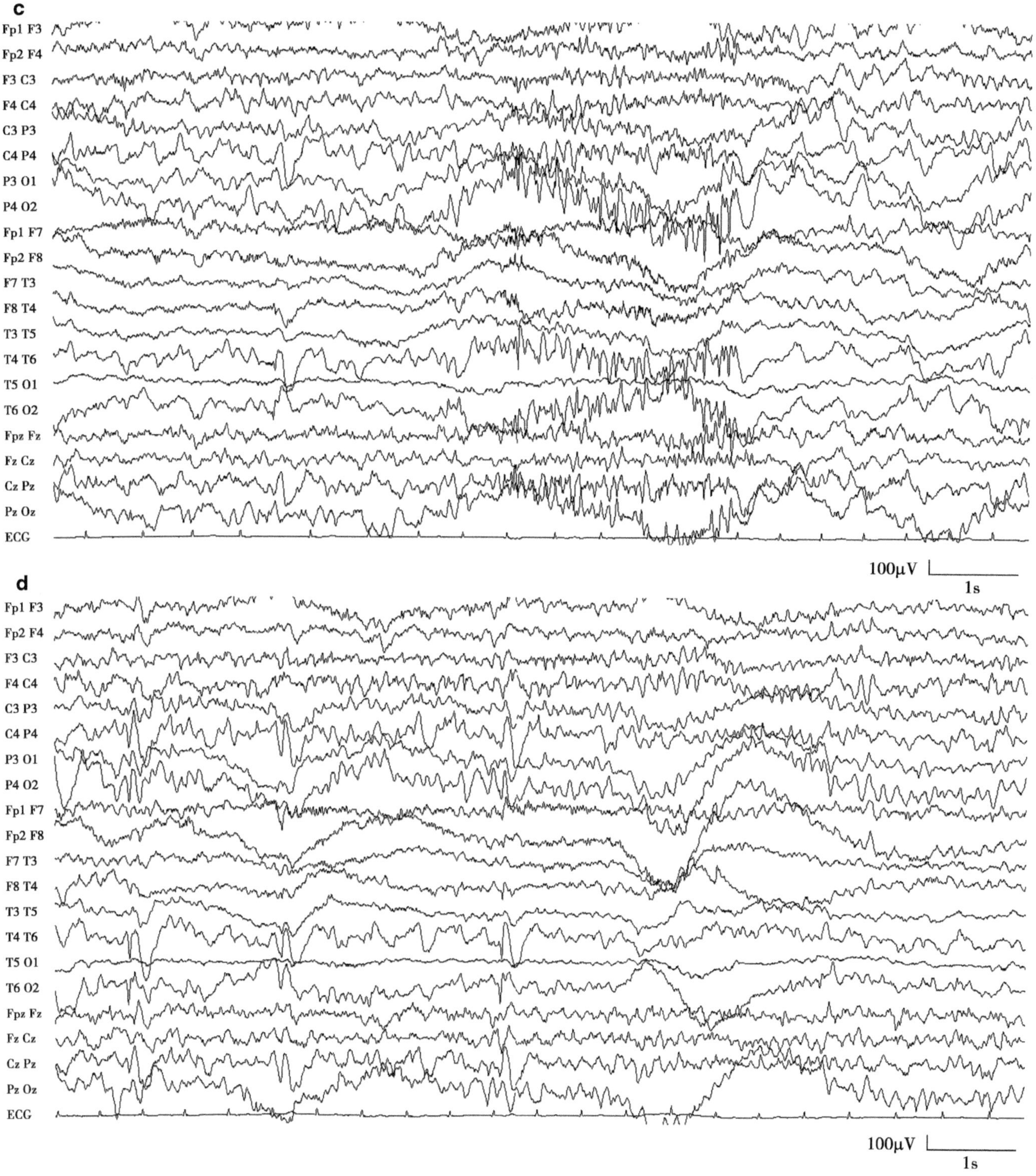

Fig. 5.17 (continued)

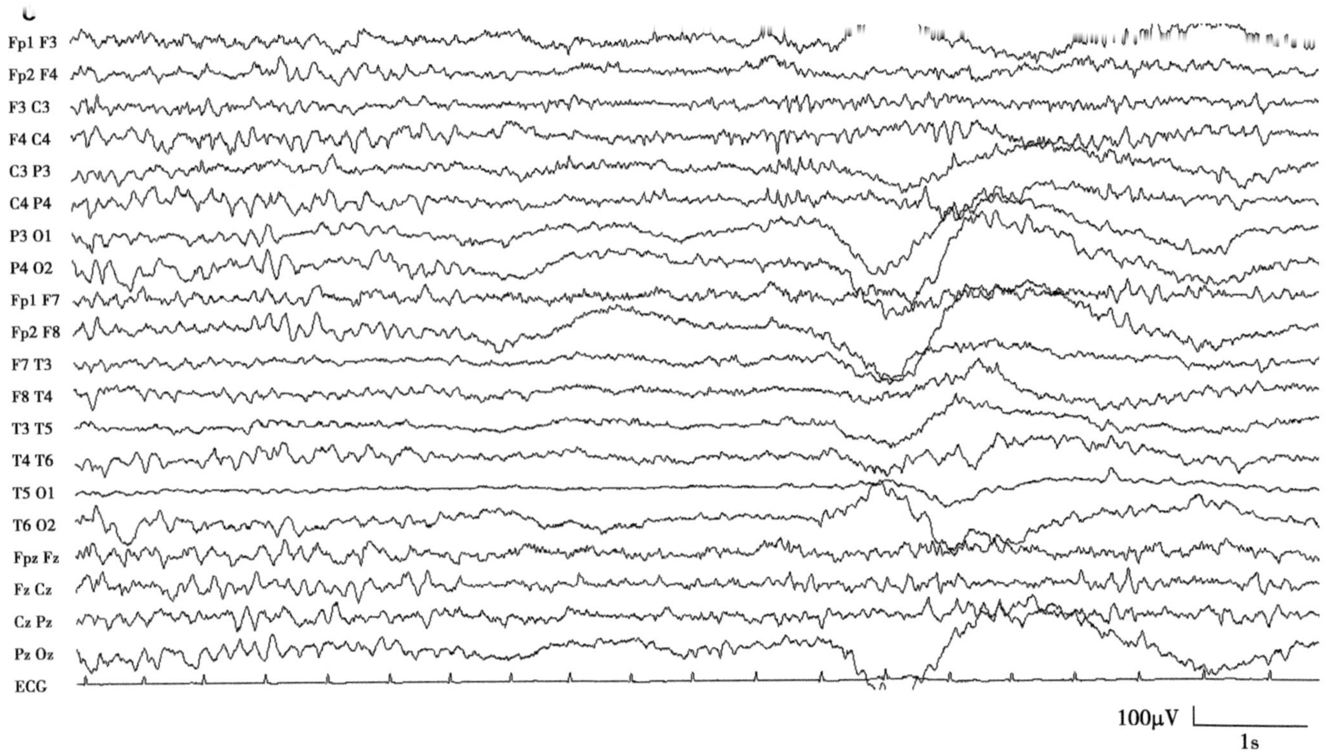

Fig. 5.17 (continued)

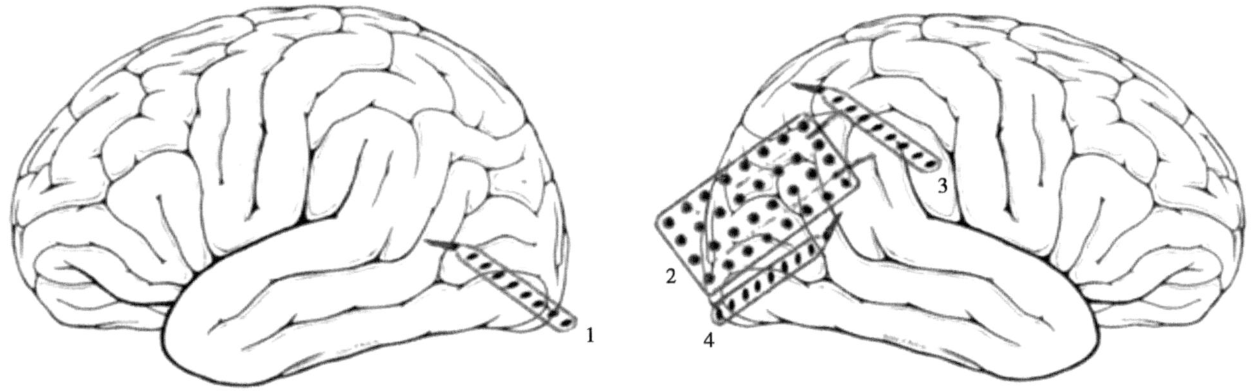

Fig. 5.18 Scheme of intracranial electrodes
Strip electrode 1: left occipital pole (8 contacts)
Grid electrode 2: right lateral occipital region (32 contacts)
Strip electrode 3: right parietal region (8 contacts)
Strip electrode 4: right occipital pole (8 contacts)

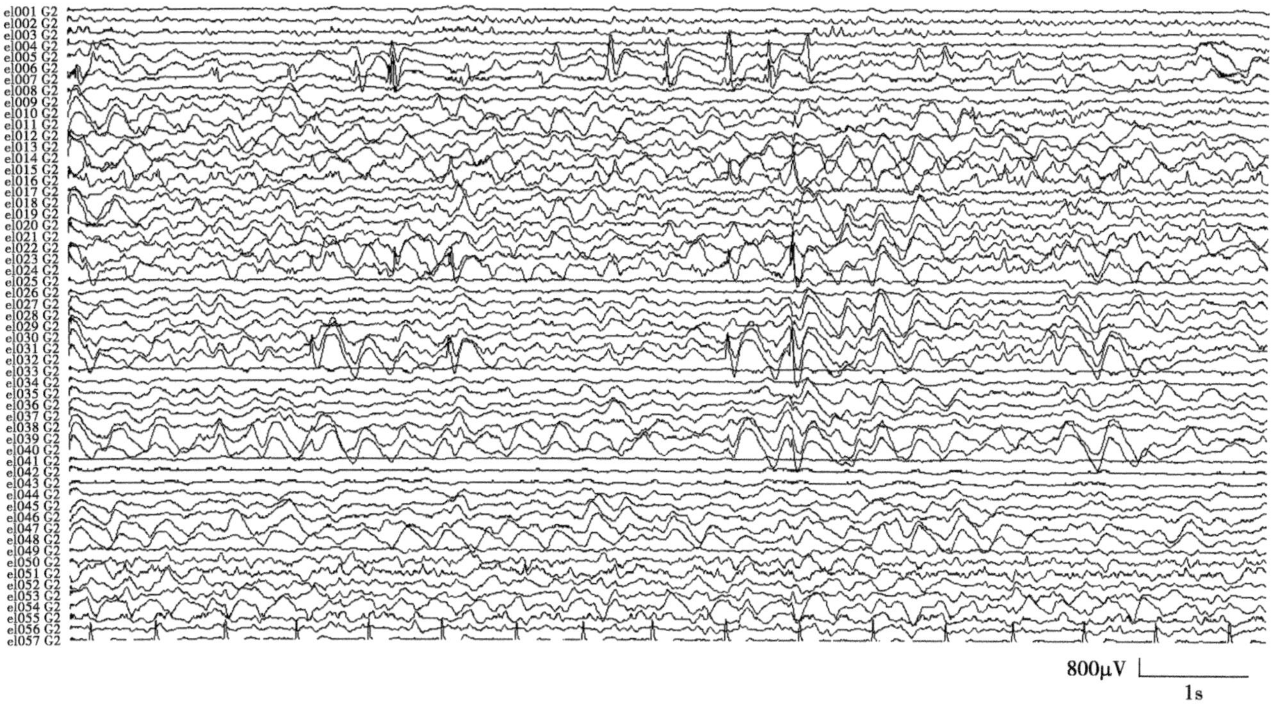

Fig. 5.19 Interictal intracranial EEG
Paroxysmal high-amplitude spike-and-wave complexes over the left occipital region (contact numbers el005, el006, el007) and right occipital region (contact numbers el015, el016, el023, el024, el031, el032, el039, el040). The discharge was asynchronous between left and right hemisphere

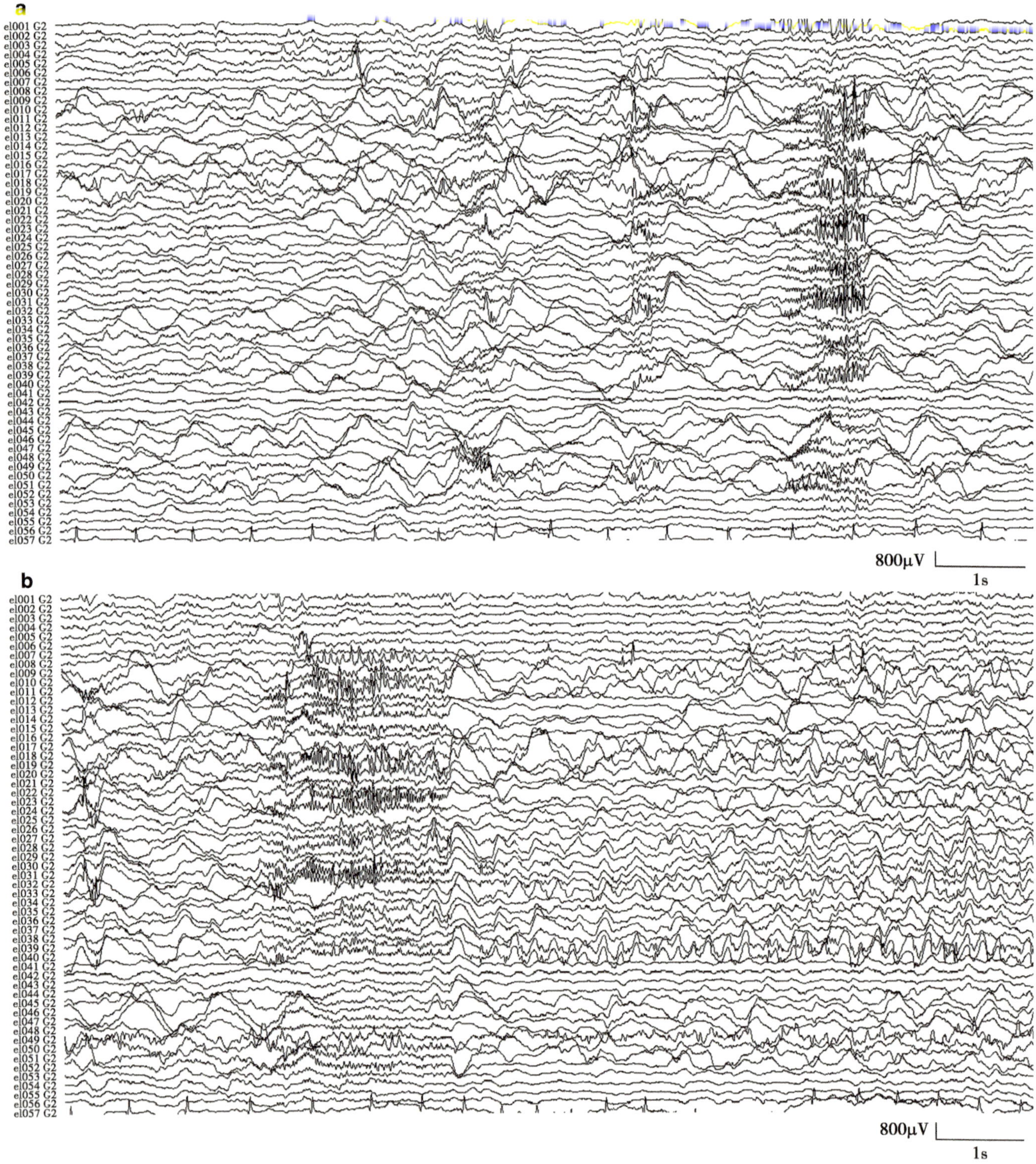

Fig. 5.20 Ictal intracranial EEG. (**a**) Before the seizure onset, the patient was sleeping in left lateral position. Paroxysmal medium-to high-amplitude spike rhythm was seen over the right occipital region (contact numbers el009, el010, el011, el012, el013, el014, el017, el018, el019, el023, el027, el031, el032, el036, el039, el040, el049, el050, el051). (**b**) The patient opened the eyes and the body slightly turned to the left with both upper limbs flexion. The IEEG showed low amplitude fast activities, followed by spikes, irregular slow waves over the right occipital region. (**c**) The patient stared with unresponsiveness. The IEEG showed intensified spike rhythm with wave amplitude gradually increasing. Then the wave rhythm propagated to multiple channels over the right occipital region. 2.0–3.0 Hz δ wave rhythm was observed over the right occipital region (contact numbers el009, el010, el011, el017, el018, el019, el020). (**d**) The patient's head slowly turned to the right with eyes gazing to the right side. The IEEG showed δ activity over the right occipital region and then propagated to the right hemisphere with mixed low-amplitude spikes. (**e**) At the end of the seizure, the patient returned to left position and fell into sleep again. The irregular slow waves gradually decreased

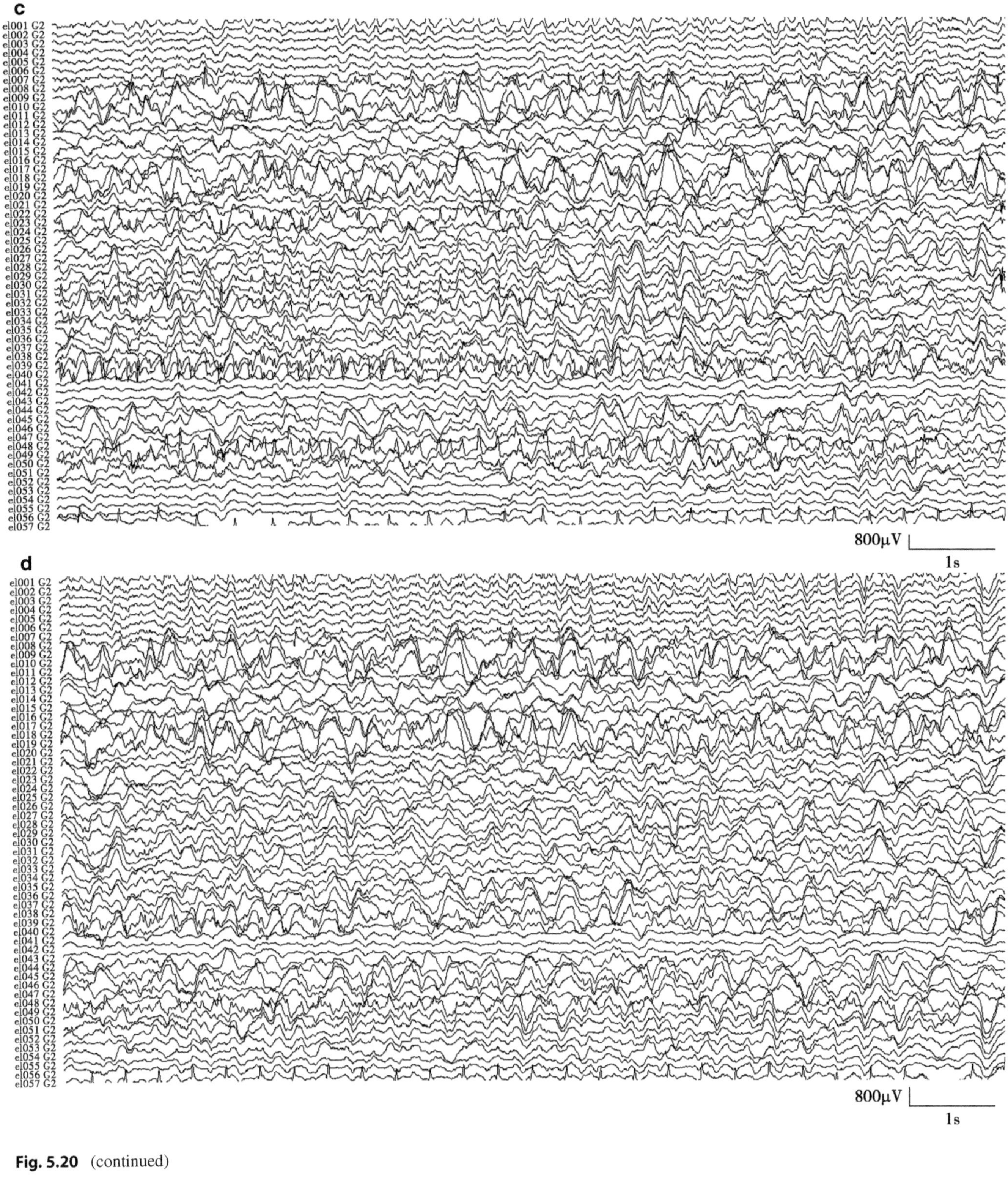

Fig. 5.20 (continued)

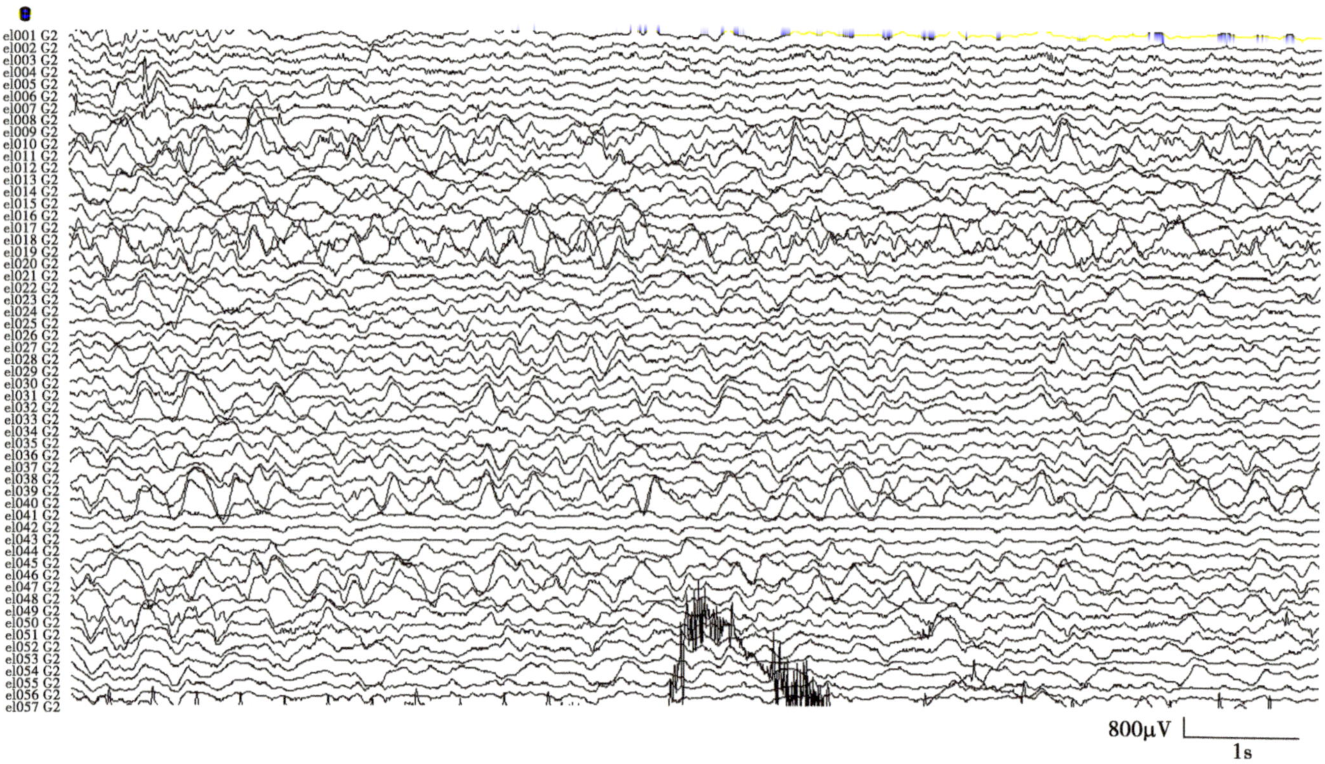

Fig. 5.20 (continued)

[Case Review]

In this case, the cortical atrophy was located in left parieto-occipital region. However, the interictal and ictal scalp EEG showed that the abnormal activities were significant over the right hemisphere. In order to further determine the origin of seizure, intracranial electrodes were implanted in bilateral occipital lobes. The IEEG showed that the origin of seizure was located in the cortex of occipital lobe on the side opposite to the focus. The patient underwent right occipital region resection and was followed up for 5 years. He was seizure free.

Case 5.5 Occipital Lobe Epilepsy

[Abstract of Medical Records]
Male, 30 years old.

1. *Chief complaint*: Paroxysmal loss of consciousness with limbs clonus for 22 years.
2. *History of present illness*: The patient accidentally experienced a drowning asphyxia 22 years ago (at 8 years old). Half a year afterwards, he underwent a sudden seizure with gazing to the right and loss of consciousness. The symptoms relieved after about 2 min. The patient could not recall the episode after the seizure, and there was no seizure in the following half year. About 21 years ago (at 9 years old), he experienced recurrent seizures with head turning to the right and loss of consciousness. The seizure lasted for about 2 min. The auras were dizziness and blurred vision. The seizures also included abrupt falling, rightward deviation of head and eyes, trismus, and subsequent limbs clonus, vocalization, and foaming at mouth. The seizure frequency varied from 1 or 2 times a week to several times a day. In most cases, the seizures were clustered in several days. Diurnal seizures were most common. The patient was orally taking multiple antiseizure medications, but the treatment results were unsatisfactory. He was taking magnesium valproate, 1200 mg/d, and carbamazepine, 600 mg/d. But the control of symptoms was poor, and the patient still had several episodes a month.
3. *Past history*: The patient was born at full-term by normal delivery and had a history of drowning asphyxia at 8 years old.
4. *Physical examination*: Examination of visual field revealed visual field defects in lower right quadrant of both eyes.
5. *Imaging examination*: MRI revealed abnormal signals over the left occipital lobe.
6. *EEG*: For details, see Figs. 5.21, 5.22, 5.23, 5.24, and 5.25.

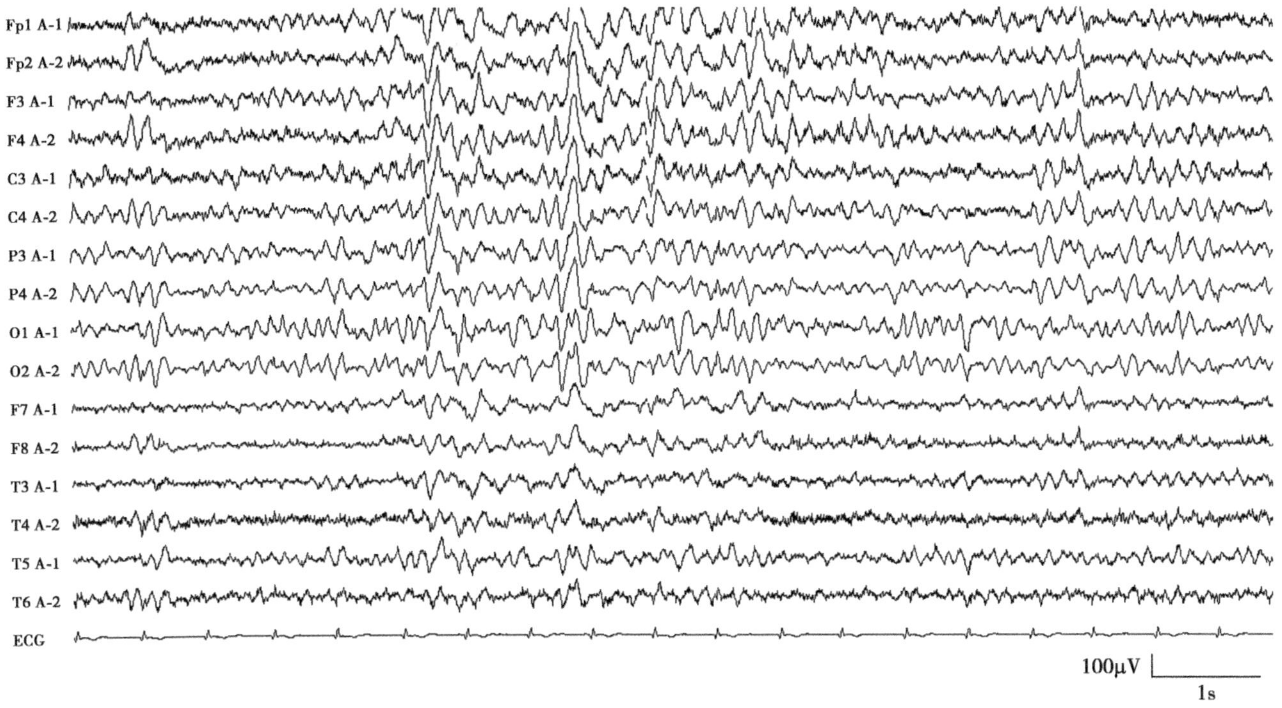

Fig. 5.21 Interictal scalp EEG
The EEG showed basic rhythm 8.0 Hz and paroxysmal medium-to high-amplitude 4.0–5.0 Hz slow wave rhythm over the bilateral hemispheres

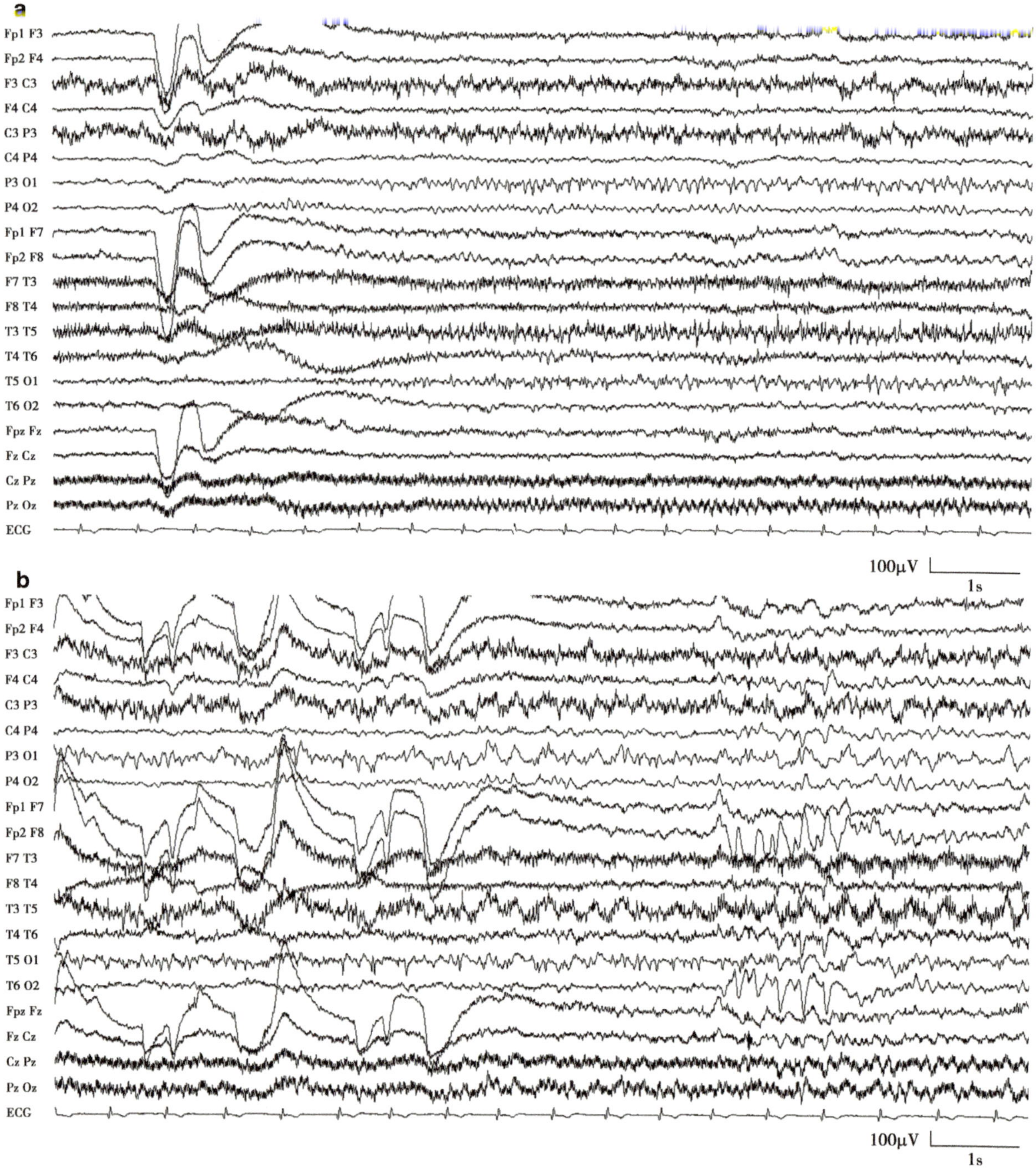

Fig. 5.22 Ictal scalp EEG. (**a**) Before the seizure, the patient was in supine position. The EEG showed fast activity over the left occipital region (P3 O1, T5 O1). The left central region and temporal region mixed many EMG artifacts, and the parietal midline and the occipital midline regions showed artifacts caused by poor contact of electrodes. (**b**) The patient opened eyes for several seconds and then closed eyes again. The EEG showed increased amplitude of spikes over the left occipital region, lasting for about 10 s. Then paroxysmal spike-and-wave complexes occurred over the right frontal (Fp2 F8) and posterior temporal occipital regions (T6 O2); EMG artifacts were identified over the left central region (F3 C3, C3 P3) and temporal region (F7 T3, T3 T5). (**c**) The patient opened eyes and sighed. EEG signals were mixed with numerous wobbling artifacts and EMG artifacts. (**d**) The patient did not respond to questions with hands automatisms. The EEG characteristics were the basically same as **c**. (**e**) Head turned to the right with rightward gazing of eyes, and he raised his right upper limb. Numerous EMG artifacts were observed. (**f**) The patient manifested with left upper limb flexion, right upper limb extension, bilateral lower extremities flexion, limbs clonus, and vocalization. The EEG presentation was the same as **e**. (**g**) The patient's limbs were abducted while been tonic and clonic. The EEG characteristics were the same as **e**. (**h**) The patient manifested with mild tonic limbs and slowed clonus. The EEG characteristics were the same as **e**. (**i**) The patient showed clonus of limbs. EMG artifacts appeared at a rhythm of 2.0–3.0 Hz. (**j**) The patient manifested with mild clonus of limbs with coarse wheezing and then clonus stopped. EEG signals were mixed with numerous EMG artifacts that incorporated high-amplitude sharpened slow waves. (**k**) The seizure ended after 1.5 min. EEG signals were mixed with numerous EMG artifacts

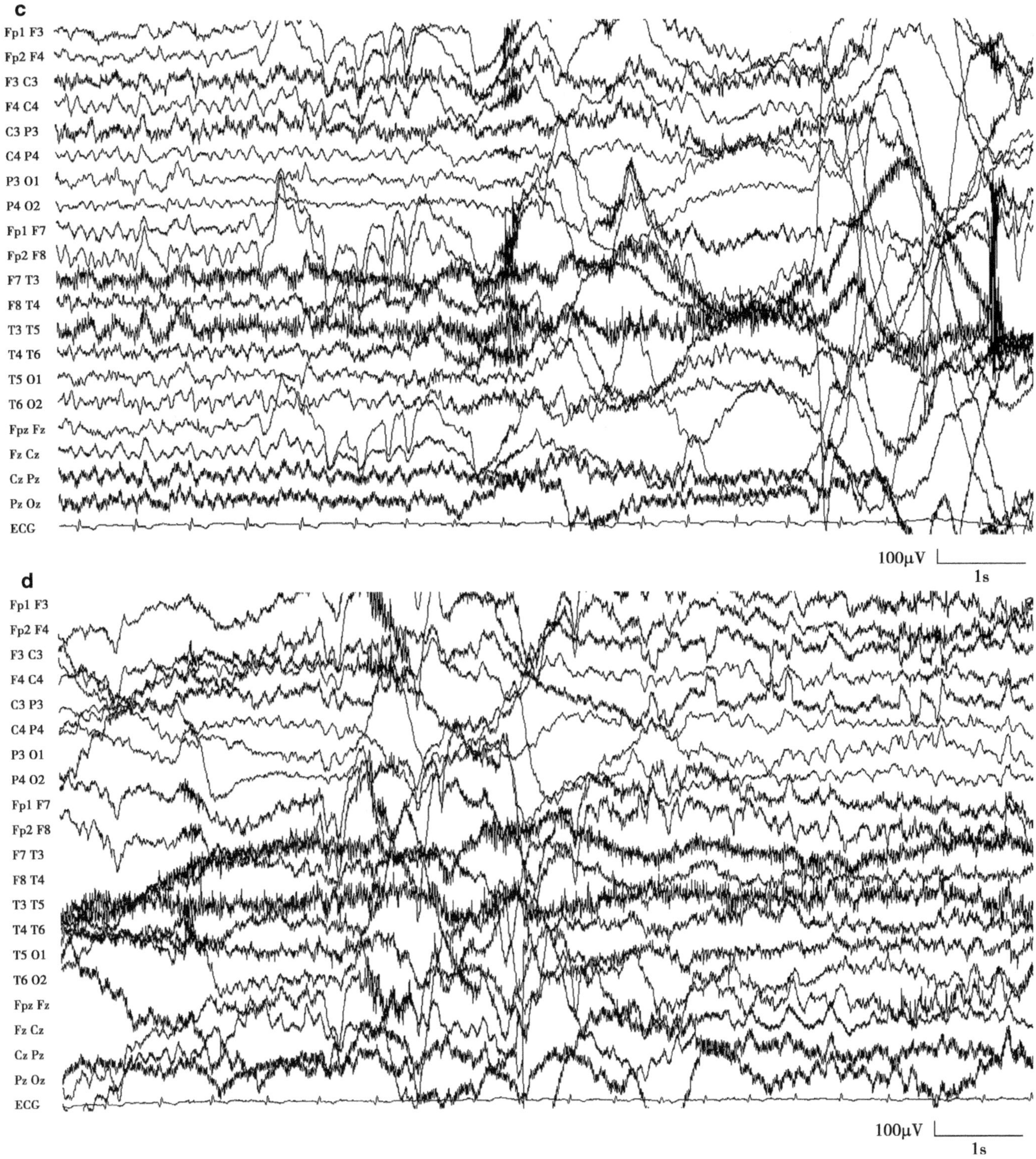

Fig. 5.22 (continued)

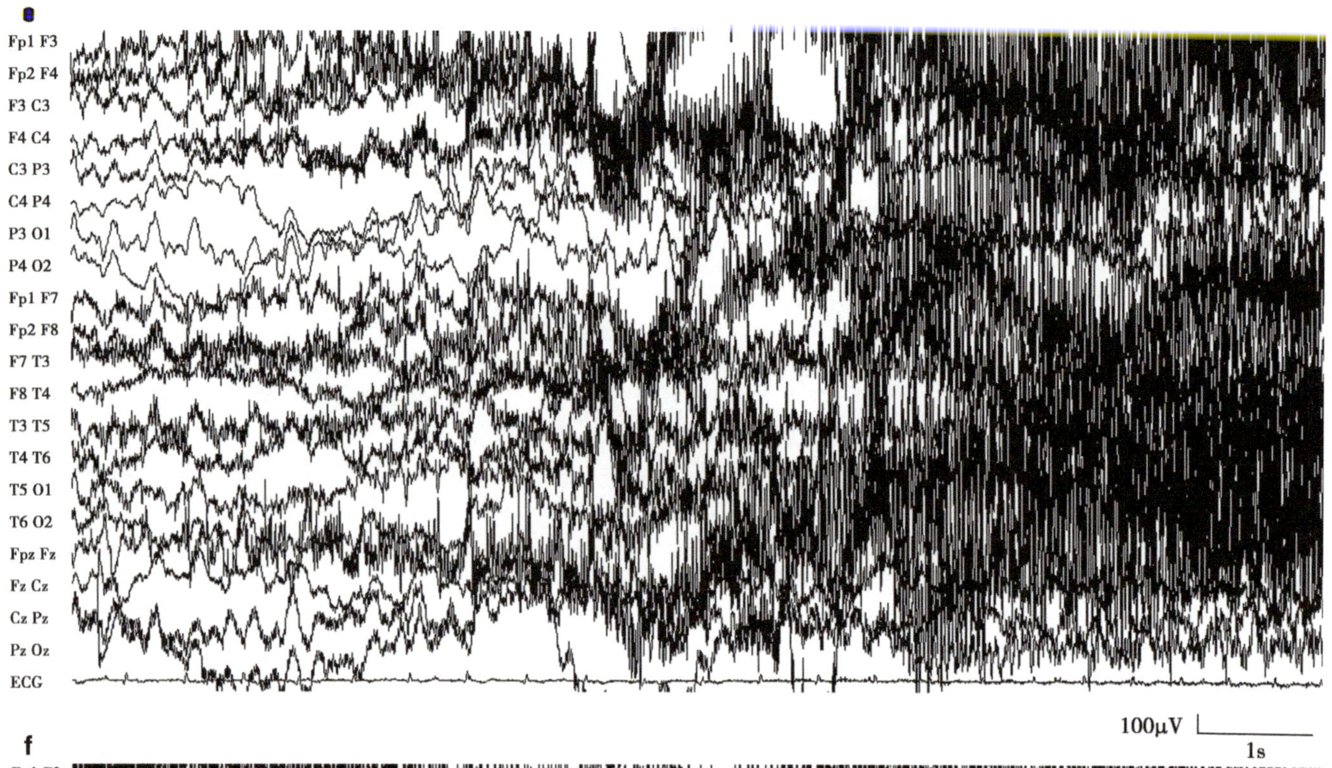

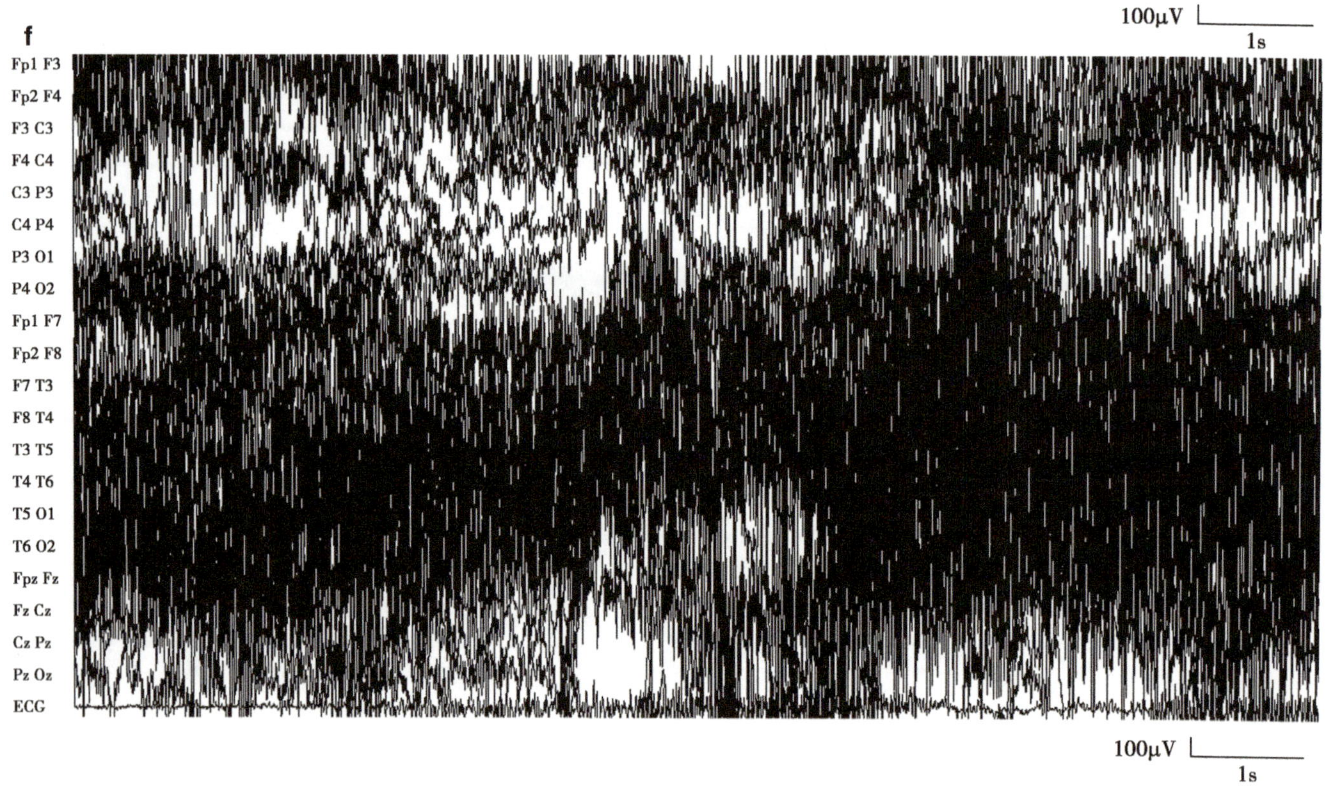

Fig. 5.22 (continued)

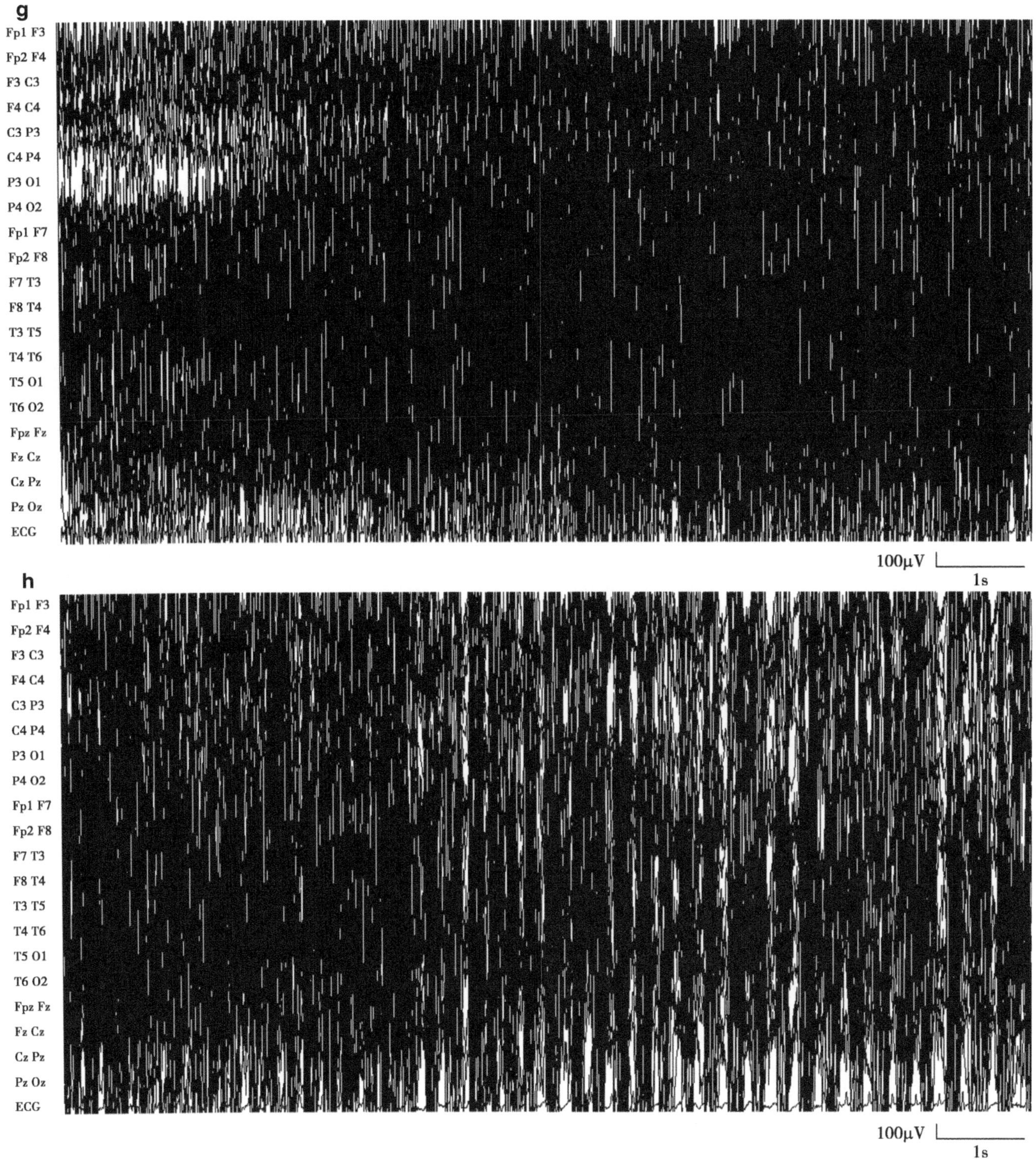

Fig. 5.22 (continued)

i

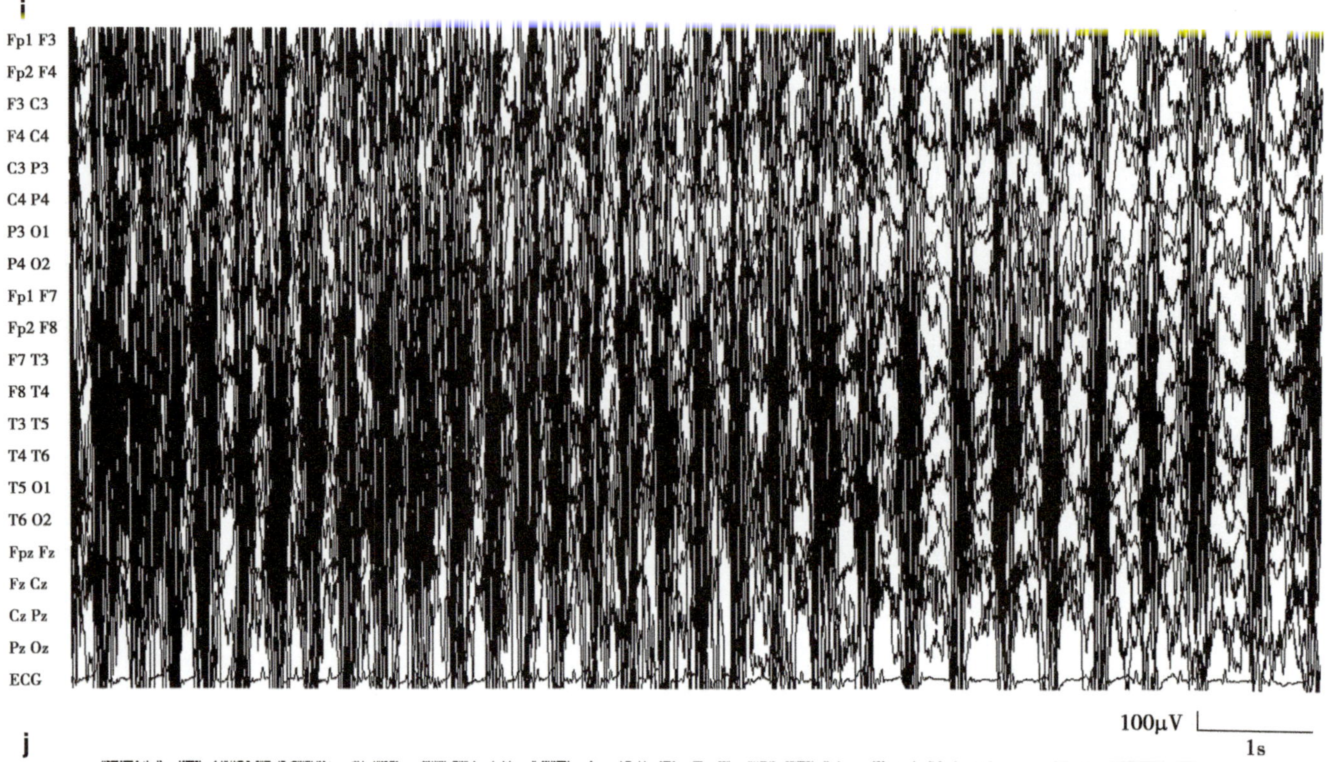

j

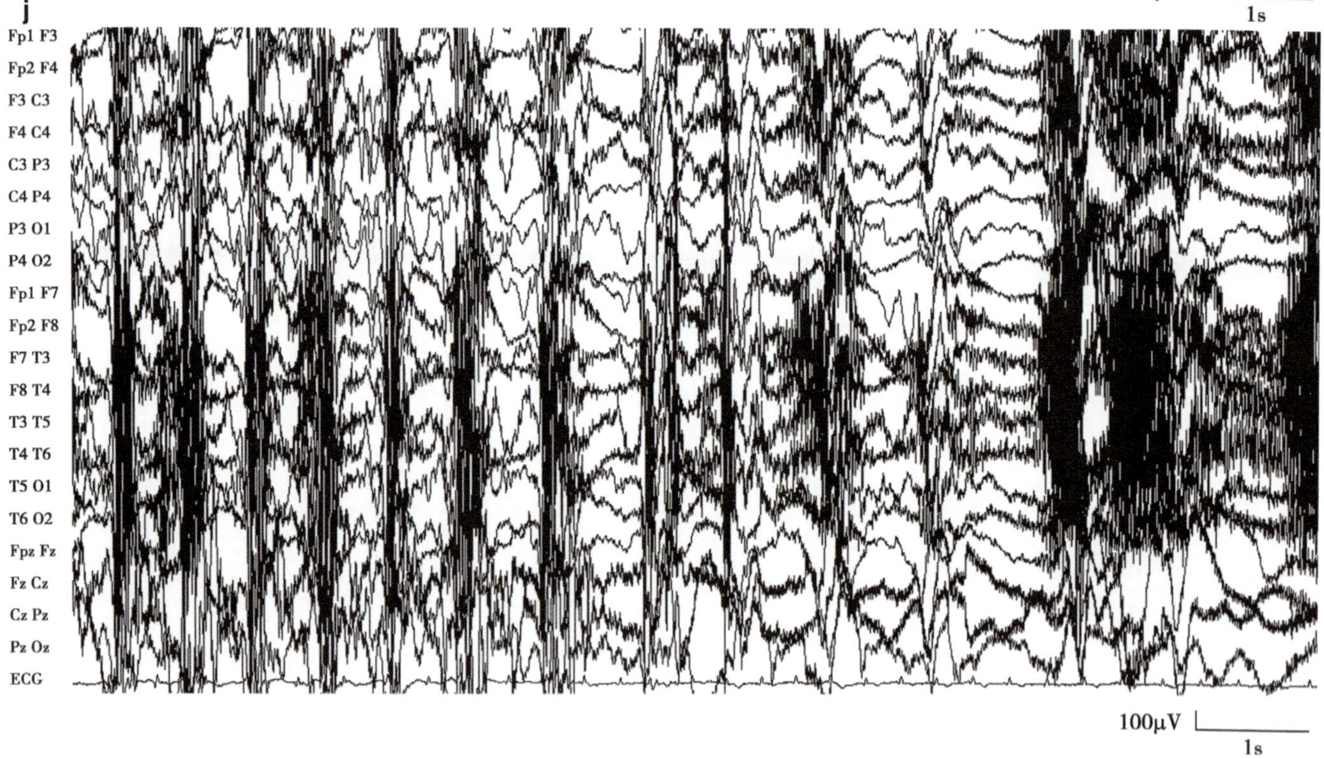

Fig. 5.22 (continued)

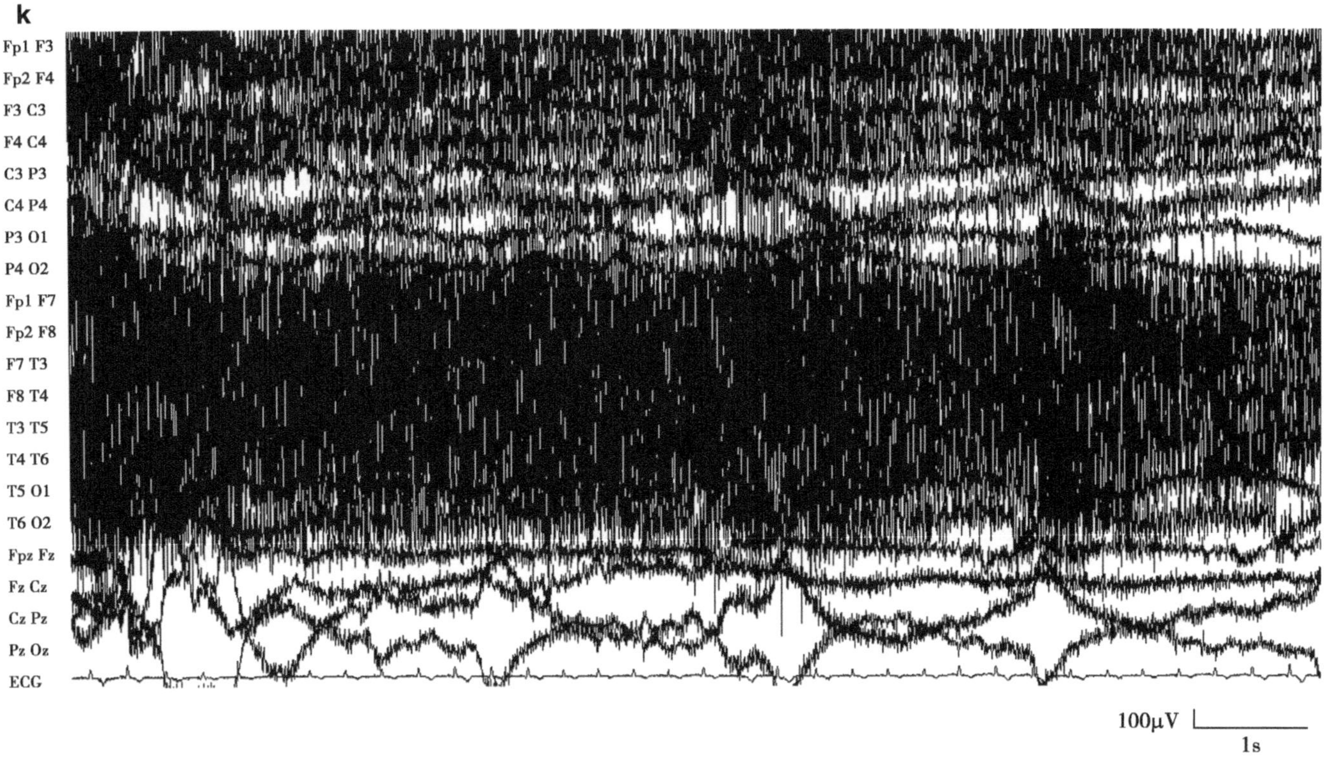

Fig. 5.22 (continued)

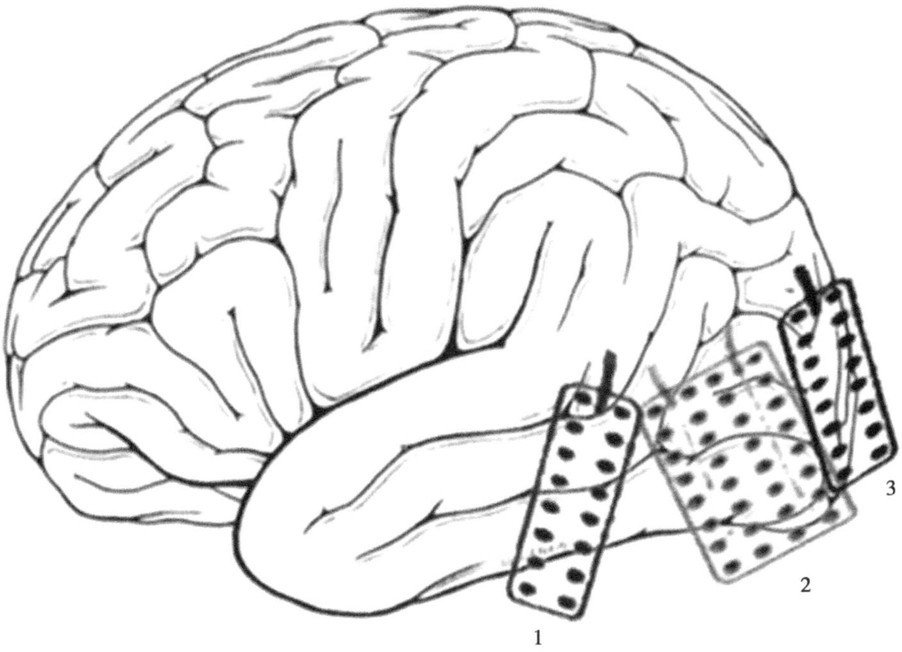

Fig. 5.23 Scheme of intracranial electrodes
Grid electrode 1: left posterior temporal region (16 contacts)
Grid electrode 2: left basal occipital lobe (32 contacts)
Grid electrode 3: left medial occipital lobe (16 contacts)

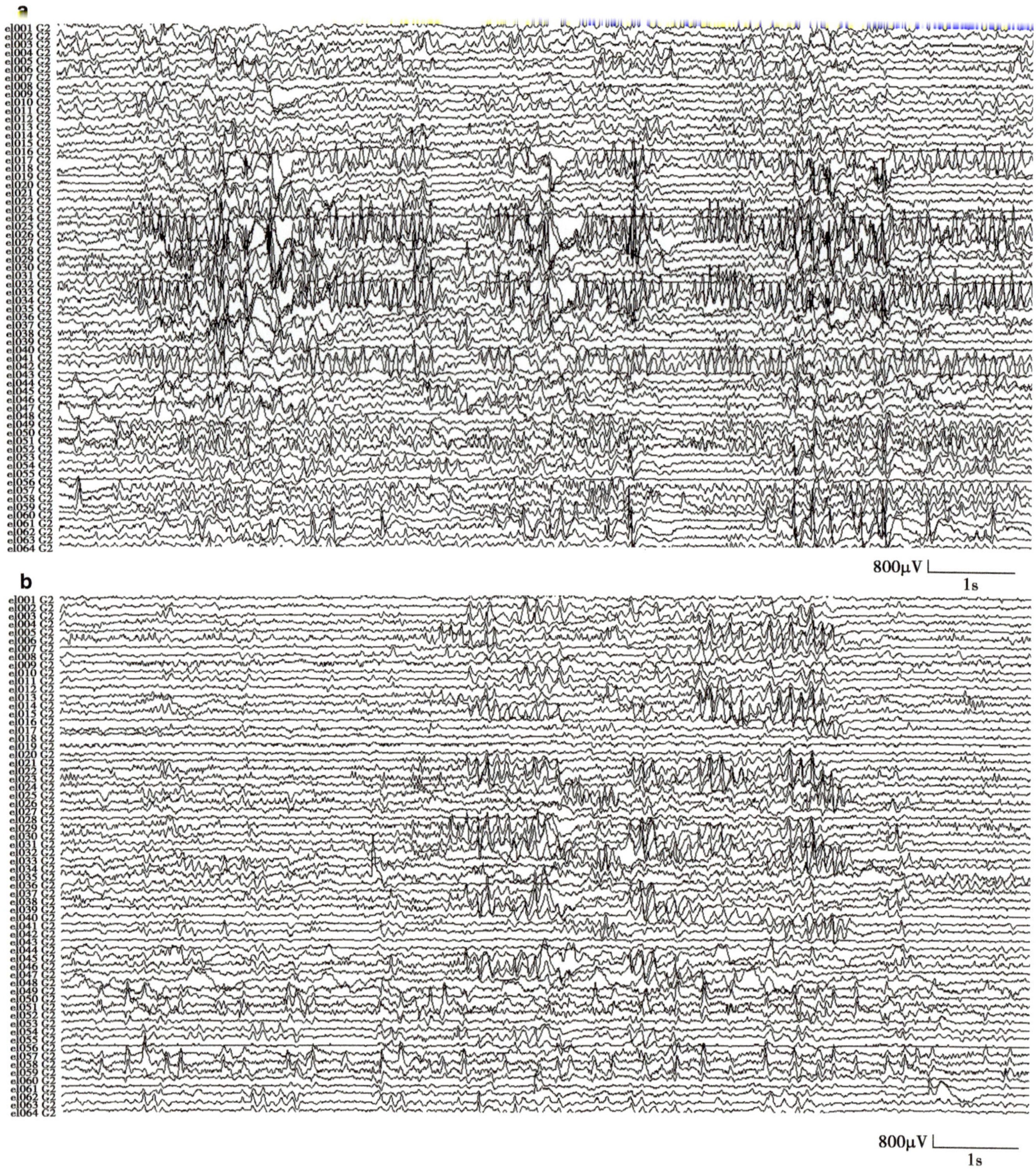

Fig. 5.24 Interictal intracranial EEG. (**a**) High-amplitude spike rhythm was seen over the left basal occipital lobe (contact numbers el017, el018, el025, el026, el029, el030, el033, el034, el038, el039, el041, el042) and posterior medial occipital region of interhemispheric fissure (contact numbers el053, el054, el055, el061, el062, el063), mainly the basal occipital lobe (contact numbers el017, el018, el025, el026, el029, el030, el033, el034, el038, el039, el041, el042). (**b**) The patient remained eyes closing; medium- to high-amplitude sharp wave rhythms were observed over the left posterior temporal region (contact numbers el005, el006, el007, el008, el013, el014, el015), basal occipital lobe (contact numbers el022, el023, el024, el029, el030, el031, el032, el038, el039). Medium-amplitude rhythmic spikes were observed over the left posterior medial occipital part of interhemispheric fissure (contact numbers el050, el051, el058, el059)

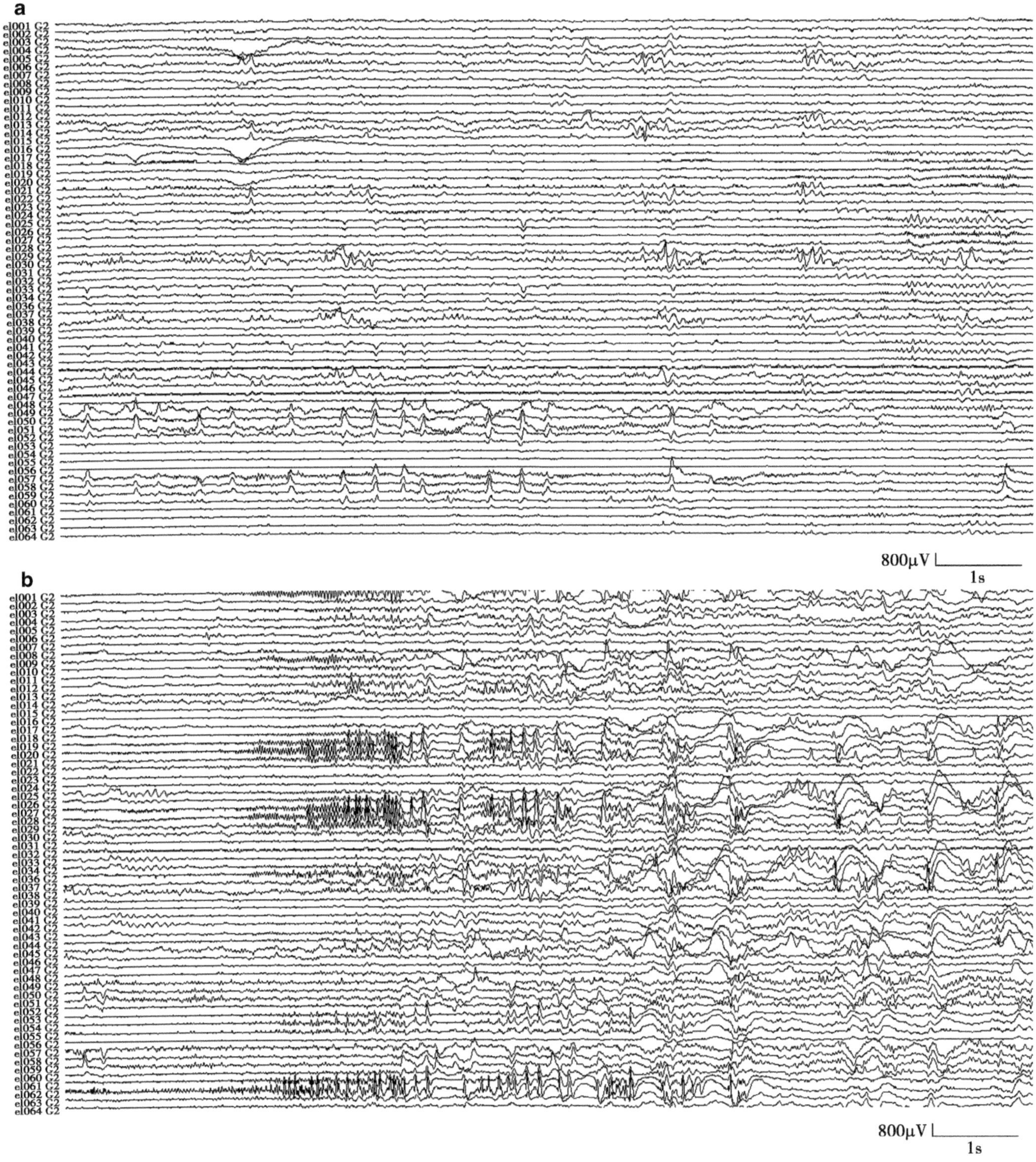

Fig. 5.25 Ictal intracranial EEG. (**a**) Before the seizure, the patient was in supine position. The IEEG showed low amplitude fast activity over the left basal occipital lobe (contact numbers el017, el018, el019, el020, el025, el026, el027, el028, el033, el034, el036). (**b**) He closed eyes and breathed deeply and slowly. The IEEG showed fast activity over the left basal occipital lobe, posterior basal temporal lobe (contact numbers el001, el009, el012, el013) and posterior medial occipital region of interhemispheric fissure (contact numbers el061, el062) with increased rhythm and amplitude. (**c**) The patient opened eyes occasionally without limb clonus and did not answer questions. The IEEG showed the rhythmic spikes over the left basal occipital lobe (contact numbers el020, el021) and posterior medial occipital region of interhemispheric fissure (contact numbers el050, el051, el057, el058, el059). (**d**) The seizure ended. The IEEG characteristics were the same as shown in **c**

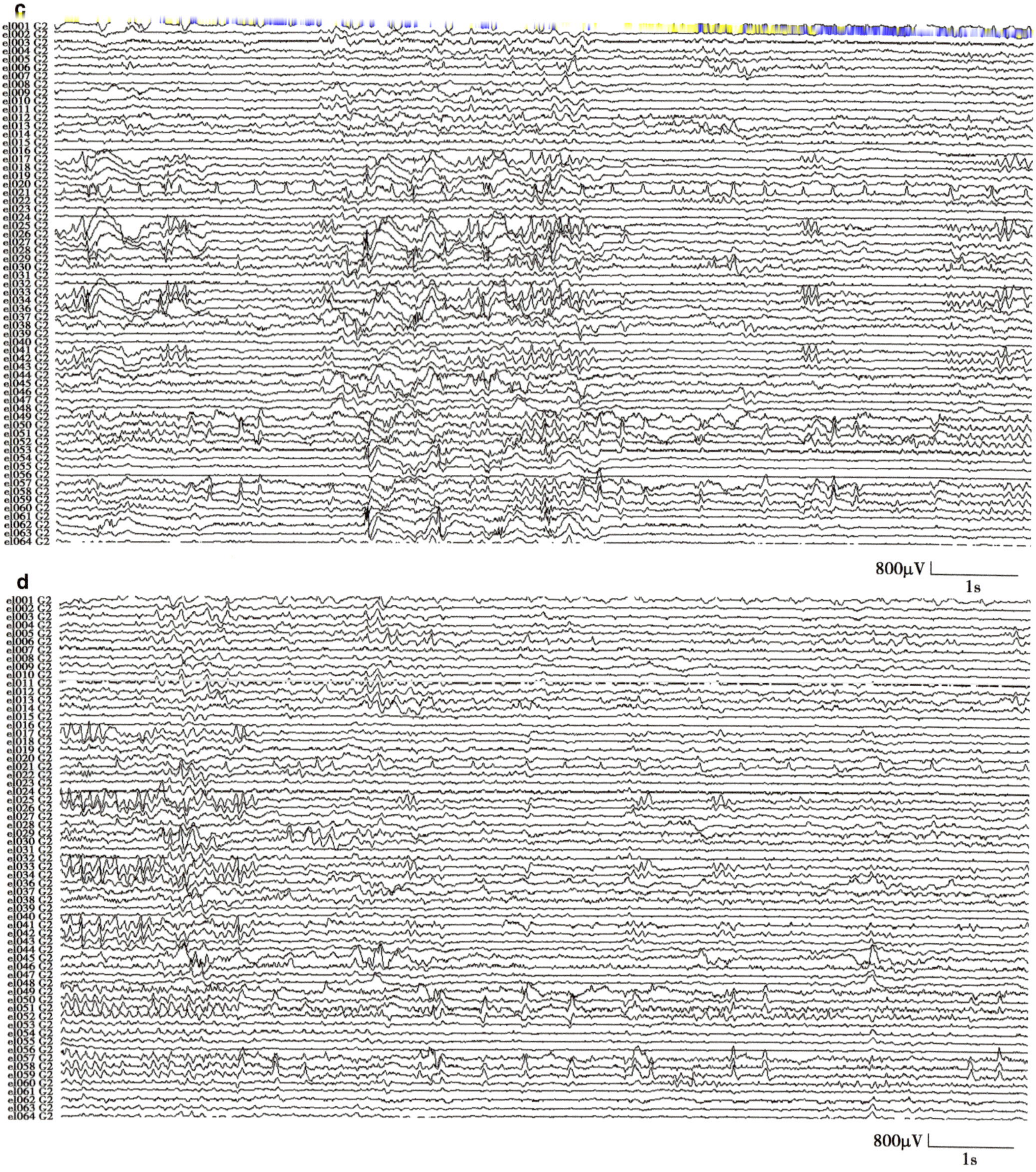

Fig. 5.25 (continued)

[Case Review]

The patient had aura of visual hallucination. The intracranial EEG showed localized low-amplitude fast activities. Surgical resection of the local originating zone could improve the prognosis. One year after the left occipital region resection, the patient voluntarily discontinued his drug therapy and had seizures. Afterwards, the patient took the antiseizure medications and the seizure frequency reduced 80%.

Cases of Insula-opercular Epilepsy

6

Xu Cuiping, Yu Tao, Zhang Mengyao, and Hao Wensi

Overview of Insula-opercular Epilepsy

Due to the unique anatomical location of the insula, seizure originating from the insula-opercular region is still poorly understood, and it is difficult to localize the epileptogenic zone during presurgical evaluations. With the application of intracranial recording, especially stereotactic electroencephalography (SEEG), and the accumulation of clinical experience, insula-opercular epilepsy has received increasing attention. From a surgical perspective, insular epilepsy is defined as seizures originating from insular identified by intracranial electrodes or the presence of an insular lesion.

Anatomy of Insula-opercula

The insula is on the deep side of the vascular wall within the lateral fissure and is separated from the frontal, parietal, and temporal lobes by the anterior, superior, and inferior circular sulcus. The central sulcus of insula divides the insula into two parts, i.e., the anterior insular lobule and the posterior insular lobule. The anterior insular lobule is divided into three short gyri, and the posterior insular lobule is divided into two long gyri. The opercula, consisting of frontal opercula, parietal opercula, and temporal opercula, is the gray matter that covers insula around the lateral fissure. The white matter fibers in the deep of the insula are the extreme capsule and the external capsule. The main long fasciculi associated with insula include uncinate fasciculus, arcuate fasciculus, inferior-fronto-occipital-fasciculus, temporal stem, and optic radiation. The deep posterior superior insula, directly adjacent to the pyramidal tract, is a risk area for surgery. In a Meta-analysis of fMRI studies on the insula, Kurth et al. divided the insula into four functional regions, namely, the social-emotional region around the insula pole, cognitive region in the dorsal part of the anterior short gyrus and the middle short gyrus, olfactory-gustatory region in the middle short gyrus, and sensorimotor region in the posterior short gyrus—the upper posterior long gyrus.

Localization of Epileptic Foci in the Insula-opercular Region

1. *Symptomatology*: The functional connectivity of the insula is complex. The symptomatology of epileptic seizures originating from the insula and peri-insular cortices is also complex and can be summarized in the following categories: (1) Somatosensory symptoms, mainly manifesting as a painless tingling sensation, electrified sensation, or a feeling of warmth distributed in restricted areas of the skin (perioral, facial, hands, upper limbs) or wide areas. Other somatic sensations include tightness, a sense of tremor, and throbbing sensations. (2) Somatic motor symptoms, such as hypermotor symptoms, or asymmetrical tonic gesture, lateral dystonic postures, etc. (3) Autonomic symptoms, mainly referring to heart rate changes (too fast, too slow, cardiac arrest) and skin changes (pallor, flushing, piloerection) during the seizure, as well as nausea, rising epigastric sensation, vomiting, etc. (4) Abnormal symptoms of throat and chest, such as tightness in the throat and chest, which may manifest as dyspnea and asphyxia in severe cases. (5) Oroalimentary automatisms, associated with oropharyngeal movements, such as chewing, smacking lips, swallowing, etc. (6) Special sensations, including special gustatory and auditory symptoms, and vestibular symptoms, such as a sensation of rotation, floating or falling, and dizziness. (7) Language dysfunction in the conscious state. These auras and ictal symptoms may suggest the involvement of insula-opercula during the seizure.
2. *Imaging examination*: High-resolution MRI is an important basis for the localization and diagnosis of insular epi-

X. Cuiping (✉) · Y. Tao
Department of Neurosurgery, Beijing, China

Z. Mengyao · H. Wensi
Department of Neurology, Beijing, China

Y. Wang (ed.), *Electroencephalogram for Presurgical Epilepsy Evaluation*, https://doi.org/10.1007/978-981-95-8003-3_6

lepsy. Insular epilepsy can often be diagnosed by lesions in the insular region displayed by MRI. However, due to a large number of cortical folds in the insula-opercular region, it is difficult to scan along the sulcus gyrus in parallel even with thin-layer MRI, making it hard to identify small cortical dysplasia. If MRI does not clearly show a localized focus, the diagnosis of insula epilepsy will be extremely challenging. PET examination may contribute to suggest insula-opercular epilepsy, especially when combined with MRI, which often reveals the hypometabolic regions of the localized cortex. Ictal SPECT may also definitely help to locate insula-opercular epilepsy.

3. *Electroencephalography and magnetoencephalography*: The scalp electroencephalography (EEG) of insula-opercular epilepsy is not specific and can show localized abnormal discharges over the frontal, temporal, and central parietal regions or widespread abnormal activities or may fail to record obviously abnormal discharges. It is difficult to localize insula-opercular epilepsy with either interictal or ictal scalp EEG.

   Compared with scalp EEG, magnetoencephalography (MEG) has significant advantages in localizing insula-opercular epilepsy. MEG actually measures the magnetic field generated by currents in the postsynaptic potentials that are tangential to the brain surface. Therefore, MEG is more sensitive for measuring abnormal discharges in the cerebral cortex within the sulci and fissure. MEG is particularly sensitive to abnormal discharges of insular epilepsy, particularly those in the opercular cortex that folds back within the lateral fissure. It is especially useful for cases with negative MRI. Depending on MEG findings, some patients can directly receive a surgical resection of epileptic foci without the implanting of intracranial electrodes for monitoring, while for some patients, the implantation scheme of intracranial electrodes may be adjusted according to the MEG findings to avoid the missed diagnosis of insula-opercular epilepsy.
4. *Intracranial electrode recording*: A definitive diagnosis of insula-opercular epilepsy often requires the intracranial electrode recording. Due to the specific anatomical location of the insula, it may be difficult to clearly localize insula-opercular epilepsy even with cortical electrodes. Hence, it often requires the combined application of deep electrodes or the separation of the lateral fissure to embed intracranial electrodes in the insula and opercular cortices. In contrast, stereotactic deep electrodes are very useful in localizing insula-opercular epilepsy. SEEG electrodes can be implanted in different parts of the insula-opercula to pinpoint the seizure onset zone or allow for the application of cortical electrical stimulation to induce clinical seizures and assist in identifying the epileptic focus. As SEEG has been maturely applied, the understanding of insula-opercular epilepsy increasingly deepens. Some poorly localized or surgically unsuccessful cases have been confirmed as insula-opercular epilepsy.

Cases of Insula Epilepsy

Case 6.1 Insula Epilepsy

[Abstract of Medical Records]
Male, 20 years old.

1. *Chief complaint*: Episodic loss of consciousness with limbs jerks for 15 years.
2. *History of present illness*: The patient developed episodic loss of consciousness with limbs jerks 15 years ago with no marked inducement and was diagnosed with epilepsy in a local hospital. The effect of oral administration of multiple antiseizure medications was not good. Four years ago, he received the treatment with gamma knife in a hospital, but the effect was poor. Three years ago, he received the implantation of electrodes in bilateral frontal and temporal regions and then received left frontal lobectomy. No seizures occurred within 1 year after the operation. Two years before admission, the patient had epileptic seizures again with the same pattern, but with a significantly reduced frequency, with 3–4 seizures lasting about 1 min every 6 months, which often occurred during sleep at night. The patient fell asleep after the seizures. Throat itching often occurred before the seizure. The patient was orally taking carbamazepine at a dose of 400 mg at night, lamotrigine at a dose of 50 mg once in the morning and in the evening, and sodium valproate at a dose of 400 mg in the morning and 600 mg in the evening. There are 3–4 seizures every 6 months.
3. *Physical examination*: Clear-minded and fluent in speech, slightly decreased memory and ability to calculate; all remaining items were normal.
4. *Past history*: *He underwent* left frontal lobectomy 3 years ago.
5. *Personal and family history*: No history of associated diseases.
6. *Imaging examination*: MRI revealed changes after left frontal lobectomy.
7. *EEG*: For details, see Figs. 6.1, 6.2, 6.3, 6.4, and 6.5.

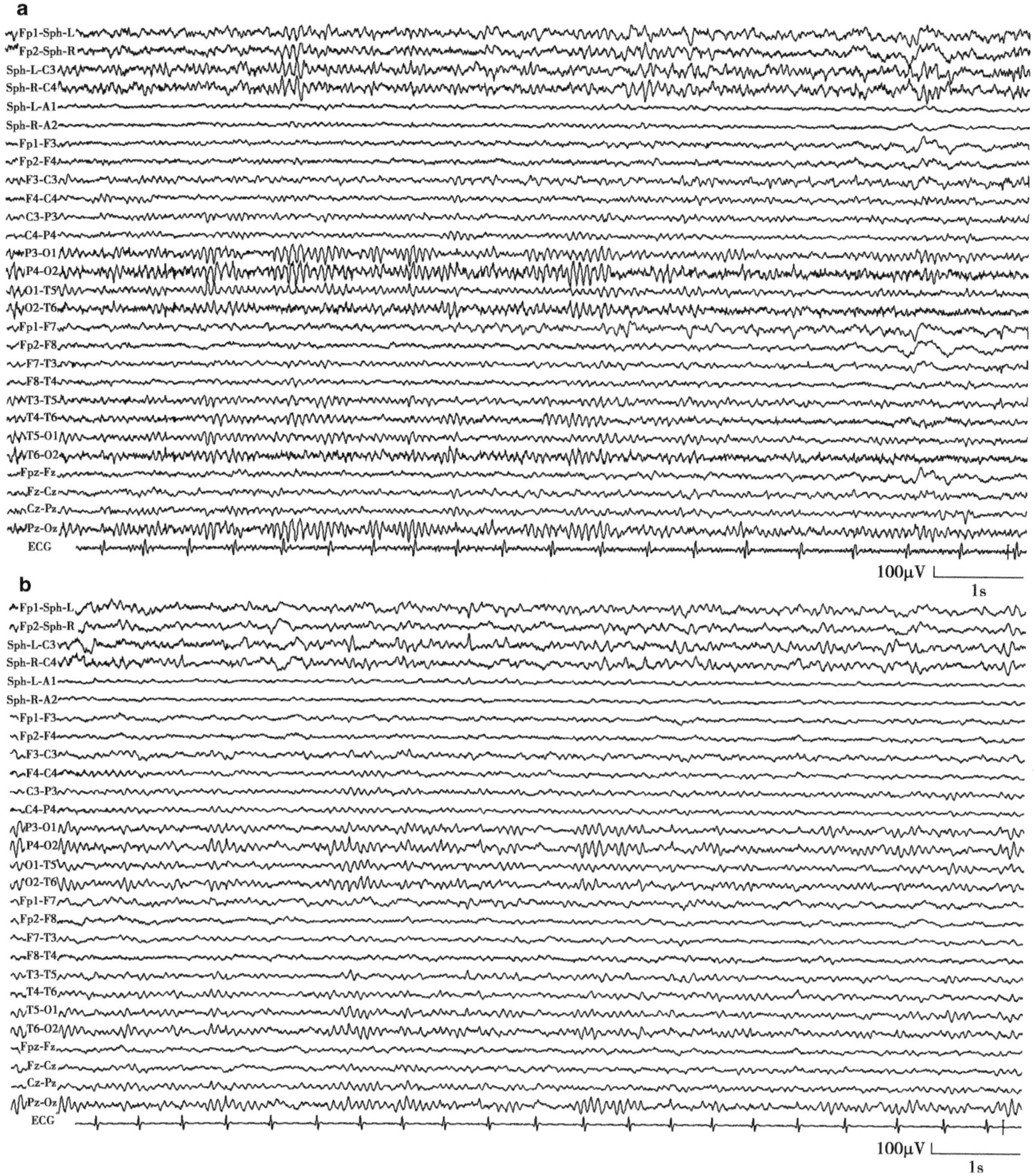

Fig. 6.1 Interictal scalp EEG. (**a**) The patient was awake, and the background activity of EEG was alpha wave of 9.0–10.0 Hz over the occipital regions. (**b**) The EEG showed low amplitude sharp waves over the left sphenoidal electrode. (**c**) The patient was asleep. The EEG showed spike-and-wave complexes over the left frontal and temporal regions. (**d**) The patient was asleep. The EEG showed spike-and-wave complexes or polyspike and wave complexes over the left frontal and temporal regions

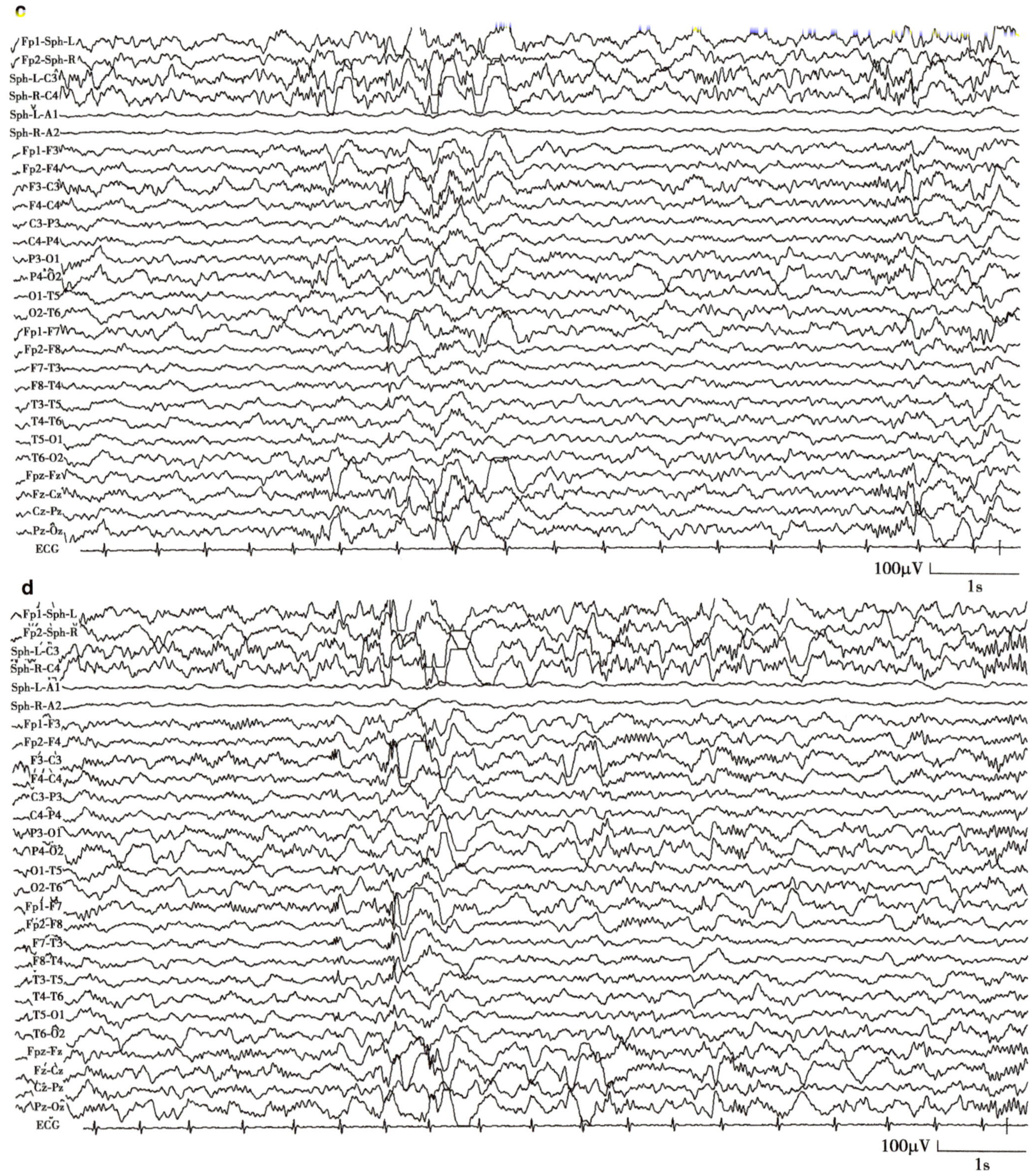

Fig. 6.1 (continued)

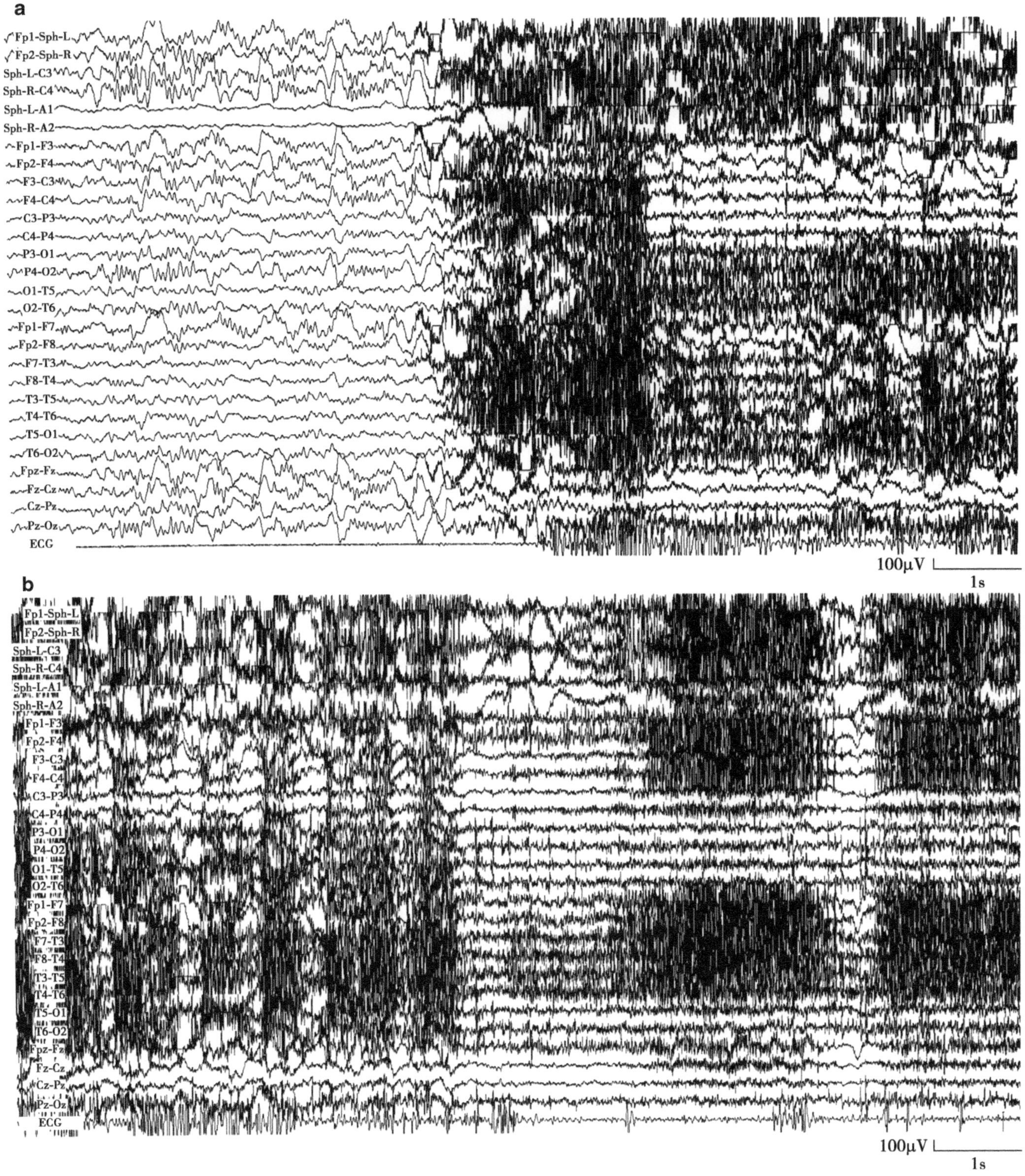

Fig. 6.2 Ictal scalp EEG. (**a**) The patient was asleep and had a sense of itching in the throat before the seizure. EMG artifacts were seen. (**b**) The patient suddenly sat up and pouted, followed by retching. Mixed EMG artifacts were seen. (**c**) The patient's seizure ended. Mixed EMG artifacts were seen, which recovered to the background wakeful EEG at the end of seizure

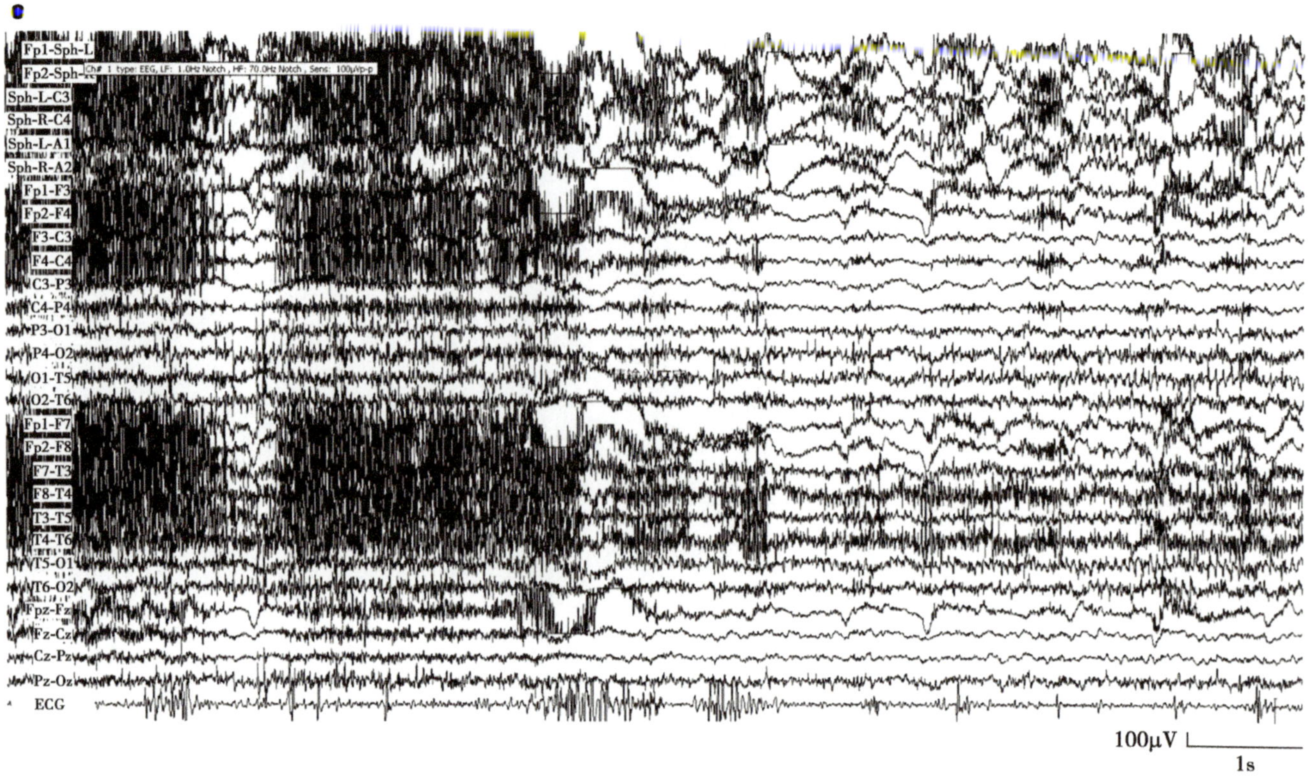

Fig. 6.2 (continued)

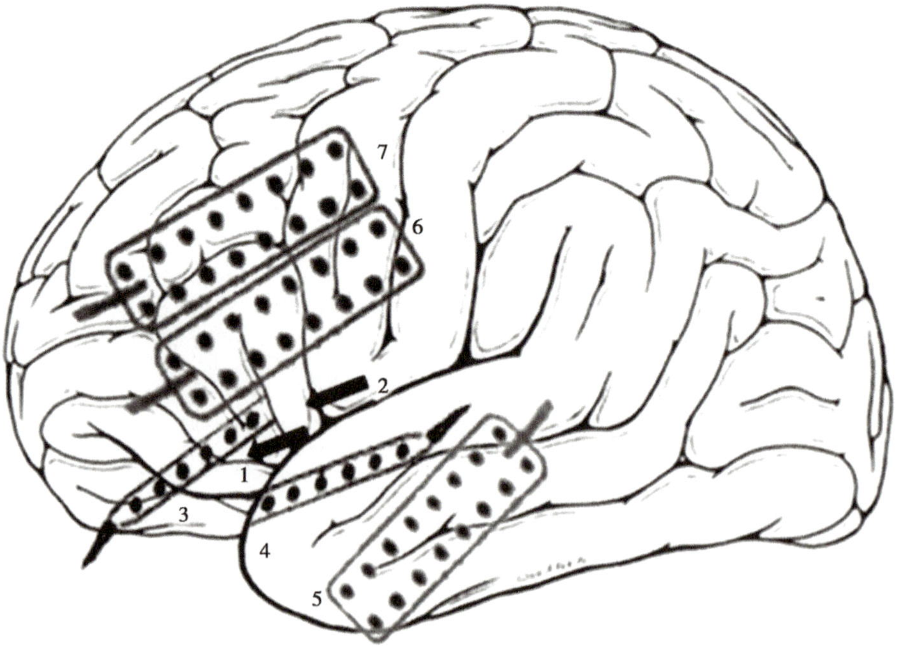

Fig. 6.3 Scheme of intracranial electrodes
Intracranial electrode 1 (deep): the anterior part of the left insula long gyrus (4 contacts)
Intracranial electrode 2 (deep): the posterior part of the left insula long gyrus (4 contacts)
Intracranial electrode 3 (strip): the left frontal operculum (6 contacts)
Intracranial electrode 4 (strip): the left temporal operculum (6 contacts)
Intracranial electrode 5 (grid): the left temporal base (16 contacts)
Intracranial electrode 6 (grid): the posterior part of the left inferior frontal gyrus and the central region (16 contacts)
Intracranial electrode 7 (grid): the posterior part of the left middle frontal gyrus and the central region (16 contacts)

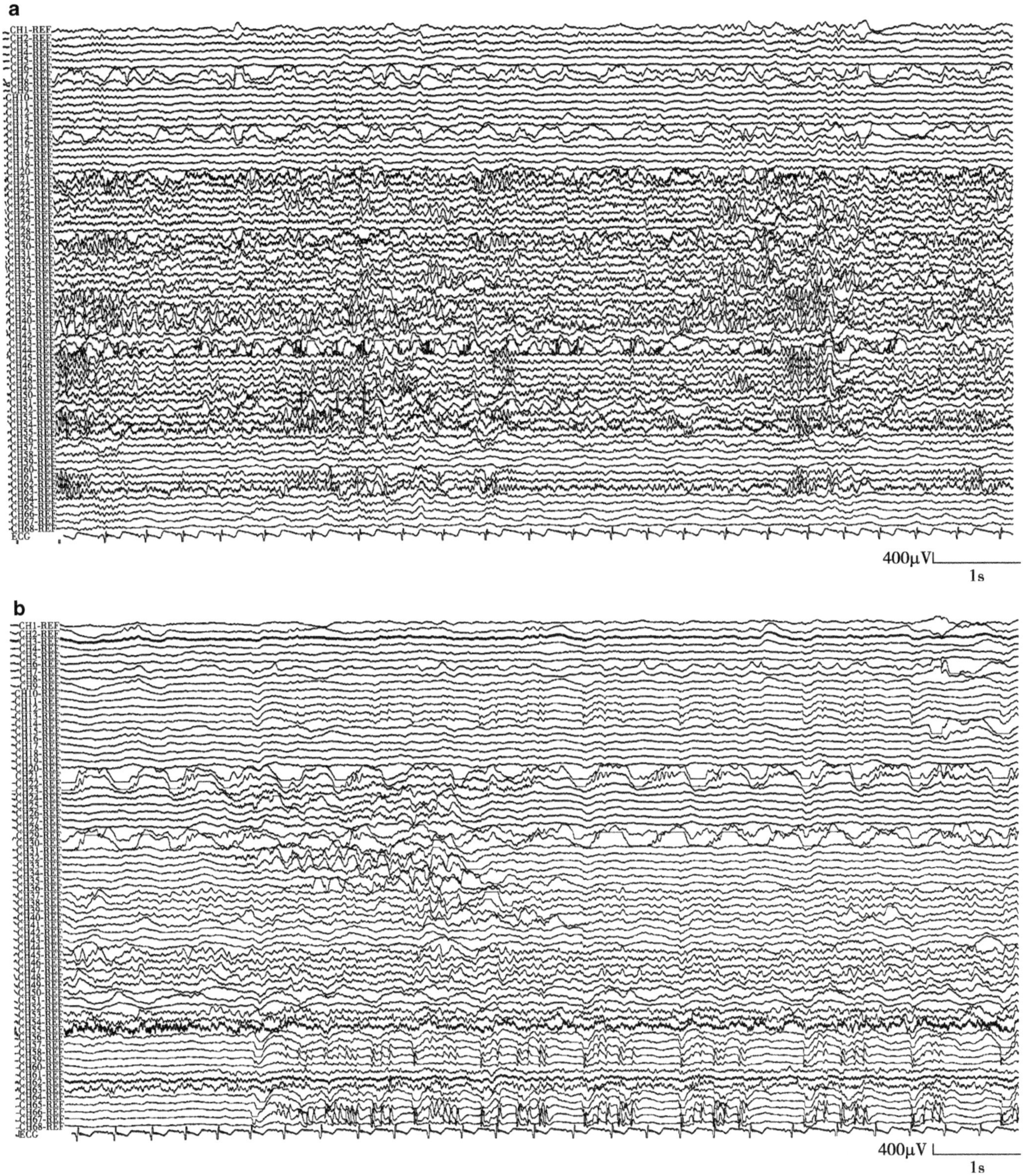

Fig. 6.4 Interictal intracranial EEG. (**a**) The IEEG showed spike over the left inferior frontal gyrus (contact numbers CH51 and CH52). (**b**) The IEEG showed the paroxysmal sharp waves rhythm over the left middle and inferior frontal gyrus (contact numbers CH57, CH58, CH59, CH60, CH65, CH66, CH67 and CH68). (**c**) The IEEG showed spike-and-wave complexes over the left insula long gyrus (contact numbers CH7 and CH8)

c

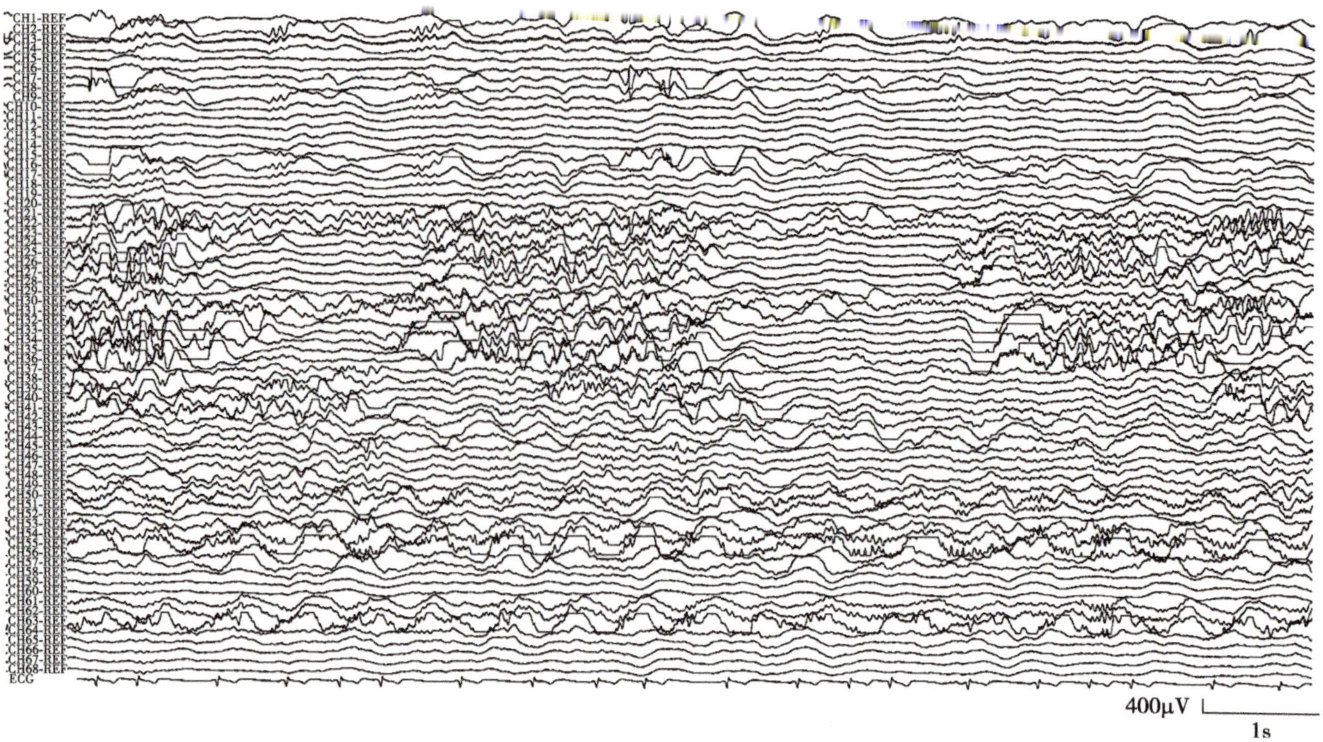

Fig. 6.4 (continued)

a

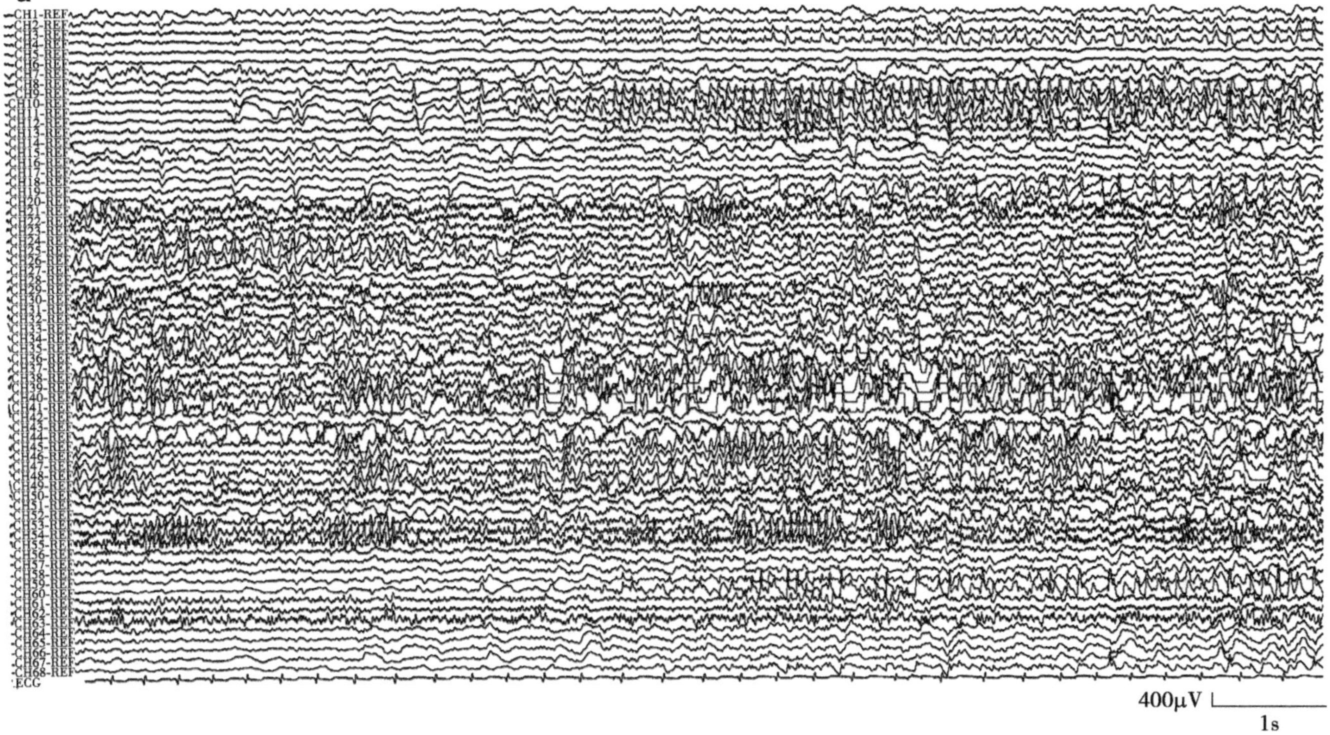

b

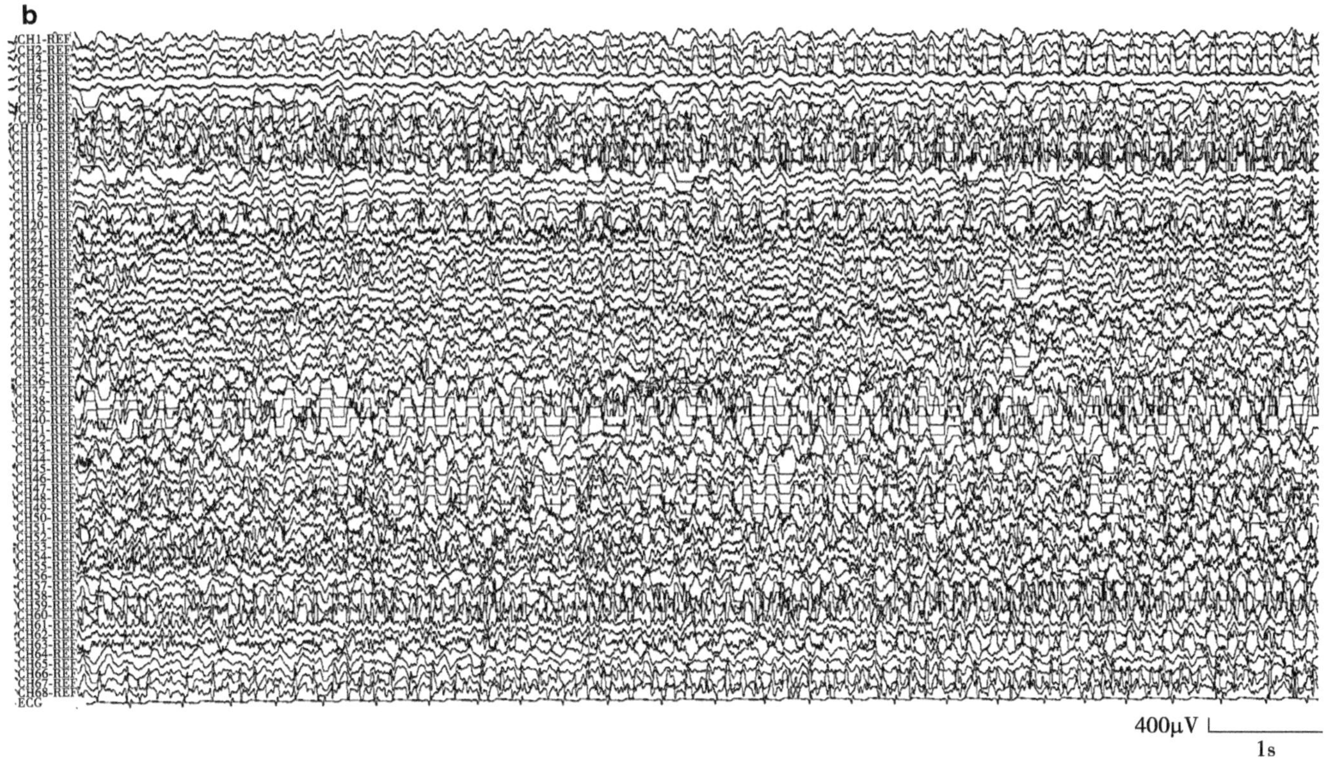

Fig. 6.5 Ictal intracranial EEG. (**a**) The patient was awake and had a sense of itching in the throat before the seizure. The IEEG was the background IEEG, followed by the sharp wave rhythm over the left frontal operculum (contact numbers CH9, CH10, CH11 and CH12) and the sharp wave rhythm over the left middle and inferior frontal gyrus (contact numbers CH59, CH60, CH66, CH67 and CH68. (**b**) The patient felt that the itching in the throat was becoming severe. The IEEG showed the sharp wave rhythm over the left frontal operculum (contact numbers CH9, CH10, CH11 and CH12), the left inferior frontal gyrus and the central area (contact numbers CH59, CH60, CH66, CH67 and CH68), which gradually spread to the nearby cortex, and then the rhythm of spike-and-wave complexes occurred over the anterior part of the left insula long gyrus (contact numbers CH3 and CH4), the left frontal operculum (contact numbers CH9, CH10, CH11, CH12, CH13 and CH14), the left temporal operculum (contact numbers CH19 and CH20), the posterior part of the left inferior frontal gyrus and the

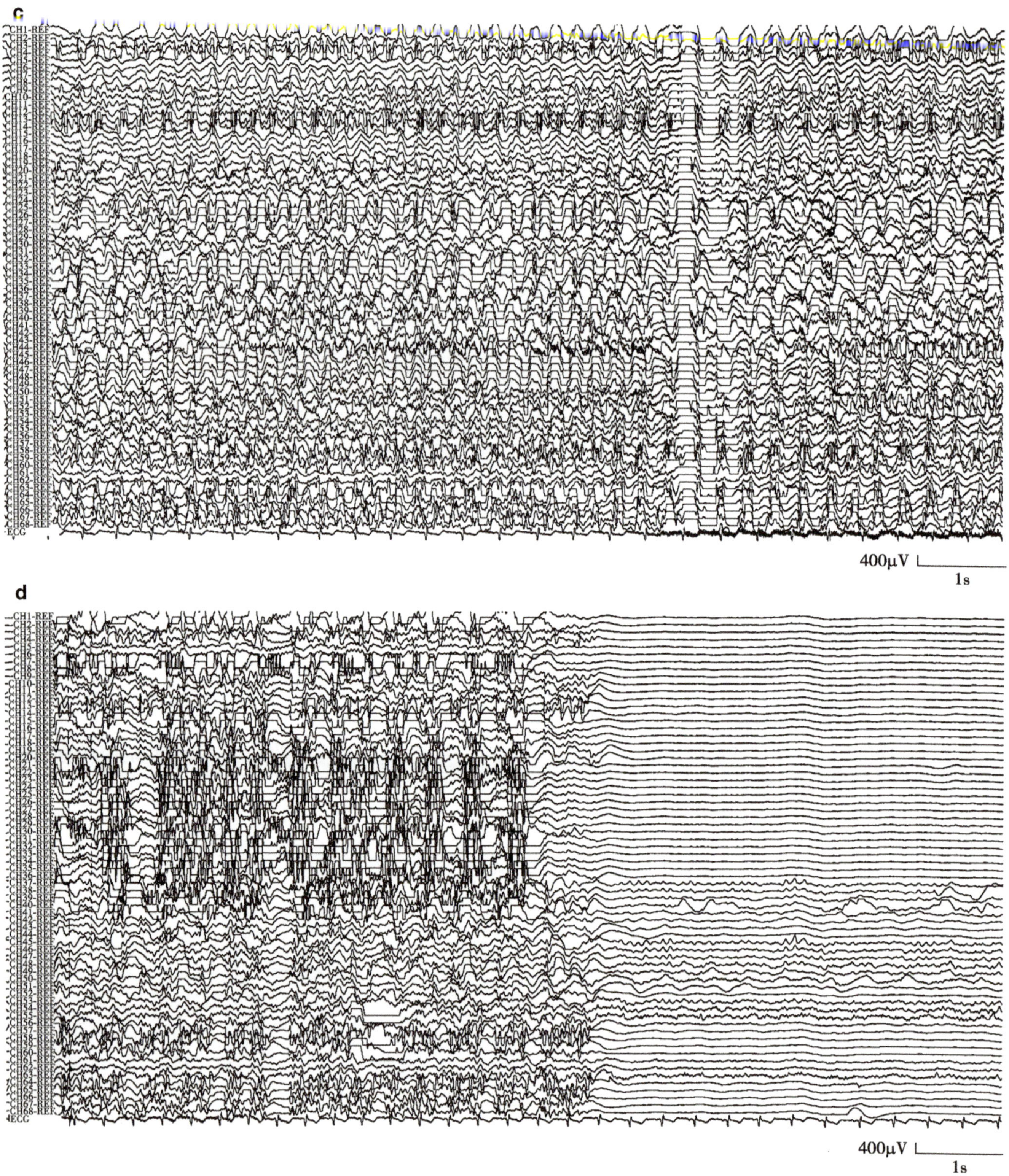

Fig. 6.5 (continued) central area (contact numbers CH38, CH39, CH40, CH41, CH51 and CH52) and the posterior part of the left middle frontal gyrus and the central area (contact numbers CH58, CH59, CH60, CH66, CH67 and CH68). (**c**) The patient developed oropharyngeal automatism followed by retching. The IEEG showed the spike-and-wave complexes rhythm over the anterior part of the left insular long gyrus (contact numbers CH3 and CH4), the left frontal operculum (contact numbers CH9, CH10, CH11, CH12, CH13 and CH14), the left temporal operculum (contact numbers CH19, CH20, CH24, CH25, CH26, CH27, CH31, CH32, CH33 and CH34), the left inferior frontal gyrus (contact numbers CH38, CH39, CH40, CH41, CH51, CH52, CH58 and CH59) and the left middle frontal gyrus (contact numbers CH60, CH63, CH64, CH65, CH66, CH67 and CH68). (**d**) The patient lay quietly and was immobile after the seizure. The IEEG showed the rhythm of spike-and-wave complexes over the posterior part of the left insula long gyrus (contact numbers CH7 and CH8), the left frontal operculum (contact numbers CH13 and CH14), the left middle temporal region and the left inferior frontal gyrus (contact numbers CH21 - 42, CH51 and CH52) and the left middle frontal gyrus (contact numbers CH58, CH59, CH60, CH64 - 68)

[Case Review]

1. *Case Characteristics*
   (a) *Seizure characteristics*: (1) Episodic loss of consciousness with generalized tonic clonic seizure. (2) There was a clear aura, i.e., throat itching.
   (b) *Characteristics of medical history*: The patient received left frontal lobectomy and was seizure free 1 year after this operation.
   (c) *Imaging characteristics*: MRI revealed changes after left frontal lobectomy.
   (d) *EEG characteristics*: The EEG showed low amplitude sharp waves over the left sphenoidal electrode and the left temporal region when the patient was awake; the ictal EEG was mixed with EMG artifacts and did not show a clear seizure onset zone.
2. *Diagnosis and treatment strategy and follow-up results*: The patient had an aura of throat itching before the seizure, a symptom highly suggestive of the seizure originating from the insula. The interictal EEG showed the abnormal discharges over the left frontal and temporal regions. Then it was decided to implant intracranial electrodes over the left frontal region, temporal region and insula. The ictal IEEG showed that the seizure started from the left frontal operculum and rapidly spread to the left insula and left middle and inferior frontal gyrus. After the left insula and frontal operculum were resected, no seizure occurred in the postoperative follow-up. The patient had a satisfactory postoperative outcome because the seizure aura was clear and consistent with the characteristics of insular seizures, the EEG presentation was consistent with the seizure symptoms, and the focus was completely resected.

Case 6.2 Insula Epilepsy

[Abstract of Medical Records]
Female, 12 years old.

1. *Chief complaint*: Repeated episodic crying for more than 8 years.
2. *History of present illness*: The patient suddenly cried without marked inducement 8 years ago, with few tears, no limbs stiffness or twitches, no response to calls, and no incontinence, lasting about 10 s. The seizures occurred during the day and night, and 10–20 times every day. She took the oral solution of sodium valproate at a dose of 3 mL b.i.d. No further seizures occurred after this treatment. Five years ago, after gradual discontinuation of the drug, the symptoms occurred again, with right-sided limb flexion, clenched right fist, and no response to call, but after the seizure, the patient could recall the situation of the seizure, and there was no incontinence, which lasted 20–30 s. She continued to take sodium valproate with poor effect. Two years ago, she changed to take oxcarbazepine at a dose of 450 mg bid but still had 4–5 seizures per day. Since the onset of the disease, she had a good spirit, normal diet, good sleep, and normal bladder and bowel function.
3. *Past history*: No significant past history.
4. *Personal history*: The patient was delivered by cesarean section at full term without a history of asphyxia or febrile convulsions.
5. *Physical examination*: The patient had a blood pressure of 110/70 mmHg, was conscious and articulate, and had normal higher cortical functions. Neurological examination was normal. Right handedness. Muscular strength and muscular tone were normal. The tendon reflexes were normal and the pathological signs were negative. Both of the superficial and deep sensation and the coordinate movement were normal.
6. *Neuropsychological examination*: The patient had a moderate (normal) intelligence with VIQ = 93, PIQ = 104, FIQ = 98.
7. *Imaging examination*:
   (a) MRI revealed abnormal signal foci in the left frontal lobe and insula, without any enhancement.
   (b) MEG revealed spike dipoles over the left frontal lobe and insula.
8. *EEG*: For details, see Figs. 6.6 and 6.7.

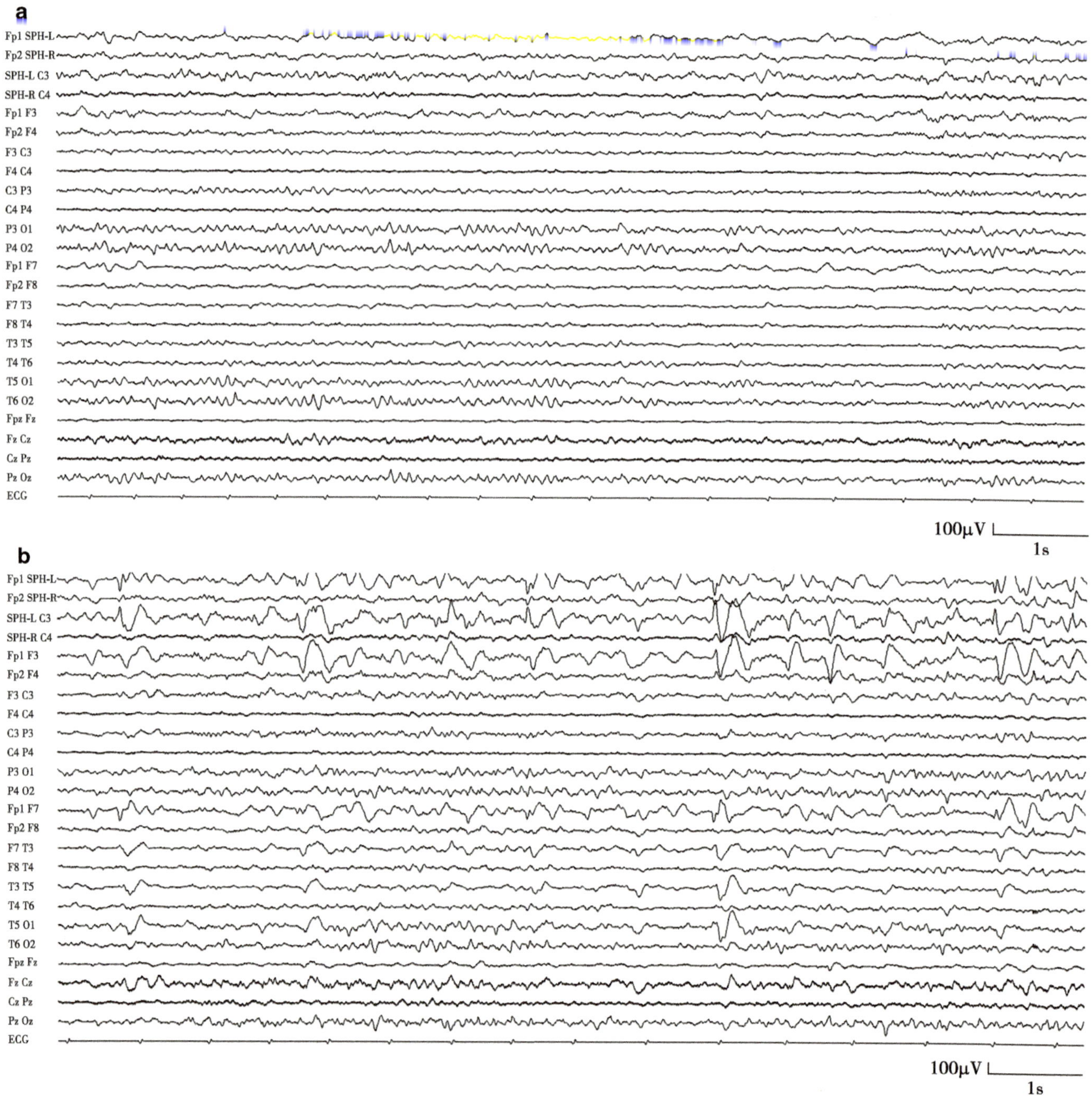

Fig. 6.6 Interictal scalp EEG. (**a**) Background EEG during wakefulness. (**b**) The EEG showed slow waves over the left frontal and temporal regions, sharp-and-wave complexes over the left frontal pole, and sharp waves over the left sphenoidal electrode. (**c**) C The EEG showed sharp-and-waves complexes over the left frontal, central, parietal, and temporal regions; and sharp waves over the left sphenoidal electrode

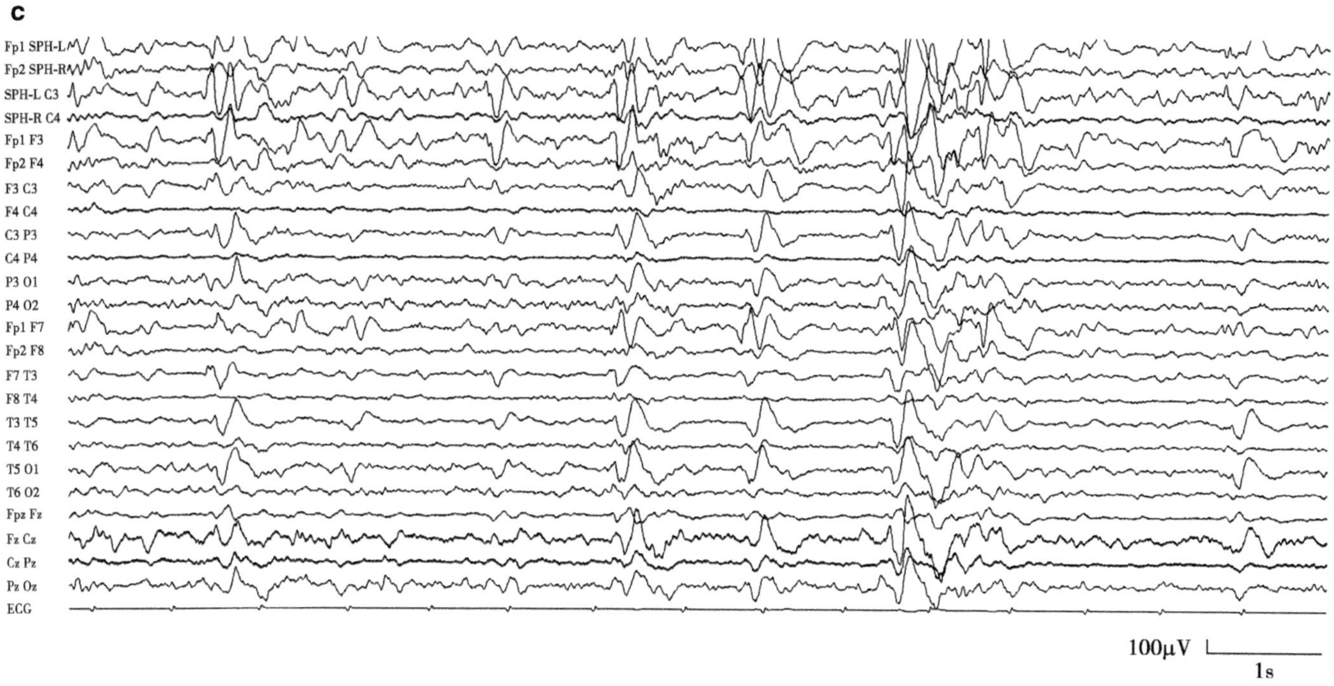

Fig. 6.6 (continued)

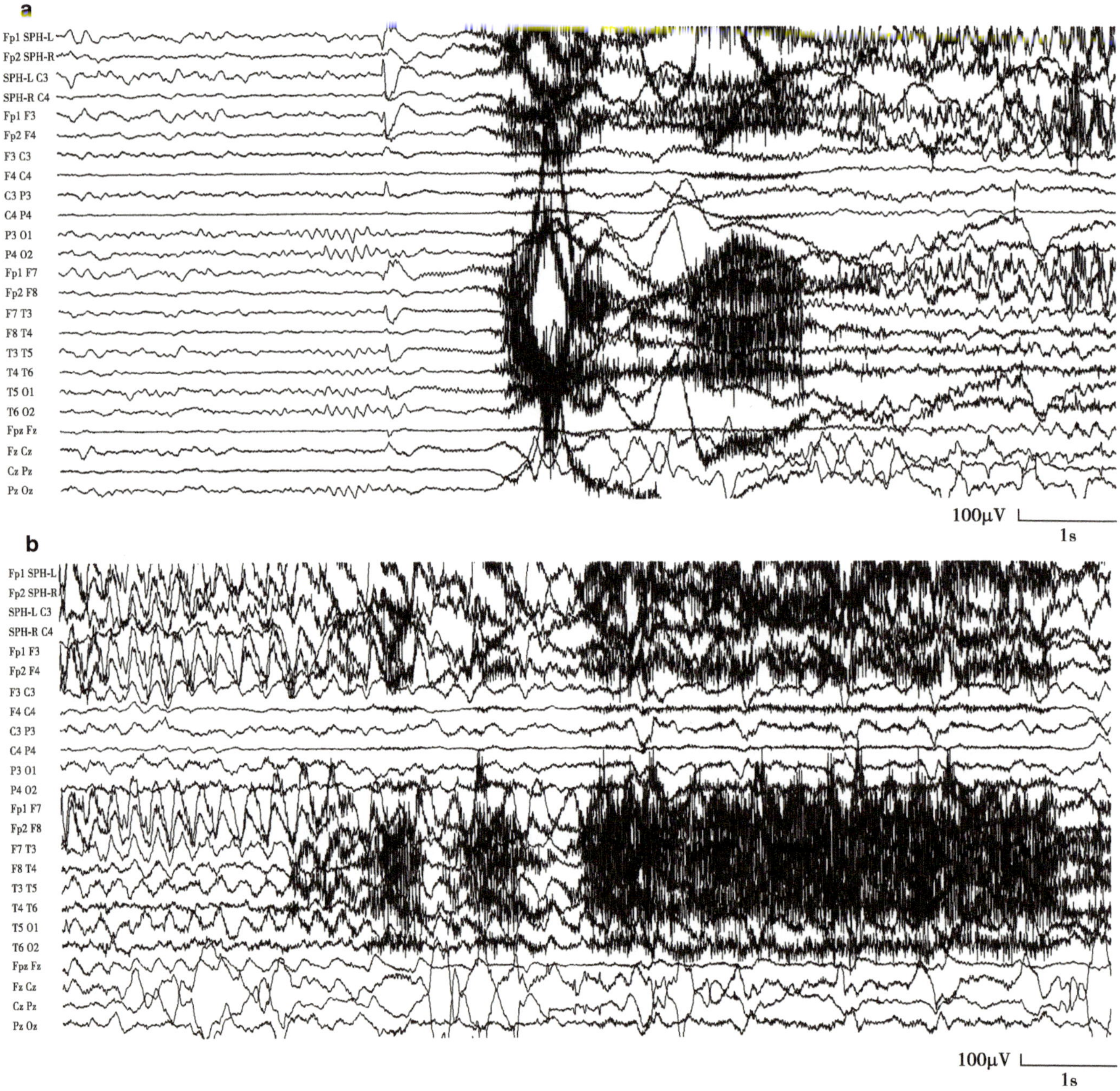

Fig. 6.7 Ictal scalp EEG. (**a**) The patient tightly closed eyes after waking, having a painful expression and clenching the right hand. The EEG showed low amplitude fast activity over the left frontal and temporal regions before the seizure, followed by mixed EMG artifacts and the slow waves rhythm over the left temporal region. (**b**) The patient's right upper limb was stiff and elevated, with painful facial expression. The EEG showed rhythm of the spike-and-wave complexes over bilateral frontal regions, mainly on the left side, and the slow wave rhythm was seen over the left temporal and parietal regions. (**c**) The patient sat up and regained consciousness. The EEG showed the slow wave rhythm over the left hemisphere, and then mixed EMG artifacts

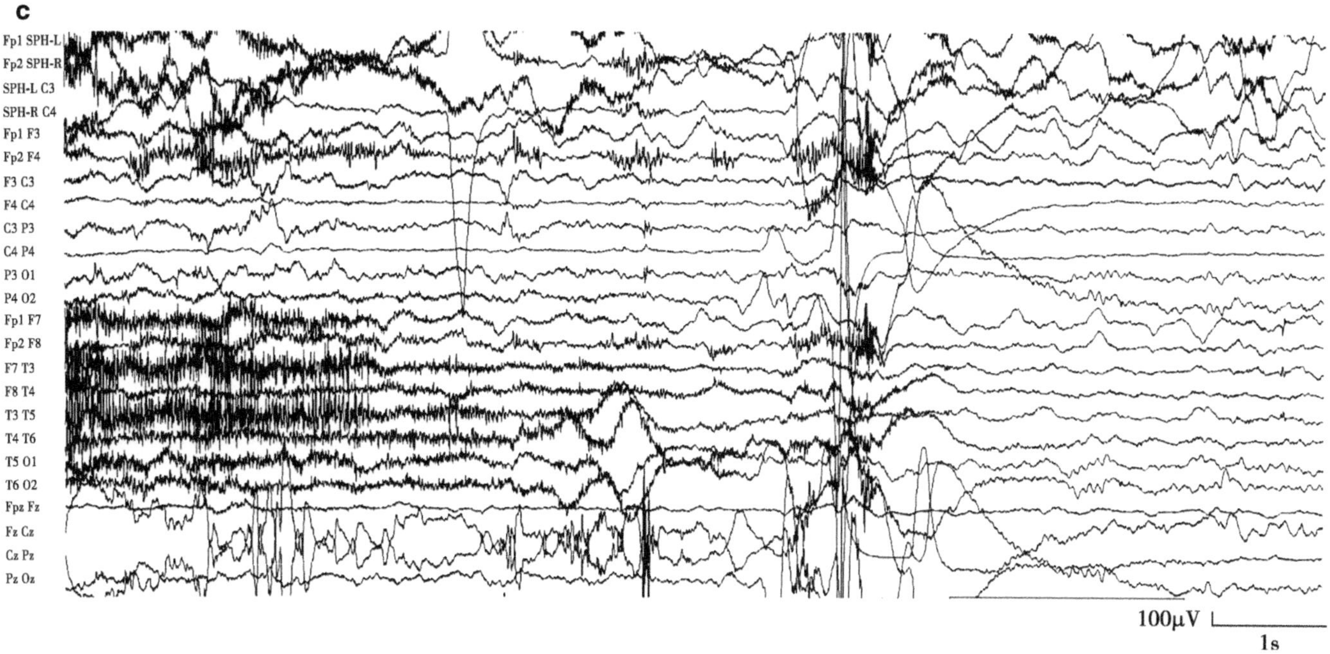

Fig. 6.7 (continued)

[Case Review]

1. *Case Characteristics*
   (a) *Seizure characteristics*: (1) Episodic crying with few tears, which lasted for about 10 s and then resolved. (2) Frequent seizures at a frequency of 4–5 times per day.
   (b) *Imaging characteristics*: (1) MRI revealed the abnormal signals over the left frontal lobe and insula. (2) MEG revealed spike dipoles over the left frontal lobe and insula.
   (c) *EEG characteristics*: Interictal EEG during wakefulness showed slow waves over the left frontal and temporal regions, sharp-and-wave complexes over the left frontal region, and sharp waves over the left sphenoidal electrode. The EEG during sleep showed sharp-and-wave complexes over the left frontal, central, parietal, and temporal regions. The ictal EEG showed sharp waves over the left sphenoidal electrode, the frontal, central, and temporal regions, and low amplitude fast activity over the left frontal and temporal regions.
2. *Diagnosis and treatment strategy and follow-up results*: According to the patient's seizure symptoms of right-hand clenching and stiffened and lifted right upper limbs, the epileptic focus was considered to be on the left side, but the exact location could not be determined. The interictal EEG showed extensive abnormal discharges, mainly over the left frontal and temporal regions, and the ictal EEG was the same as the interictal EEG. The specific site of the epileptic focus could not be determined according to the seizure symptoms and EEG features. However, the MRI showed clear abnormal signals over the left frontal region and insula, and MEG also suggested spike dipoles over the left frontal and insular regions. The seizure symptoms and EEG presentation were not contradictory to the lateralization of focus showed by MRI. Therefore, the resection of the left frontal and insula foci may be considered. During a 2-year follow-up after the surgical resection of the left inferior frontal gyrus and insula, the seizure disappeared. The patient had a favorable postoperative outcome because the MRI showed definite foci, the seizure symptoms and EEG presentation were not contradictory to the side of the foci, and the foci were completely resected.

Case 6.3 Insula Epilepsy

[Abstract of Medical Records]
Female, 18 years old.

1. *Chief complaint*: Episodic downward twisting of mouth corners for 12 years.
2. *History of present illness*: 12 years ago (at the age of 6), the patient suddenly felt tight in facial muscles without any inducement, with Chapeau de Gendarme, both upper limbs piloerection, fear, and tachycardia, which lasted for more than 10 s. During the seizures, the patient was conscious without a tightening sensation in the throat. The seizures occurred repeatedly, occasionally with shouting and loss of consciousness in severe situation. She was diagnosed with epilepsy at a local hospital and treated with sodium valproate and lamotrigine (oral); the effect was good. Seizures occurred once within several years. Three months ago, due to menstrual disorders, she planned to discontinue sodium valproate and additionally take topiramate. However, during the course of taking topiramate, the seizure frequency increased significantly. The patient developed episodic auditory hallucinations and hence took levetiracetam. She took lamotrigine at a dose of 100 mg every 12 h and levetiracetam at a dose of 1500 mg every 12 h, which failed to effectively control the seizure. In the past 2 months, the seizures occurred frequently, more than 10 times a day, mostly during the daytime or when she was about to wake up, while there were no seizures after she fell asleep.
3. *Past history*: The patient was delivered at full term, with normal motor, language, and intellectual development.
4. *Personal history*: The patient was intellectually competent and is a freshman. Right handedness.
5. *Family history*: No history of associated diseases.
6. *Physical examination*: The neurological examination was normal.
7. *Imaging examinations*:
   (a) MRI did not show any significant abnormality.
   (b) MEG showed the spike dipoles over the left anterior insula.
8. *EEG*: For details, see Figs. 6.8, 6.9, 6.10, 6.11, and 6.12.

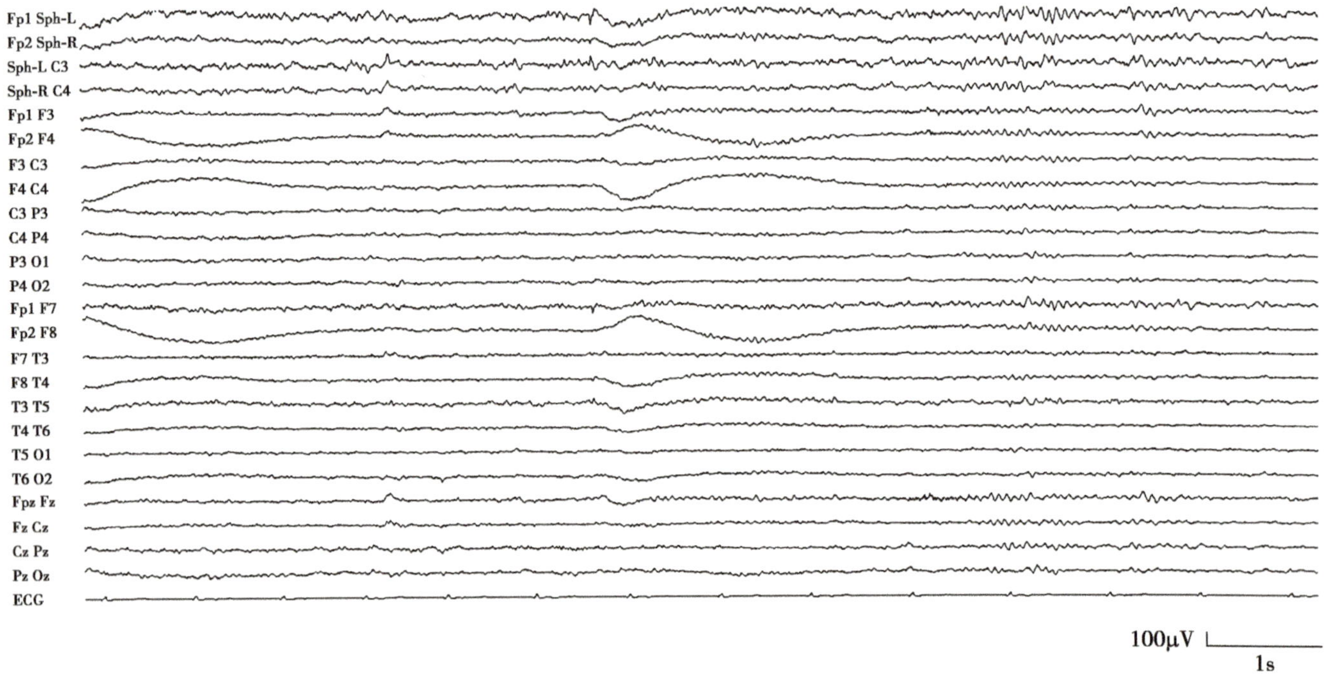

Fig. 6.8 Interictal scalp EEG. Low amplitude sharp waves over the left sphenoidal electrode and the left anterior temporal region

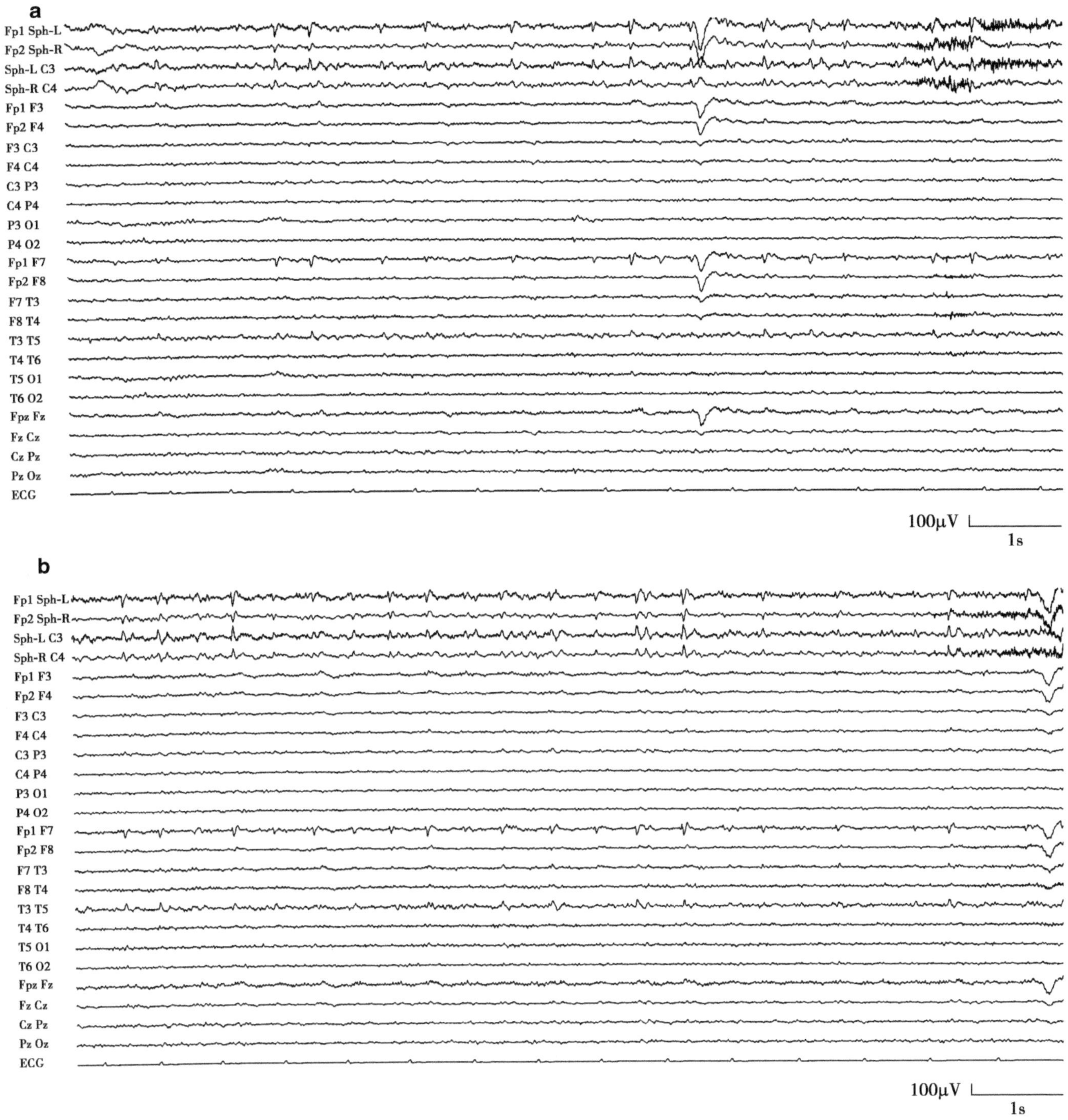

Fig. 6.9 Ictal scalp EEG. (**a**) Before seizure, the EEG showed frequent low amplitude sharp waves over the left sphenoidal electrode and the left temporal region. (**b**) The EEG showed frequent sharp waves over the left sphenoidal electrode and the left temporal region. (**c**) The EEG showed rhythmic sharp waves over the left sphenoidal electrode and the left temporal region. (**d**) The EEG showed rhythmic sharp waves over the left sphenoidal electrode and the left temporal region. (**e**) The patient was awake and lying position. During the seizure, the mouth corners were bilaterally twisted downward, manifesting as "Chapeau de Gendarme". She first lay on the left and then on the right. Before the onset of clinical symptoms, the EEG showed the sharp wave rhythm over the left sphenoidal electrode and the temporal region. Mixed EMG artifacts can be seen at the onset of clinical symptoms. (**f**) The patient developed both hands automatism, and then sat up while breathing heavily. She then lay in a supine position while covering her mouth and nose with the left hand. The EEG showed the sharp wave rhythm over the left anterior temporal region, and mixed EMG artifacts can be seen over the remaining regions. (**g**) The patient sat up and panted. The EEG showed the sharp wave rhythm over the left anterior temporal region

c

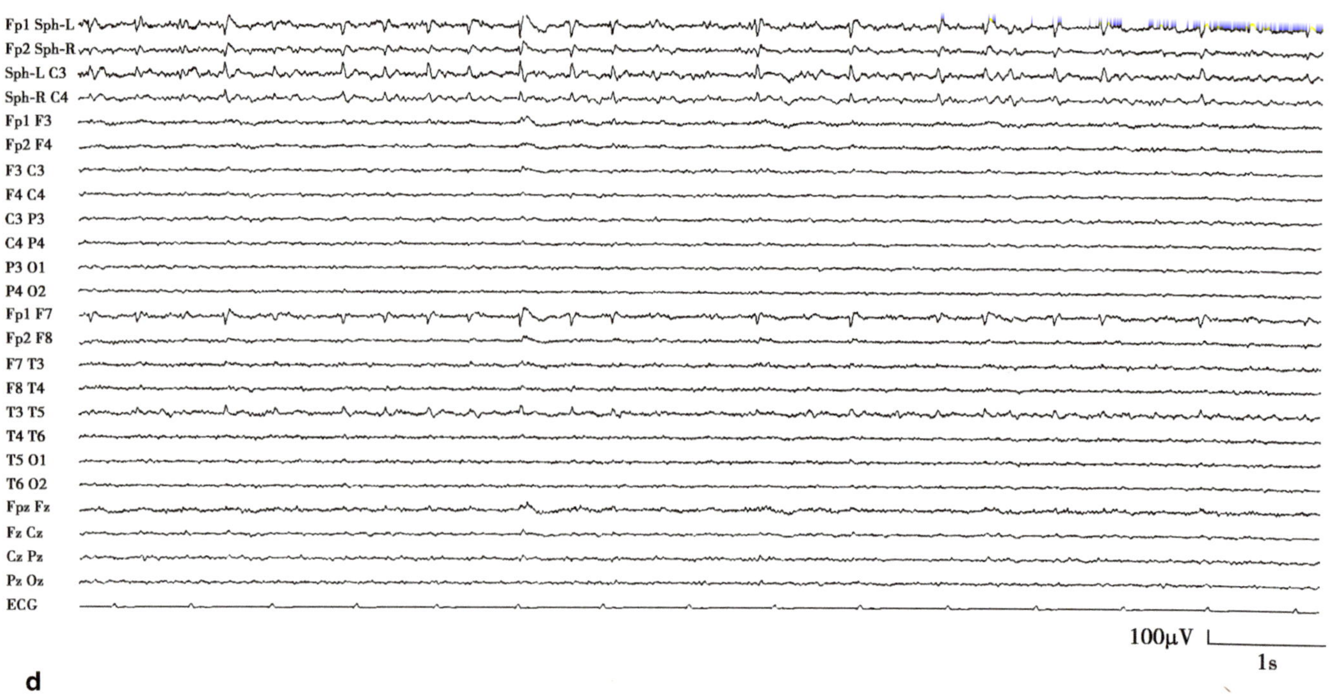

d

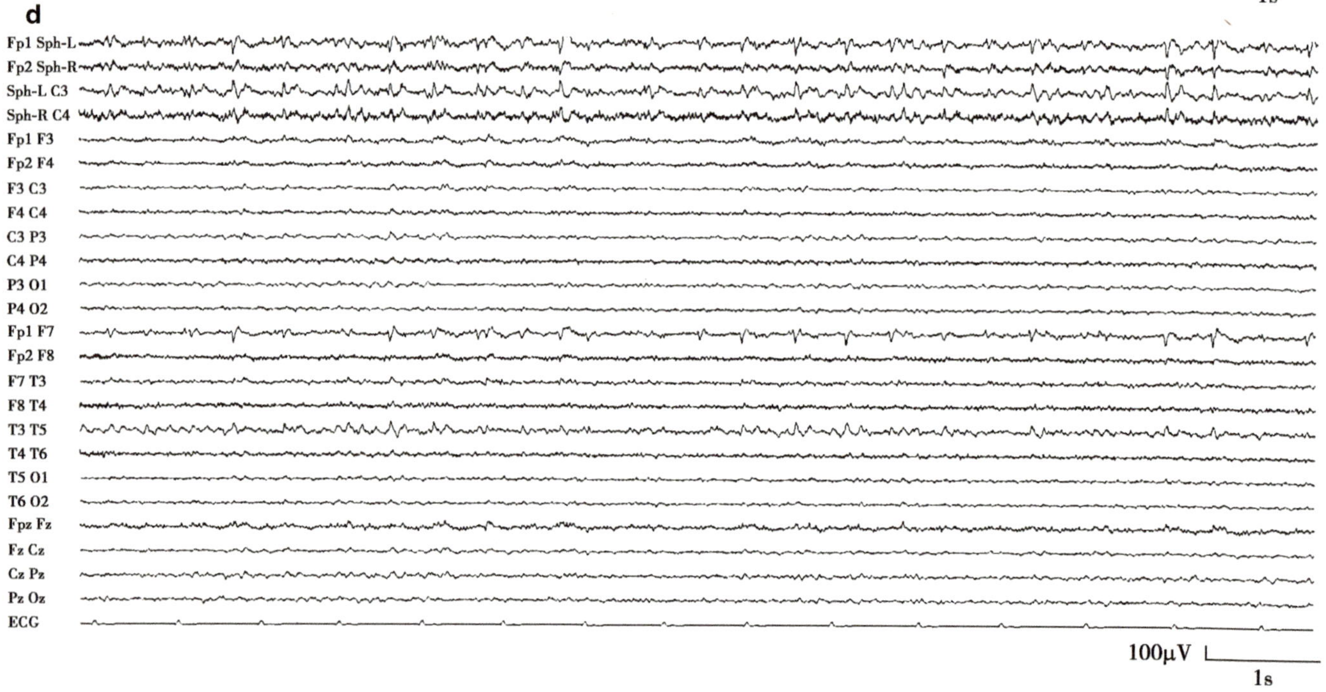

Fig. 6.9 (continued)

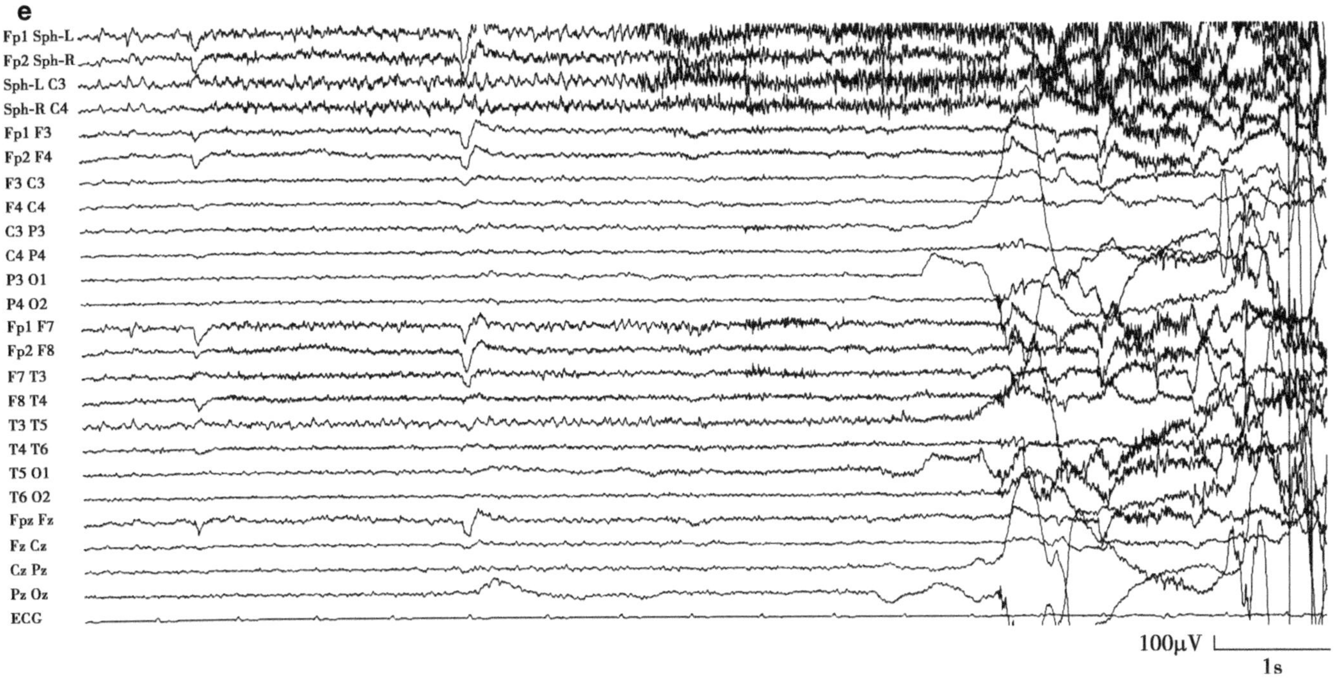

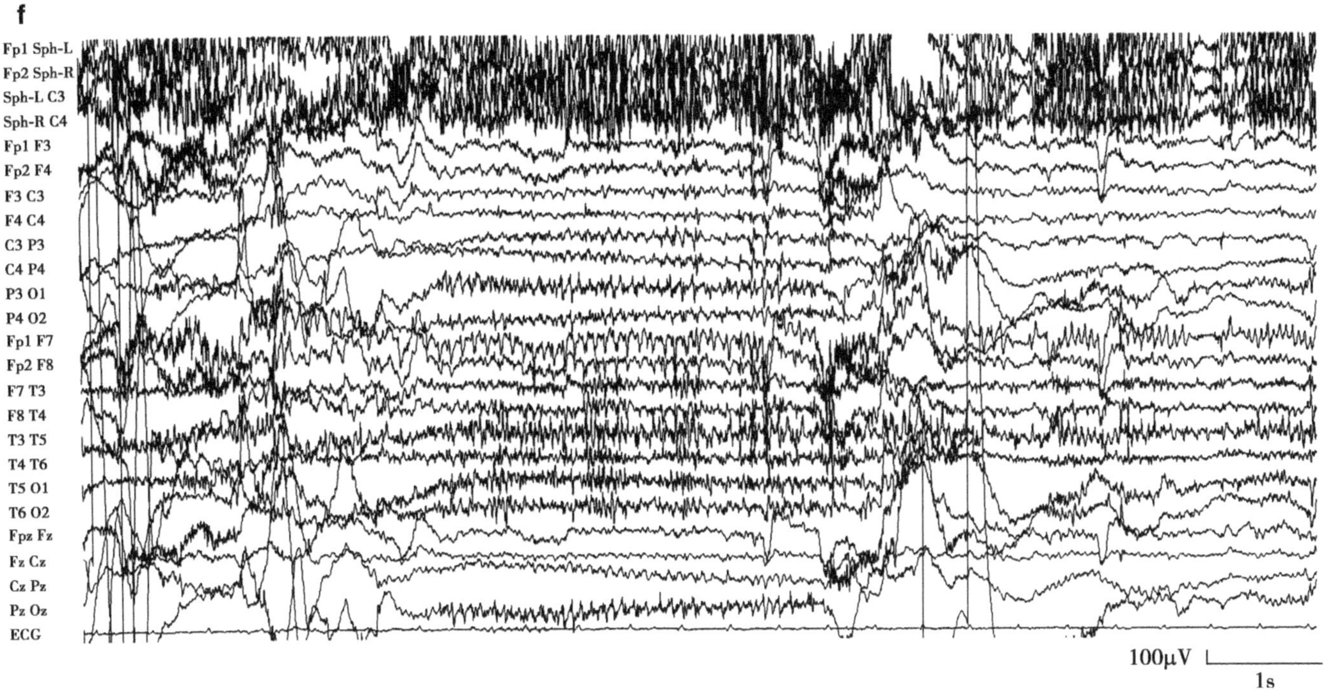

Fig. 6.9 (continued)

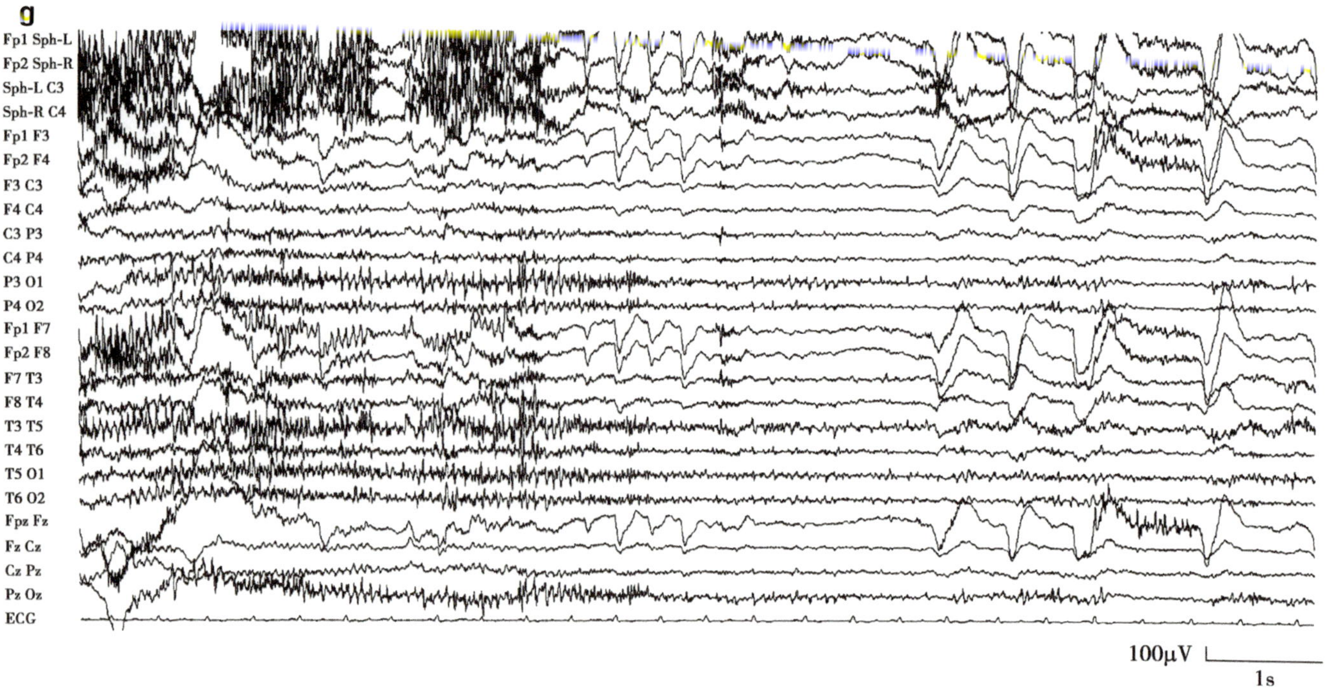

Fig. 6.9 (continued)

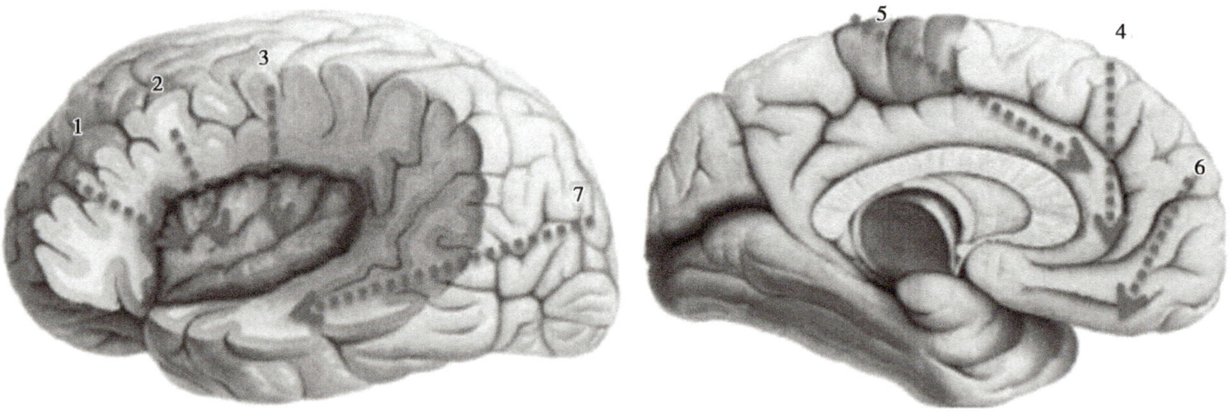

Fig. 6.10 Scheme of intracranial electrodes
Depth electrode 1: the anterior part of left middle frontal gyrus → the anterior part of insula (12 contacts)
Depth electrode 2: the anterior part of left inferior frontal gyrus → the anterior part of insula (12 contacts)
Depth electrode 3: the middle part of left middle frontal gyrus → the middle part of insula (10 contacts)
Depth electrode 4: the anterior part of the left superior frontal gyrus → the lower part of the anterior cingulate cortex (12 contacts)
Depth electrode 5: the posterior part of the left middle frontal gyrus → the upper part of the anterior cingulate cortex (12 contacts)
Depth electrode 6: the end of the left inferior frontal sulcus → the orbitofrontal region (10 contacts)
Depth electrode 7: the left occipital region → hippocampus (16 contacts)

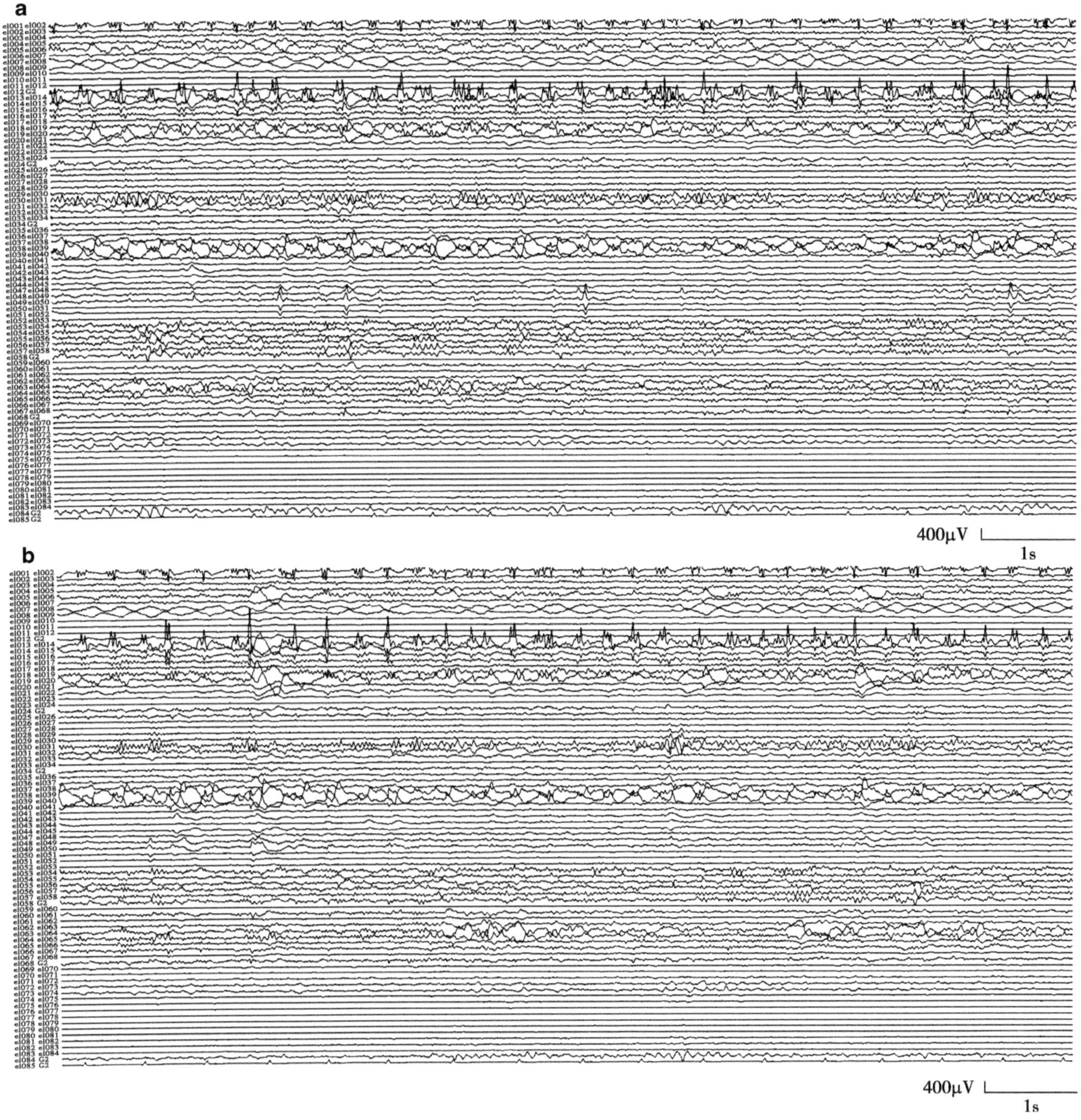

Fig. 6.11 Interictal intracranial EEG. (**a**) The IEEG showed polyspikes and spike-and-wave complexes over the anterior part of insula (contact numbers el001 and el013) and spike-and-wave complexes over the lower part of the anterior cingulate cortex (contact number el039). (**b**) The IEEG showed polyspikes and spike-and-wave complexes over the anterior part of insula (contact numbers el001 and el013) and spike-and-wave complexes over the lower part of the anterior cingulate cortex (contact number el039)

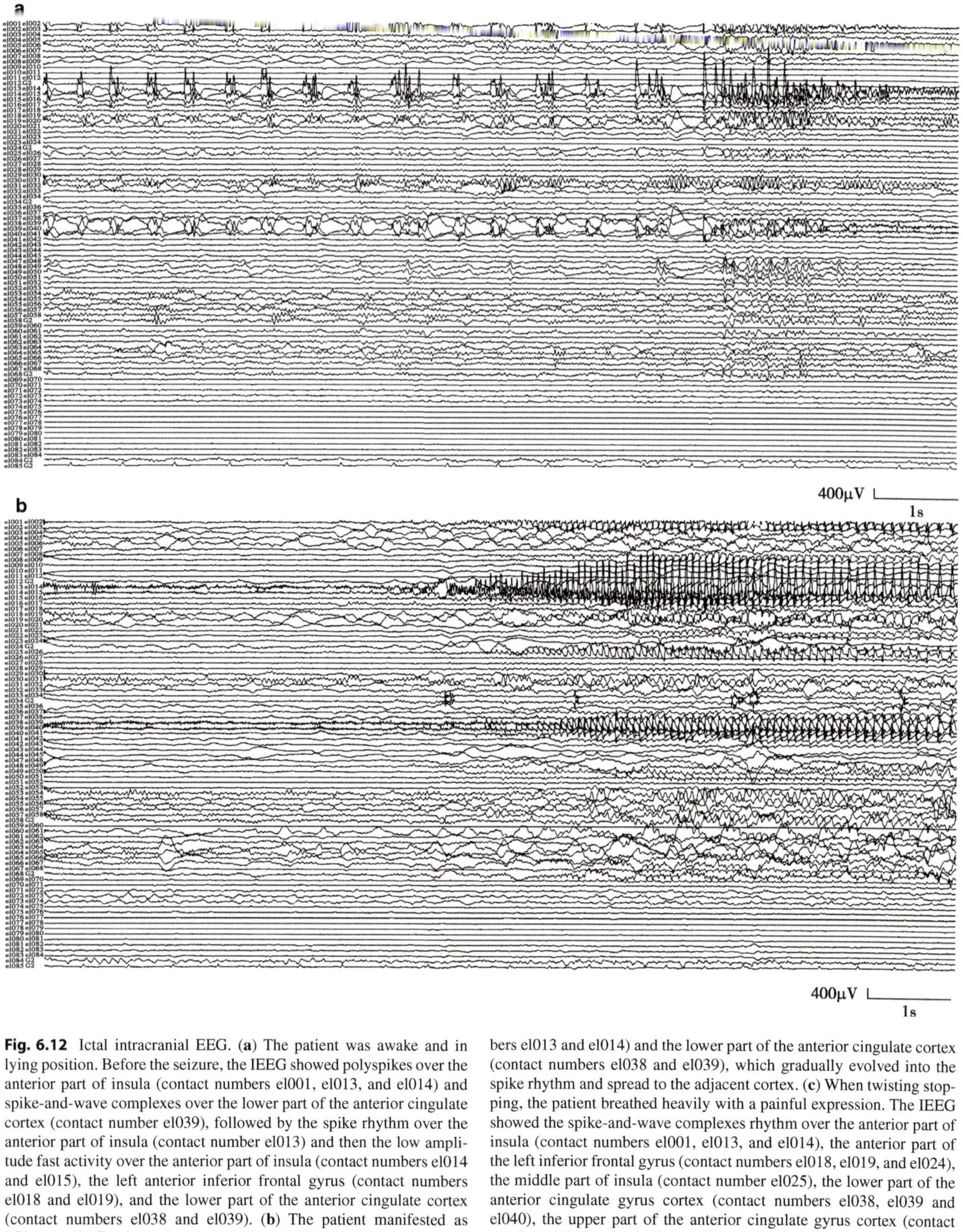

Fig. 6.12 Ictal intracranial EEG. (**a**) The patient was awake and in lying position. Before the seizure, the IEEG showed polyspikes over the anterior part of insula (contact numbers el001, el013, and el014) and spike-and-wave complexes over the lower part of the anterior cingulate cortex (contact number el039), followed by the spike rhythm over the anterior part of insula (contact number el013) and then the low amplitude fast activity over the anterior part of insula (contact numbers el014 and el015), the left anterior inferior frontal gyrus (contact numbers el018 and el019), and the lower part of the anterior cingulate cortex (contact numbers el038 and el039). (**b**) The patient manifested as "Chapeau de Gendarme," and the body twisted. The IEEG showed the low amplitude fast activity over the anterior part of insula (contact numbers el013 and el014) and the lower part of the anterior cingulate cortex (contact numbers el038 and el039), which gradually evolved into the spike rhythm and spread to the adjacent cortex. (**c**) When twisting stopping, the patient breathed heavily with a painful expression. The IEEG showed the spike-and-wave complexes rhythm over the anterior part of insula (contact numbers el001, el013, and el014), the anterior part of the left inferior frontal gyrus (contact numbers el018, el019, and el024), the middle part of insula (contact number el025), the lower part of the anterior cingulate gyrus cortex (contact numbers el038, el039 and el040), the upper part of the anterior cingulate gyrus cortex (contact numbers el048 and el049), and the orbitofrontal region (contact numbers el061, el062, el067 and el068)

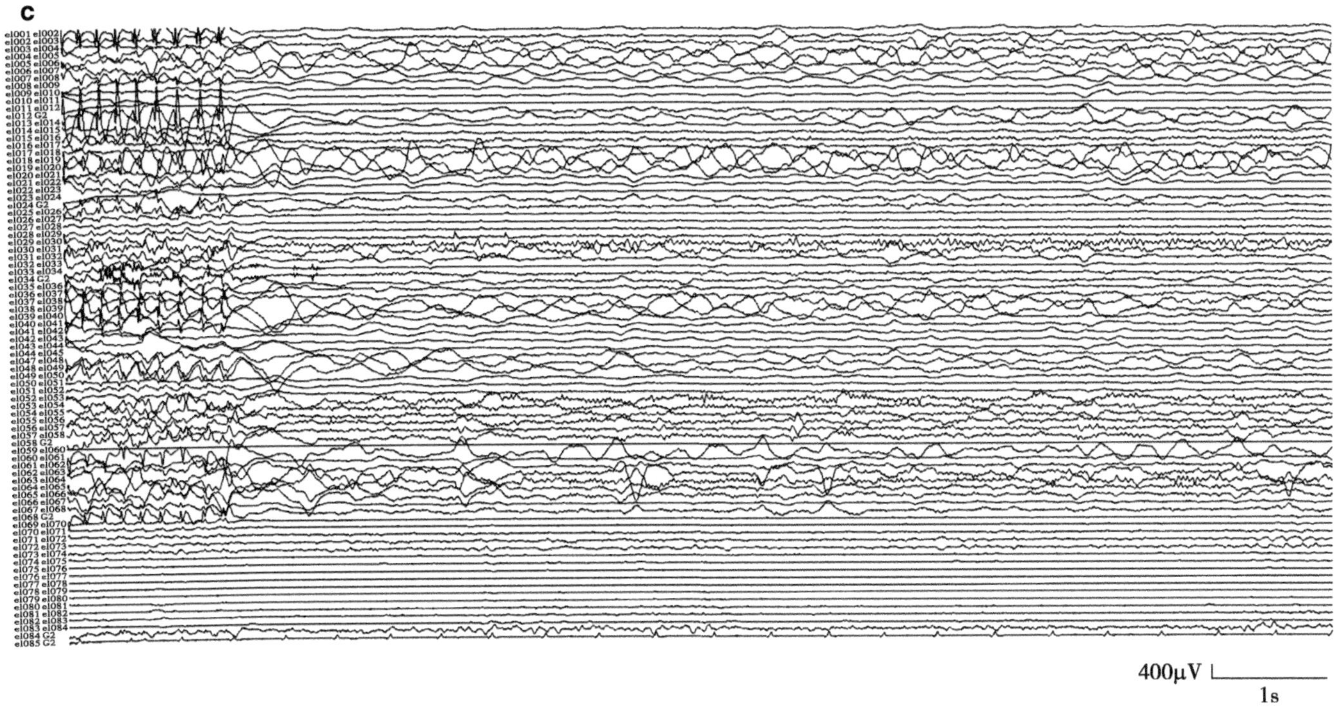

Fig. 6.12 (continued)

[Case Review]

1. *Case Characteristics*
   (a) *Seizure characteristics*: (1) Chapeau de Gendarme, and then piloerection on the upper limbs, with fear and tachycardia. (2) Without loss of consciousness during the seizure. (3) Seizures were frequent, more than 10 times per day.
   (b) *Imaging characteristics*: (1) MRI showed no obvious abnormalities. (2) MEG showed that the spike dipoles were located in the left anterior insula.
   (c) *EEG characteristics*: Interictal EEG showed sharp waves over the left sphenoidal electrode and the left anterior temporal region; ictal EEG showed the rhythmic sharp waves over the left sphenoidal electrode and the left temporal region.
2. *Diagnosis and treatment strategy and follow-up results*: According to the seizure symptoms such as "Chapeau de Gendarme," "piloerection," and fear and the ictal EEG features, the epileptic focus was first considered to be the cingulate cortex and the temporal region. It may be necessary to cover the insula with electrodes based on the MEG findings. The interictal IEEG showed persistent abnormal discharges over the interior part of the insula, and the ictal IEEG showed the seizure onset zones were the anterior part of insula and the anterior part of the inferior frontal gyrus. During a 4-year follow-up after the surgical resection of the left orbital-frontal and frontal operculum, the seizure disappeared. The definite seizure onset zone and the complete resection of the epileptic focus made the surgical outcome favorable.

Cases of Epilepsy with Severe Hemispheric Lesions

7

Du Wei, Zhang Xiating, Zhang Guojun, Ni Duanyu, and Wei Min

Overview of Epilepsy with Severe Hemispheric Lesions

Hemispherectomy was performed by Dandy for the treatment of diffuse hemispheric glioma in 1928 and by McKenzie for refractory epilepsy in 1938. Since then, this procedure has been applied in clinical practice for the treatment of refractory epilepsy associated with severe hemispheric lesions. The procedure has evolved into a variety of techniques, including anatomic hemispherectomy, functional hemispherectomy, and multi-lobe disconnection, etc. Such cases are characterized by varied and complex types of clinical symptoms, frequent seizures and even mostly status epilepticus, poor response to drug therapy, and significant impact on patients' activities of daily living.

Indications for Hemispherectomy

Patients with extensive, multifocal epileptic lesions in one hemisphere (e.g., traumatic brain injury, cerebral hemorrhage, perinatal disease) that have caused severe dysfunction in the contralateral limbs; patients with progressively worsening underlying disease in unilateral hemisphere that has caused epileptic seizures.

1. Patients with extensive cerebral atrophy in either hemisphere after cerebral hemorrhage
2. Patients with extensive encephalomalacia in either hemisphere after encephalitis
3. Patients with extensive hemispheric lesions due to specific causes, such as Sturge-Weber syndrome and Rasmussen's encephalitis
4. Patients with seizures originating from the lesion side and with compensated function
5. Frequent seizures, poor response to drug therapy, possible effects on the development and function of the healthy hemisphere

Preoperative Evaluation for Hemispherectomy

1. *Type, frequency, and severity of seizures and medication*: Due to extensive lesions, patients may have various types of seizures, including focal seizures with or without impairment of consciousness, focal status epilepticus, and even generalized tonic-clonic seizures. Patients often have frequent seizures (up to dozens of seizures per day) and poor response to drug therapy and may suffer from significant impact on patients' activities of daily living.
2. *EEG*: Abnormal EEG background is associated with different courses of disease and the severity of hemispheric lesions, which is manifested as diffuse slow activity, rhythmic delta or theta activity, or bilateral diffuse abnormalities (often asymmetrical). During the interictal stage, the patient may have multifocal or diffuse discharges over the unilateral hemisphere, or simultaneous discharges over the bilateral hemispheres; significant epileptiform discharges may not be detected in ictal EEG, possibly due to limitation of discharge origin, lower voltage, or failure

D. Wei · Z. Guojun · N. Duanyu (✉)
Department of Neurosurgery, Beijing, China

Z. Xiating · W. Min
Department of Neurology, Beijing, China

Y. Wang (ed.), *Electroencephalogram for Presurgical Epilepsy Evaluation*, https://doi.org/10.1007/978-981-95-8003-3_7

of scalp electrodes to record EEG signal due to discharge origin in the deeper sulci. As the disease progresses, independent epileptiform discharges may be detected over the contralateral hemisphere. EEG may be inconsistent with clinical symptoms and imaging findings.

3. *General physical conditions*: As hemispherectomy is relatively major invasion to patients, the patient's general physical conditions must be adequate to tolerate the procedure.
4. *Neurological examination and psychological assessment*: Neurological examination includes limb motor function, sensory function, language function, etc., and must be conducted in a careful and sufficient manner. Special attention should be paid to the possibility of progressive worsening of hemispheric function. Most of these patients have cognitive impairment.
5. *Functions of the hemisphere with lesions*: It is particularly important to figure out whether the hemisphere with lesions still has basic motor, sensory, and language functions. Examinations include functional magnetic resonance imaging (fMRI), motor evoked potentials (MEP), and sensory evoked potentials (SEP). MRI shows changes in the cerebral peduncle, and the size comparison of the right and left cerebral peduncles is also important indicator.

Prognosis

Of patients who have undergone hemispherectomy, 75–90% are seizure-free. Some patients still have seizures in the early period postoperation or even an increase in seizures. However, seizures are gradually controlled in most cases during the follow-up of 1 year.

The improvement in postoperative limb motor deficit is related to the timing of surgery and the age of the patient at the time of surgery. In general, the younger the patient, the more adequately the motor and sensory functions of the limb are compensated. Those with preoperative hemiparesis may also get improved to a certain degree with postoperative rehabilitation. Post-operative behavioral abilities such as cognitive function and attention may also get improved.

Cases of Epilepsy with Severe Cerebral Hemispheric Lesions

Case 7.1 Hemispheric Damages

[Abstract of Medical Records]
Female, 20 years old.

1. *Chief complaint*: Paroxysmal limb convulsion for 8 years.
2. *History of present illness*: 8 years ago, when the patient woke up in the morning, she had a sudden loss of awareness, with the head turning to the right and the right limb convulsion, which lasted for about 10 min and then resolved, followed by a twilight state. The symptoms above reoccurred in a fixed pattern later. The patient once visited a hospital and was initially diagnosed as having epilepsy and then treated with sodium valproate, the effect of which was poor. The present type of seizure is relatively fixed, mainly manifested as sudden head deviation to the right when waking up, right limb convulsion, especially in the right upper limb. The convulsions are clustered, with each convulsion lasting dozens of seconds and reappearing after an interval of 10 s or so. In the early stage of convulsion, the patient is conscious and can communicate with her family members briefly but loses consciousness in the late stage of convulsion. The seizures usually occur when the patient wakes up, and the patient is easily irritated thereafter. The patient is currently taking oral lamotrigine at 100 mg per dose every 12 h for an average of 2–4 episodes per day.
3. *Past history*: No febrile convulsions.
4. *Physical examination*: The patient's right hand was claw-shaped, with atrophy of the thenar and hypothenar muscles, and no hypalgesia or thermohypesthesia. The proximal muscle strength of the right upper limb was of Grade 4; the distal muscle strength was of Grade 2; the proximal muscle strength of the right lower limb was of Grade 4; the distal muscle strength was of Grade 2, and the remaining muscle strength was normal.
5. *Imaging examination*: MRI revealed encephalomalacia in the left basal ganglia region.
6. *EEG*: For details, see Figs. 7.1 and 7.2.

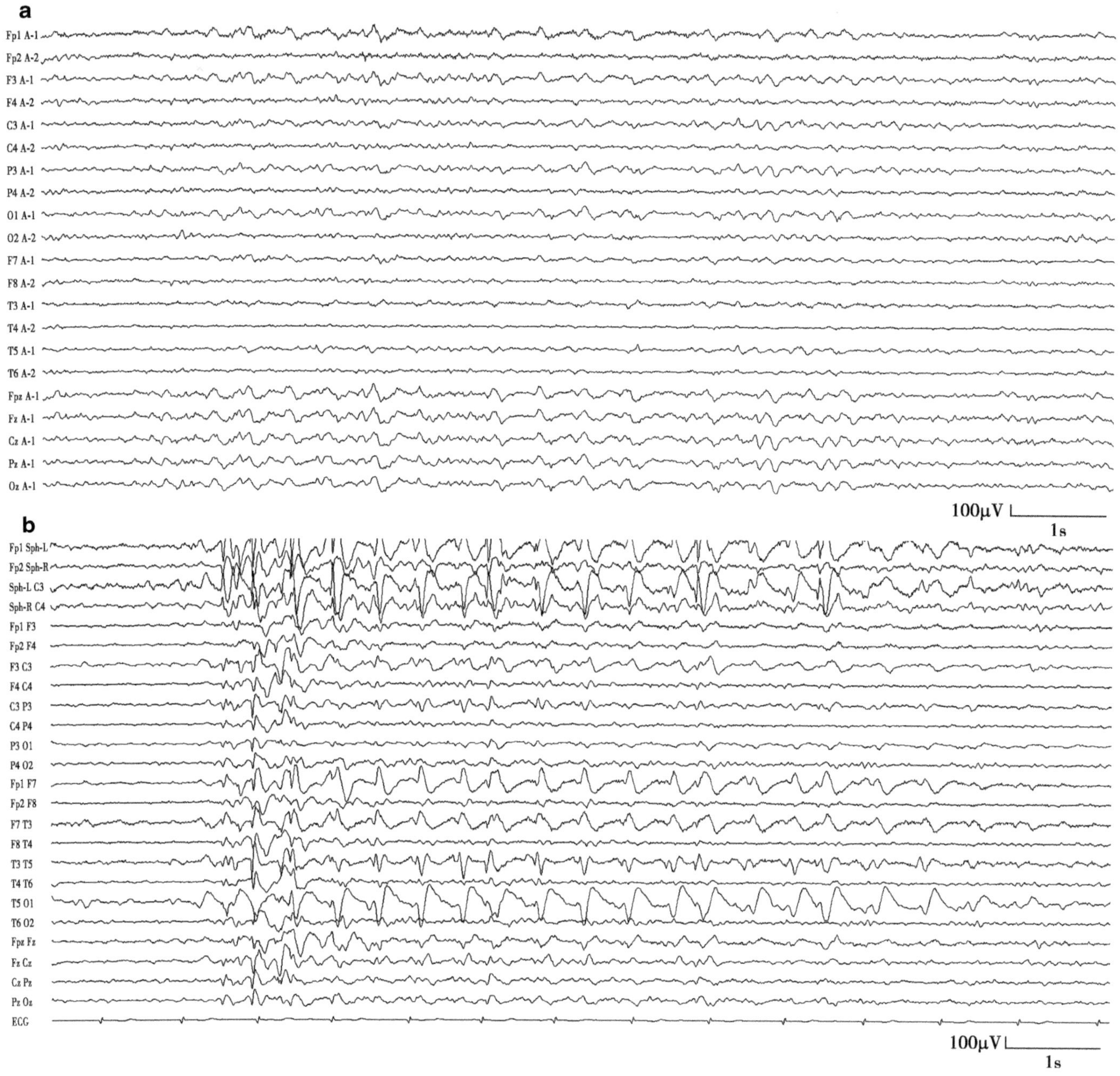

Fig. 7.1 Interictal scalp EEG. (**a**) Irregular slow sharp waves over the left leads are seen on the EEG. (**b**) Rhythmic slow sharp-and-wave complexes and sharp waves were seen over the left hemisphere, prominent with the left frontal and temporal regions

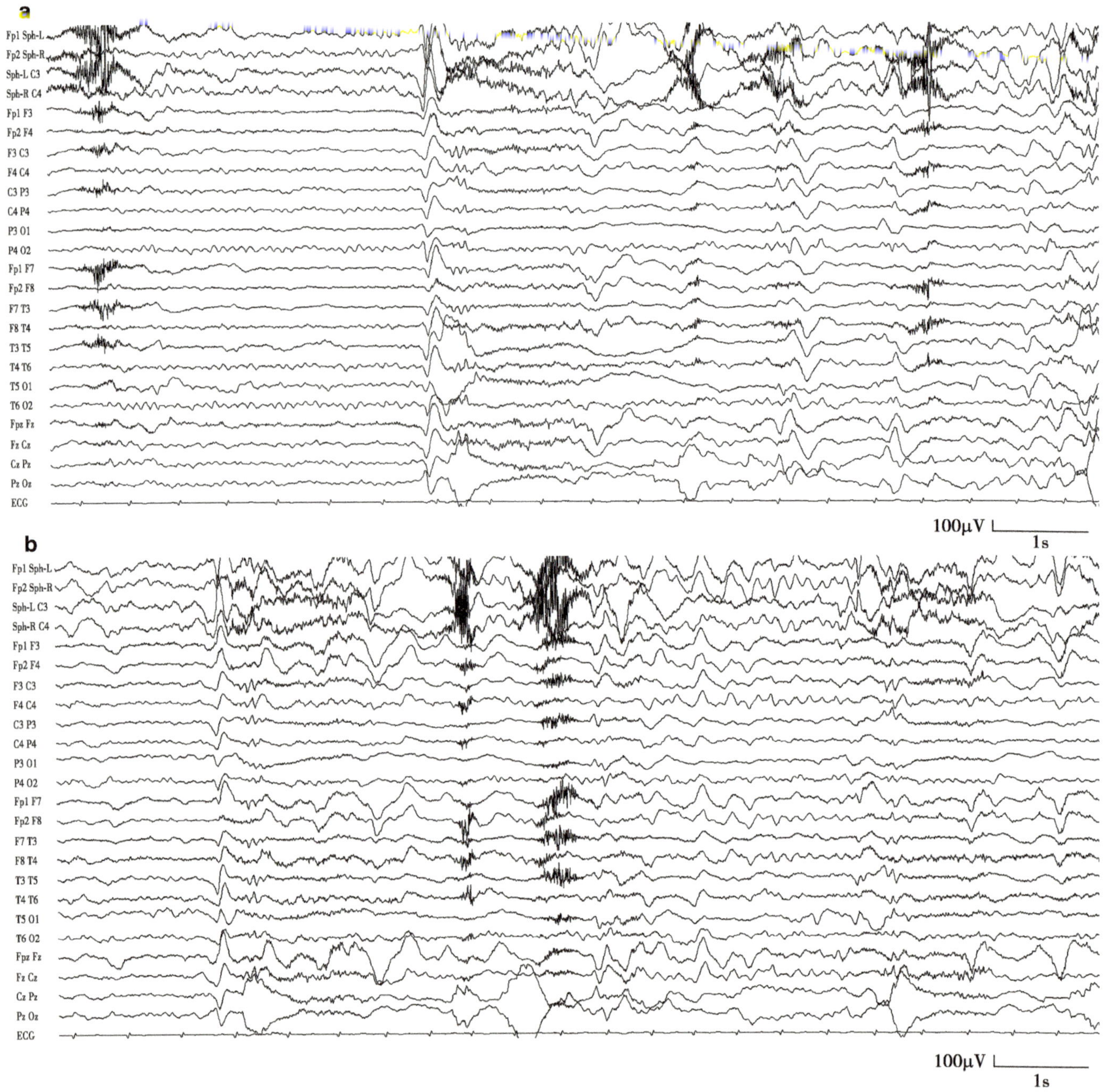

Fig. 7.2 Ictal scalp EEG. (**a**) The patient was in a supine position, with the right upper limb elevating with tonicity. The EEG shows high-amplitude sharp waves (Fp1 F3, Fp2 F4, F3 C3, F4 C4, C3 P3, Fp1 F7, Fp2 F8, T3 T5, T4 T6, T5 O1, Fpz Fz, Fz Cz), followed by fast activity and then slow waves over the left hemisphere. (**b**) The patient was in a supine position, with the right upper limb elevating with tonicity, which reoccurred after an interval of 8 s. The EEG shows high-amplitude slowed sharp waves (Fp1 F3, Fp2 F4, F3 C3, C3 P3, Fp1 F7, Fp2 F8, T3 T5, T4 T6, T5 O1, Fpz Fz, Fz Cz), followed by fast activity and then slow waves over the left hemisphere

[Case Review]

1. *Case Characteristics*
   (a) *Seizure characteristics*: The patient had an onset at 12 years old, with a medical history of 8 years and habitual seizure of right limb convulsion.
   (b) *Imaging characteristics*: MRI revealed encephalomalacia in the left basal ganglia region.
   (c) *EEG characteristics*: Interictal EEG showed rhythmic slow sharp waves as well as sharp-and-wave complexes over the left leads; ictal EEG showed abnormal discharges mainly over the left side.
2. *Diagnosis and treatment strategy and follow-up result*: The EEG, seizure symptoms, and MRI information were consistent, and the epileptic seizure origin was located in the left hemisphere. It was decided to perform a multilobar disconnection of the left hemisphere with preservation of the functional area, resulting in proper control of the seizures post operation.

Case 7.2 Hemispheric Damages

[Abstract of Medical Records]
Male, 6 years old.

1. *Chief complaint*: Paroxysmal limb convulsion for 2 years.
2. *History of present illness*: The patient experienced right limb convulsion without obvious cause 2 years ago, which lasted 2–3 min, without loss of awareness. The patient visited a local hospital and was orally administered with sodium valproate (500 mg per dose, b.i.d.) and topiramate (100 mg in the morning, 50 mg in the afternoon, and 100 mg in the evening), resulting in appropriate control. The patient had frequent seizures in recent months, including right limb convulsion, sometimes followed by generalized convulsions, 3–4 times per month.
3. *Past history and family history*: No history of associated diseases.
4. *Physical examination*: No neurological abnormalities were found.
5. *Imaging examination*: MRI revealed hypoplasia of the left cerebral hemisphere.
6. *EEG*: For details, see Figs. 7.3 and 7.4.

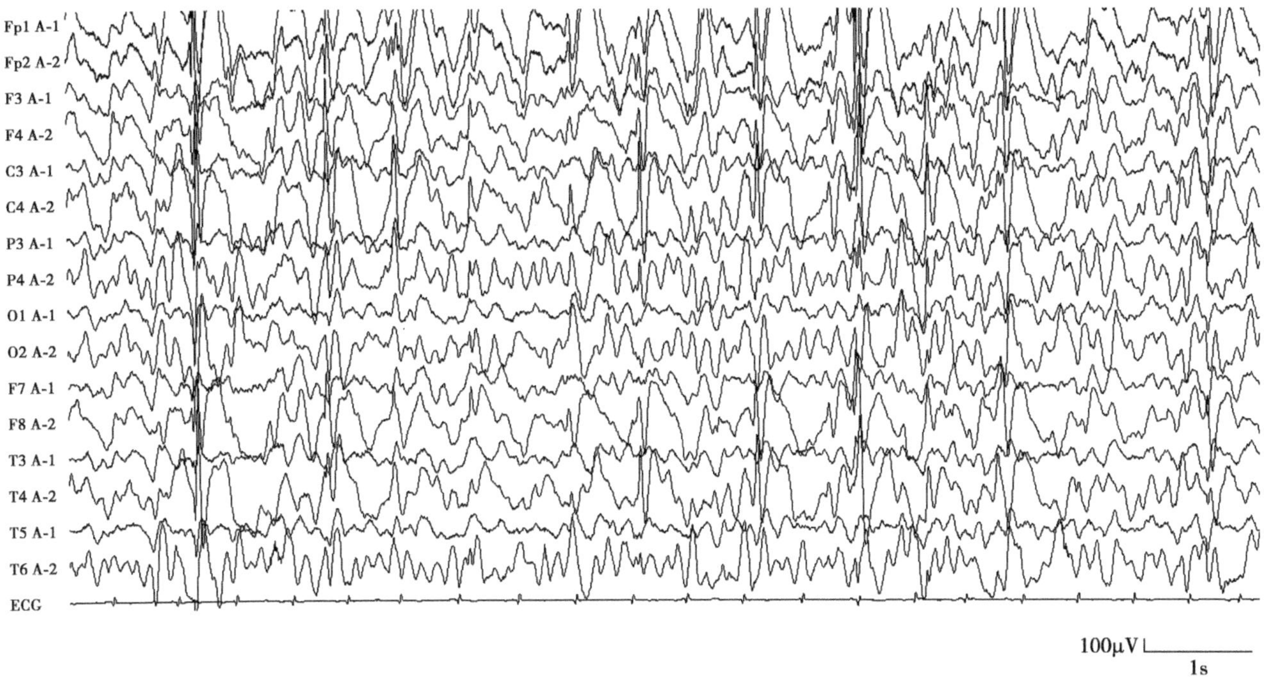

Fig. 7.3 Interictal scalp EEG. Basic rhythms 7 Hz, with higher amplitude over the right side than on the left side; more medium- and high-amplitude slow spike-and-wave complexes were seen over the right hemisphere (Fp2, F4, C4, P4, O2, F8, T4, T6)

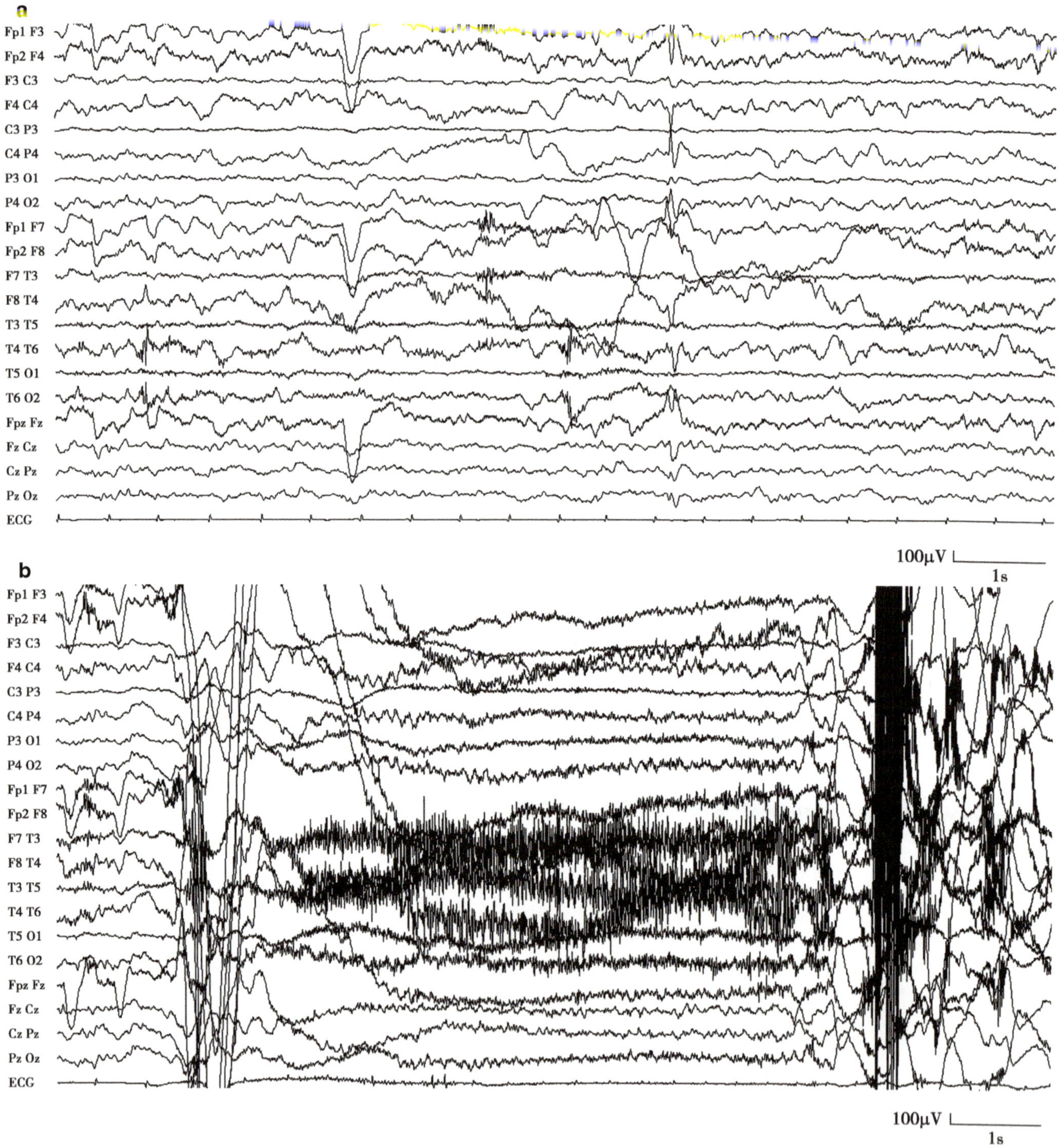

Fig. 7.4 Ictal scalp EEG. (**a**) The patient was playing in the position of right lateral decubitus before the seizure. EEG showed oculomotor artifacts over the bilateral frontal (Fp1 F3, Fp2 F4, Fp1 F7, Fp2 F8, Fpz Fz) regions, inversion of spikes in the right central (C4) region, and scattered spikes over the bilateral frontal (Fp1 F3, Fp2 F4, Fp1 F7, Fp2 F8, Fpz Fz) regions, right temporal (F8 T4, T4 T6) region, and parietal (P4) region. (**b**) During the seizures, the patient's upper limbs were suddenly raised and abducted with tonicity, with lower limbs flexed and elevated. His body turned left to a supine position, with his head turning to the right. The origin of the abnormal discharge was unclear. There were many EMG artifacts over the leads in the bilateral temporal regions (F7 T3, F8 T4, T3 T5, T4 T6), and 6.0–7.0 Hz θ waves over the right central region and parietal region (F4 C4, C4 P4). (**c**) The tonic movements of upper limbs of the patient were mitigated, with intermittent limb clonus and making "humming" sounds. Electrode wobble artifacts and EMG artifacts can be seen. (**d**) The patient's limb movements stopped, but he was still making "humming" sounds and breathing heavily. His family member patted his body to soothe him. EEG showed many irregular medium- and high-amplitude slow waves over the right leads (Fp2 F4, F4 C4, C4 P4, P4 O2, Fp2 F8, F8 T4, T4 T6, T6 O2) and midline leads (Fpz Fz, Fz Cz, Cz Pz), mixed with electrode wobble artifacts. (**e**) After the seizure, the patient returned to the position of right lateral decubitus. EEG showed slow wave rhythms over all electrodes (Fp2 F4, F4 C4, C4 P4, P4 O2, Fp2 F8, F8 T4, T4 T6, T6 O2) over the right region and midline leads (Fpz Fz, Cz Pz, Pz Oz) and then gradually recovered to the background EEG

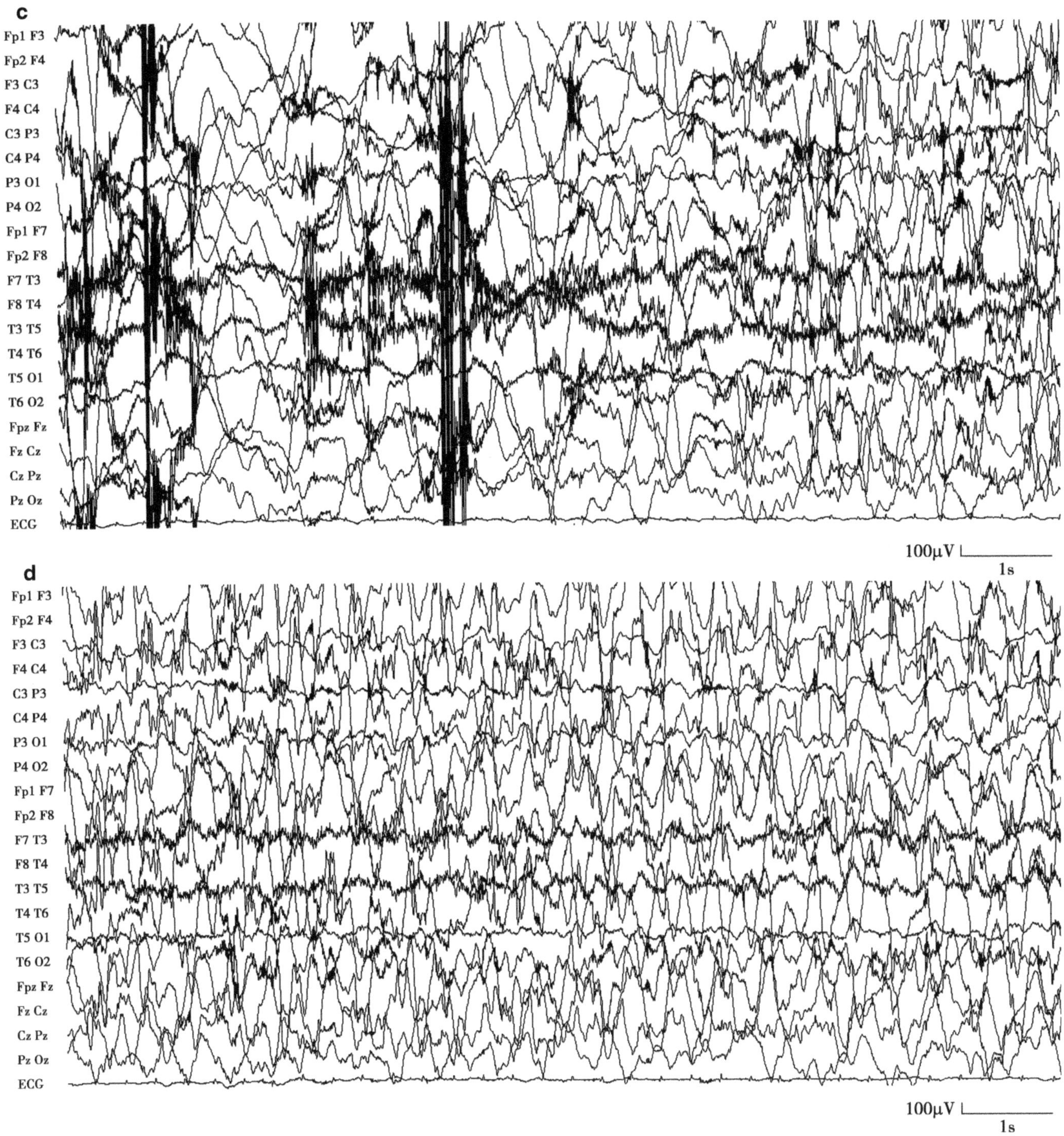

Fig. 7.4 (continued)

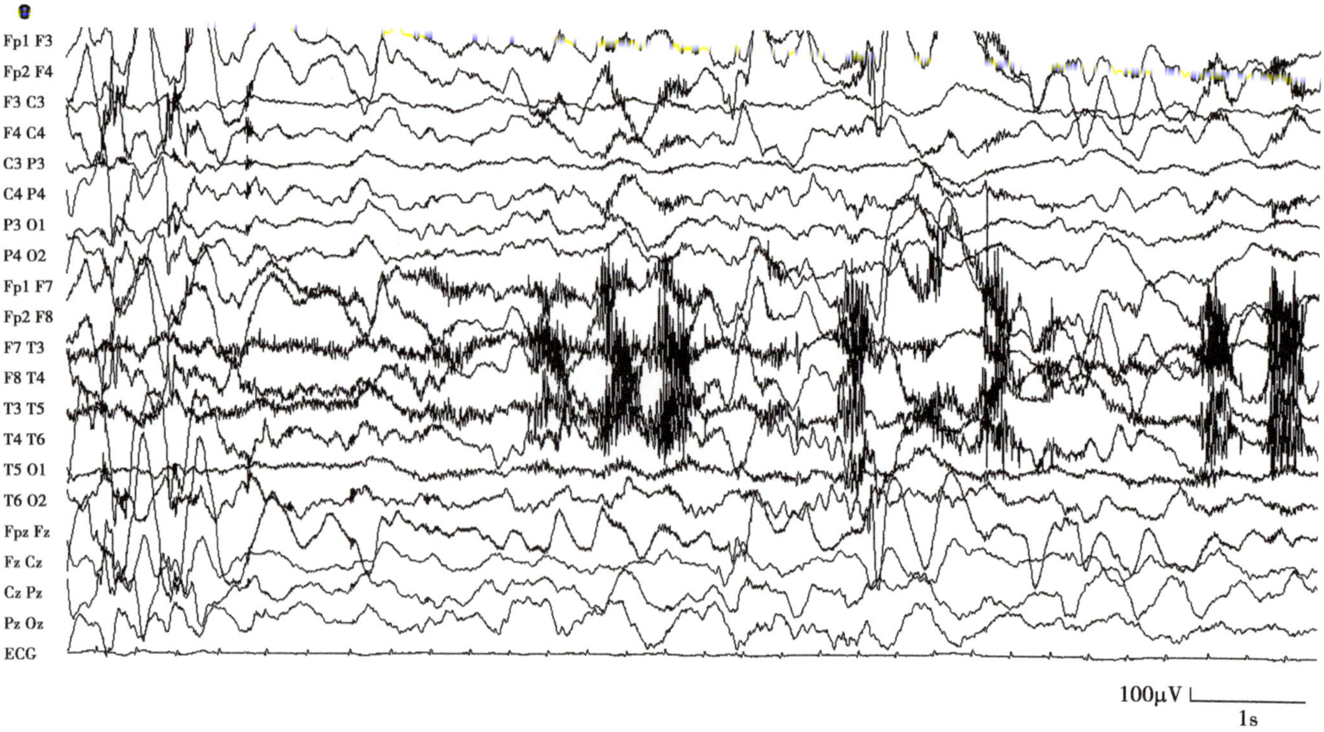

Fig. 7.4 (continued)

[Case Review]

1. *Clinical Characteristics*
   (a) *Seizure characteristics*: (1) The patient had a seizure onset at 4 years old, with a medical history of 2 years. (2) His habitual seizure was right limb convulsion.
   (b) *Imaging characteristics*: MRI revealed hypoplasia of the left cerebral hemisphere.
   (c) *EEG characteristics*: EEG showed the presence of bilateral basic rhythm, with higher amplitude over the right side than the left side; interictal EEG showed extensive high-amplitude slow waves over many leads over the right region; the origin of brain electricity on the ictal EEG was unclear; slow wave rhythms were seen over multiple leads over the right region.
2. *Diagnosis and treatment strategy and follow-up result*: The EEG presentation was inconsistent with the symptoms during seizures and the lesions showed in MRI. It was probably due to cortical atrophy of the left cerebral hemisphere and weak discharging that could not be easily detected by scalp EEG, while the abnormal discharging on the right side could be caused by long-term seizures. According to the symptoms of habitual seizure (right limb convulsion) and the imaging examinations (apparent and extensive brain atrophy in the left cerebral hemisphere), the origin of seizure was located in the left hemisphere. The limb movements of the patient were generally normal, and motor evoked potentials and functional magnetic resonance imaging (fMRI) revealed the presence of functions in the left hemisphere. To control the epileptic seizures, it was decided to perform a multilobar disconnection of the left hemisphere with preservation of the functional area. The epileptic seizures were well controlled post operation, with no limb motor impairment. In patients with extensive hemispheric lesions, EEG abnormalities tend to be diffuse. If the lesioned side is severely atrophied, the abnormal discharges may not be obvious. Due to long-term epileptic seizures, frequent abnormal discharges may occur in the contralateral hemisphere. In conclusion, in patients like this, one should never locate the origin of the seizure solely on the abnormal discharges shown on the EEG during a localization diagnosis.

Case 7.3 Hemispheric Damages

[Abstract of Medical Records]
Male, 19 years old.

1. *Chief complaint*: Paroxysmal left limb convulsion for 17 years.
2. *History of present illness*: After asphyxia due to dystocia at birth, the patient experienced left limb convulsion, without loss of awareness, at 2 years old, which lasted from a few

seconds to a few minutes. The frequency of seizures ranged from 1 to 2 times a month to several times a day. The patient once took carbamazepine and nitrazepam but discontinued them due to side effects. The patient had a delayed development of intellectual and motor functions and could not walk and talk until 2 years old. The muscle strength of the distal left upper limb was of Grade 4.

3. *Imaging examination*: MRI revealed abnormal development of the right cerebral hemisphere.
4. *EEG*: For details, see Figs. 7.5 and 7.6.

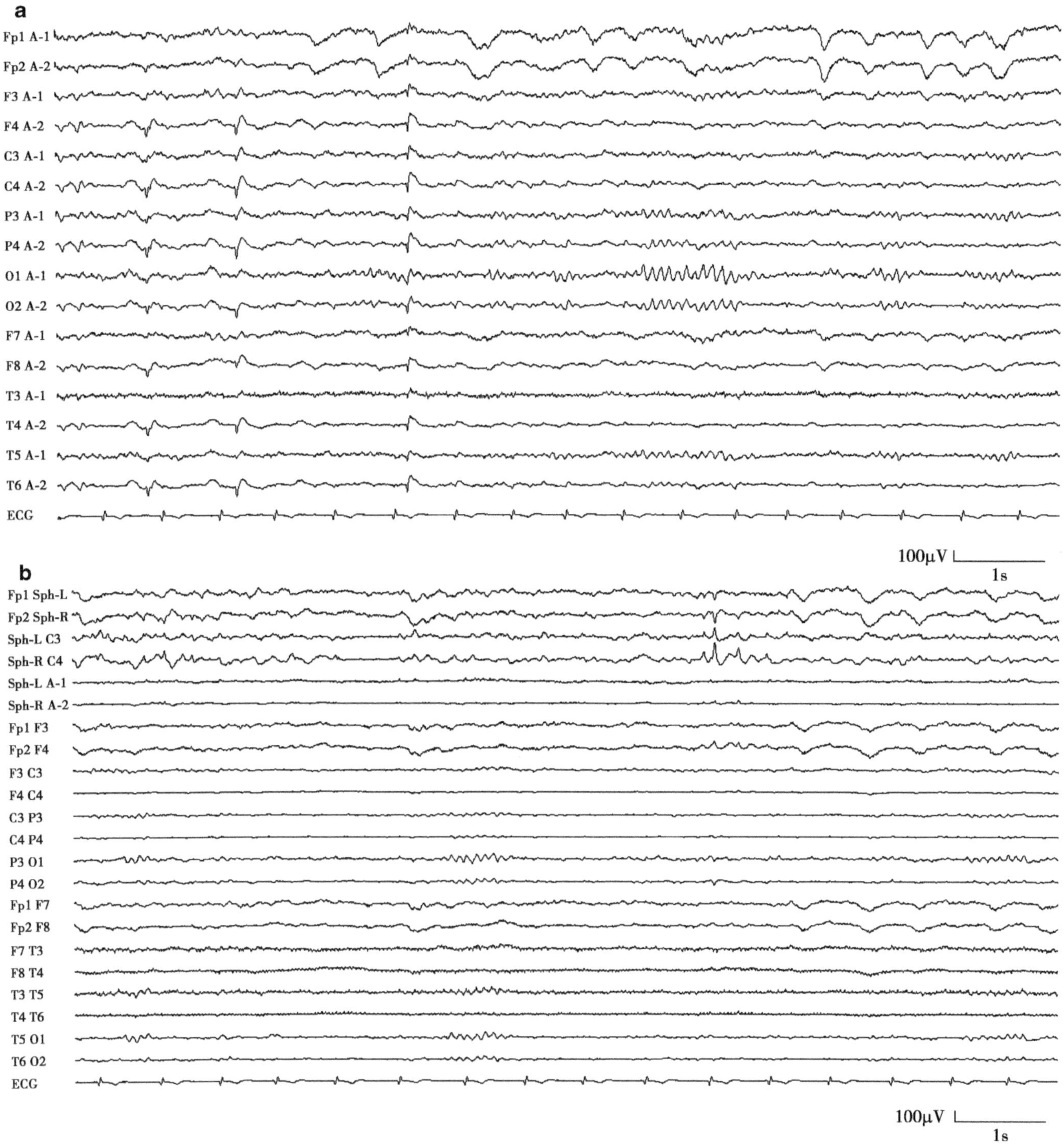

Fig. 7.5 Interictal scalp EEG. (**a**) The basic rhythm was 8.0 Hz, and scattered positive sharp waves (earlobe electrode activation) were seen over the bilateral leads, especially the right side. (**b**) EEG shows scattered sharp waves over the right sphenoid electrode (Sph-R)

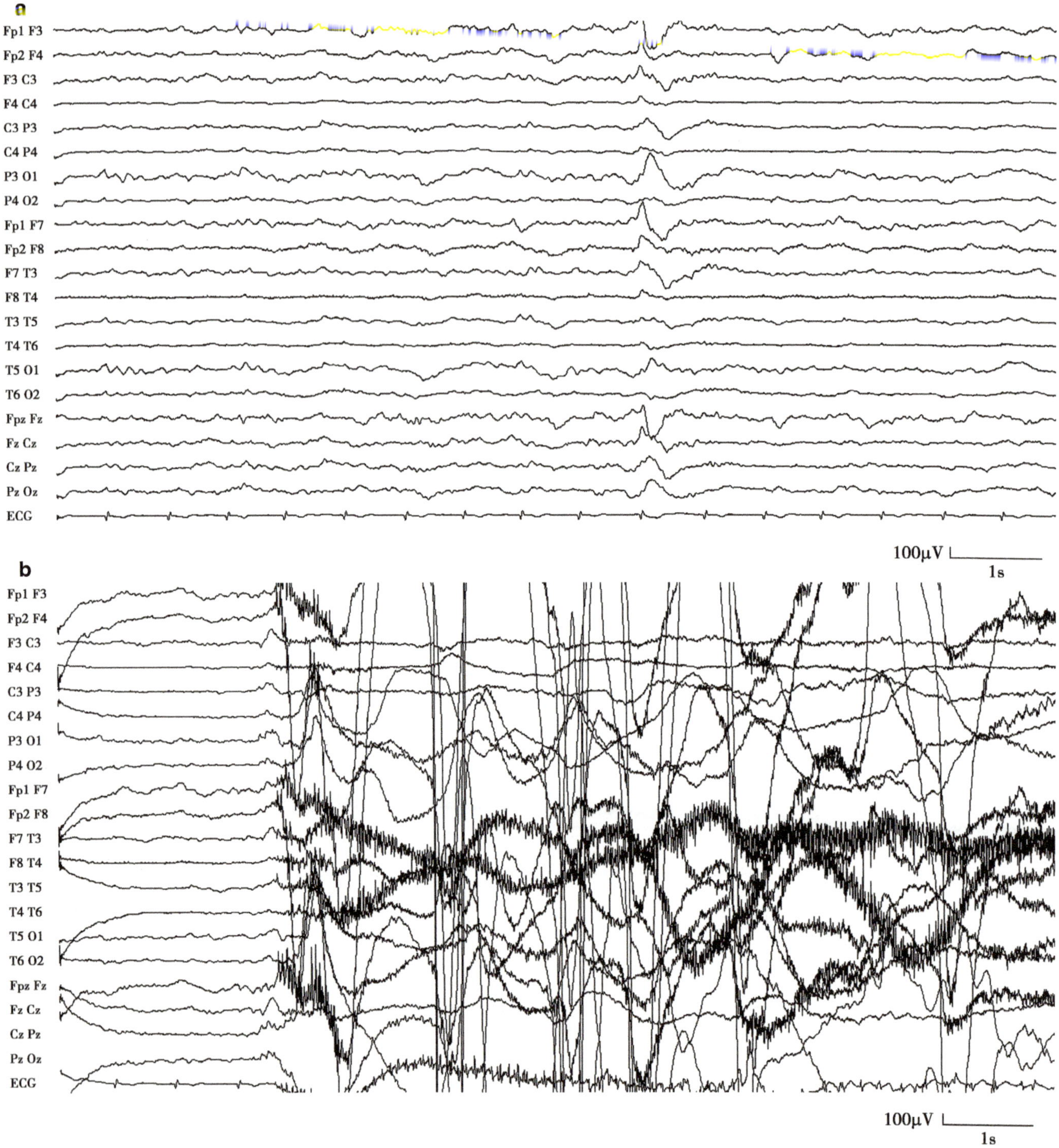

Fig. 7.6 Ictal scalp EEG. (**a**) The patient was asleep before the seizure. The EEG is a background EEG when the patient was in stage II of sleep, showing basically symmetrical bilateral spindle waves. (**b**) When the seizure attacked, the patient suddenly opened his eyes with a painful expression, with his right upper limb raising to his head and his left upper limb flexed with clonic jerks, which lasted for about 15 s. 3 s before the seizure, the EEG showed low-amplitude θ waves (4.0–5.0 Hz) over the left frontotemporal region (Fp1 F3, Fp1 F7, F7 T3, T3 T5, T5 O1) and the frontal midline (Fpz Fz); when the seizure occurred, the EEG showed electrode wobble artifacts and significant EMG artifacts over the bilateral frontotemporal regions (Fp1 F3, Fp2 F4, Fp1 F7, Fp2 F8, F7 T3, F8 T4, T3 T5, T4 T6) and the frontal midline (Fpz Fz). (**c**) The seizure ended. EEG gradually recovered to the background EEG, with EMG artifacts visible over the bilateral frontotemporal regions (Fp1 F3, Fp2 F4, Fp1 F7, Fp2 F8, F7 T3, F8 T4, T3 T5, T4 T6) and frontal midline regions (Fpz Fz)

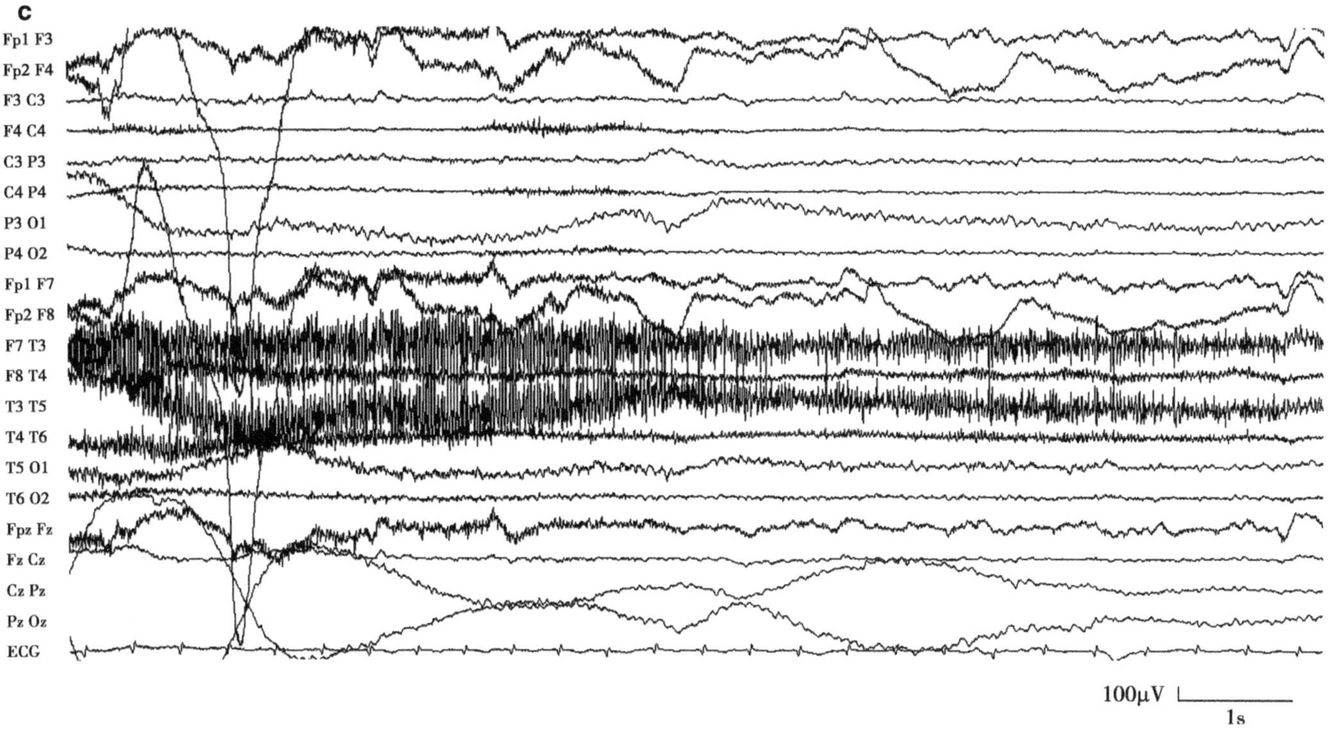

Fig. 7.6 (continued)

[Case Review]

1. *Clinical Characteristics*
   (a) *Characteristics of medical history*: The patient had a seizure onset at 2 years old, with a history of 17 years and a history of asphyxia at birth.
   (b) *Seizure characteristics*: The main symptom of seizure was left limb convulsion, which lasted 10 s or so to resolve.
   (c) *Imaging characteristics*: MRI showed abnormal development of the right cerebral hemisphere.
   (d) *EEG characteristics*: In consideration of the interictal occasional sharp discharges and the ictal insignificant abnormal discharges on the EEG, it was believed that the cortical discharges were too weak to be detected by the scalp EEG as the right hemisphere was extensively and severely atrophied.
2. *Diagnosis and treatment strategy and follow-up result*: According to seizure symptoms and significant imaging manifestations of MRI, the epileptic seizure origin was located in the right hemisphere. It was hence decided to perform a hemispherectomy to the right cerebral hemisphere. After surgery, the epileptic seizures disappeared, without new limb motor impairment. In this case, the origin was on the left side shown on the ictal EEG and the lesion was on the right side. The epilepsy focus was located mainly based on MRI examinations.

Case 7.4 Hemispheric Damages

[Abstract of Medical Records]
Female, 12 years old.

1. *Chief complaint*: Paroxysmal limb convulsion for 10 years.
2. *History of present illness*: The patient had intracranial hemorrhage 40 days after birth, frequent febrile convulsions from 1 to 5 years old, and convulsions without fever from 5 years old onward, manifested by twisting of the body to the left side, head turning to the left, upward gaze of eyes, and tonicity of the left upper limb without loss of awareness, sometimes accompanied by generalized tonic and clonic seizures, lasting from a few seconds to several minutes, with varying frequency. The patient was diagnosed as having epilepsy at a local hospital and was treated with valproamide and sodium valproate, which were not effective. After 9 years old, the patient was treated with topiramate (50 mg in the morning and 100 mg in the evening) in combination with sodium valproate (200 mg per dose, tid), and seizures were controlled. After 3 years of no seizures, the dose was reduced. When sodium valproate was reduced to 100 mg per dose tid, seizures attacked again. Then the dose was recovered to the original one, while the seizures could not be controlled. At admission, the dosage was 250 mg (morning)

and 500 mg (evening) for sodium valproate and 50 mg (morning) and 100 mg (evening) for topiramate. Now the seizures attacks 2–3 times a day in a type same as before, sometimes accompanied by hand numbness or amaurosis after the seizure.

3. *Physical examination*: The left upper limb and left facial muscles had atrophy and hypoesthesia in the left limbs.
4. *Imaging examination*. MRI revealed extensive lesions in the right cerebral hemisphere.
5. *EEG*: For details, see Figs. 7.7 and 7.8.

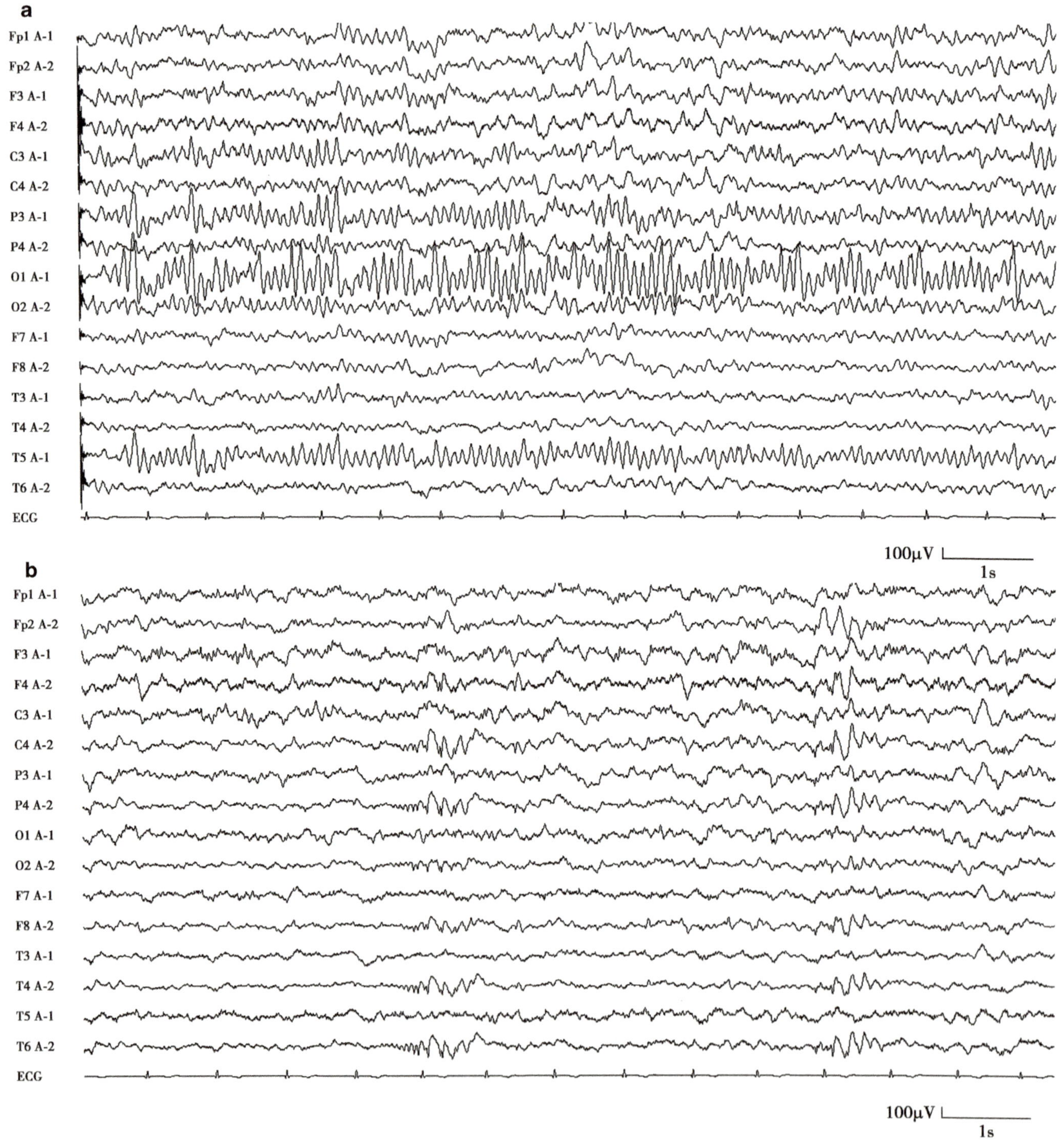

Fig. 7.7 Interictal scalp EEG. (**a**) The EEG basic rhythm was 10.0 Hz, and the left wave amplitude was higher than the right side. (**b**) Spikes and sharp waves over the right hemisphere are seen on the EEG (Fp2, F4, C4, P4, T4, T6). (**c**) Polyspikes over the right hemisphere (F4, C4, P4, T4, T6) are seen on the EEG

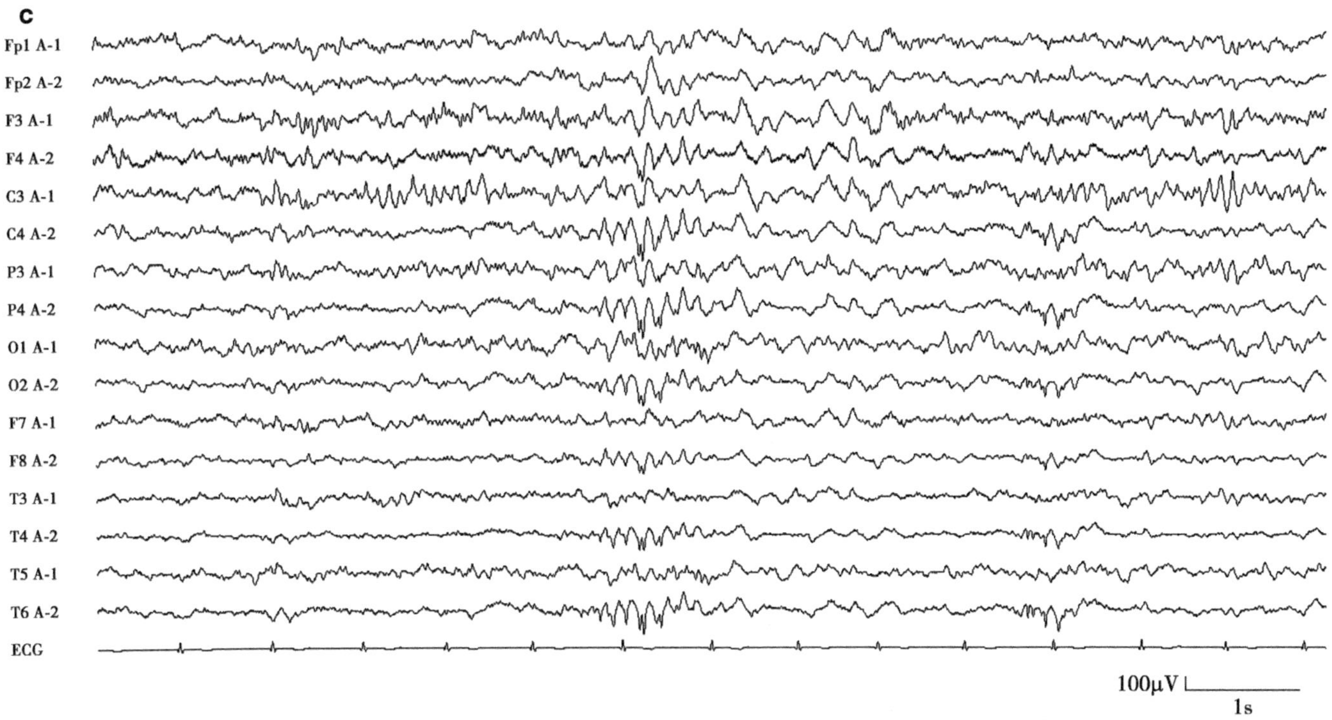

Fig. 7.7 (continued)

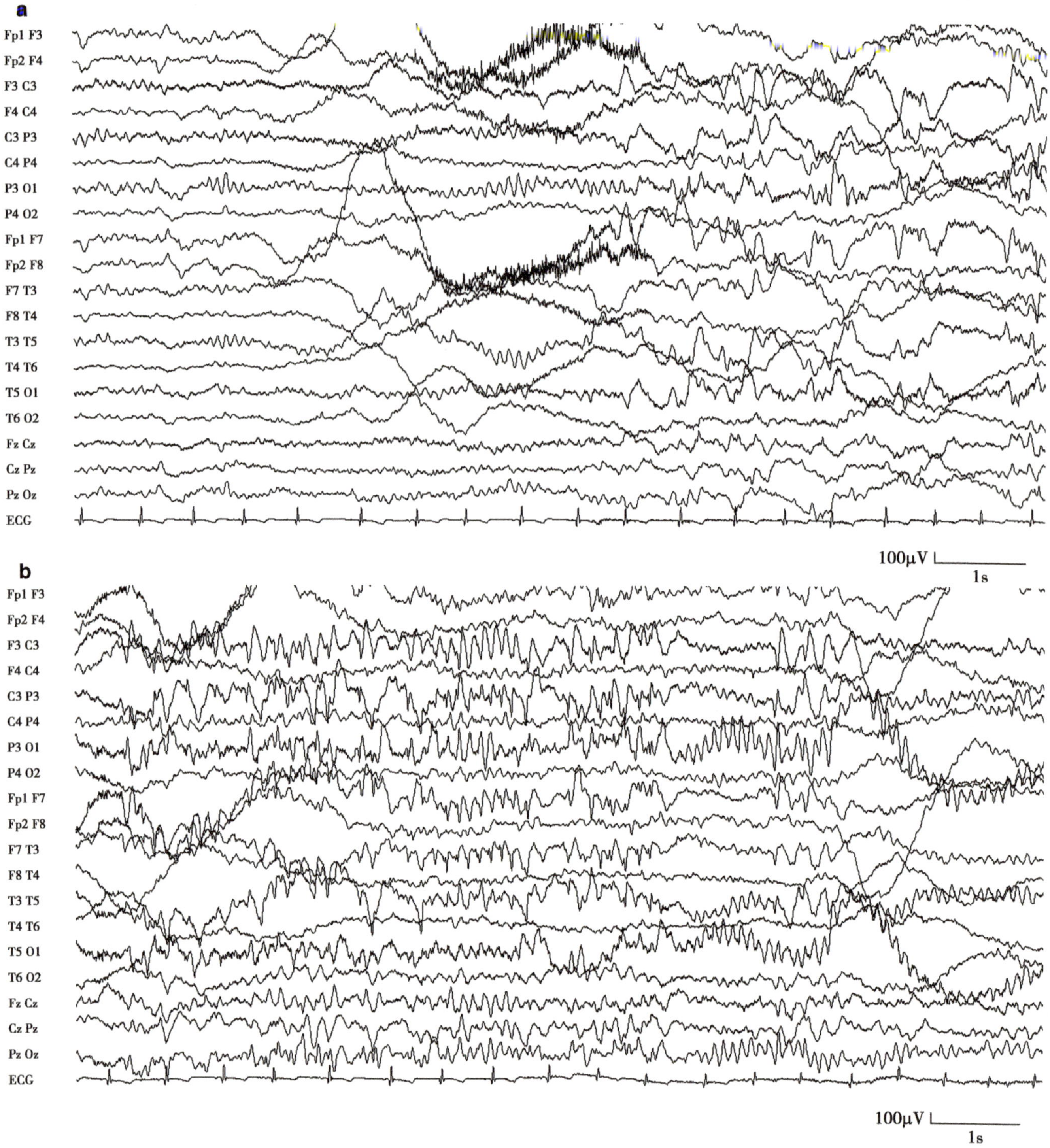

Fig. 7.8 Ictal scalp EEG. (**a**) The patient was in a supine position. EEG showed sharp waves and slow waves over the left side (Fp1, F3, C3, P3, T3, T5), especially over the anterior regions. (**b**) The patient elevated upper limbs followed by left upper limb clonus. The EEG showed the rhythm of sharp waves over the left side. (**c**) The patient had clonus in the left upper limb and tonicity in the left lower limb. The EEG showed the rhythm of sharp waves over the left central region (C3), parietal region (P3), and temporal region (T5), followed by the rhythm of sharpened slow waves over the left central region (C3). (**d**) At the end of clonus, the patient began to cry. The EEG showed EMG artifacts and wobble artifacts and then gradually recovered to the background EEG

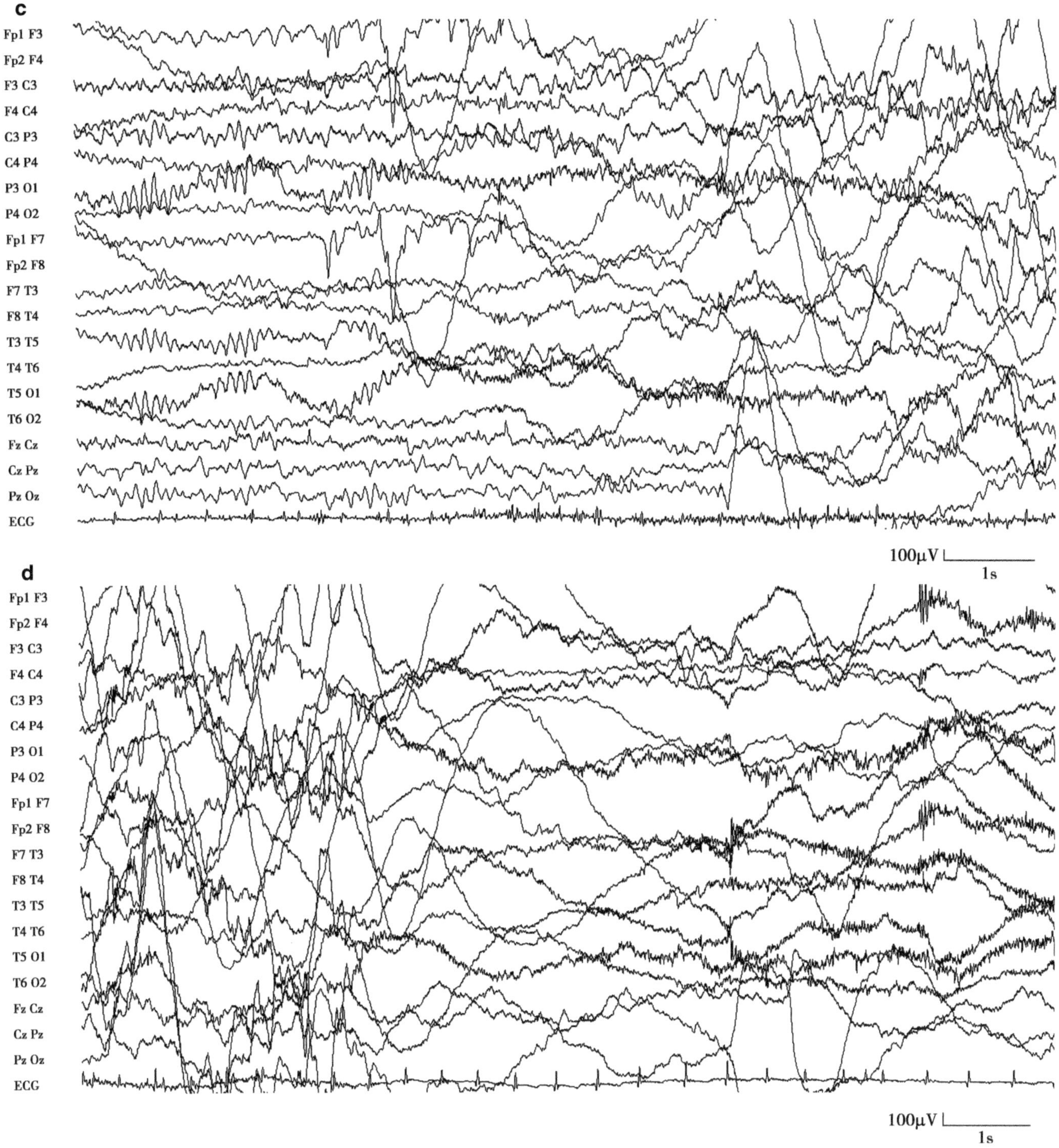

Fig. 7.8 (continued)

[Case Review]

1. *Case Characteristics*
   (a) *Characteristics of medical history*: The patient experienced intracranial hemorrhage 40 days after birth followed by seizures.
   (b) *Seizure characteristics*: The seizure was manifested as body twisting to the left side and tonicity of the left upper limb.
   (c) *Imaging characteristics*: MRI showed extensive lesions in the right cerebral hemisphere.
   (d) *EEG characteristics*: Interictal EEG showed spikes and sharp waves over the right leads.
2. *Diagnosis and treatment strategy and follow-up results*: MRI showed extensive lesions in the right cerebral hemisphere, and the seizure symptoms and abnormal interictal epileptic discharges were consistent with the MRI findings. The lesions in the right cerebral hemisphere were extensive, and the seizures were frequent, accompanied by left limb and facial muscle atrophy, which were difficult to be controlled by medication. It was diagnosed as epilepsy induced by the lesions in the right cerebral hemisphere with clear seizure patterns. A hemispherectomy was performed to the right hemisphere. For patients of this kind, the diagnosis was clear and the epileptic seizures were obviously related to the lesion. Therefore, early surgery should be performed for the benefit of epileptic seizure control, limb function recovery and cognitive function protection. The seizures disappeared during a 2-year follow-up after surgery.

Cases of Epileptic Syndrome

8

Li Liping, Liu Jing, Du Wei, Zhang Xiating, Xu Cuiping, Ni Duanyu, and Sun Ying

Overview of Surgical Treatment of Epileptic Syndrome

Epilepsy is a chronic neurological disorder characterized by recurrent seizures, with multiple clinical causes and complex and diverse seizure symptoms. Epilepsies with the same etiology and similar clinical features are called epileptic syndrome. The diagnosis of epileptic syndrome is based on the age of onset, etiology, and type of seizure. The most common syndromes include West syndrome, Lennox-Gastaut syndrome, and a group of epilepsies with myoclonic seizures. For most epileptic syndromes, a surgical treatment is not considered because of their complex etiology, which is mostly genetic and metabolic. However, a small number of catastrophic epileptic syndromes are symptomatic, for which a surgical treatment may be considered, including epileptic spasms, a group of epilepsies with myoclonic seizures, Rasmussen's encephalitis, Sturge-Weber syndrome, Tuberous sclerosis complex, and Lennox-Gastaut syndrome. With the improvement of localization techniques and the increasing understanding of epilepsy in recent years, some epilepsy syndromes are considered to be focal epilepsy, which could be treated by surgery.

Sturge-Weber Syndrome

Sturge-Weber syndrome, commonly known as encephalofacial angiomatosis, is mainly manifested as a red facial vascular nevus and ipsilateral encephalofacial angiomas mainly located around the orbito-frontal area on one side. The encephalofacial angiomas are mostly located in the pia mater and commonly seen in the parieto-occipital region on one side, accompanied by underlying cortex atrophy and often by calcification. Epileptic seizures, intellectual impairment, and paralysis contralateral to the angioma are often clinically present, sometimes accompanied by glaucoma. Most patients have no abnormalities in the first few months, even years of life and develop febrile convulsions and hemiparesis at 2–3 years old. Epileptic seizures occur in 72% of patients with unilateral facial angioma and 93% of patients with bilateral facial angiomas. The seizure type is usually focal motor seizures, which may be followed by generalized tonic-clonic seizures. Individual children are manifested as infantile spasms, myoclonus, and atonic seizures.

The EEG shows asymmetric background, with localized voltage reduction at the lesion site, dysrhythmias, and discharges of spikes. A few patients show multifocal spikes, high arrhythmias or extensive spike-and-wave complexes, or polyspike and wave complexes, which are often prominent in the occipital region. Resection of the occipital region can control the seizures in some patients. A hemispherectomy may be performed at early stage for severe children younger than 1 year old with extensive lesions.

Tuberous Sclerosis Complex

Tuberous sclerosis complex (TSC) is an autosomal dominant genetic disorder that can involve multiple organs of the body. Its main clinical manifestations include epileptic seizures, mental retardation, and skin damage. 80–90% of patients with TSC have seizures, among which 67% have seizures at 1 year old or younger and 80% have seizures at 3 years old or younger. In addition, about 12% of patients have an onset of epileptic seizures in adulthood, suggesting that patients with TSC are at high risk for seizures throughout their lives. In most patients, their EEGs show abnormalities, such as diffuse slow waves, focal spikes, or multifocal spikes. Infantile spasms may occur in 20–30% of patients in infancy, but 70% of patients do not have a highly dysrhythmic EEG. In 95% of patients with TSC, MRI shows multiple nodules. In some

L. Liping · L. Jing · Z. Xiating · S. Ying (✉)
Department of Neurology, Beijing, China
e-mail: Sunying@xwhosp.org

D. Wei · X. Cuiping · N. Duanyu
Department of Neurosurgery, Beijing, China

Y. Wang (ed.), *Electroencephalogram for Presurgical Epilepsy Evaluation*, https://doi.org/10.1007/978-981-95-8003-3_8

patients, the site of cortical nodules on MRI is consistent with the ictal EEG characteristics, but in some other patients, the information is inconsistent. The key to successful surgery is to identify the epileptogenic nodules. Often, cortical nodules in the parietal or occipital lobe may be closely associated with infantile convulsive seizures.

Lennox-Gastaut Syndrome

The onset of Lennox-Gastaut syndrome reaches the peak at the ages between 3 and 5 years old. The main clinical manifestations are various patterns of seizures and mental retardation. The most common types of seizures are tonic seizures, atypical absence seizure, and myoclonus and atonic seizures. Among them, tonic seizures are the most characteristic one of LGS, with a 92% occurrence rate. The interictal EEG showed slow sharp-and-wave complexes slower than 2.5 Hz, and the bursts of rhythm of spikes can be seen during sleep; the EEG during the tonic seizures showed the low amplitude fast activities or spikes. The effect of drug treatment is poor.

Cases Receiving Surgical Treatment of Epileptic Syndrome

Case 8.1 Sturge-Weber Syndrome

[Abstract of Medical Records]
Female, 25 years old.

1. *Chief complaint*: Paroxysmal convulsion for 24 years.
2. *History of present illness*: The patient had febrile convulsions 24 years ago (at 4 months old), manifested as head and eyes turning to the left, left limb flexion and convulsions, and subsequent left tonicity and loss of awareness. Each seizure lasted 1–2 min. The patient began to have seizures mostly during sleep 5 years ago, with tonicity of the left hand and vocalization in the throat, followed by tonicity of the limbs and loss of awareness. After a few minutes, the patient started to fumble for the covers. At the end of the seizure, the left limbs were paralyzed for a few minutes. Before the seizure, the patient's eyes saw a flash or amaurosis and felt blurred (especially in the left visual field). The patient fell asleep after the seizure, which often occurred in the daytime. The patient had been treated with carbamazepine, phenytoin sodium, phenobarbital, and sodium valproate, with poor effects. The patient had a right facial angioma since birth.
3. *History of growth and development*: The patient was born at term with a right facial angioma. After treatment with coagulant injections 15 years ago, the patient had a reduced vision in the right eye and is now blind. The patient received prefrontal dermatoplasty on the right side 2 years ago.
4. *Physical examination*: The right eye was blind, and the left eye had a visual acuity of 0.12. Visual field examination showed a large number of dark spots in the center and periphery of the left eye. The muscle strength of the left upper limb was slightly poor, and the left side showed pathological reflex (positive).
5. Imaging examination:
   (a) CT revealed calcified foci in the right temporal and occipital lobes.
   (b) MRI revealed diffuse atrophy of the right cerebral hemisphere.
6. *EEG*: For details, see Figs. 8.1, 8.2, and 8.3.

[Case Review]

1. Case Characteristics
   (a) The patient had seizures since her childhood and the seizures exacerbated in the last 5 years. She took various medications with unfavorable results.
   (b) The angioma located over the right face.
   (c) The CT revealed calcified foci in the right temporal and occipital lobes. The MRI revealed diffuse atrophy of the right hemisphere.
   (d) The interictal EEG showed slow waves, sharp-and-wave complexes over the right hemisphere, especially over the right parietal and posterior temporal regions.
   (e) The symptoms included head turning to the left, looking to the left, and late-stage left corner of mouth twitching with the left upper limb clonus.
2. Diagnosis and treatment strategy and follow-up results. The clinical symptoms, the interictal and ictal EEG, the CT and the MRI revealed consistent abnormalities. One stage resection is the best treatment. She underwent right functional hemisphere resection. She was seizure free after 2 years of postoperative follow-up.

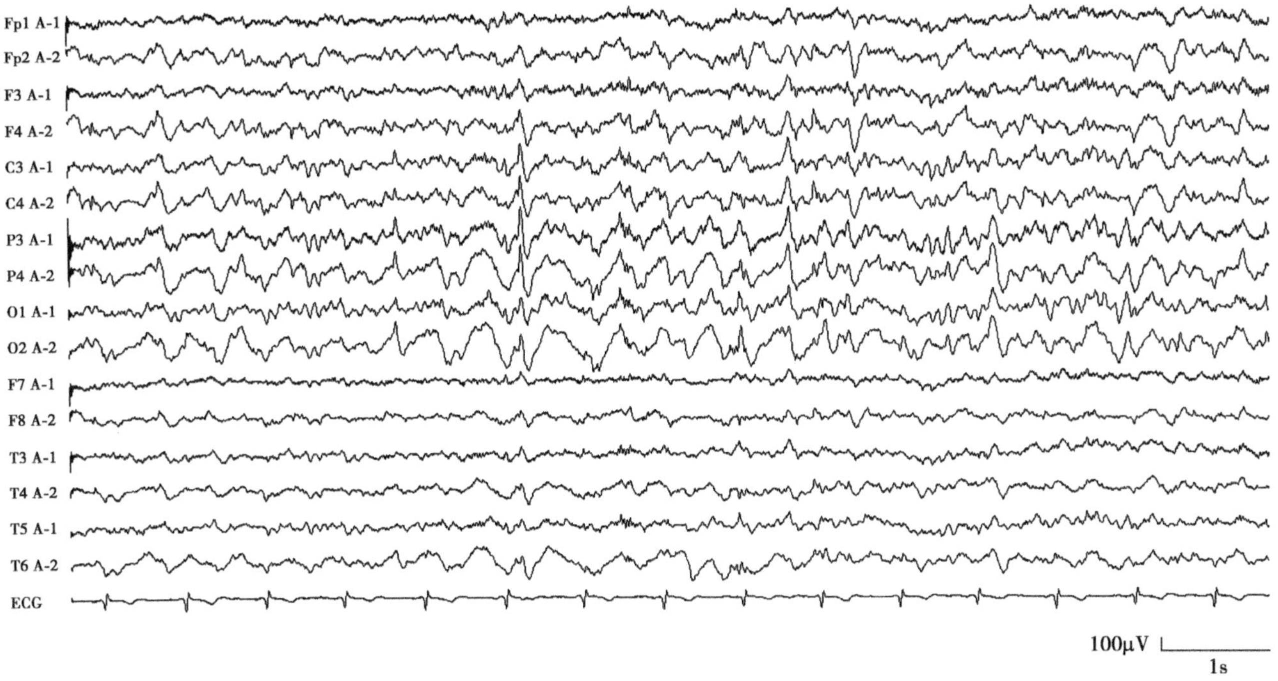

Fig. 8.1 Interictal scalp EEG. The basic rhythm is 10 Hz. The EEG showed spikes, spike-and-wave complexes over the bilateral central (C3, C4), parietal (P3, P4) and right occipital (O2) regions. The rhythm of medium- and high-amplitude 2–3 Hz slow activities occurred over the right posterior temporal (T6), parietal (P4), and occipital (O2) regions

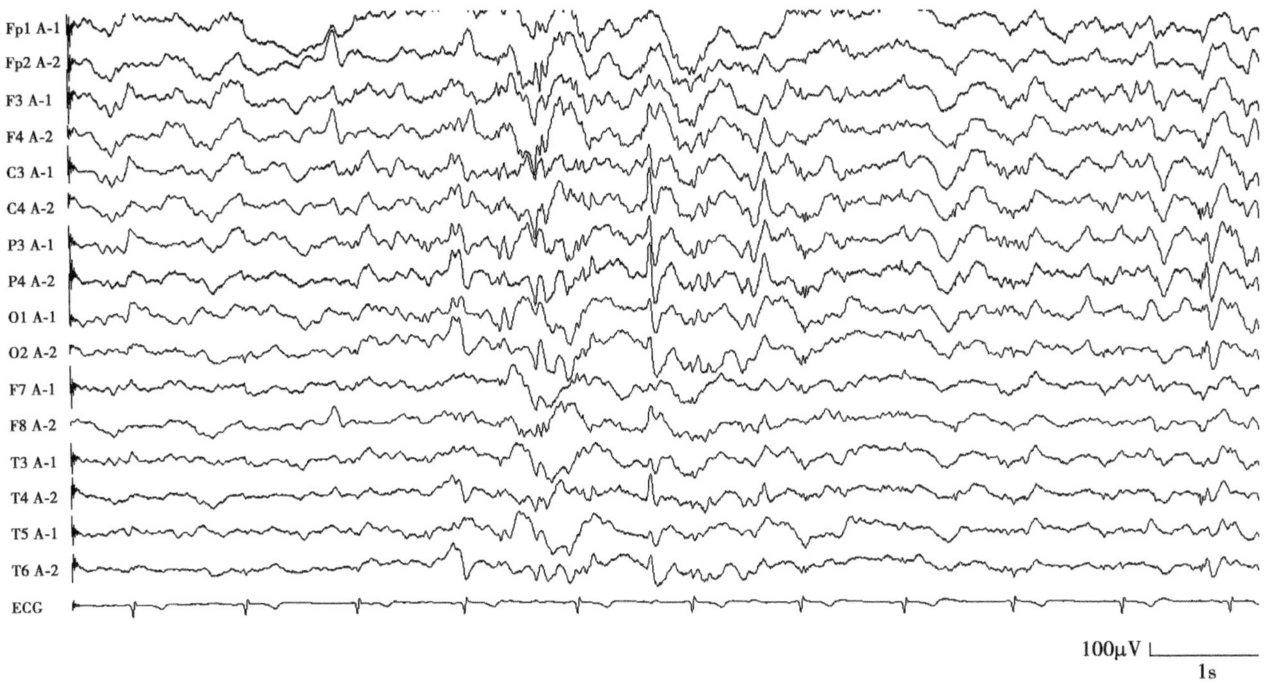

Fig. 8.2 Interictal scalp EEG. The background EEG of stage II showed symmetrical bilateral spindle waves. The spike-and-wave complexes can be seen over the right hemisphere (Fp2, F4, C4, P4, O2, F8, T4, T6), especially the central (C4), parietal (P4), and the posterior temporal (T4, T6) regions

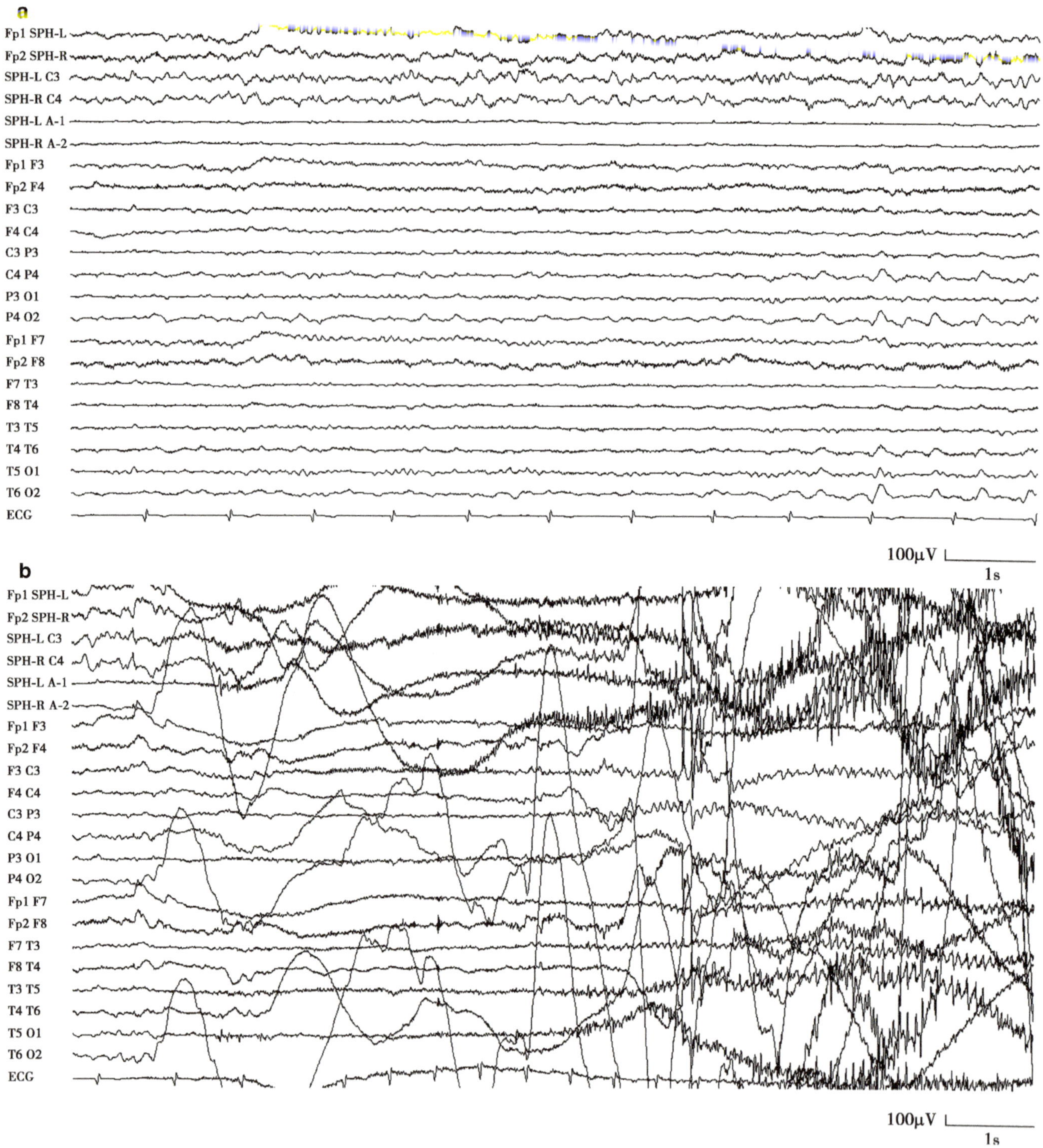

Fig. 8.3 Ictal scalp EEG. (**a**) Before the seizure, the patient was sleeping in the position of right lateral decubitus. The EEG showed α activity dissociation, and 2.0–3.0 Hz slow waves can be seen over the right parietal (C4 P4, P4 O2) and posterior temporal (T4 T6, T6 O2) regions 3 s before the seizure. (**b**) During the seizure, the patient suddenly opened the eyes and gazed the left side with the left upper limb tonic jerks and the body turning to the left, accompanied by the loss of consciousness. The amplitude of the EEG was low for about 6 s, followed by 8.0–9.0 Hz activities over the left central and parietal regions, accompanied by bilateral frontotemporal EMG artifacts. The wobble artifacts can be seen over the right occipital region. (**c**) The patient's mouth was tilted to the left. The right upper limb was flexed in front of the chest, and the left upper limb was tonic. EMG artifacts were seen over the EEG. (**d**) The body slowly turned to the right with the right upper limb extending and the limbs tonic-clonic. Mixed EMG artifacts were seen over the EEG. (**e**) The patient had tonic-clonus. Mixed EMG artifacts were seen over the EEG. (**f**) The patient had tonic-clonus. Mixed EMG artifacts were seen over the EEG. (**g**) The patient had tonic-clonus. Mixed EMG artifacts were seen over the EEG. (**h–m**) The patient's limbs gradually relaxed and clonus slowly resolved. The patient was heavily wheezing and salivating. The EEG showed a rhythmic 4 Hz spike-and-wave complexes over the bilateral hemispheres with the left slightly higher wave amplitude than the right. (**n, o**) At the end of the seizure, the patient was still unconscious. The EEG showed an amplitude decrease over all channels, manifested as irregular 2–4 Hz slow waves

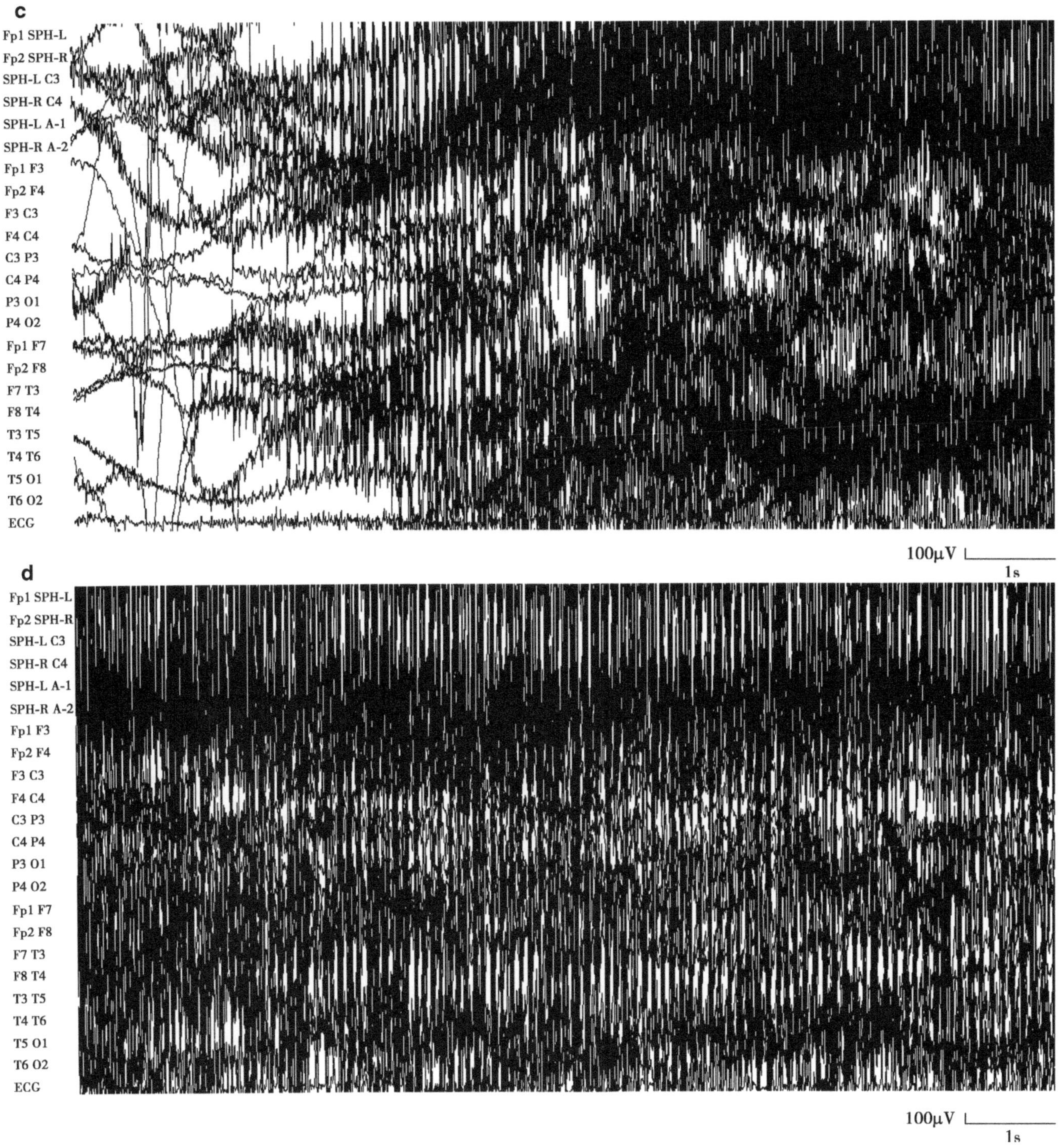

Fig. 8.3 (continued)

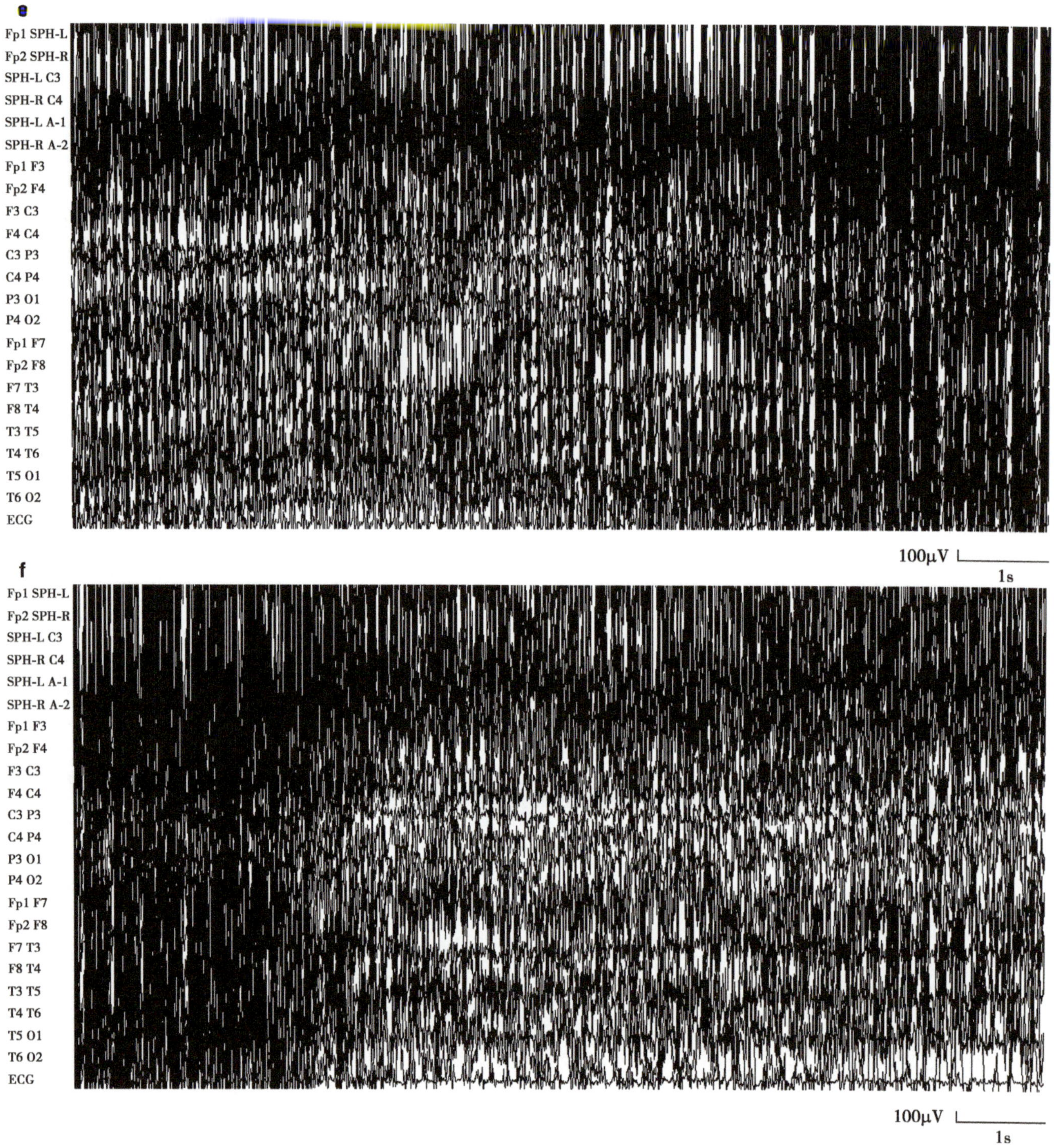

Fig. 8.3 (continued)

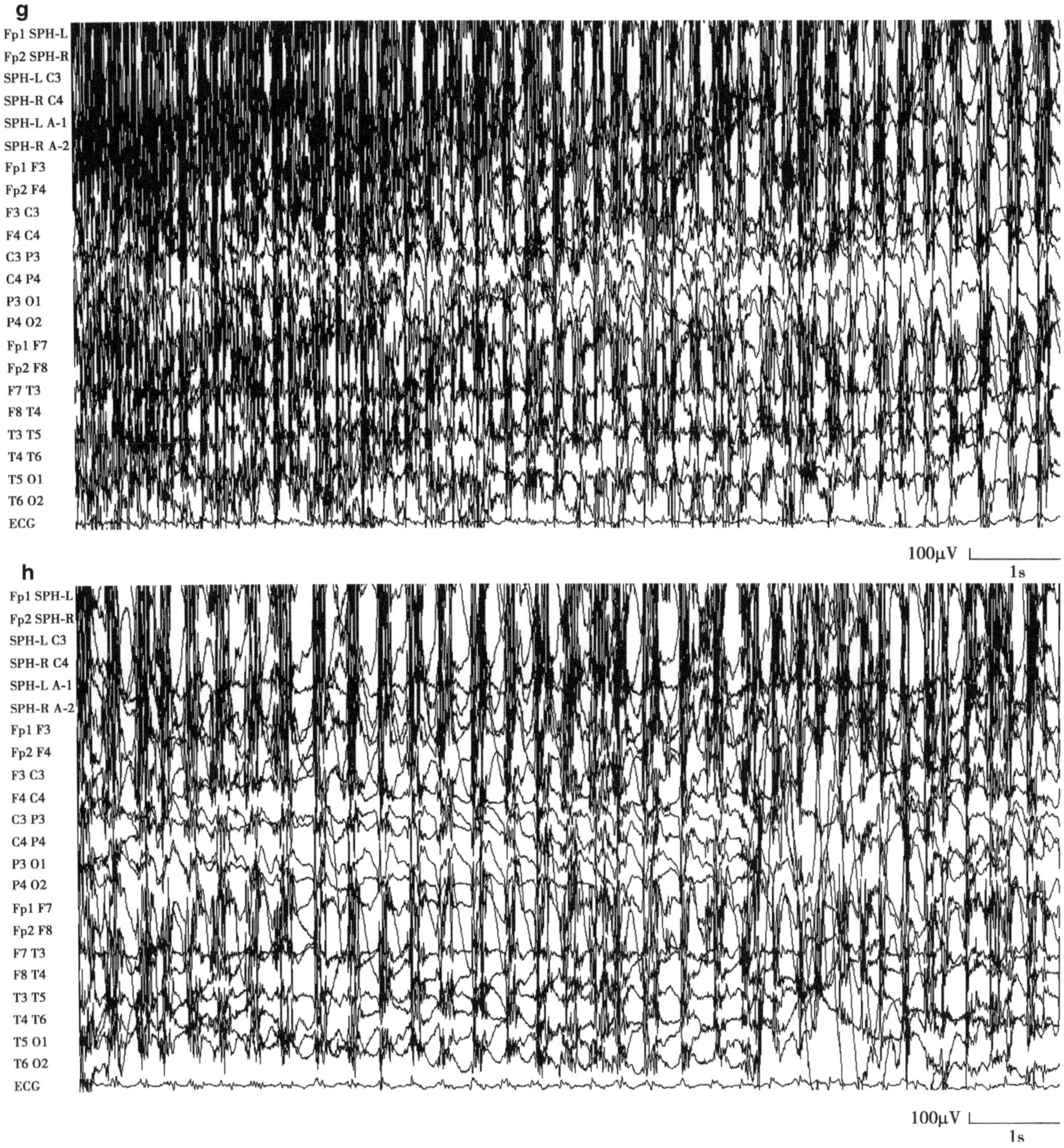

Fig. 8.3 (continued)

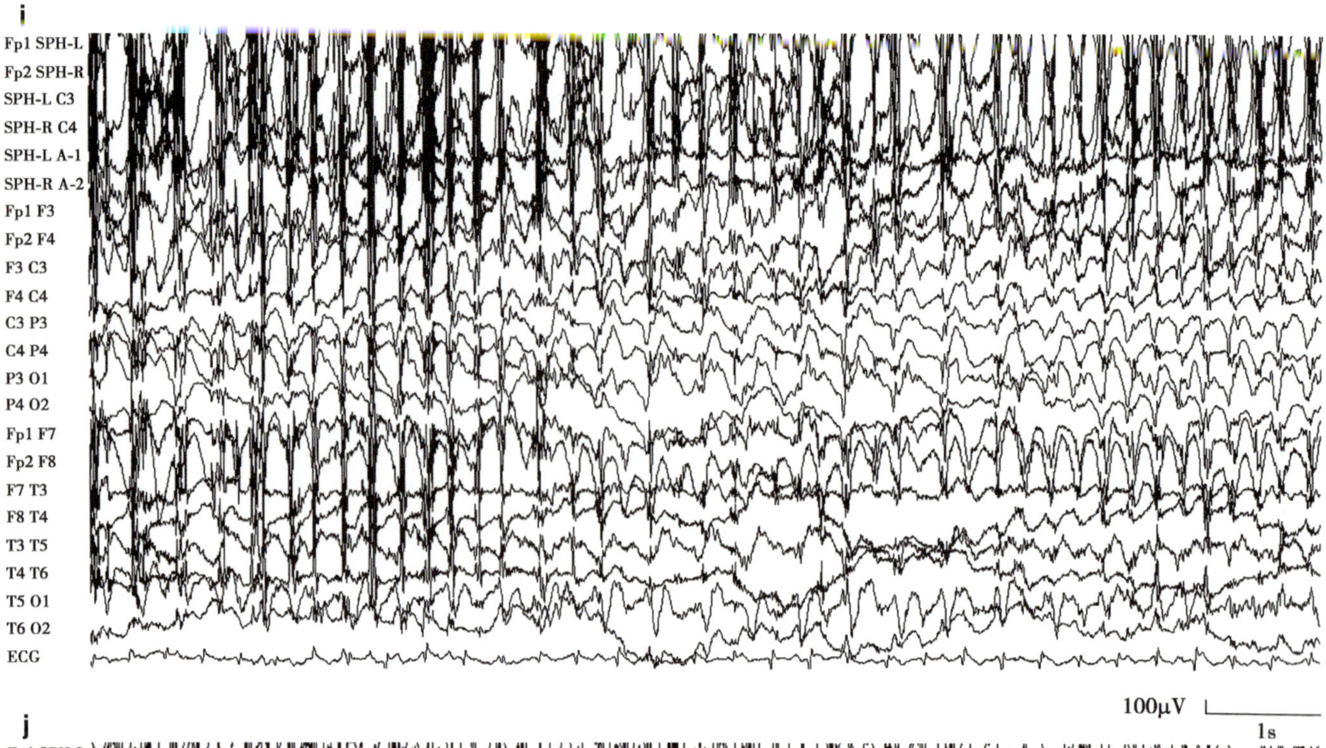

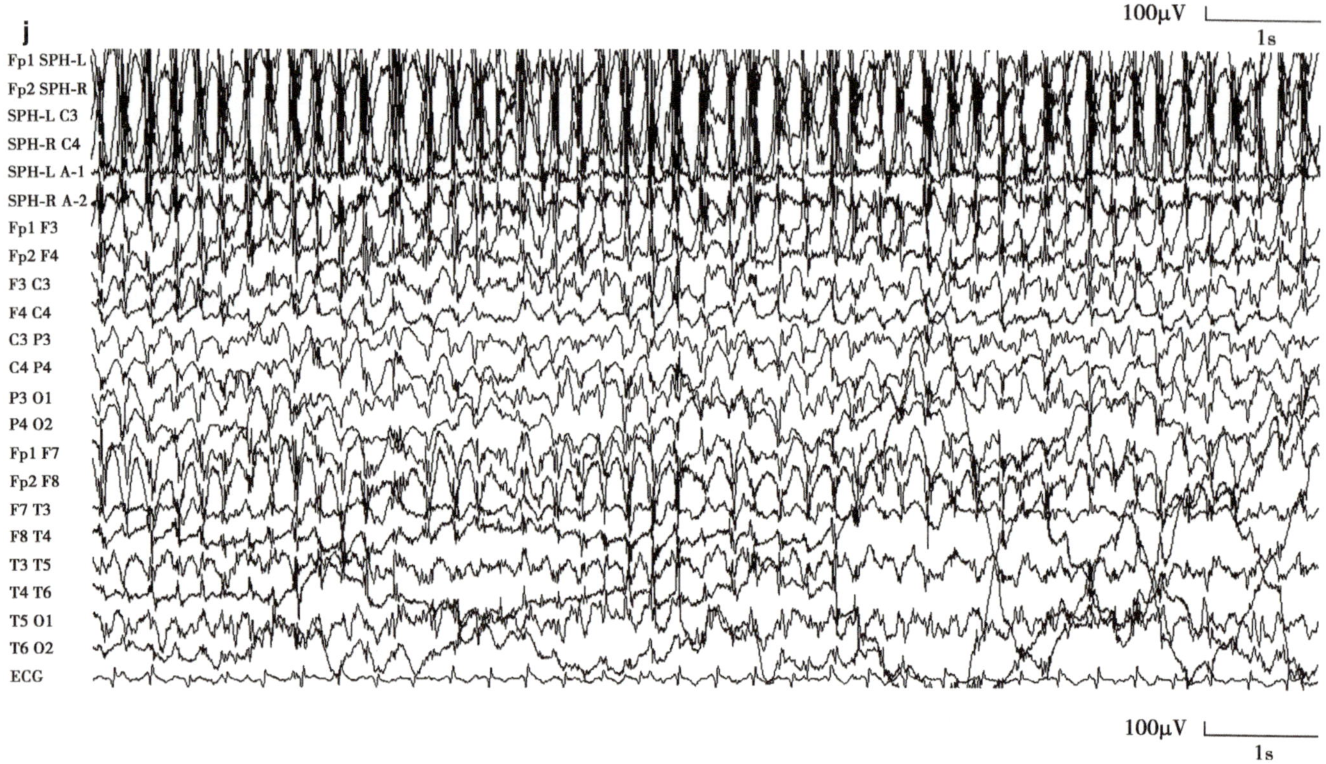

Fig. 8.3 (continued)

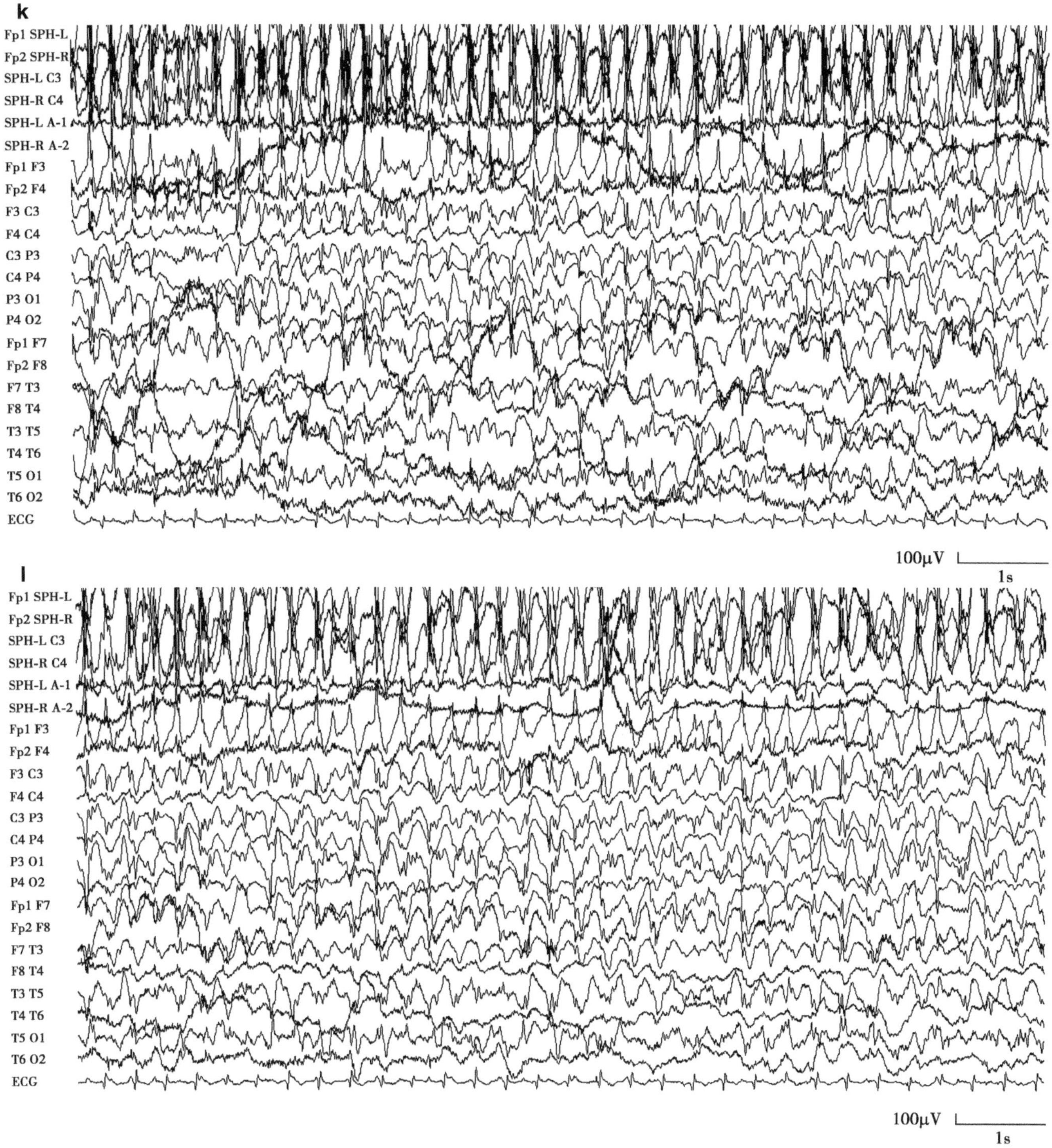

Fig. 8.3 (continued)

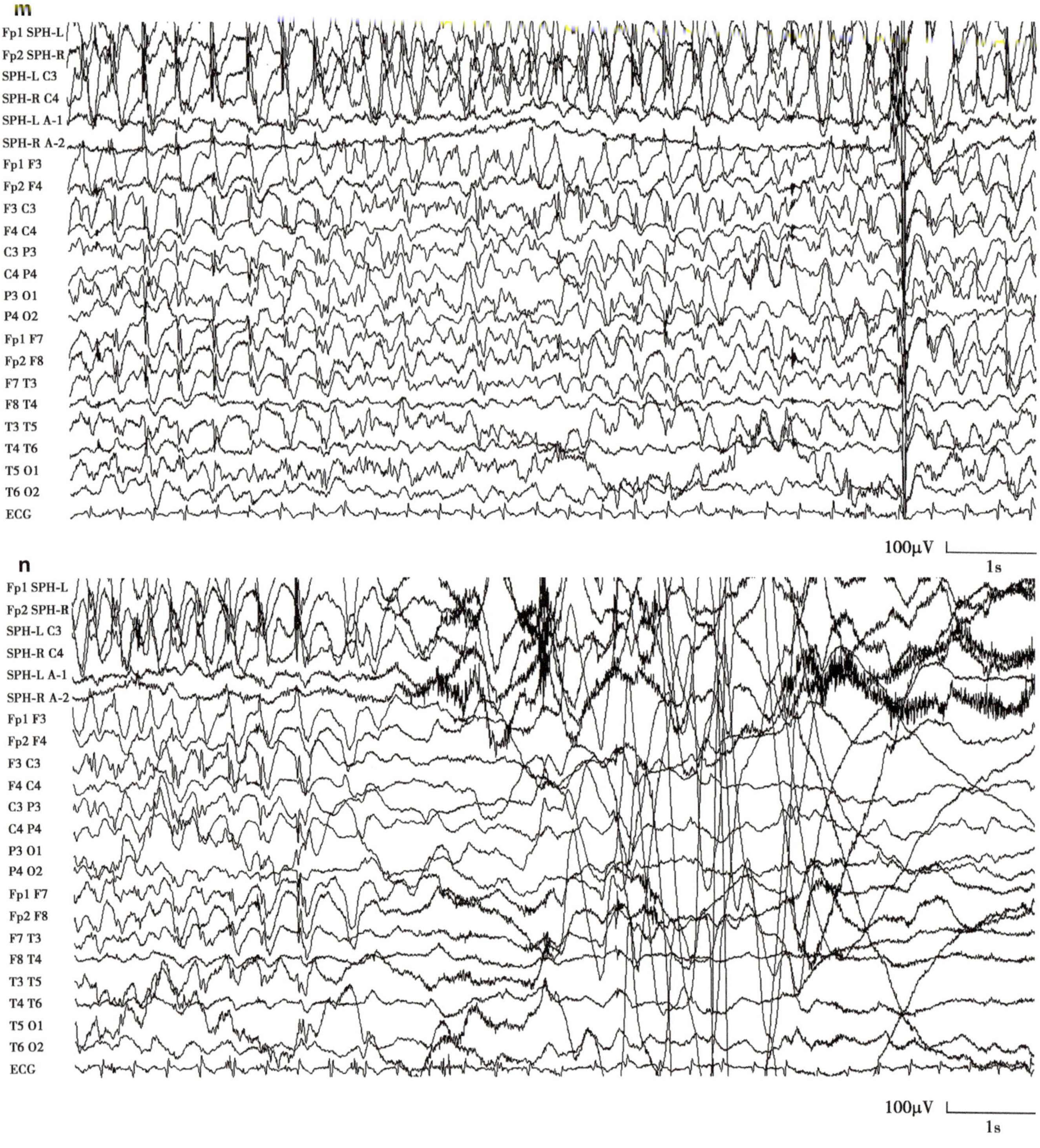

Fig. 8.3 (continued)

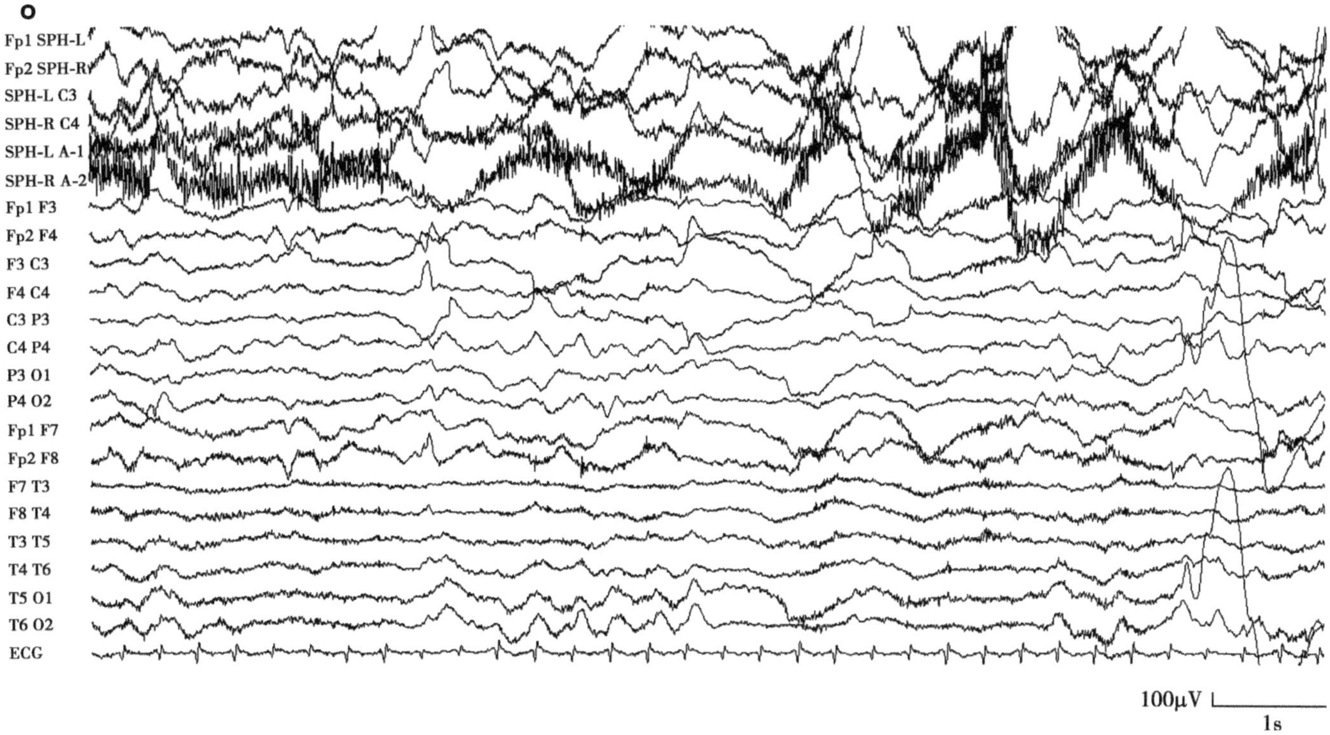

Fig. 8.3 (continued)

Case 8.2 Sturge-Weber Syndrome

[*Abstract of Medical Records*]
Female, 14 years old.

1. *Chief complaint*: The patient had paroxysmal loss of consciousness for 5 months and paroxysmal limbs clonus for 2 months.
2. *History of present illness*: Five months ago, the patient suddenly screamed in sleep and then loss of consciousness with her eyes looking to the left, head turning to the left, and mouth corners tilting to the left, which lasted for about 10 min before resolution. Four months ago, she suddenly had a hallucination, followed by head and eyes turning to the left and limb weakness during a class, which resolved after 4–5 min. One month ago, she suddenly developed confusion, followed by loss of consciousness and head and eyes turning to the left, which resolved after about 1 min. The frequency was once a month. The CT suggested calcified foci over the right prefrontal lobe.
3. *Physical examination*: Right facial angioma. No neurological abnormalities were found
4. Imaging Examination:
   (a) The MRI showed abnormal signals in the right frontal cortex.
   (b) The CT suggested calcification in the right frontal lobe.
5. *EEG*: See Figs. 8.4, 8.5, and 8.6 for details.

[*Case Review*]

1. Case Characteristics
   (a) The patient had a short course with frequent focal seizures. The symptoms included head turning to the left, the corners of the mouth tilting to the left, and the eyes constantly turning to the left and the upwards.
   (b) She had right facial angioma.
   (c) The CT and MRI both showed focus in the right frontal cortex.
   (d) The interictal EEG showed slow waves and sharp waves predominantly in the bilateral frontal regions, which sometimes extended to all leads. The ictal EEG showed the rhythmic slow waves and spike-and-wave complexes over the bilateral frontal regions.
2. *Diagnosis and Treatment Strategy and Follow-up Results*: The seizure symptoms were consistent with the EEG features and the localization revealed by the MRI. She underwent right frontal epileptic focus resection. The seizures disappeared after 1 year of postoperative follow-up. The structural abnormality is the most important factor in the localization of the epileptogenic focus.

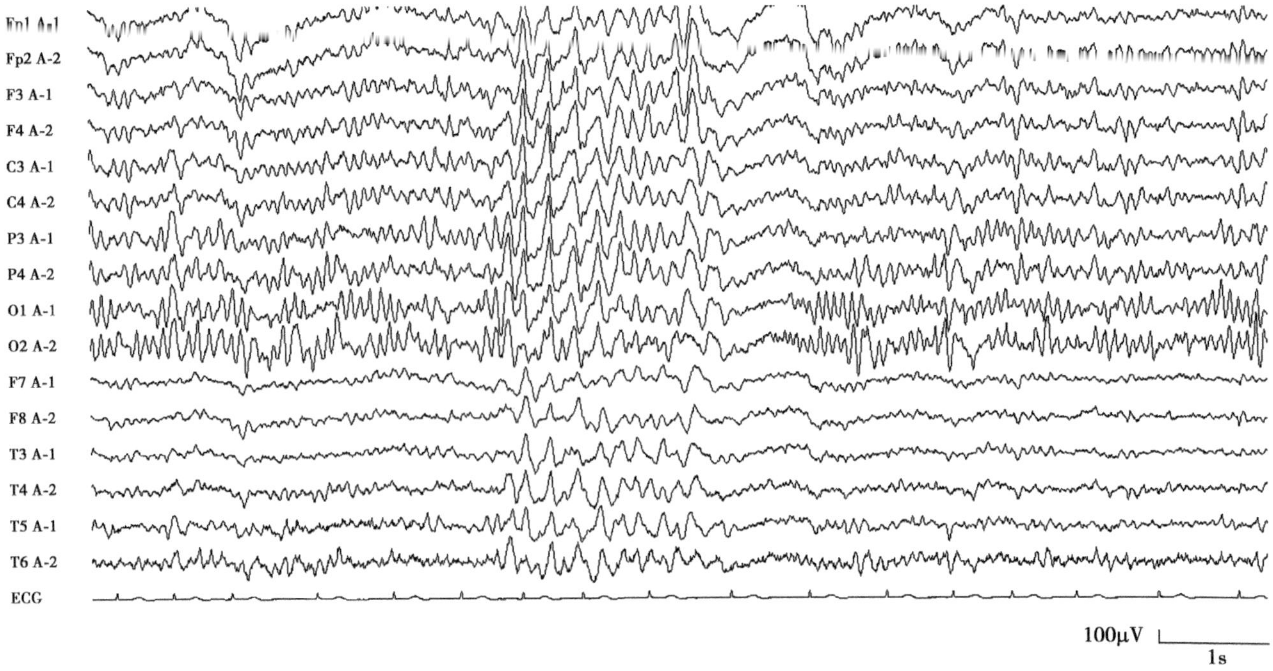

Fig. 8.4 Interictal scalp EEG 1. The basic rhythm was 9–10 Hz. Paroxysmal high-amplitude sharpened slow wave rhythm was seen over the bilateral hemisphere

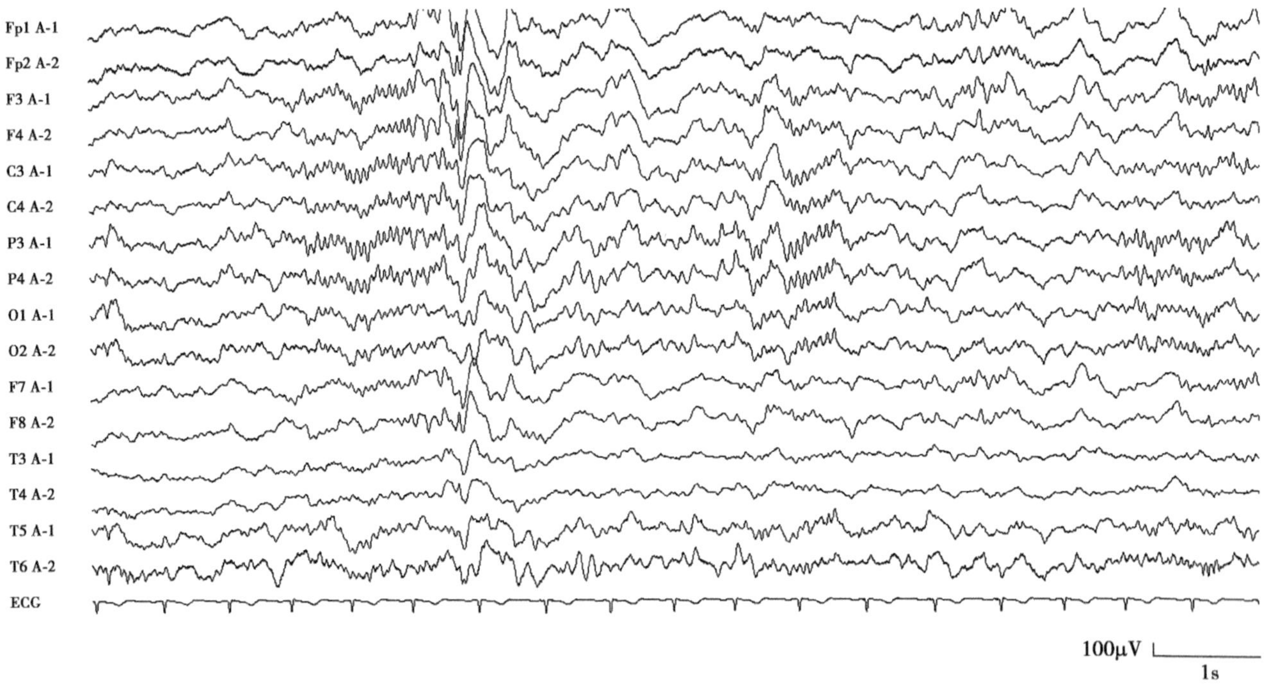

Fig. 8.5 Interictal scalp EEG 2. The stage II sleep EEG showed symmetrical bilateral spindle activity. The spike-and-wave complexes were seen over the right frontal region and anterior temporal region

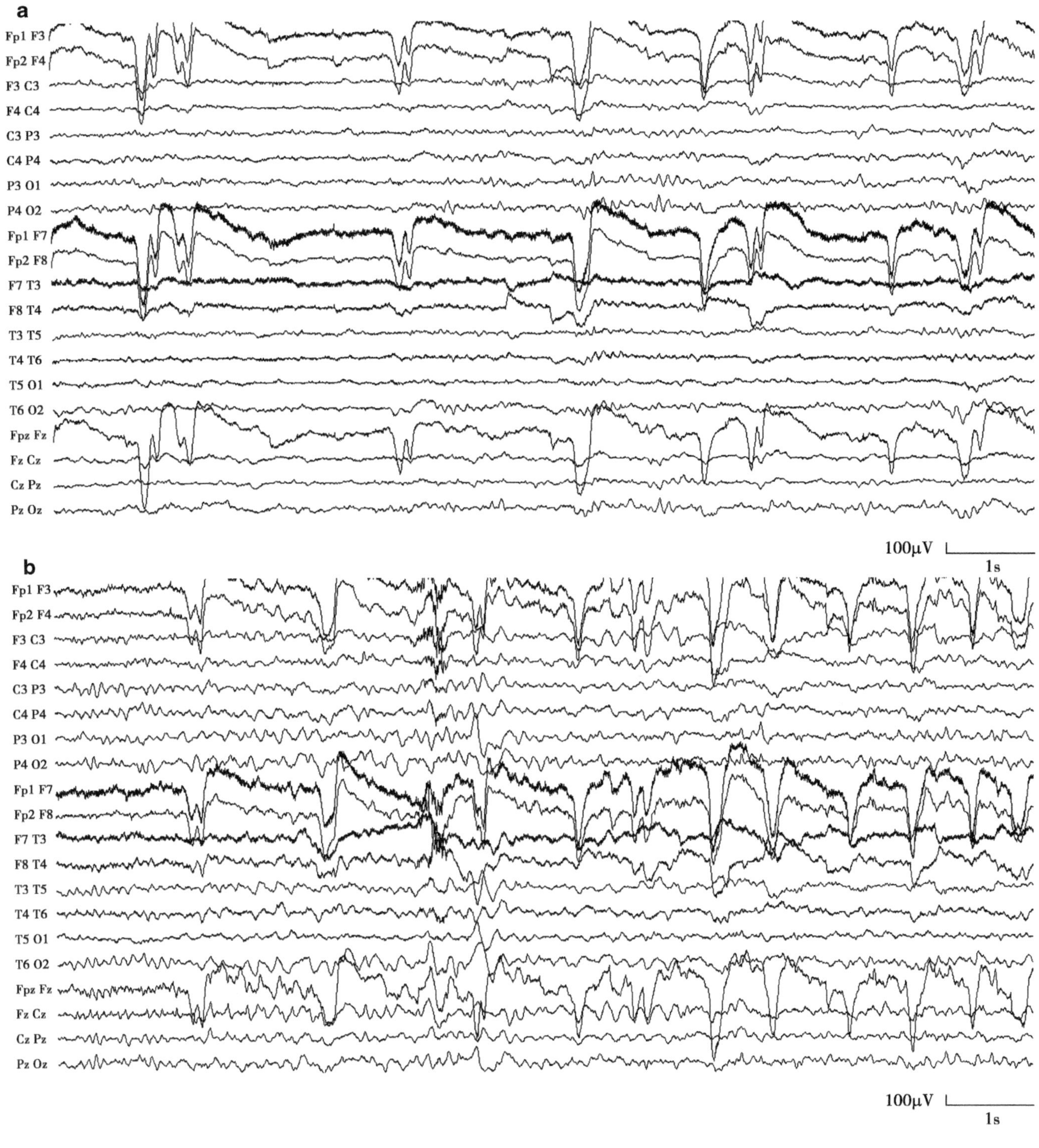

Fig. 8.6 Ictal scalp EEG. (**a**) Prior to the seizure, the patient was in supine position. The EEG showed α activity suppression and more oculomotor artifacts over the frontal pole region. (**b**) During the seizure, the patient's eyes frequently turned to the upper left and upper right, accompanied by rapid eyelid blinking. The EEG showed 5–6 Hz low amplitude slow waves over the bilateral occipital and temporal regions and plenty of oculomotor artifacts over the bilateral frontal pole regions. (**c**) The patient did not respond to questions and rapidly blinked the eyelids. The EEG showed a gradual increase of slow wave amplitude bilaterally, with the higher wave amplitude in right hemisphere. The 3.5–4.0 Hz high-amplitude slow wave rhythms or spike-and-wave complexes were seen over the bilateral frontal pole regions. (**d**) The clinical symptoms and the EEG presentation were same as **c**. (**e**) At the end of the seizure, the patient recovered consciousness. The EEG recovered to the awake background EEG

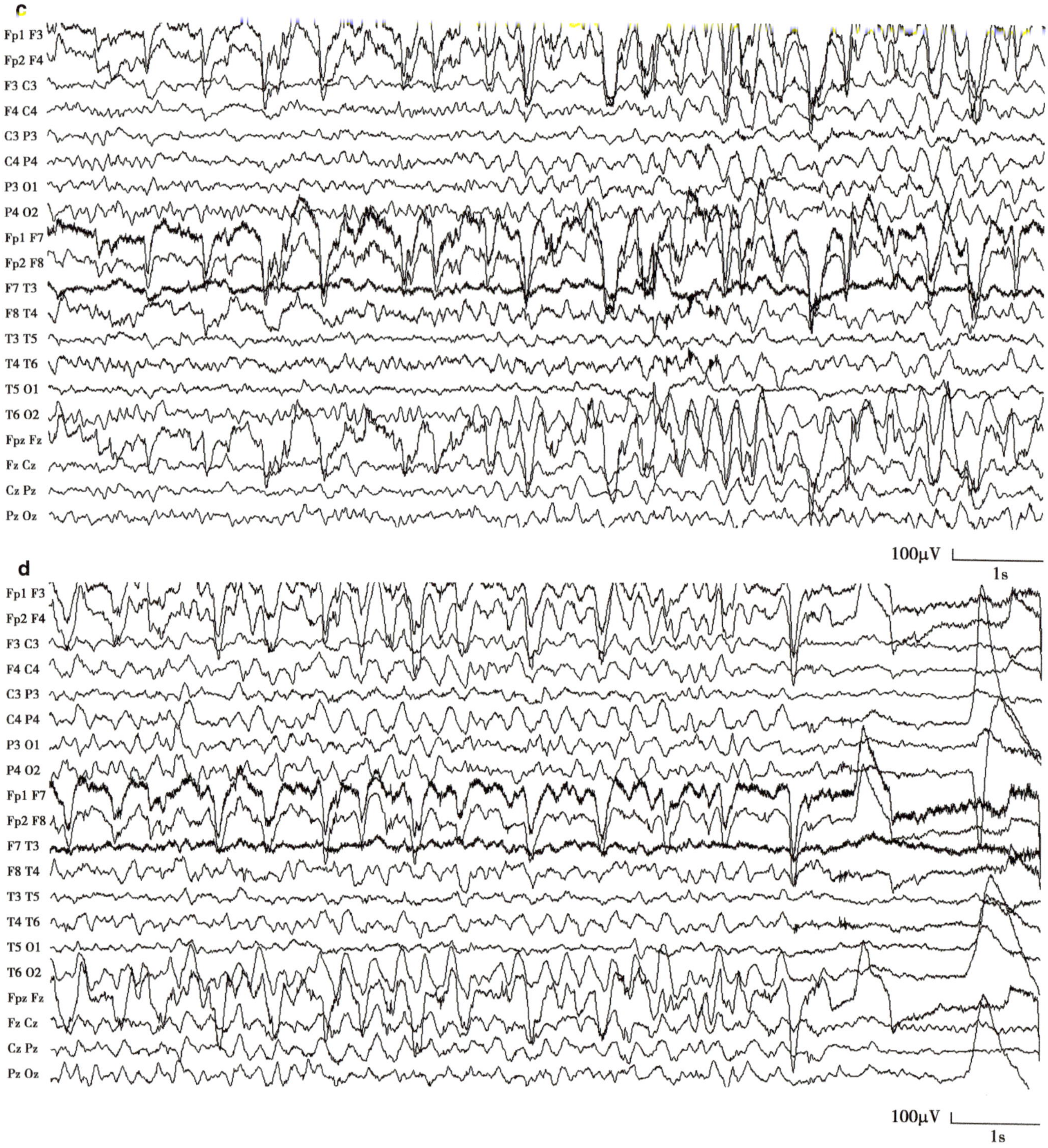

Fig. 8.6 (continued)

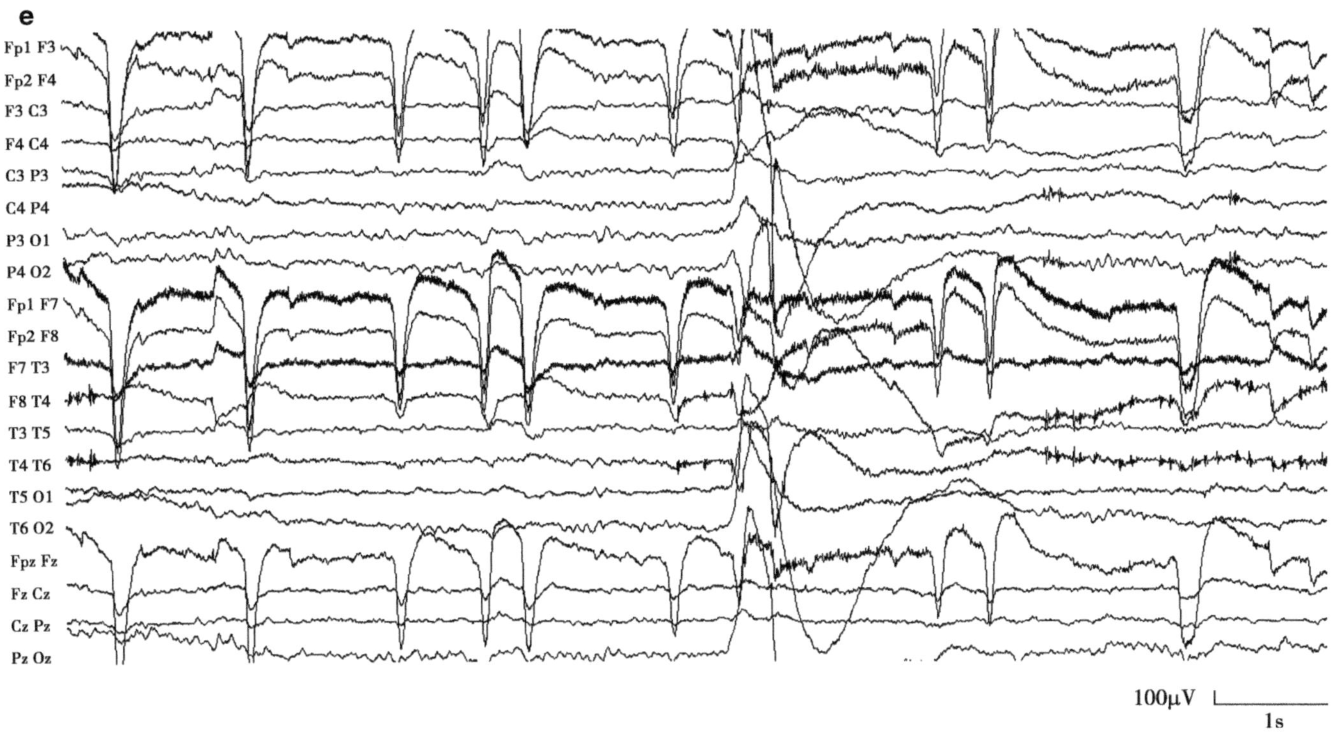

Fig. 8.6 (continued)

Case 8.3 Tuberous Sclerosis Complex

[*Abstract of Medical Records*]
The patient was male and 15 years old.

1. *Chief complaint*: Recurrent episodes of unconsciousness with limbs clonus for 10 years.
2. *History of present illness*: The patient had episodic loss of consciousness with limbs clonus 10 years ago. The seizures were recurrent, stereotypical, and mostly occurred during sleep. In the past 4 years, the patient experienced an aura of numbness in the right hand followed by limbs clonus 4–7 times a day. Currently, the seizures mostly manifested as numbness spreading from right hand to right upper arm followed by right hand clonus, with clear consciousness, which lasted for 1–2 min. The patient received sodium valproate, 800 mg/d and clonazepam, 1 mg per night.
3. *Physical examination*: The patient was conscious but not articulate and experienced right hand hypoactivity and reduced sensation in the right hand. He was left-handed and had a Grade 5 muscle strength in the right hand and Grade 5 muscle strength for other limbs, showing unstable and inaccurate movement in finger-nose-test in the right hand. The patient showed negative pathological signs and right eye poor visual acuity.
4. *Neuropsychological examination*: VIQ < 43, PIQ = 45, FIQ = 37, moderate dysgnosia and mental retardation.
5. *Imaging Examination*:
   (a) The CT revealed calcified foci in the left parietal lobe.
   (b) The MRI revealed multiple small patchy abnormal signals at the edges of the ventricles bilaterally and abnormal signals in the left parietal and temporal cortical regions.
   (c) SPECT suggested poor perfusion of the whole cerebral cortex with multiple areas of hypoperfusion.
6. *EEG*: See Figs. 8.7, 8.8, 8.9, 8.10, 8.11, and 8.12 for details.

[*Case Review*]

1. Case Characteristics
   (a) Characteristics of medical history: He had epileptic seizure for about 10 years.
   (b) EEG characteristics: The interictal EEG showed spike-and-wave complexes and slow waves over the left central, parietal, occipital, and posterior temporal regions.
   (c) Seizure characteristics: The aura was numbness in the right hand, and the seizure symptom was right upper limb clonus. The EEG recorded the slow wave rhythm over the left central, parietal, and posterior temporal regions.

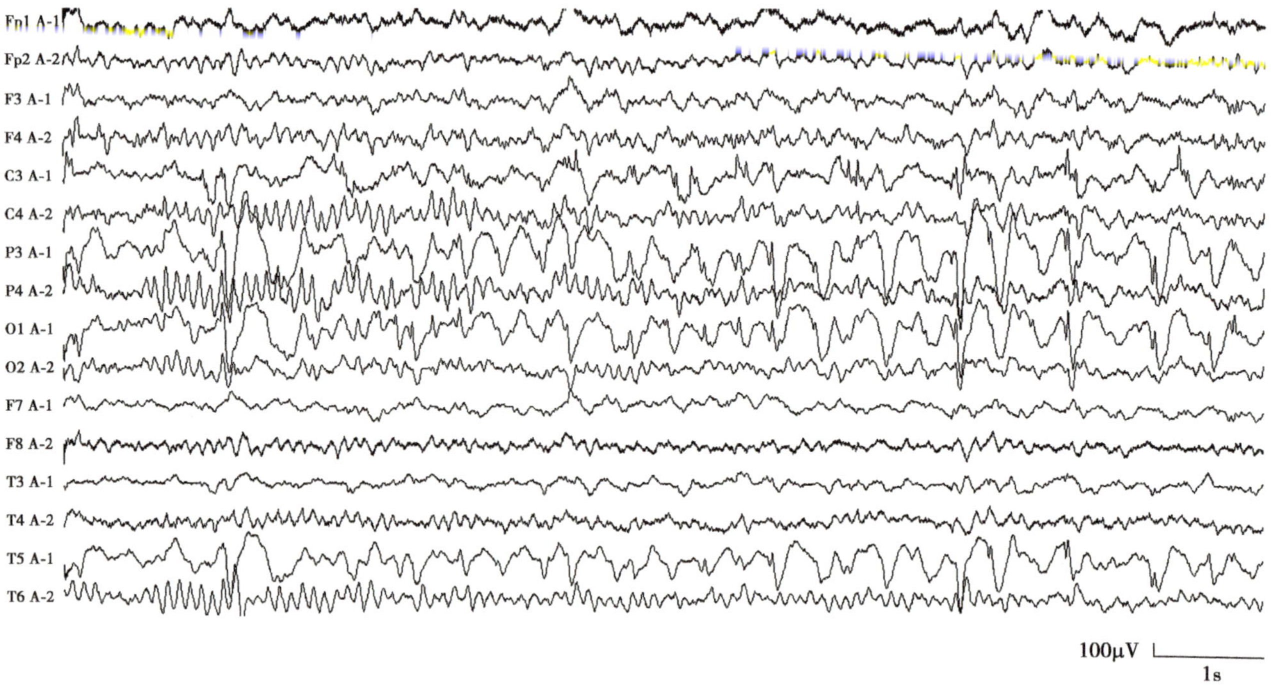

Fig. 8.7 Interictal scalp EEG 1. The basic rhythm was 8–9 Hz. Spike-and-wave complexes and slow waves can be seen over the left central, parietal, occipital, and posterior temporal regions

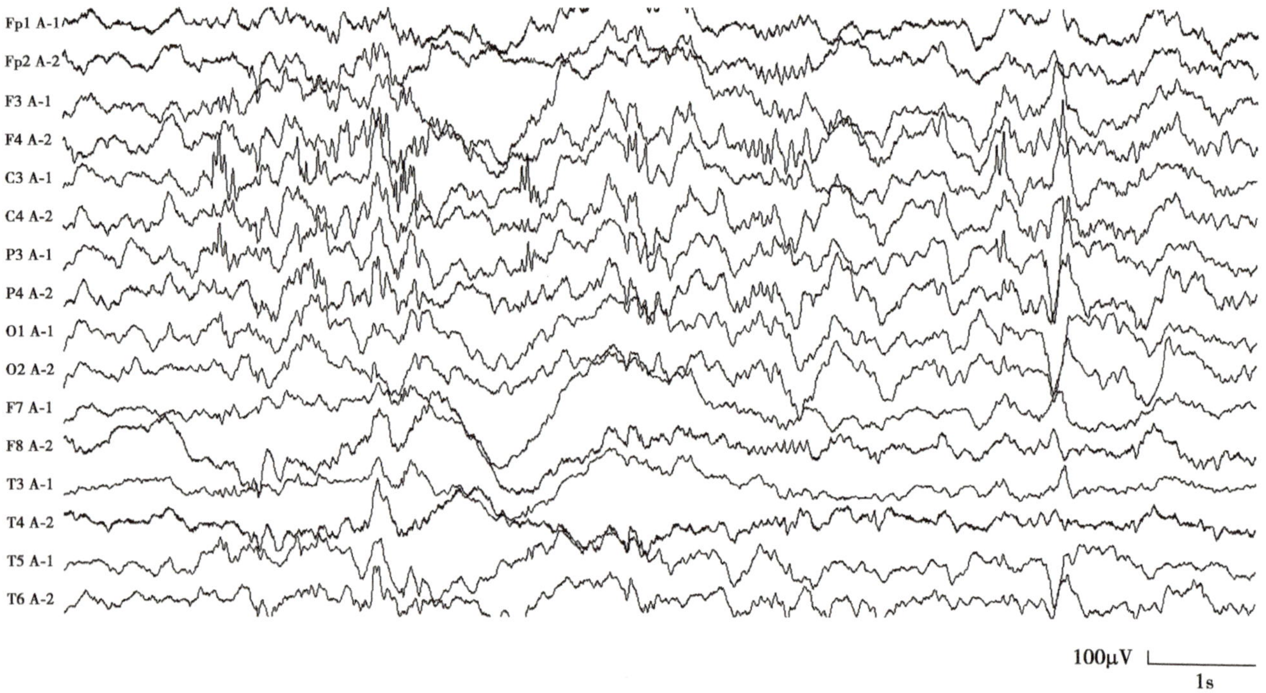

Fig. 8.8 Interictal scalp EEG 2. The EEG of stage II of sleep showed the spikes and spike-and-wave complexes over the left central and parietal regions

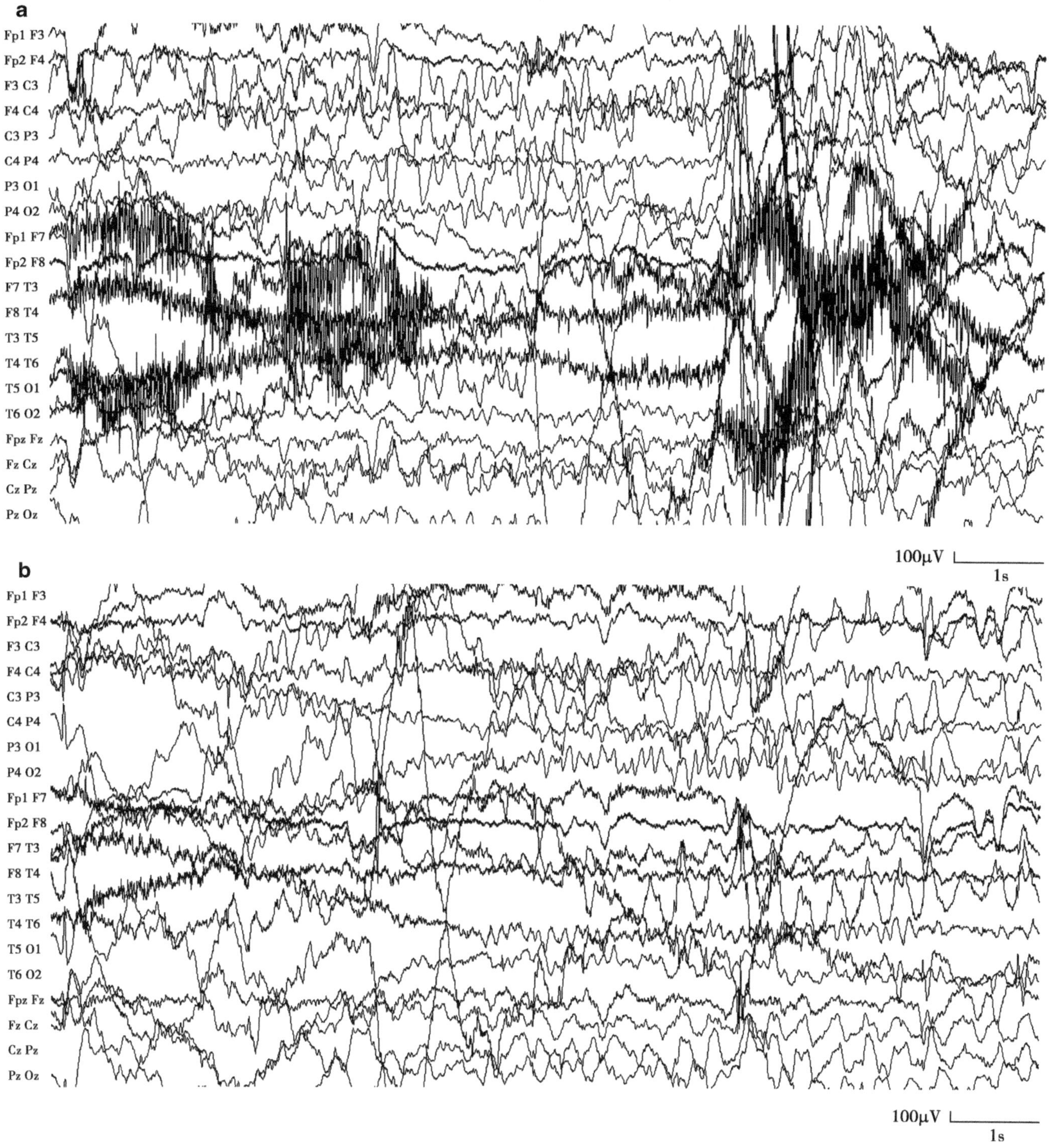

Fig. 8.9 Ictal scalp EEG. (**a**) Prior to the seizure, the patient was in supine position and happily talking with his families. The EEG showed a mixture of EMG artifacts and electrode wobble artifacts when the patient was awake. (**b–e**) The patient's right upper limb shook involuntarily during the seizure, lasting about 50 s, with intervals ranging from 1 to 5 s. The EEG showed 3–4 Hz low-amplitude slow waves rhythm over the left hemisphere, especially the central, parietal, and posterior temporal regions. Scattered sharp waves were seen over the left central region, and EMG and electrode wobble artifacts were still visible over all channels. (**f**) The patient's upper right limb stopped shaking when the seizure ended. The EEG recovered to the background EEG

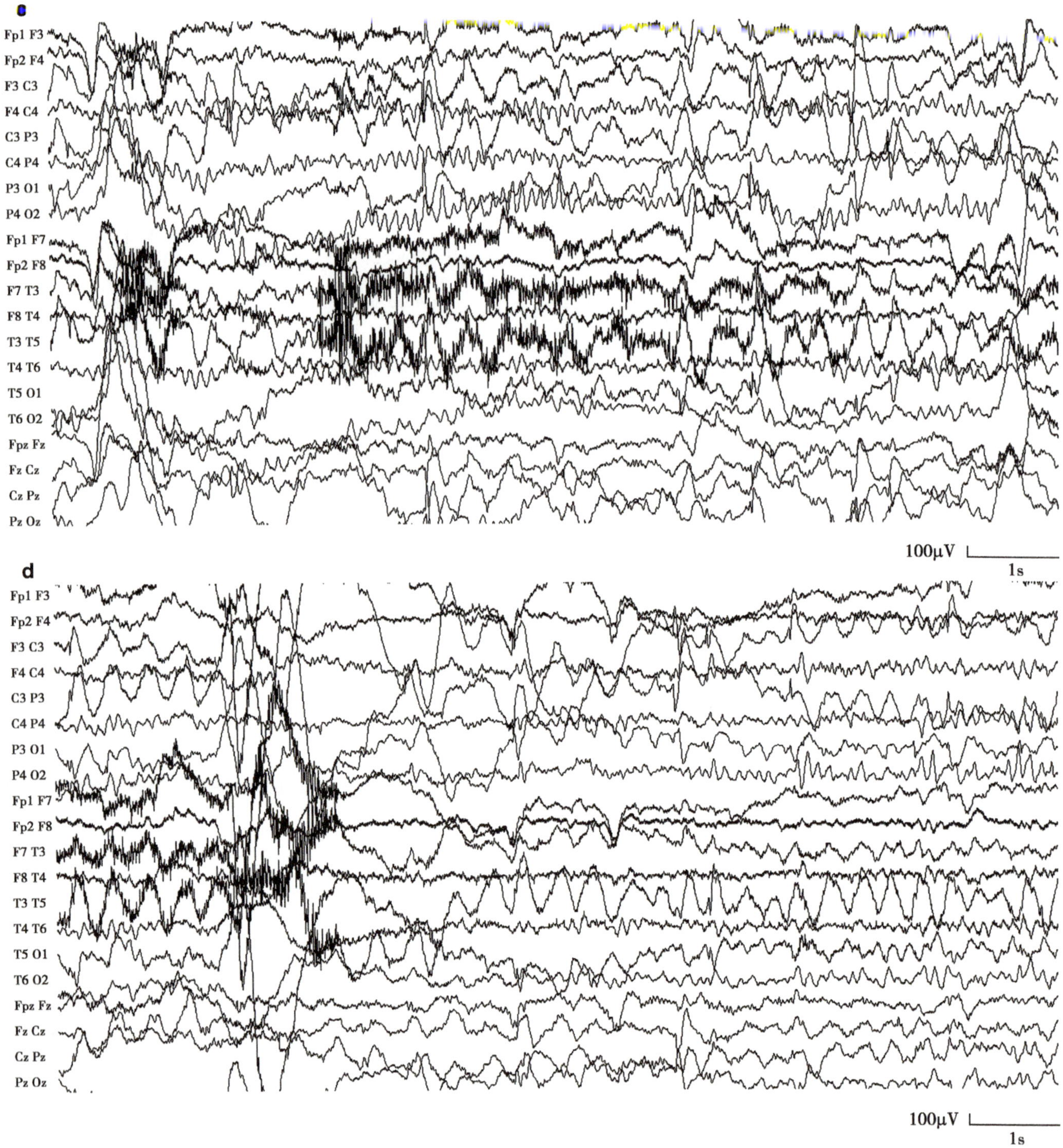

Fig. 8.9 (continued)

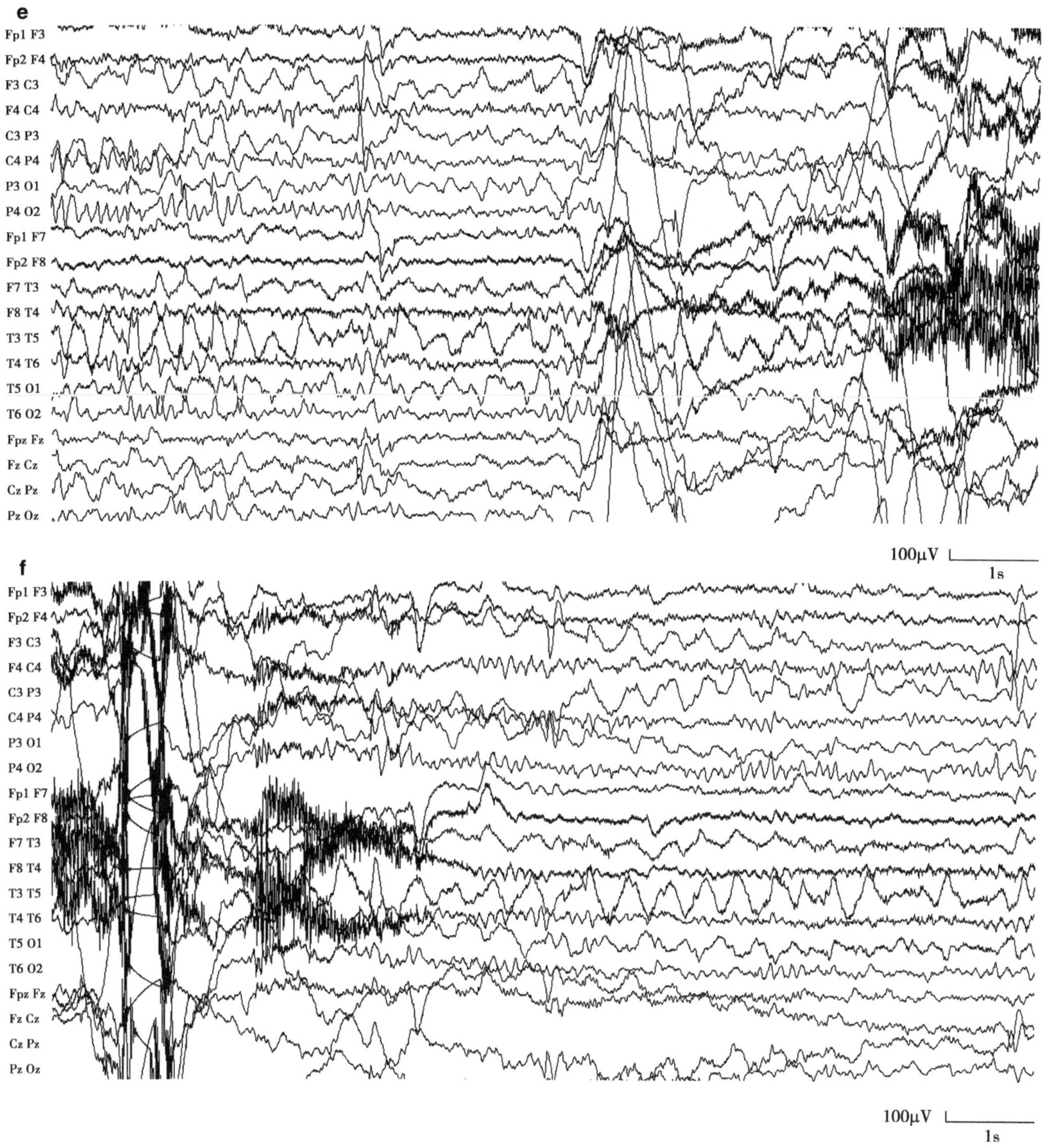

Fig. 8.9 (continued)

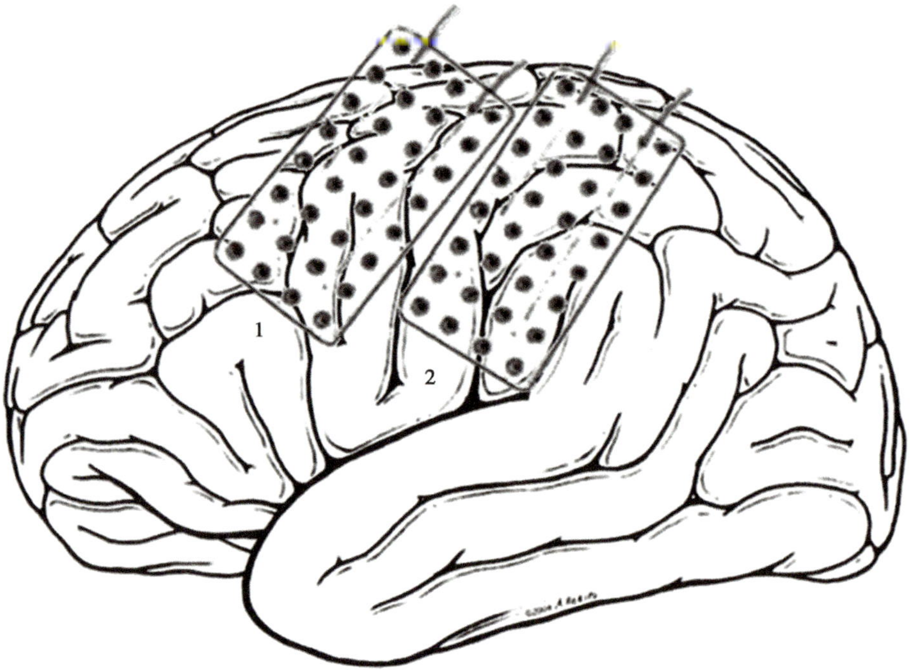

Fig. 8.10 Scheme of Intracranial Electrodes
Grid electrode 1: the left posterior frontal region and the precentral gyrus (32 contacts)
Grid electrode 2: the left posterior central gyrus and the parietal region (32 contacts)

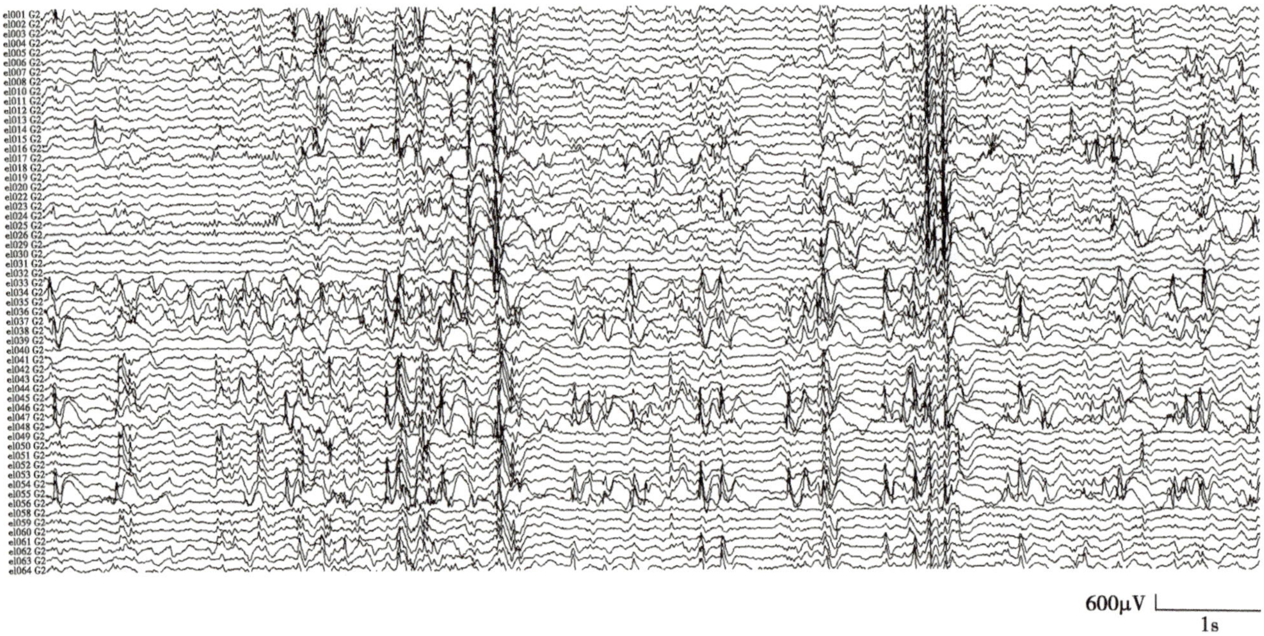

Fig. 8.11 Interictal intracranial EEG. Diffuse spikes and spike-and-wave complexes were seen over all channels

(d) Imaging characteristics: The CT and MRI revealed multiple intracranial calcification and cortical abnormal signals in the left parietal and temporal lobes.

2. *Diagnosis and treatment strategy and follow-up result*: The epileptic focus was near to the left central region. To avoid damaging motor function, grid electrodes were embedded in the left posterior frontal region and the frontoparietal region. The electrical stimulation was applied to determine the relationship between motor function and the epileptic focus. He underwent left postcentral gyrus resection. The seizures disappeared in 2 years of postoperative follow-up. The MRI showed multiple foci. The key focus was defined according to the symptoms and the EEG. In addition, the electrical stimulation, which was applied to determine the motor function, was the key to a successful surgery.

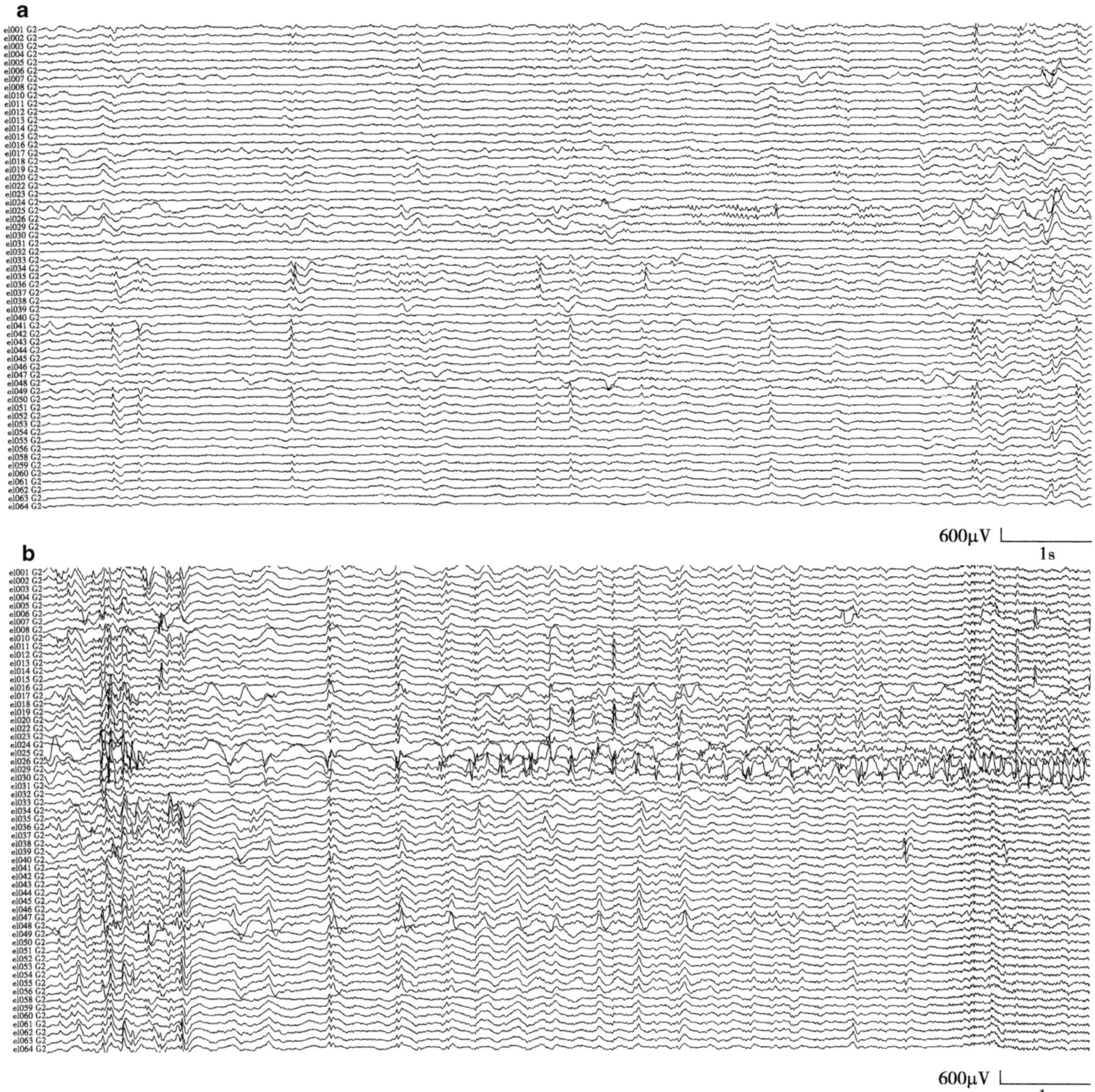

Fig. 8.12 Ictal intracranial EEG. (**a**) The IEEG showed low amplitude fast activities over the left posterior frontal region and precentral gyrus (contact numbers el025, 026, 029, 030), followed by the slow wave rhythm over the left posterior frontal region and precentral gyrus (contact numbers el025, 026, 029, 030), and sharp waves over the left posterior central gyrus and parietal region (contact numbers el034–037, el041–045, el049–053, el058–061). (**b**) The IEEG showed paroxysmal spikes over all channels followed by the spike-and-wave complexes rhythm over the left posterior frontal region and precentral gyrus (contact numbers el025, 026, 029, 030). (**c**) The IEEG showed periodic sharp waves over the left posterior frontal region and precentral gyrus (contact numbers el007, 008, 015, 016), the spike-and-wave complexes rhythm over the left posterior frontal region and precentral gyrus (contact numbers el019–023, el025, 026, 029, 030) and the posterior central gyrus and the parietal regions (contact numbers el039, 040), and the sharp wave rhythm over the posterior central gyrus and parietal regions (contact numbers el047, 048). (**d**) The IEEG showed the spike-and-wave complexes rhythm over the left posterior frontal region and precentral gyrus (contact numbers el019, 020, 022, 023, 025, 026, 029, 030) and rhythmic spikes over the posterior central gyrus and parietal regions (contact numbers el039, 040, 047, 048). (**e**) The patient was lying asleep and slowly turned the head to the right after turning awake, with the lower right limb tonic. The IEEG was same as **d**. (**f**) The patient turned the body to the right with the lower right limb obviously tonic. The IEEG was same as **d**. (**g**) The patient experienced generalized tonic-clonic seizure. The IEEG showed spike-and-wave complexes rhythm over the left posterior frontal region and the precentral gyrus. (**h**) The patient experienced a generalized tonic-clonic seizure. The IEEG was same as **g**. (**i**) The patient had generalized tonic-clonic seizures. The IEEG showed spike-and-wave complexes rhythm over the left posterior frontal region and the precentral gyrus, involving the left posterior central gyrus and the parietal region

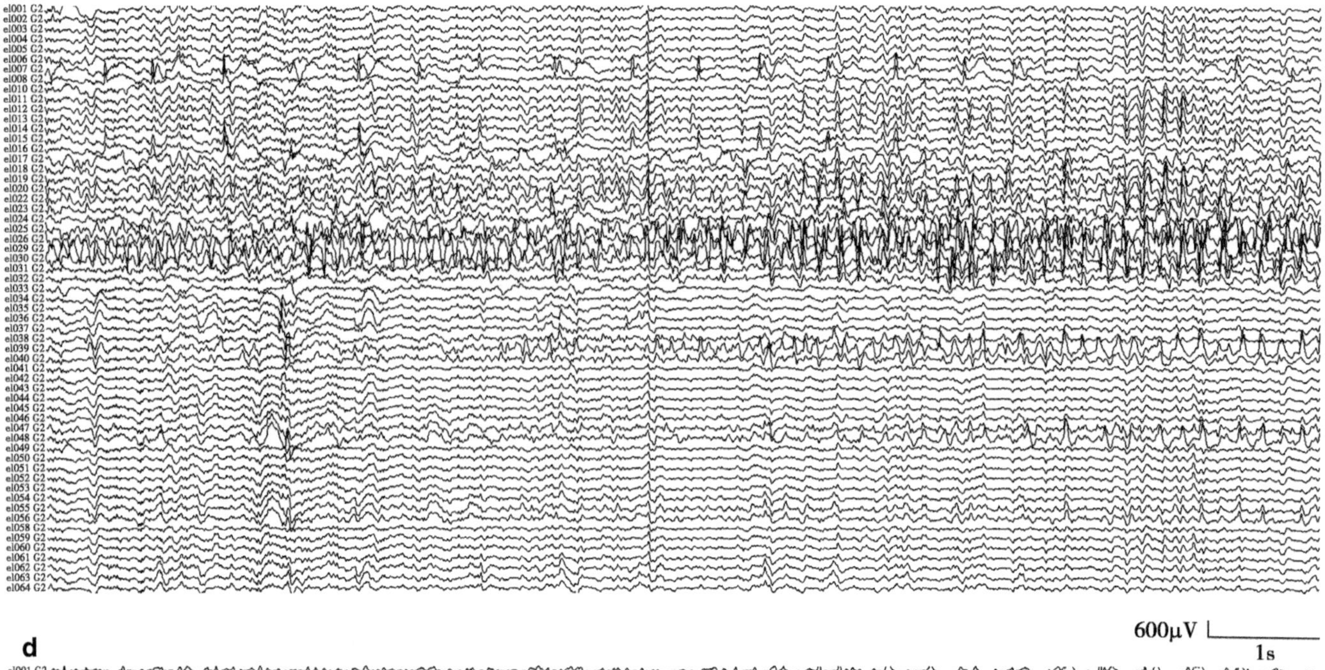

d

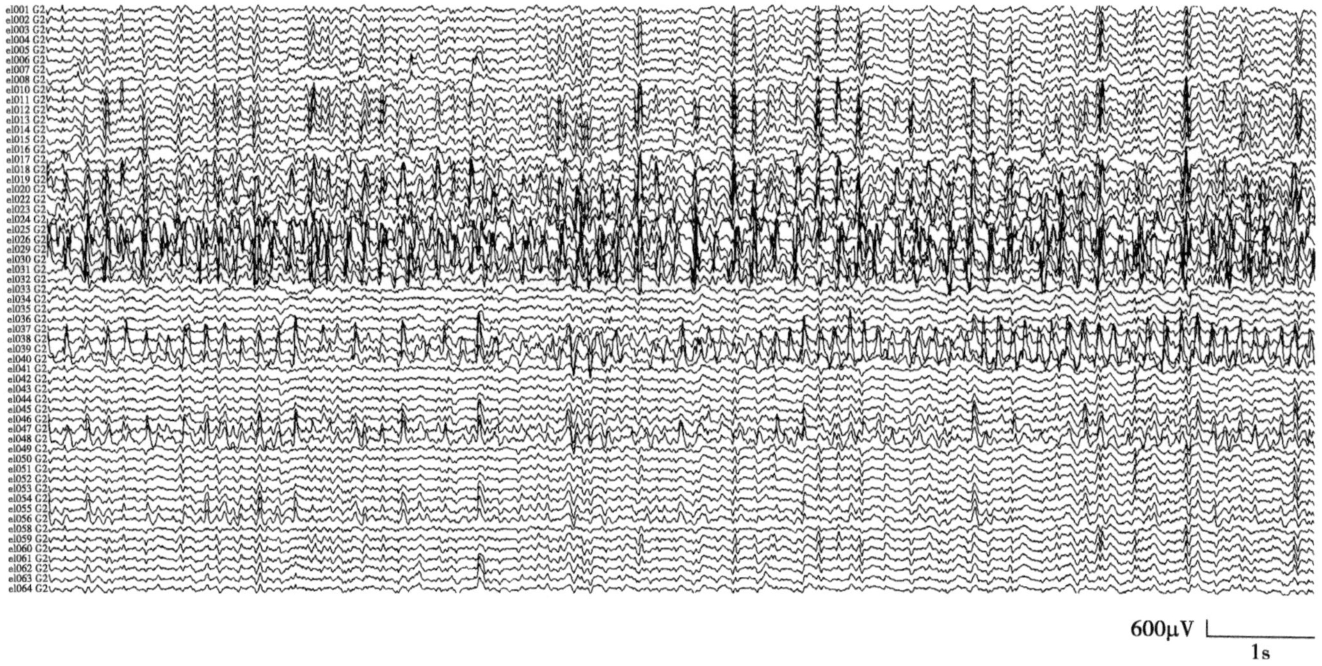

Fig. 8.12 (continued)

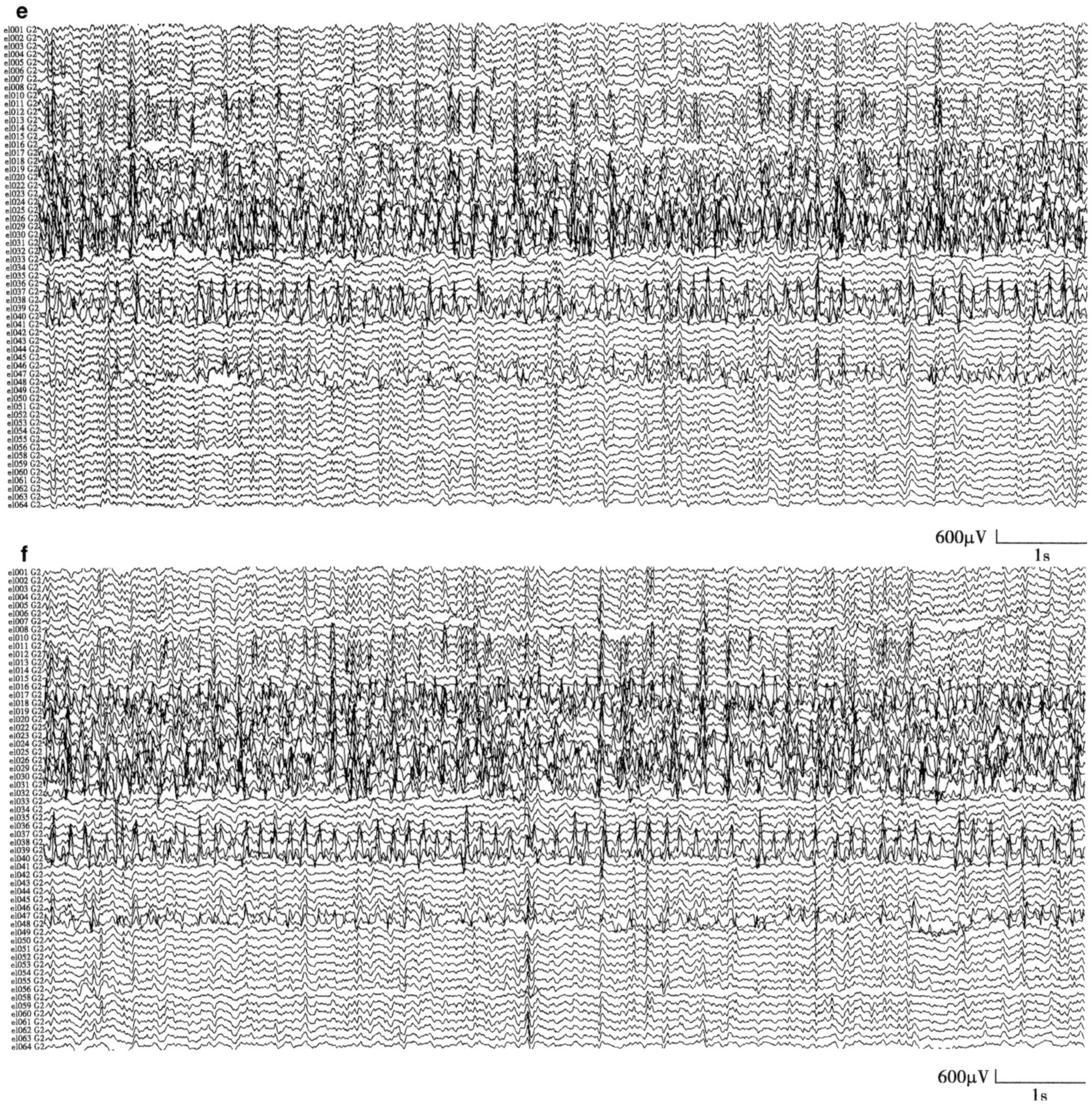

Fig. 8.12 (continued)

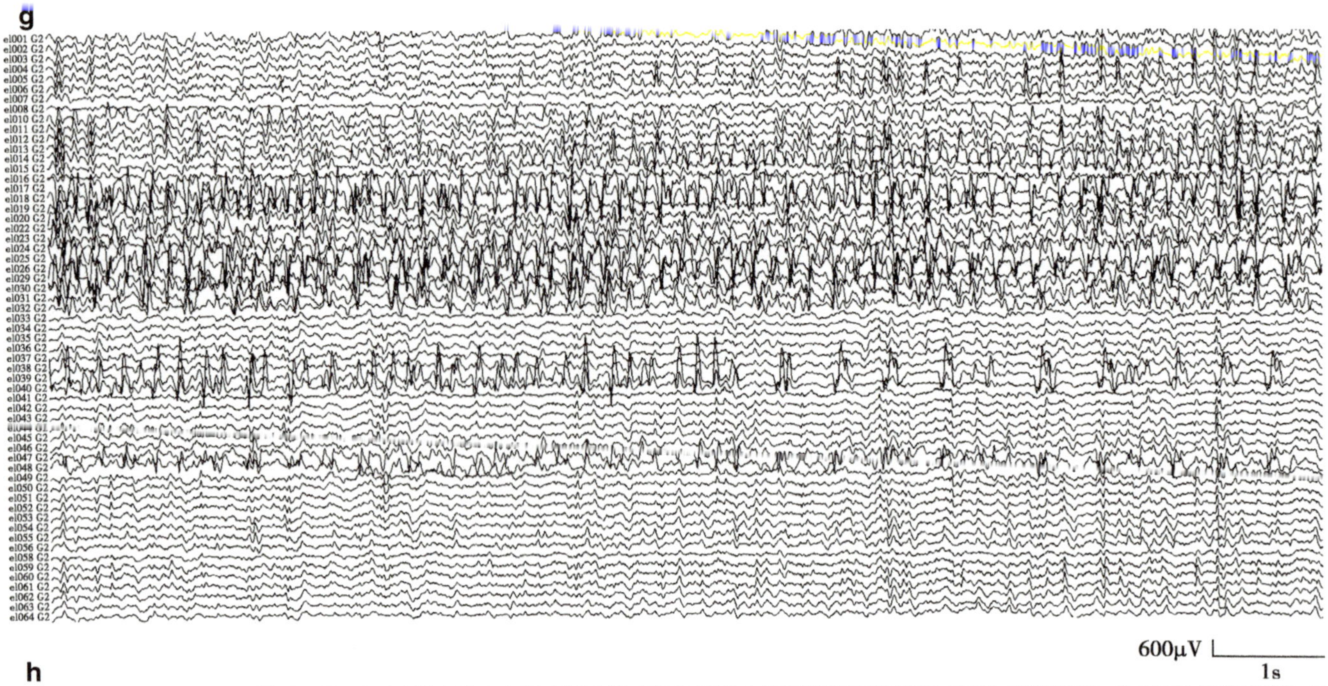

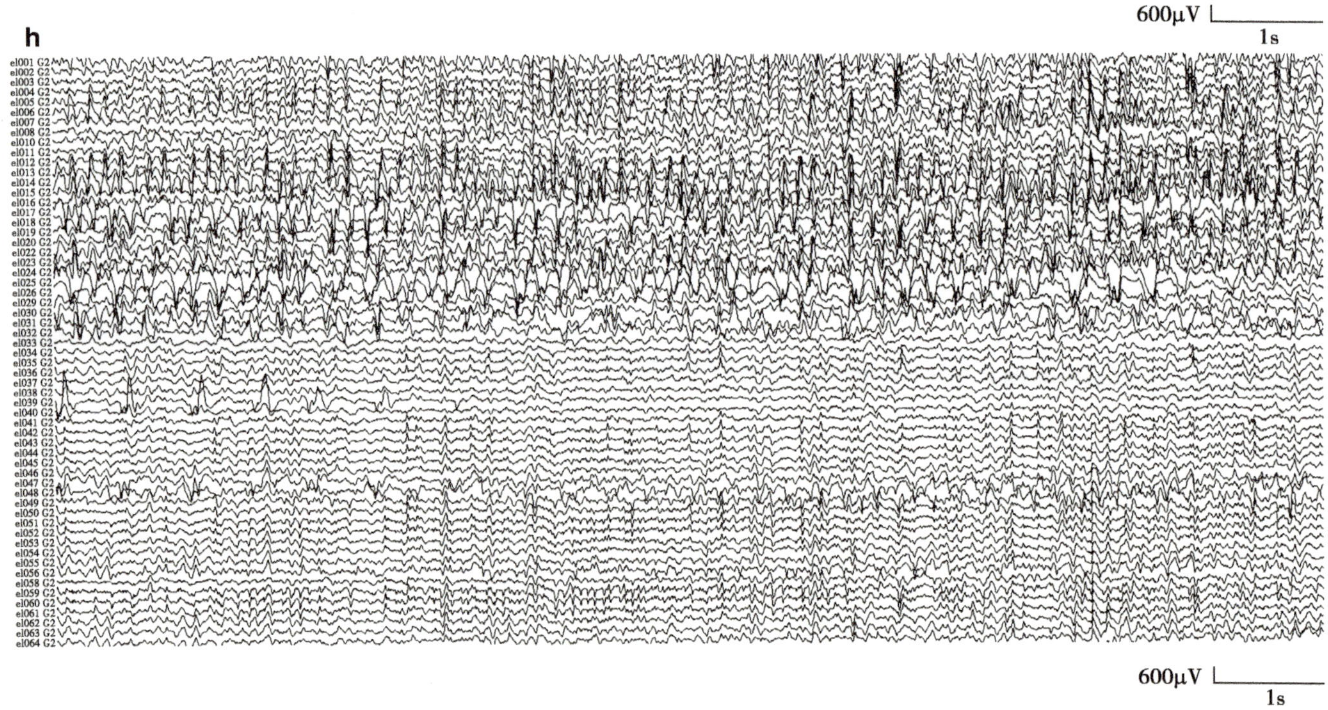

Fig. 8.12 (continued)

i

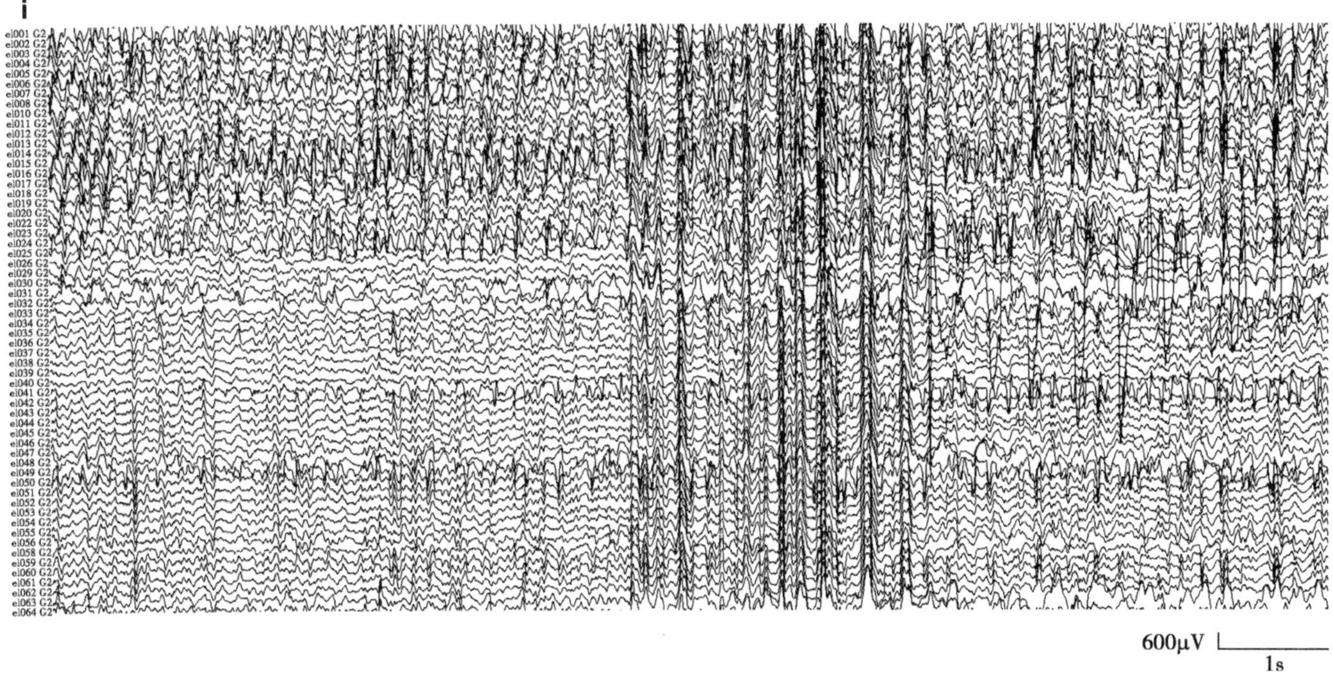

Fig. 8.12 (continued)

Case 8.4 Lennox-Gastaut Syndrome

[Abstract of Medical Records]
The patient was male and 17 years old.

1. *Chief complaint*: Paroxysmal convulsion with loss of consciousness for 8 years.
2. *History of present illness*: Eight years ago, the patient suddenly lost consciousness, foamed at the mouth, and suffered from limbs tonic-clonic, which resolved after about 3 min. The patient has experienced recurrent episodes since then, sometimes manifesting as dialeptic seizure. The treatment with phenytoin sodium and nitrazepam was ineffective with one seizure every 1–2 weeks. He started taking sodium valproate and carbamazepine orally 4 years before admission but still had frequent seizures, 7–8 times a day. The seizures could not be controlled despite several drug adjustment during this period.
3. *Personal and family history*: No history of associated diseases.
4. *Examination of nervous system*: No neurological abnormalities were found.
5. *Imaging examination*: The MRI suggested the atrophy of left hippocampus.
6. *EEG*: See Figs. 8.13, 8.14, 8.15, 8.16, 8.17, and 8.18 for details.

[*Case Review*]

1. Case Characteristics
   (a) The patient had seizures at his childhood.
   (b) The interictal EEG showed comprehensive rhythmic slow sharp/spike-wave complexes.
   (c) He had multiple seizures and tonic seizure is common. The EEG showed the spike rhythm over all channels during tonic seizure, which lasted about 6 s.
2. *Diagnosis and treatment strategy and follow-up results*: The patient was diagnosed with Lennox-Gastaut syndrome, with frequent seizures and poor effects after the treatment of multiple drugs. The patient had an urgent desire for surgical treatment. Based on the analysis of his seizure symptoms, it could be seen that the patient had asymmetrical movements of upper limbs during seizures and slight clonus in the left limb. Therefore, a local resection of the right frontal lobe was performed, but with poor outcomes. The intracranial electrodes should be used to further precisely localize the epileptogenic focus before resection, which could improve the surgical prognosis.

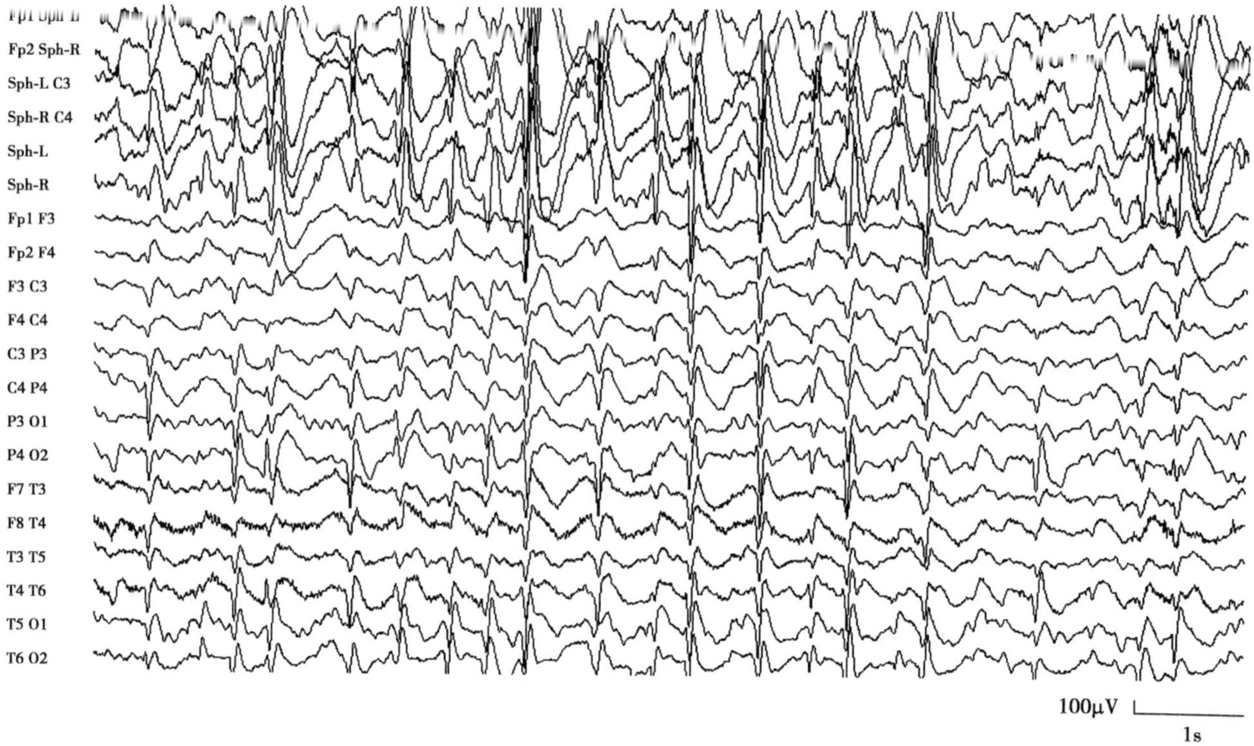

Fig. 8.13 Interictal scalp EEG 1. Slow sharp-and-wave complexes of 2–3 Hz were seen over all channels, especially the right side

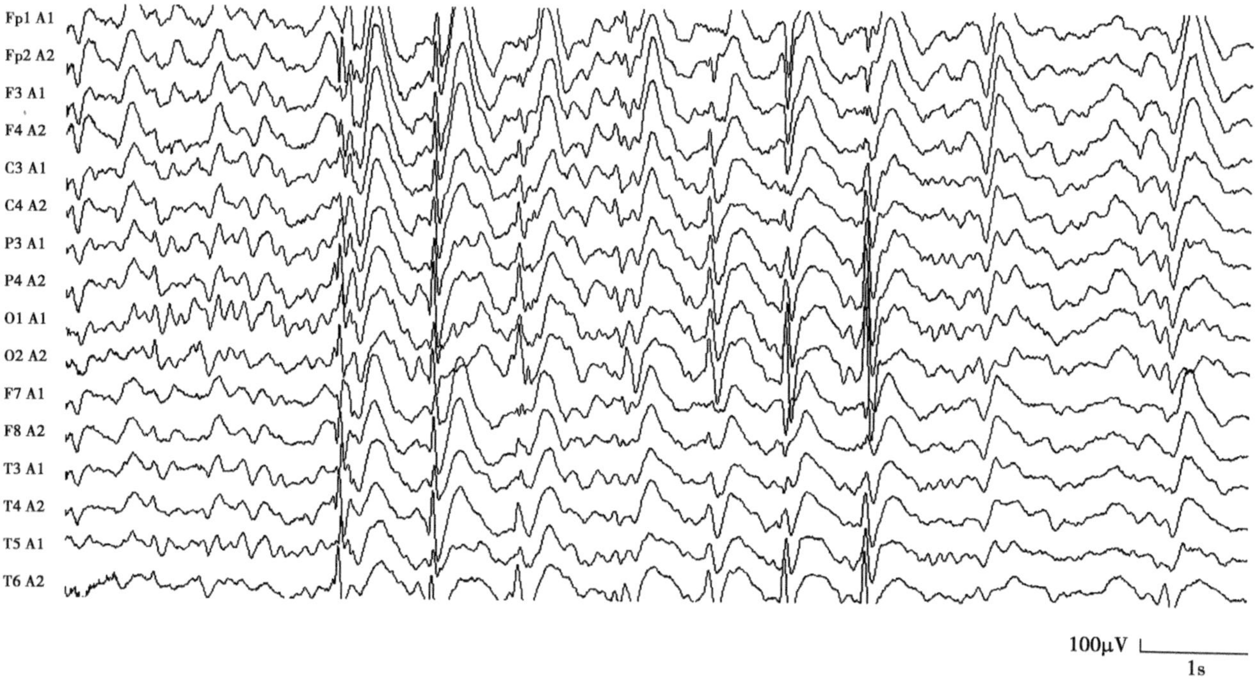

Fig. 8.14 Interictal scalp EEG 2. 1.5–2.5 Hz high-amplitude sharps or spike-and-wave complexes were seen over all channels when the patient was asleep, especially the right side

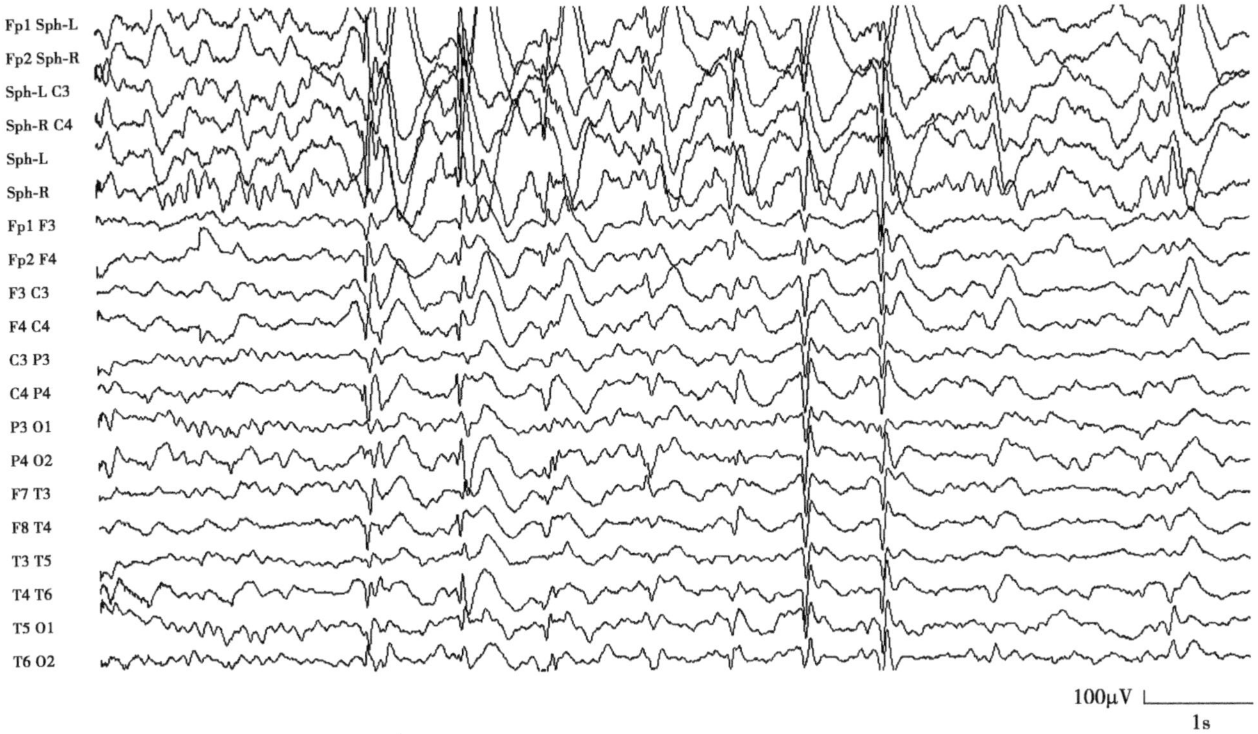

Fig. 8.15 Interictal scalp EEG 3. Comprehensive sharps or spike-and-wave complexes were seen when the patient was asleep, especially the right side

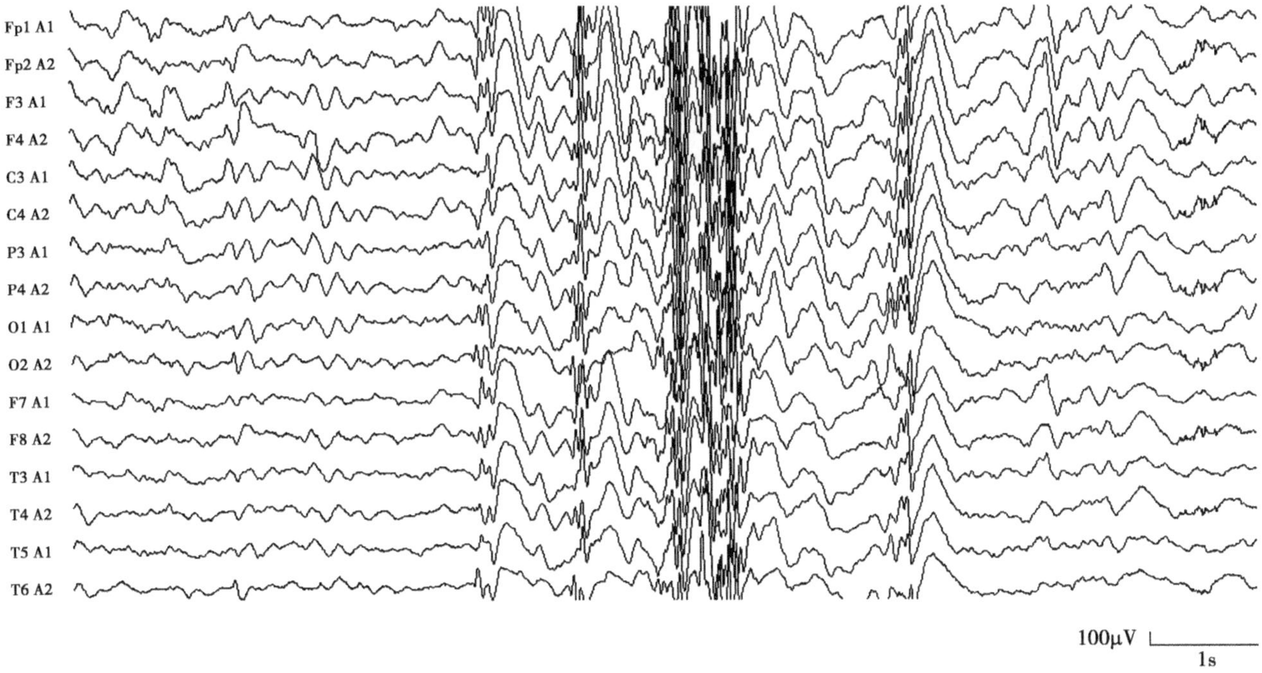

Fig. 8.16 Interictal scalp EEG 4. The burst of spikes, polyspikes or spike-and-wave complexes were seen over all channels when the patient was asleep, especially the right side

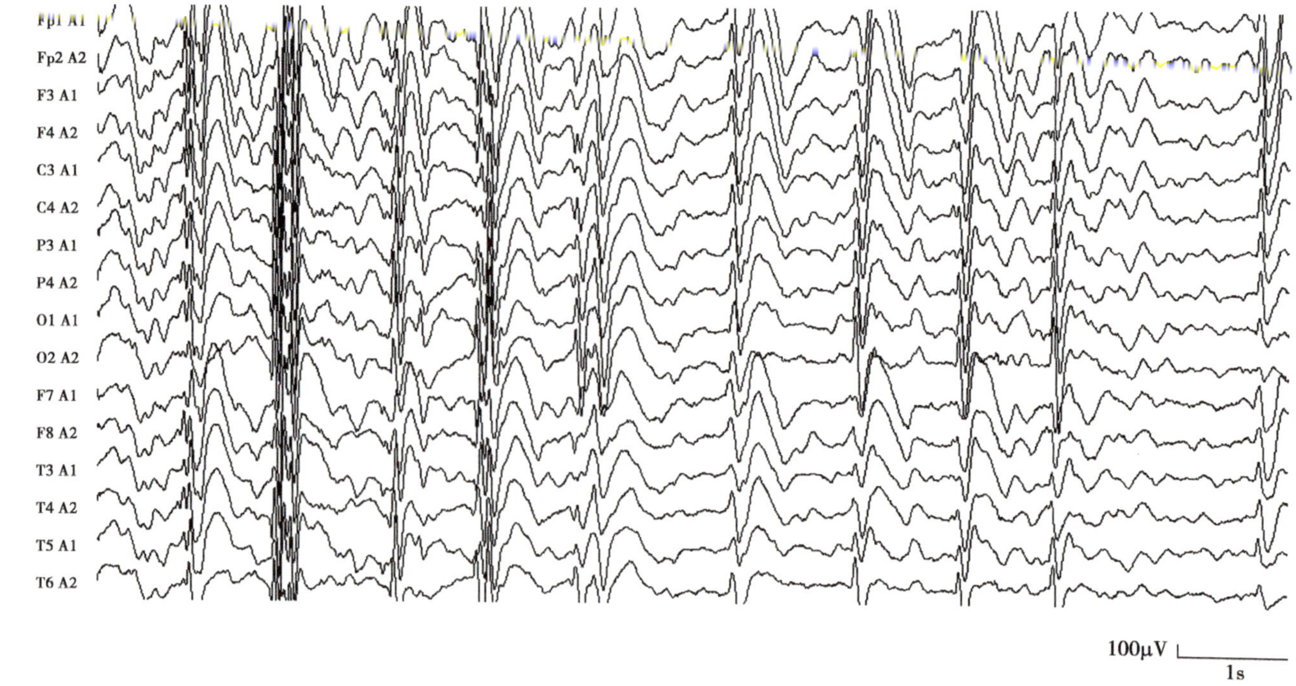

Fig. 8.17 Interictal scalp EEG 5. The periodic sharp/spike-and-wave complexes and polyspike and wave complexes were seen over all channels at a frequency of 1.0–1.2 Hz

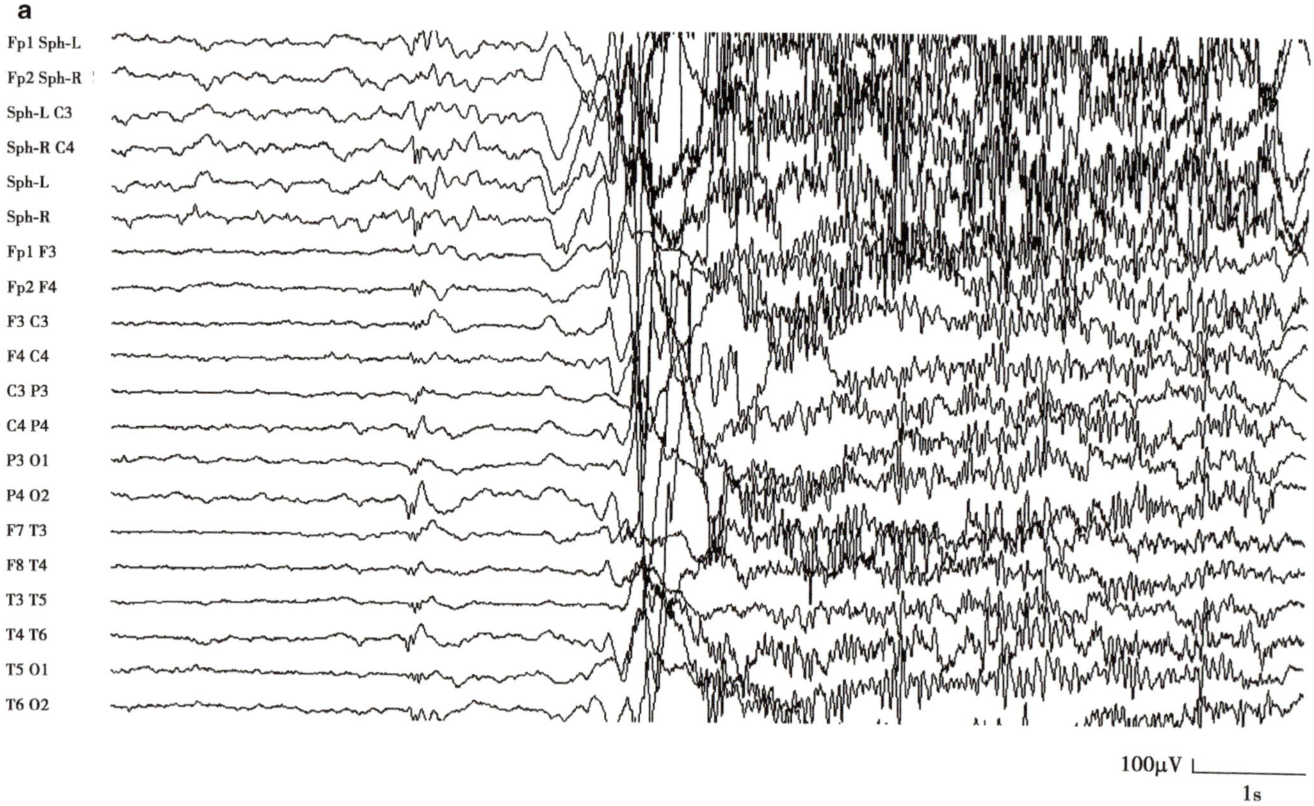

Fig. 8.18 Ictal scalp EEG. (**a**) The patient raised upper limbs, opened eyes, and raised his head, followed by slight twitches in the left upper limb. The EEG showed the high-amplitude spike rhythm over all channels, which disappeared after 6 s. (**b**) The patient lowered the upper limbs and the seizure ended. The EEG showed slow waves over all channels, followed by spike-and-wave complexes

b

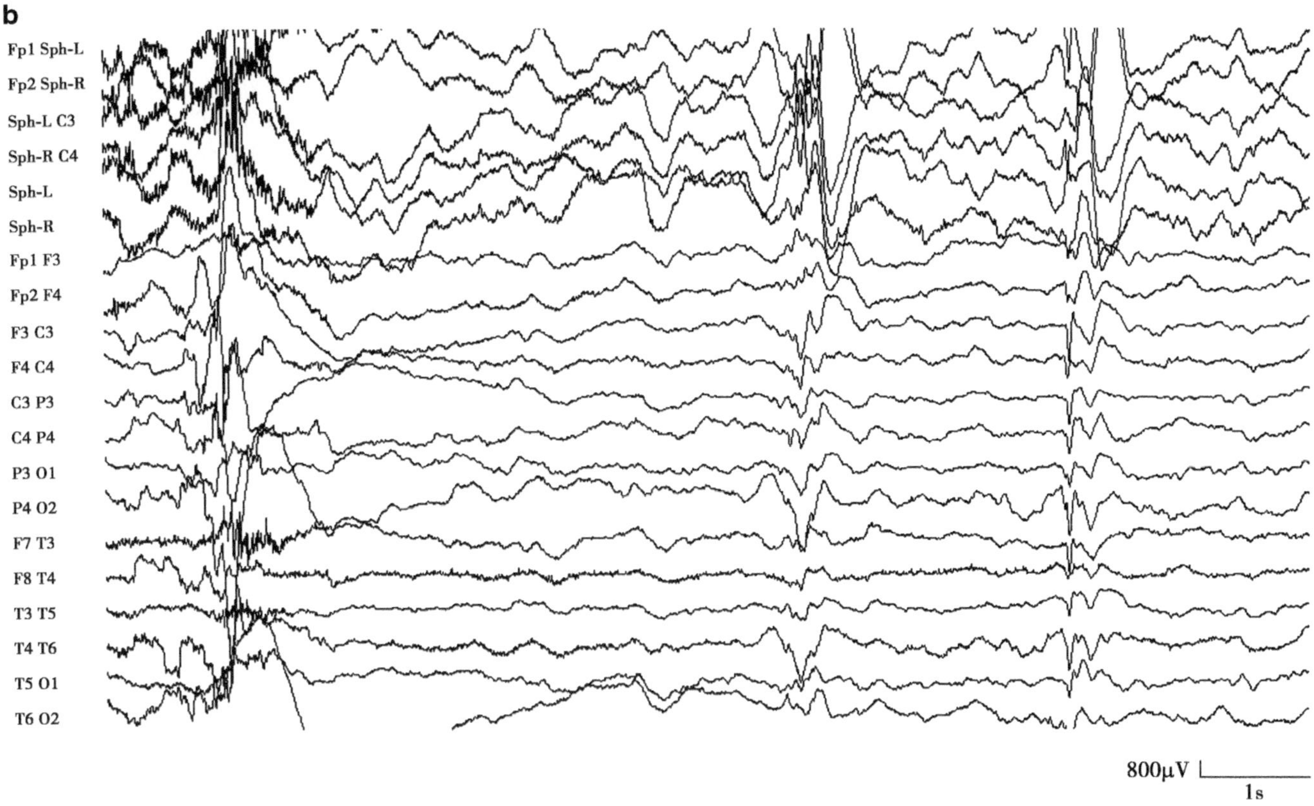

Fig. 8.18 (continued)

GPSR Compliance

The European Union's (EU) General Product Safety Regulation (GPSR) is a set of rules that requires consumer products to be safe and our obligations to ensure this.

If you have any concerns about our products, you can contact us on ProductSafety@springernature.com

In case Publisher is established outside the EU, the EU authorized representative is:

Springer Nature Customer Service Center GmbH
Europaplatz 3
69115 Heidelberg, Germany

Batch number: 10890033

Printed by Printforce, the Netherlands